Hepatitis C Virus-Host Interactions and Therapeutics: Current Insights and Future Perspectives

Authored By

Imran Shahid

Department of Pharmacology and Toxicology, Faculty of Medicine, Umm-Al-Qura University, Makkah, Saudi Arabia

&

Qaiser Jabeen

Department of Pharmacology, Faculty of Pharmacy, The Islamia University of Bahawalpur, Bahawalpur, Pakistan

Hepatitis C Virus-Host Interactions and Therapeutics: Current Insights and Future Perspectives

Authors: Imran Shahid and Qaiser Jabeen

ISBN (Online): 978-981-5123-43-2

ISBN (Print): 978-981-5123-44-9

ISBN (Paperback): 978-981-5123-45-6

First published in 2023.

Bentham Science Publishers Pte. Ltd.
80 Robinson Road #02-00
Singapore 068898
Singapore
Email: subscriptions@benthamscience.net

BENTHAM SCIENCE

CONTENTS

FOREWORD

Virus-host interactions (dependencies) and their intricate interplay are always phenomenal and of paramount interest to investigate molecular epidemiology and pathogenesis of all viral infections. However; complex cross-talks between hepatitis C virus (HCV) and host cells involving a plethora of genes and cell signaling pathways leading asymptomatic acute hepatitis C infection to chronic hepatitis C (CHC) and further durable, sustained, and insidious extrahepatic manifestations are still mysterious, murky, inconclusive, and even more, remains to elucidate. The world has always seen paradigms in HCV infection biology and therapeutics since its discovery in the late 1980s by gene cloning methods instead of the use of conventional tissue culture, or classical virological techniques. We can say that the world could not be able to see this revolutionary advancement in molecular biology techniques, state-of-the-art diagnostic tools, sophisticated protocols of clinical trials, astute knowledge of molecular drug targets, and serendipitous design and development of drug molecules without HCV discovery that once labeled as the 'silent epidemic' afflicting even more than 58 million peoples around the globe nowadays. Before the advent and approval of all oral interferon-free direct-acting antivirals, the gold standard of care, a combination therapy including pegylated interferon plus ribavirin achieved sustained clearance of HCV and subsequent improvements in liver disease in only 60% of treated patients. It has been a long haul, a big haul, but we've made it with the current landscape of HCV therapeutics to cure harder-to-treat special HCV subpopulations including cirrhotic, decompensated cirrhotic, HCV/HIV or HCV/HBV co-infections, and liver transplant or post-transplant patients with virus recurrence. Despite oral direct-acting antivirals having started to bear fruit in real-world clinical settings against HCV, unmet challenges, barriers, and hurdles in HCV diagnostics and treatment accessibility still prevail that need to surmount and overcome to reduce the global healthcare burden of HCV and to achieve WHO striving goal of HCV elimination by 2030.

This thought-provoking book tends to cover a comprehensive and up-to-date overview of the latest advancement in HCV infection biology, perplexing molecular clinical pathology, novel diagnostic tools, fortuitous anti-HCV therapeutic options on the horizons, management of difficult-to-treat subpopulations, and imperative compensatory therapies against hepatitis C infection in the late stage of their development. The book intends to cover the latest guidelines issued by the US FDA, AASLD/IDSA (American Association for the Study of Liver Diseases/Infectious Diseases Society of America), ECDC (European Center for Disease Prevention and Control), and NYSDOH-AI (New York State Department of Health Aids Institute) on HCV screening, diagnosis, treatment and management for the clinicians, physicians, infectious disease experts, and primary care providers (nurses and paramedics). The contents of the book not only provide ABC of HCV infection, diagnostic tools, and treatment strategies to common and interested readers but also address current information about some pretty mind-boggling aspects of hepatitis C biology, immunology, pharmacology, therapeutics, and vaccinology to obtain relevant answers with thoughtful explanations of some outstanding problems in the field nowadays. The book also covers up-to-date guidelines about patient screening, treatment protocols, and optimization of therapy in real-world clinical settings.

The book also summarizes unanswered questions currently faced by investigators in the intriguing molecular pathogenesis of CHC in humans, and physicians, clinicians, hepatologists, and healthcare officials are concerned with HCV clinical diagnosis and therapeutics. I hope that this book will also be a valuable addition to hepatology for curious undergraduate and postgraduate students pursuing a new career in HCV medicine or newcomer in hepatitis C research to broaden their knowledge and gain a wide perspective of the field. The multi- and interdisciplinary presentation of information in this book would open a new school of thought for postdoctoral fellows to search for new horizons and milestones in hepatitis C research. The book closes while shedding light on remarkable and amalgamated efforts by the World Health Organization (WHO), health policymakers, and public healthcare providers to a proper ending of this 'silent epidemic' from the world by 2030.

Both authors of the book (Imran Shahid and Qaiser Jabeen) are agile, bright, and very active investigators in the concerned field of hepatitis C research with more than 10 and 20 years of experience respectively. I wish that this web-based, as well as hard copy format book, would rapidly become an international referral and guideline in hepatitis C infection biology, diagnostics, and therapeutics.

Sajida Hassan
Senior Research Scientist III
Viral Hepatitis Program, Laboratory Medicine
University of Washington
Seattle, WA, USA

PREFACE

The public health care burden of hepatitis C virus infection remains significant despite the remarkable progress in HCV therapeutics during the last decade, as around 58 million people are currently having the virus and almost 4,00,000 deaths are reported annually due to hepatitis C-induced hepatocellular carcinoma. The advent and approval of a dozen oral interferon-free direct-acting antivirals have revolutionized the treatment paradigms for hepatitis C infection while achieving higher sustained virologic response rates (>95%) in treated individuals. Analogously, HCV and host interactions to map networks in disease progression, extrahepatic manifestations, and virus invasion strategies to the host immune system are still enigmatic to fully understand. Albeit, ample understanding of HCV life cycle *in vitro* and transient *in vivo* replication models, provide valuable insights towards the viral entry, genome replication, virion formation, and host infection involving a highly orchestrated series of molecular and cellular events, including a plethora of genes and cell signaling cascades. However, questions remain to answers regarding the virus clearance without any therapeutic intervention in some HCV-infected populations, molecular pathogenesis of infection transforming the acute hepatitis C infection to end-stage liver disease, post-viral eradication, hepatocellular carcinoma, and the fate of the immune system once the virus eliminates from the body.

This book intends to provide insights into what has been achieved in HCV infection biology, virus-host interactions, molecular epidemiology of the infection, and the full spectrum of immune responses to hepatitis C, either the involvement of innate or adaptive immune responses in the first three chapters. The following chapters 4 and 5 comprehensively illustrate the simplified HCV diagnostic solutions, predictive barriers, and future perspectives for general, as well as vulnerable HCV infected populations, along with the up-to-date procedural and protocol guidelines for HCV diagnosis. Book Chapter 4 also highlights the strides toward a better understanding of HCV screening and diagnostic strategies for high throughput anti-HCV screening and diagnosis, applications for risk prediction tools, and cost-effective analysis of current diagnostic in the hepatitis C cascade of care. The next four book chapters (from chapters 6 to 9) precisely and comprehensively illustrate the current landscape of HCV treatment, their administration, consensus treatment guidelines for their recommendations, and their real-world treat outcomes. These book chapters also provide the probable answers to some fundamental questions like why some HCV-infected populations are nonresponsive to IFN-free DAAs, the phenomena behind viral relapse, and reasons behind treatment failure in harder-to-treat specific HCV subpopulations. Within those book chapters, chapter 9 also emphasizes real-world challenges in HCV therapeutics to unleash certain barriers while making it possible to expand the scale of therapy, and the cascade of care, and bridge existing gaps in hepatitis C care between developed and poor nations. Chapter 10 of the book overviews the emerging anti-HCV treatment strategies in the pipeline and explains the efforts to do while refocusing on anti-mRNA-based treatment strategies and nanomedicine-based approaches used in conjunction with DAAs for hepatitis C. The book chapter also portrays some glimpses into the future for the design of controlled animal and human HCV infection models for the design of an appropriate but effective prophylactic or protective anti-hepatitis C vaccine model. The last two book chapters (chapters 11 and 12) discuss the goals, policy implementation, and progress of the Global Health Sector Strategies (GHSS) 2016-2021 on HCV worldwide in the last decade as well as the cross-cutting barriers to break and actions to be taken in this decade while achieving the global goal of HCV elimination by 2030. The final chapter of the book also describes the strategies to opt at hospitals, community services centers, health care service providers, and government levels to prevent new HCV incidences and reduce HCV-related morbidities and mortalities with concrete efforts, collective will, and public health notes to galvanize the efforts to eradicate this epidemic worldwide by 2030.

Overall, this well-written book provides from simple, accessible introduction to a complex hepatology field, and in-depth information about HCV basics, clinical diagnostics, and therapeutic knowledge to all stakeholders involved in HCV screening, diagnosis, treatment, and management. Without being exhaustive or redundant, it can be easily accessed to concepts by extensive cross-referenced studies. We hope that this book will enhance the knowledge of a common reader about hepatitis C infection, its diagnosis, and treatment, and provide answers to the physicians, clinicians, hepatologists, infectious disease experts, health care providers, and investigators to some of the outstanding problems in the ever-changing field of hepatitis C research.

CONSENT FOR PUBLICATION

Not applicable.

CONFLICT OF INTEREST

The authors declare no conflict of interest, financial or otherwise.

ACKNOWLEDGEMENT

Declared none.

Imran Shahid
Department of Pharmacology & Toxicology
Faculty of Medicine
Umm-Al-Qura University
Makkah, Saudi Arabia

&

Qaiser Jabeen
Department of Pharmacology
Faculty of Pharmacy, The Islamia University of Bahawalpur
Bahawalpur, Pakistan

DEDICATION

Dedicated to one of my beloved teachers who told me that "To be a star in real-life, you will have to do a lot".

CHAPTER 1

HCV-Host Interactions: A Plethora of Genes and their Intricate Interplay Part 1: Virus Specific Factors

Abstract: Hepatitis C virus (HCV) interaction with host cells is pivotal for natural disease course starting from asymptomatic acute infection to progress into persistent chronic infection and subsequent extrahepatic manifestations, including fibrosis, cirrhosis, and hepatocellular carcinoma (HCC). The HCV infection biology in infected host cells *via* virus attachment, virus genome replication, mRNA translation, new virion formation, and egress from infected cells involves highly coordinated participation of the virus- and host-specific proteins, a plethora of genes, and cell signaling cascade. The progression of persistent chronic hepatitis C (CHC) infection to hepatic fibrosis, cirrhosis, and HCC involves viral invasion strategies against host immune system defense mechanisms as well as impeding healthy metabolic and signaling networks of the liver cells. Thereby, HCV-induced liver injury *via* chronic inflammatory processes that fail to resolve is responsible for decompensated cirrhosis and on occasion, hepatocarcinogenesis in infected individuals. With the latest advancement and rapid expansion of our knowledge in hepatology, the human liver is deciphered as an immunologically distinct organ with its specialized physiological niche. The relationship between human hepatocytes and different components of the immune system is quite complex and dynamic. The immunopathogenesis of various viral infections demonstrates that the immune system plays an essential role to determine the progression of many hepatic diseases through immune cell communication and cell signaling networks. In this book chapter, we overview HCV-host interactions and their intricate interplay with complex crosstalk to propagate less fetal acute HCV infection to CHC and subsequent hepatocarcinogenesis (*i.e.* HCC) in infected individuals.

Keywords: Acute hepatitis C, Chronic hepatitis C, Cirrhosis, Cell communication, Cell signaling, Core protein, Envelope glycoproteins, Fibrosis, Genome organization, Hepatocytes, HCV life cycle, Hepatocellular carcinoma, Immunopathogenesis, Molecular pathogenesis, Nonstructural proteins, RNA polymerase, Replication, Structural proteins, Translation, Virus-host interaction.

Imran Shahid and Qaiser Jabeen

INTRODUCTION

Hepatitis C Virus Taxonomy

HCV belongs to the *Flaviviridae* family of viruses which is divided into three genera: flavivirus, pestivirus, and hepacivirus [1].

Flaviviruses include yellow fever virus, dengue fever virus (DENV), Japanese encephalitis virus, and Tick-borne encephalitis virus [2]. Pestiviruses include the bovine viral diarrhea virus, classical swine fever virus, and Border disease virus [1]. HCV, with 8 genotypes (GTs) and numerous subtypes (around 70), is a member of the *hepacivirus* genus, which includes tamarin virus and GB virus B (GBV-B) and is closely related to human virus GB virus C (GBV-C) [3]. All currently identified HCV GTs and subtypes are hepatotropic, which means that they preferentially infect hepatocytes and cause liver inflammation, broadly known as viral hepatitis C infection [3]. However, viral infectivity and pathogenicity do vary at GTs and subtypes level, which may variably influence the progression of HCV infection from the acute phase to chronicity and subsequent hepatic-comorbidities in infected individuals [4]. Interestingly, all members of the *Flaviviridae* family of viruses shares and resembles several basic structural and virological characteristics [1]. At the genome level, all *Flaviviridae* viruses are single-strand RNA viruses from 9600 to 12,300 nucleotides (nts) in length, with an open reading frame (ORF) encoding a polyprotein of 3000 amino acids (aa) or more [5]. The viral genome is flanked by a 5' untranslated region (5' UTR) upstream to the structural part of the ORF of 95-555 nts and a 3' untranslated region (3' UTR) of 114-624 nts in length adjacent to nonstructural proteins [5]. Structurally, the HCV virus is enveloped in a lipid bilayer in which two or more envelope glycoproteins (*i.e.* E1 and E2) are anchored [6]. The virus envelope surrounds the nucleocapsid, which is composed of viral antigen protein (*i.e.* core or C; multiple copies of a small basic protein) and the viral RNA genome [6]. The viral structural proteins (*e.g.*, C, E1, and E2) are encoded by the N-terminal part of the ORF, whereas the 7 nonstructural proteins (*e.g.* P_7, NS1, NS2, NS3, NS4A, NS4B, NS5A, and NS5B) are constituted by the remaining portion of the ORF [6]. Surprisingly, motifs-conserved across RNA protease helicase (*i.e.* nonstructural protein; NS3) and RNA replication enzyme (*i.e.* nonstructural protein NS5B; an RNA-dependent RNA polymerase (RdRp)) are found in similar locations in the polyproteins of all of the *Flaviviridae* viruses [6]. In addition to that, the hydropathic profile of polyproteins is much closer/identical between flaviviruses and hepaciviruses than pestiviruses [1].

Likewise, with the above-mentioned similarities, HCV exhibits several virological, epidemiological, and pathophysiological differences from the other members of the *Flaviviridae* genera [1]. Flavivirus translation is cap-dependent, *i.e.* it is mediated by a type 1 cap structure located in the 5' UTR (m^7GpppAmp), followed by the conserved AG sequence and a relatively short stretch upstream of the polyprotein coding region [7]. In contrast, HCV translation is cap-independent, where the 5' UTR is uncapped and folds into a complex RNA secondary structure adjacent to a portion of the core-coding domain [7]. Almost all 5' UTR and a few upstream nucleotides of the core-coding domain are occupied by several stem-loops (SLs) of internal ribosome entry sites (IRES) which span a region of ~341 nts and mediate direct binding of ribosomal subunits and cellular factors and initiate subsequent translation [6]. 3' UTR of the other members of flavivirus is highly structured, however; HCV 3' UTR is relatively short, less structured, and contains a poly-uridyl tract that varies in length and plays a central role in HCV replication [6].

HCV: Route of Transmission

The major route of HCV transmission is exclusively through direct blood-to-blood contact between humans which signifies its narrow tissue tropism and host specificity for HCV infection [8]. However, some other body fluids and tissue specimens are also capable of transmitting HCV infection (Table **1**). Flaviviruses principally infect a broad range of vertebrate animals by using mosquitoes or ticks as a virus vector, and humans are dead-end host that does not participate in the perpetuation of virus transmission [9]. Pestivirus can rarely infect humans and no known insect vector has been identified until now [10]. Most of the infections caused by flaviviruses are acute-limited in vertebrate animals whereas HCV in humans has a high chronicity rate (50%-80%) depending on the age at infection [11]. Protection and recovery of flavivirus and pestivirus infections are entirely dependent on strong and adapted humoral and cellular immune responses [10]. However; in CHC and subsequent extrahepatic manifestations of HCV infection (*i.e.* cirrhosis, HCC), virus-induced host-immune responses fail to confer protection and prevention to reinfection with homologous and heterologous strains of HCV in the infected individuals [11].

HCV Genome Organization

HCV is a positive-sense single-stranded RNA virus of approximately 9600 nucleotides in length [7]. The viral genome flanks by highly conserved 5' and 3' UTRs along with a single ORF of 3010 to 3037 amino acids polyprotein [7]. Both 5' and 3' UTRs are pre-requisite for virus replication and mRNA translation and signals required for both these phenomena are coordinated in a highly orchestrated manner within viral and cellular proteins and between these two regions of the HCV genome (*e.g.*, molecular interaction of IRES domain IIId, stem-loop (SL) -II and SL-III of 3' UTR and *cis*-acting replication elements (CRE)/region at 3' end of NS5B is key for genome replication)) [5, 6]. The precursor polyprotein is post-translationally processed by cellular and host proteases into an initial structural region encoding three proteins including core (C), E1, and E2, and a nonstructural region of 4 nonstructural proteins (NS2 to NS5) after a cap-independent IRES translation mechanism mediated by an IRES structure within the 5' UTR (Fig. **1**) [12].

Table 1. Fluids and tissue specimens capable of transmitting hepatitis C infection [52].

Fluid, Tissue Specimens	HCV Transmission
Lab specimens containing concentrated HBV, HCV, or HIV	Yes
Blood, serum, plasma, or other biological fluids visibly contaminated with blood	Yes
Pleural, amniotic, pericardial, peritoneal, synovial and cerebrospinal fluids	Yes
Semen, vaginal secretions	Yes
Saliva	No, unless contaminated with blood
Breastfeeding	Biologically plausible, particularly if nipples are cracked or bleeding
Organ and tissue transplants	Yes
Screened donated blood & manufactured blood products	Minimal risk

These secondary and tertiary structures (*i.e.* 5' UTR, IRES, 3' UTR) are also essential for the proper binding and positioning of HCV RNA within the host cell's protein translation machinery [5]. The 3' UTR is a tripartite structure located at the end of the viral genome and is indispensable for HCV replication [5] (Fig. **1**).

HCV MOLECULAR BIOLOGY

HCV replicates in the cytoplasm of hepatocytes with a very high replication rate producing approximately 10^{12} virions daily with a short turnover reaching a maximum time of three hours [13]. The host cells' immune responses are triggered to neutralize viral translation and polyprotein processing, however; the extraordinary ability of the virus to mutate because of poor fidelity and error-prone nature of RdRp enzyme during virus replication as well as lack of RNA repair mechanism, those mutations are accumulated within the HCV genome [14]. Consequently, HCV circulates as a population of closely related but diverse viral sequences in infected individuals referred to as quasispecies [14, 15]. Persistent infection, resistance to therapy, and variable treatment outcomes are believed to be attributed to the quasispecies dynamics of HCV isolates circulating in an infected individual [13]. Viral genetic heterogeneity is also a consequence of those accumulated mutations by which different HCV isolates display significant nucleotide variability within different genome regions [6]. The envelope glycoproteins (*i.e.*, E1 and E2) and some nonstructural proteins (*e.g.*, NS3, NS5A, and NS5B) are significantly variable, whereas 5' UTR, Core, and 3' UTR are highly conserved regions [6]. The evolution of six HCV GTs and more than 70 subtypes is also based on the accumulation of mutations in the HCV genome over time (Fig. **2**) [7]. HCV replication and translation both occur simultaneously in the hepatic cytoplasm, which makes it an ideal candidate to elucidate HCV infection biology and molecular pathogenesis mechanisms [13]. However, HCV-host intricate interplay involving many viral and host-specific proteins and their overlapping signaling cascade during viral replication is not fully understood [7]. Surprisingly, much is known about virus-host interactions during viral translation and polyprotein processing. The lack of an inefficient cell culture system also hampers carrying on HCV infection biology studies in the long-term perspective of the molecular pathogenesis of the infection [16].

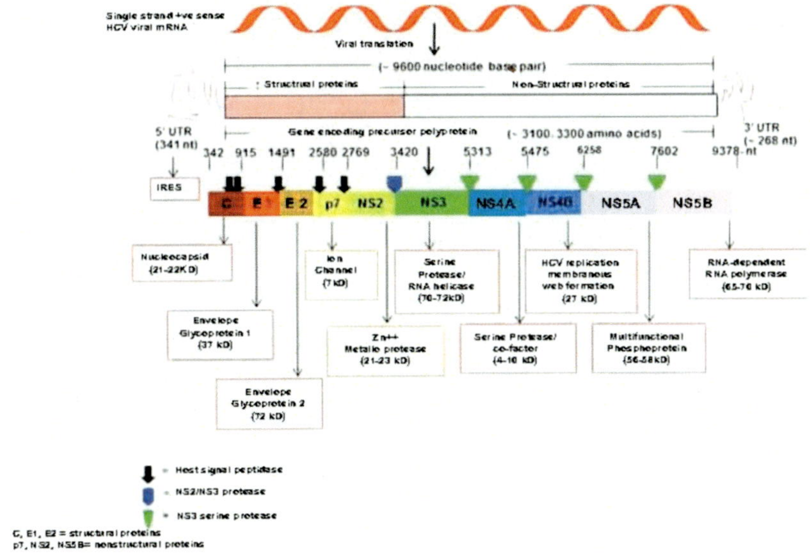

Fig. (1). Genome organization of HCV. HCV genome is a linear, positive-sense single-strand RNA(+ssRNA) of 9.6 kb in size. The viral genome is flanked by 5' and 3' untranslated regions (UTRs). The genomic mRNA encodes for three structural and seven nonstructural proteins upon primary translation, which is post-translationally modified by viral proteases and host cellular peptidases into mature proteins. Each viral protein is specific for its role (indicated in a red rectangular box with its estimated weight) in the virus life cycle to produce new viral progeny. Generally, HCV structural proteins are essential for viral infectivity and the production of new virions, while viral nonstructural proteins are pivotal for HCV replication and translation. UTR; untranslated region, IRES; internal ribosome entry site, kD; kilo Dalton.

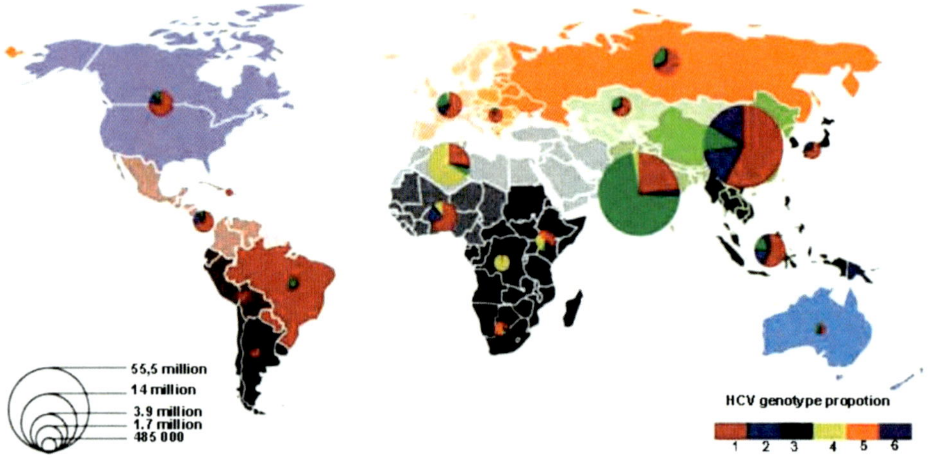

Fig. (2). Global distribution of HCV genotypes [51].

HCV MOLECULAR VIROLOGY

HCV-host interactions start as the virus attaches to the host cell surfaces (mostly hepatocytes; albeit HCV also infects some dendritic and lymphocytic cells, please see chapter 2 for more details) while binding to one or more cellular receptors organized as a receptor complex [17] (Fig. **3**). The cellular membranes of envelope glycoproteins E1 and E2 support the deliverance of nucleocapsids to the cytoplasm during pH-dependent virion fusion into hepatocytes. After decapsidation the viral genome is translated, leading to the production of a precursor polyprotein [18].

The precursor polyprotein is post-translationally processed by both cellular and viral proteases into 3 structural (C, E1, and E2) and 6 nonstructural proteins (NS2-NS5B) [18]. HCV replication takes place in the endoplasmic reticulum (ER)-derived membrane spherules (*i.e.* membranous web) in the cytoplasm *via* the synthesis of full-length negative-strand RNA intermediates [19]. During the assembly of progeny virions from cytoplasmic vesicles, the core (C) protein is released and transferred from the lipid droplets to form nucleocapsids that with the assistance of a nonstructural protein (*i.e.* NS5A) are loaded with RNA [19]. While the replicase proteins can bind to the HCV genomic RNA during replication and protein assembling process in close proximity through intracellular membranes of the membranous web (Albeit; replicase proteins are removed from maturing nucleocapsids, the intracellular sites of which might converge) [19]. HCV mature virion morphogenesis is coupled to the VLDL (very low-density lipoproteins) pathways, and new HCV particles are produced as lipoviral particles (LVPs). Mature full-length HCV virions are released into the extracellular milieu by exocytosis [18].

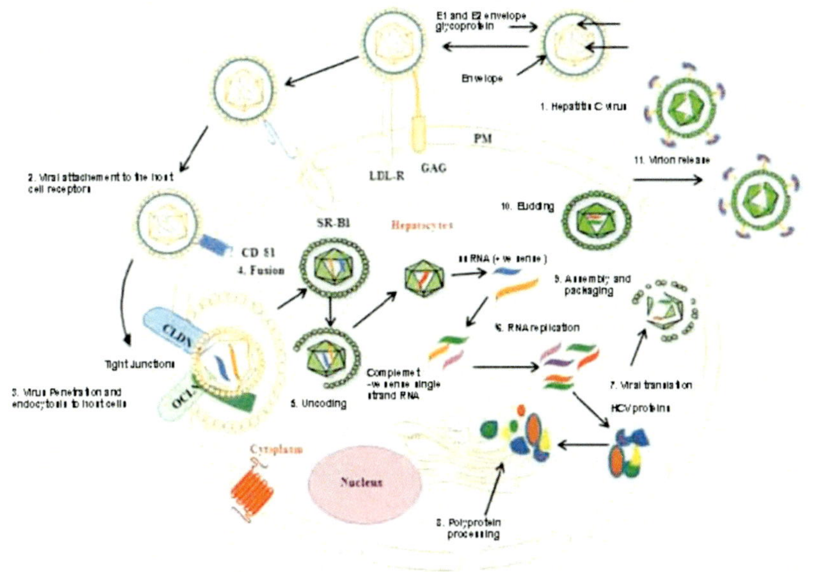

Fig. (3). HCV life cycle in host cells. HCV binds to host cell receptors (*i.e.* GAG, LDL-R, CD81, SR-B1) and with the help of tight junction-forming proteins (CLDN, OCLN) penetrates and fuses at the cellular or endosomal membrane of host cells. Following receptor-mediated endocytosis and uncoating of the virion, the +ssRNA genome is released into the cytoplasm where it is subjected to immediate translation and replication. Synthesis and post-translational modifications of structural and nonstructural proteins are processed by viral proteases and host signal peptidases that further translocate into the endoplasmic reticulum (ER) membranes. An intermediate (complement) negative-strand RNA is synthesized by viral RNA-dependent RNA polymerase (RdRp) that acts as a template for the synthesis of new viral mRNAs/new +ssRNA genomes. From ER, HCV structural and nonstructural proteins translocate to the Golgi complex. Virion assembly/packaging and budding originally initiates at the ER and completes to Golgi complex where the interaction of newly synthesized genomic RNA with viral core protein encapsidate viral genome and results in budding into the lumen of secretory vesicular compartments. Newly produced virions are released/excreted from the infected host cells by exocytosis. PM; plasma membrane, GAG; glycosaminoglycan, LDL-R; low-density lipoprotein receptor, SR-B1; scavenger receptor B type 1, CD; cluster of differentiation, CLDN; claudin, OCLN; occludin. NPCIL1; Niemann-Pick C1-like protein 1.

HEPATITIS C PROTEINS IN MOLECULAR PATHOGENESIS OF INFECTION

Almost every region of the HCV genome is crucial to play an active role in viral translation and replication regulation as well as in disease progression from asymptomatic acute infection to CHC and subsequent extrahepatic HCV manifestations [20]. Furthermore, some genome regions elicit humoral and cellular adaptive immune responses against HCV to protect infected host cells and prevent further infection transmission [18]. Some viral proteins specifically regulate host cell machinery as well as impede metabolic networks and cell signaling cascade to propagate HCV infection severity from chronicity to end-stage liver disease (ESLD) by developing cirrhosis and hepatocarcinogenesis [19].

All this happens due to an intricate interplay between hepatitis C and host cell interactions, including a plethora of genes, intracellular host cell factors regulation by viral proteins, and cell-signaling communication between infected and non-infected host cells as well as cell signaling pathways to overlap or impede between viral and host factors [21]. In the following section, we overview the contribution of viral-specific factors to disseminate HCV infection intensity from the self-limited acute phase to evolve chronic HCV infection followed by progression to severe hepatic co-morbidities (*e.g.* cirrhosis & HCC). Meanwhile, (Fig. **4**) depicts the structures of HCV structural and non-structural proteins and membrane association.

5' Untranslated Region (5' UTR)

The HCV 5' UTR spans from 332 to 343 nucleotides and contains up to 5 AUG codons depending on HCV GTs and subtypes. It is a highly conserved sequence among all HCV GTs (> 90% conservation) that folds into a complex of secondary and tertiary structures encompassing multiple SLs and two RNA pseudoknots of IRES structure [6]. However; with minor variants, it expresses quasispecies distribution in the infected populations. Quasispecies kinetics of all HCV GTs is widely based on nucleotide substitutions/mutations in one of the most conserved regions of the HCV genome like 5' UTR during viral replication [6]. These mutations provide a survival advantage or disadvantage to the mutated HCV genome in infected individuals [6]. The existence of naturally occurring variants (*i.e.* nucleotide signature sequence) within the 5' UTR region of HCV generates distinct subtype sub-populations and HCV diversification in certain HCV strains in infected human populations [5, 6]. A study demonstrates the existence of a distinct subtype 1a subpopulation in South American HCV strains which were identified by the presence of nucleotide signature sequence within the 5' UTR region of isolated strains [6]. The co-existence of multiple HCV subpopulations may occupy different regions on a fitness landscape to allow the virus to adapt rapidly to the changes in the landscape topology, which may enhance the virus settlement in its human host populations [5]. Virus particles isolated from infected host serum are likely to be released from the hepatocytes but also migrate from other cells like lymphocytes or dendritic cells, which indicates that nucleotide substitutions or sequence diversity found in 5' UTR-IRES may reflect tropism and translational activity for these compartments as well [6]. Intergenotypic and intragenotypic recombinants have also been demonstrated in some studies reported from St. Peters-burg (2k/1b), Philippines (2b/1b), Vietnam (GT-2/6), Ireland (2k/1b), France (GT-2/5), and in Peru (1b/1a) [6]. Recombination is an influencing mechanism to cause genetic diversity in some RNA viruses' families including HCV, with a potential impact on epidemiological studies, molecular pathogenesis, diagnosis, and treatment outcomes [5].

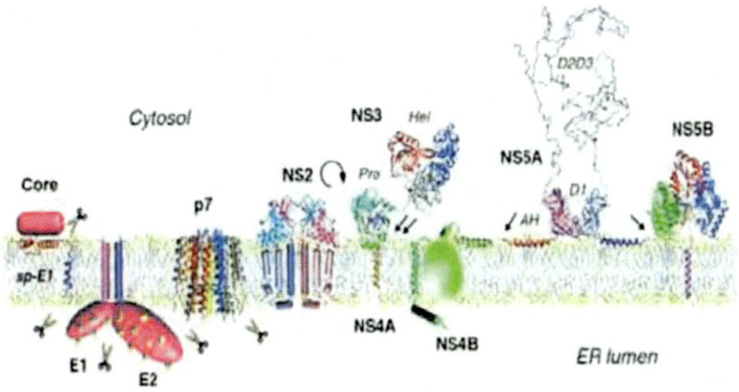

Fig. (4). HCV proteins structure and their membrane association [22]. Scissors indicate cleavage of HCV structural and nonstructural proteins by the endoplasmic reticulum (ER) signal peptidase, except on the cytosolic side where it indicates the processing of HCV core protein (antigen) by signal peptide peptidase. *The cyclic arrow* indicates the cleavage of HCV nonstructural protein NS2 by the NS2 protease. *Black arrows* indicate the cleavage of HCV polyprotein at four sites by the NS3/4A serine proteinase. The known protein structures are depicted as ribbon diagrams. HCV protein structures and the membrane bilayers are shown at the same scale. HCV proteins or protein segments whose structures are unresolved are represented as colored *spheres* or *cylinders* with their approximate sizes. HCV structural and nonstructural proteins are shown from left to right in the figure. 1) HCV core protein (red) comprises the N-terminal natively unfolded domain (D1) and two amphipathic α-helices connected by a hydrophobic loop (D2 domain) [52]. The core-E1 signal peptide (PDB entry 2KQI) is cleaved by SPP [53]. 2) HCV envelope glycoproteins (E1 and E2) heterodimer are associated by the C-terminal transmembrane domains. *Green spots* indicate glycosylation of the E1 and E2 envelope proteins. 3) Oligomeric model of HCV nonstructural protein "p7" based on the structure of the monomer solved by nuclear magnetic resonance [54] and molecular dynamics simulations in a 1-palmitoyl-2-oleoyl-sn-glycero-3-phosphocholine (POPC) phospholipid bilayer [55]. 4) The catalytic domain (dimer subunits) of HCV nonstructural protein NS2 are depicted in *blue* and *magenta* [56] which are connected to their N-terminal membrane domains constituted of three putative transmembrane segments [57, 58]. The active site residues of NS2 protein (His 143, Glu 163, and Cys 184) are shown as spheres. 5) NS3 serine protease domain (*cyan*) associated with the central protease activation and the N-terminal transmembrane domains of NS4A are depicted in *yellow*. The catalytic triad of NS3/4A serine protease (His 57, Asp 81, and Ser 139) is shown as *spheres (magenta)*. NS3 helicase domains 1,2, and 3 are represented in *silver*, *red*, and *blue* respectively. The current NS3 protein structure present in this figure [59] illustrates that the NS3 helicase domain can no longer interact with the NS3 protease domain when the latter is associated with the membrane through its amphipathic α-helix 11–21 (*green*) and the transmembrane domain of NS4A [60]. 6) The N-terminal part of NS4B includes two amphipathic α-helices of which the second has the potential to traverse the membrane bilayer [61]. The C-terminal cytosolic part includes a predicted highly conserved α-helix and an amphipathic α-helix interacting in-plane with the membrane [62]. 7) NS5A domain 1 dimer (D1) [63]; subunits colored in *magenta* and *ice blue*), as well as intrinsically unfolded domains 2 and 3 (D2D3) [64 - 67], are shown in the figure. The N-terminal amphipathic α-helix of NS5A protein in-plane membrane anchor (Penin *et al.* 2004; helices colored in *red* and *blue*) are shown in relative position to the phospholipid membrane (adapted from [63]. (8) NS5B RNA-dependent RNA polymerase (RdRp) catalytic domain [68] associated with the membrane *via* its C-terminal transmembrane segment (F.P. *et al.* unpublished data) is shown in the figure. The fingers, palm, and thumb subdomains of the catalytic domain are colored *blue*, *red*, and *green*, respectively. The catalytic site of the NS5B lies within the center of the cytosolic domain and the RNA template-binding cleft is located vertically on the right along the thumb subdomain β-fap (*orange*) and the C-terminal part of the linker segment (*silver*), connecting the cytosolic domain to the transmembrane segment (*magenta*). The cell membrane is represented as a simulated model of a POPC bilayer (http://moose.bio.ucalgary.ca/). Polar heads and hydrophobic tails of phospholipids (stick structure) are colored *light yellow* and *light gray*, respectively. The positions of the NS5A in-plane membrane helices at the membrane interface as well as that of the transmembrane domain of NS5B were deduced from molecular dynamics simulations in POPC bilayer (F.P., D.M. *et al.* unpublished data). The positioning of the NS3-4A membrane segments and of the amphipathic α-helices in the core and NS4B are tentative.

Being the most conserved region of the HCV genome, 5' UTR is mostly suited for amplification methods and contains specific sequence motifs for HCV GTs/sub-types identification [23]. Many diagnostic laboratories and most commercially available HCV typing assays target 5' UTR due to higher genotype-based assay sensitivity. However, mounting evidence suggests that direct sequencing of 5' UTR does not identify all existing HCV GT 1 subtypes in 20% of infected cases [6]. Other methods based on more variable regions of the HCV genome (*e.g.* NS5B) could be relied upon for the accurate identification of subtypes [6]. A study describes the sequencing and phylogenetic analysis of the NS5B region as the first step in molecular epidemiological studies to recognize the route of HCV transmission [14]. NS5B is an extremely preferred region for HCV subtyping, but it is not always accurately amplified because of primer-target mismatch to the highly variable nucleotide region of NS5B [14].

Interestingly, the 5' UTR role in HCV translation regulation has been studied in detail, however; its significance for RNA replication so far is not fully elucidated [6]. Previous studies demonstrate that for plus-strand RNA virus replication, signals are located in 5' UTR of the template strand where they act as promoter elements for RNA replication initiation of both minus and plus-strand RNAs [5]. But how they interact with NS5B replication machinery and 3' UTR CRE is still poorly understood. Although, RNA secondary and tertiary structure stability is regarded as a significant factor for virus genome stability, but not essential to predict virus stabilization and response to pegylated interferon (PEG-IFNα) therapy [20]. Either nucleotide variations in 5' UTR of HCV-infected treatment-naive individuals may affect viral translation or response to therapy is still unclear [20]. Previous studies show that no correlation exists between treatment outcomes and the number of viral strains and HCV genome heterogeneity in treatment-naïve patients or before initiating treatment in such populations [19]. Equivocally, treatment-experienced patients with SVRs against PEG-IFN plus RBV (ribavirin) exhibited a significant decrease in the number of viral strains as well as overall genetic diversity [19]. A significant decrease in genetic diversity was evident with increased homogenous virus population and viral clearance in patients with higher SVR rates to PEG-IFN/RBV therapy and was independent of HCV GTs [18]. Another plausible justification is the correlation between increased genetic diversity and acute hepatitis C which leads to chronic hepatitis; whereas decreased genome variations were made explicit to resolve acute hepatitis before viral clearance [18].

HCV Antigen (Core;C) Protein

HCV core protein is the first protein to be synthesized during viral translation and is considered to be the most conserved part of HCV polyprotein [24]. It is also the first protein to contact HCV-infected host cell cytoplasm contents during viral entry and nucleocapsid release [25]. In the later phase of HCV biology, it plays an important role in mature virion formation and viral assembly in the ER [26]. The core protein amino acid composition is highly conserved among different HCV GTs as compared to other HCV proteins, however; sequence variations have been reported within different domains of the protein in different HCV-induced pathological states [26]. The key function of core protein is RNA binding to encapsidation with associated membranes and with lipid droplets (LDs) to produce virus-like particles (VLPs) and infectious virion progeny [27]. However; core protein directly or indirectly interacts with host cellular factors to play an essential role in virus-mediated pathogenesis (*i.e.* oxidative stress, steatosis, insulin resistance, and hepatocarcinogenesis) [27].

HCV Core Protein Morphology

The intracellular posttranslational processing of core protein is mediated by an intramembrane protease; the signal peptide peptidase (SPP) that cleaves an immature p23 core protein (191-aa polypeptide) at the C-terminal signal peptide and releases N-terminal 173-179 aa p21 mature core protein [28]. SPP is also required to translocate E1 glycoprotein to ER during the HCV life cycle in infected host cells. The mature core protein p21 then interacts with LDs on the ER membrane (a major site of HCV particle assembly) and thus influences mature virion infectivity and morphogenesis of the viral particles [29]. p21 is found in secreted viral progeny as determined by the analysis of serum samples of HCV-infected patients [29]. The X-ray crystallography predicts that core protein consists of three domains; D1: a basic hydrophilic N-terminal region of 1-118 aa, D2: a central hydrophobic domain of 119-173 aa, and D3; the last hydrophobic signal sequence domain of 174-191 aa containing SPP [29]. The mature core protein is a 177 aa dimeric α-helical protein and acts as a membrane protein. The domain D1 is mainly involved in viral RNA binding and encapsidation of the viral genome. Domain D2 is required for proper folding and stability of D1 and association of core with ER and outer mitochondrial membranes. D3 domain along with SPP is involved in stable and infectious viral particle formation [29, 30]. HCV core protein itself is capable and sufficient to induce lipid accumulation and elicit or propagate other HCV-induced pathogenesis in infected hepatocytes that's why also named HCV 'core antigen' [30]. As a protein-protein interaction with other HCV proteins, it interacts with a non-structural NS5A phosphoprotein to form the bridge between LDs and the sites of viral RNA replication. Furthermore, it recruits other HCV non-structural proteins on LDs and this LDs and NS proteins arrangement as membrane spherules play a crucial role in viral replication and HCV particle morphogenesis [30].

HCV core interaction with host cellular factors may impede metabolic pathways of infected hepatocytes leading to hepatosteatosis, insulin resistance (IR), varied IFN response as well as affecting the transcription of cellular proto-oncogenes and other tumor suppressor genes which may progress CHC to apoptosis and hepatocarcinogenesis (*i.e.* HCC in CHC patients) [30]. However; the intensity of viral infectivity and pathogenesis may vary among different HCV strains which mainly relate to amino acids sequence variations of core protein and other viral/host factors [30]. As mentioned earlier, intergenotypic core sequences are similar, however; at subtype and quasispecies levels, the amino acid mutations or single amino acid polymorphism can modulate core protein interplay with other HCV genome proteins and host cell factors and tamper their stability to regulate normal cellular functions and metabolic pathways [30].

HCV Core Protein and Hepatic Steatosis

HCV core protein-induced hepatosteatosis (also known as liver steatosis) and oxidative stress are two preliminary pathological states which are raised due to enhanced accumulation of triglyceride-rich lipids in hepatic cells and could be used as a prognosis biomarker of CHC infection progression to hepatic fibrosis, cirrhosis, and subsequent hepatocarcinogenesis [30, 31]. Core protein causes lipid accumulation as a part of the HCV life cycle to assemble infectious virion and steatosis is the result of this lipid accumulation. Core protein upregulates the promoter activity of two major lipid synthesis enzymes in HCV-infected hepatocytes including fatty acid synthase (FAS) and sterol regulatory element-binding protein-1 (SREBP-1). The Core protein activates transcription factors, SREBP-1c4 and RXRa (Retinoid X receptor alpha), leading to enhanced activity of various enzymes involved in cellular lipid biosynthesis, and down-regulates PPAR-a (peroxisome proliferator-activated receptors alpha) and mitochondrial carnitine palmitoyl transferase-1, resulting in the reduction of fatty acid oxidation activity [32]. Hepatic cell oxidative stress is associated with core protein upregulation of the production of reactive oxygen species (ROS) from induced nitric oxide species (iNOS) by activating cyclooxygenase-2 (Cox-2) expression in hepatocyte-derived cells [33]. Another potential mechanism of HCV core-induced oxidative stress damages the mitochondrial electron transport system in core protein-expressing cells which further leads to HCC [34]. HCV GT-3 core protein has been demonstrated to induce more lipid accumulation *in vitro* than GT-1 core protein expression because of the difference of a single amino acid substitution in the D2 domain of the core protein [31]. Furthermore, core protein expression in hepatocytes of transgenic mice also resulted in steatosis and HCC development as one study expressed [33]. Very interestingly, steatosis is found more spontaneously and severely in HCV GT-3 infected patients because of the presence of specific steatogenic sequences in the core genome of this HCV GT which directly correlates to the burden of HCV viral load in hepatic cells [33]. Surprisingly, this association of high viremia to steatogenic severity is not observed in other HCV GTs-infected patients [33].

HCV Core Protein and Hepatocarcinogenesis

HCV core protein is capable to regulate the growth of hepatic cells by affecting the transcription of cellular proto-oncogenes and other tumor suppressor genes [1]. Single amino acid polymorphism or mutations within the core sequence may alter the predicted HCV RNA structures of new virion formation and can differentially regulate cellular pathways and processes that can contribute to oncogenesis [29]. In domain D3 of core protein, aa positions 70 and 91 are very much associated with anti-HCV treatment response to IFN/RBV, to induce insulin resistance (IR), apoptosis, and HCC [29]. It is beyond the scope of this book chapter to discuss in detail the intricate interplay of viral and host factors and cellular pathways involved in the pathogenesis of these hepatic comorbidities, hence we briefly overview such interactions here [32].

As previously mentioned, different domains of core protein have specific roles in HCV infection biology, therefore every domain is different to induce hepatic cell apoptosis [33]. For example, the N-terminal D1 domain is likely to be involved with a high percentage of apoptosis and necrosis than the D3 C-terminal domain, while the middle D2 domain with least induced effects [29]. The previous studies have alluded that binding interactions between HCV core and p53 protein (a tumor suppressor protein) either activation or inhibition of p53 expression resulted in consecutive anti- or pro-apoptotic effects [33]. Similarly, another study demonstrates that core protein suppresses the activation of a transcription factor NFkB (nuclear factor-kB; an inducible transcription factor and regulator of many genes involved in inflammation, immune responses, cell proliferation, and apoptosis) by inhibiting the degradation of IkBα (nuclear factor of kappa B), and activating the transcription factor activator protein-1 (AP-1) *via* JNK (c-Jun N-terminal kinase) and mitogen-activated protein kinase (MAPK) pathway that ultimate initiates anti-apoptotic or hepatocarcinogenesis effects [32]. Likewise, in spontaneous induction and severity of liver steatosis in HCV GT-3 infected patients, a similar correlation has been observed between HCC and CHC 3a subtype-infected patients in Pakistan [31]. Full-length core sequence analysis extracted from the circulating HCV RNA of HCC infected patient's serum indicates the existence of specific substitutions responsible for HCC induction as compared to patients with CHC infection only [29]. One study analyzed full-length HCV-1b sequences from HCC patients and controls and identified seven polymorphisms (nucleotide) significantly associated with increased risk of HCC

(36G/C, 209A, 271U/C, 309A/C, 435A/C, 481A, and 546A/C) [35]. Interestingly, 209A has been associated with IFN resistance and HCC induction suggesting that Core gene sequence data might provide useful information about HCC risk [32]. In one study eight mutations were found in the HCV subtype 1b core gene related to the increased risk of HCC (*i.e.*, A028C, G209A, C219U/A, U264C, A271C/U, C378U/A, G435A/C, and G481A), whereas U303C/A was found to be associated with decreased HCC risk [27]. Overall these mutations bring about four amino acid substitutions: Lys10Glu, Arg70Glu, Met91Leu, and Gly161Ser to induce HCC in CHC-infected patients [27].

Since mutations within HCV core protein or envelope glycoproteins (*i.e.* E1 and E2) may aggravate or block viral infectivity respectively, it may be assumed that those specific substitutions or mutations could be responsible for the spontaneous induction and severity of HCC in certain HCV GTs [17]. albeit; a lot of viral and host factors may incite and contribute to developing HCC, we only summarized here the polymorphism or mutations in the core gene which are associated with different pathological states leading to HCC and could be used as clinical biomarkers of HCV disease stage or development of HCC [36]. However; complete elucidation to evaluate the importance of these mutations in HCC identification/progression requires further studies. In addition to that, the identification of the molecular pathways underlying the association between certain HCV mutations and hepatocarcinogenesis also demands comprehensive virus-host interaction studies. Consequently, an ample understanding of this relationship would result in a search for novel targets for HCC therapeutic intervention.

HCV Core Protein and Insulin Resistance (IR)

HCV epidemiological data also points out a clear association between HCV infection and the development of type 2 diabetes mellitus due to the development of IR, a common metabolic disorder in the pre-diabetic state in HCV individuals [37]. The ratio of diabetes has been demonstrated more in HCV infections than in other liver diseases (*i.e.* 20–25% more in patients with HCV *vs.* 10% of those with hepatitis B) [37]. IR could be promoted by HCV viral proteins in a GT-specific mechanism (Moucari *et al.*, 2008). It has been suggested that HCV core protein leads to IR through the interference of intracellular insulin signaling, mainly by the serine phosphorylation of the insulin receptor substrate (IRS-1) pathway in HCV-infected individuals [37].

HCV Envelope Glycoproteins (E1 and E2)

HCV E1 and E2 Morphology

HCV encodes two envelope glycoproteins (E1 and E2) which are released from viral polyproteins by signal peptidase cleavage [38]. Both glycoproteins are type 1 transmembrane proteins (*i.e.* the proteins which are anchored to the lipid membrane with a stop-transfer anchor sequence and have their N-terminal domains targeted to the ER lumen during synthesis) with a highly glycosylated N-terminal ectodomain and a C-terminal hydrophobic anchor [38]. Both proteins associate with each other as noncovalent heterodimers after their synthesis. This E1-E2 heterodimer complex is necessary for HCV entry into host cells where the transmembrane domain plays an essential role in E1-E2 heterodimer assembly and subcellular localization. The transmembrane domain may also play a coordinate role to reorganize the E1-E2 protein complex for the fusion process to occur. Both proteins are retained in ER, signals for which are present in the transmembrane domains. Similarly, It has been found that the E1-E2 complex is present at the surface of HCV particles, and therefore it is an obvious candidate ligand for host cellular receptors (*i.e.* CD81[Cluster of Differentiation 81], SR-BI [Scavenger receptor class B type 1], and CLDN1 [Claudin-1]). E1 and E2 envelope glycoproteins exhibit the highest degree of genetic heterogeneity as compared to other HCV proteins, where E2 protein contains a hypervariable region 1 (HVR1), which is located at the N- terminus [38].

HVR1 of E2 Glycoprotein Modulates the Immune System

An important correlation has been found between E2 glycoprotein HVR1 sequence variation and the intensity and cross-reactivity of humoral immune responses [39]. It strongly supports the contention that HCV variant selection is driven by immune pressure. In one study, monoclonal antibodies (mAbs) generated after immunization of mice with peptides derived from the natural HVR1 sequence of HCV E2 protein were noticed to generate a neutralization response for other several HVR1 sequences, predicting the existence of conserved amino acid motifs among different HCV variants [40, 41]. This mechanism of inducting a broadly cross-reactive immune response to envelope glycoprotein E2 HVR1 could be used to generate protective immunity [41]. As the E1-E2 protein complex is exposed at the surface of the virion, this protein complex is a target for neutralizing antibodies. Antibodies to HVR1 may block viral infection by inhibiting virion binding or membrane fusion [41]. It has been attested in one study that rabbit hyperimmune serum generated against the HVR1 can neutralize the ability of HCV to infect chimpanzees [42]. Furthermore, in a lymphoid cell line, neutralizing antibodies (nAbs) were also identified by their ability to prevent

HCV replication [43]. It suggests that an HCV clone lacking E2 HVR1 is infectious and can be attenuated in an *in vivo* model (*e.g.* chimpanzees), however; HCV-infected strains in humans always contain E2 HVR1, which predicts that human intact HCV strains have HVR1 with a significant survival advantage [43]. Characterization of HCV envelope glycoproteins entry function was initially studied by the development of the HCV pseudo particle (HCVpp) models and provided useful information related to the role of this heterodimer protein complex in viral entry [43]. However, the development of a full-length HCV infectious clone (*e.g.*, JFH-1) in cell culture provided a new platform for a new generation of HCV investigations. The efficient, reproducible, and robust expression with viral infectivity of this infectious clone in permissive cell lines (*e.g.*, Huh7.5 [Human hepatoma cell line] and Huh7.5.1]) further expedited the cell culture experiments in molecular virology [44]. Consequently, the ample understanding of HCV biology in infected hosts from virus entry to new virion secretions, as well as to the development of effective antivirals was made possible and is continued.

HCV NONSTRUCTURAL PROTEINS AND THEIR ROLE IN HEPATITIS C PATHOGENESIS

HCV nonstructural proteins play essential regulatory roles in viral replication, translation, posttranslational protein modifications, and to development of antiviral drug resistance [14]. Some nonstructural proteins like NS3, NS5A, and NS5B are the potential antiviral drug targets for newly developed direct-acting antivirals (DAAs) and other anti-mRNA based treatment strategies (*e.g.*, oligonucleotides and small interference RNA, *etc.*) as well as some are acting as emerging drug targets (*e.g.* NS2 and NS4B) for the DAAs in clinical trials [14]. We briefly overview HCV nonstructural proteins' role in the viral life cycle and molecular pathogenesis of HCV infection, although most of the nonstructural proteins play regulatory roles in the viral life cycle than molecular pathogenesis of the infection.

NS2 Metalloprotease

NS2 protein along with NS3 constitutes a highly hydrophobic protease responsible for the cleavage of viral polypeptide between non-structural proteins NS2 and NS3 [45]. Three residues H143, E163, and C184 (while H952, E972, and C993 when numbered in polyprotein) constitute a catalytic triad of NS2/NS3 protease and are considered to be conserved among all HCV GTs [46]. However, many aspects of NS2/NS3 protease's role in HCV infection biology and viral life cycle are still controversial or unknown [45]. Some studies project its role as either cysteine or metalloprotease, albeit; its sequence homology is not significant to proteases of known function. Similarly, some studies demonstrate its pivotal role for persistent infection in a chimpanzee, however; not fully elucidated in an *in vitro* system to study all aspects of HCV replication. Interestingly, some recent studies have alluded to the possible role of cleaved NS2 protein in the modulation of host cell gene expression and apoptosis [45].

NS3/4A Serine Protease/Helicase

NS3 acts as a serine protease as well as an RNA helicase/NTPase during HCV polyprotein processing and viral replication [47]. It is a non-covalent heterodimer consisting of a catalytic subunit (the N-terminal one-third of NS3 protein) and an activating cofactor (NS4A protein) and is responsible for cleavage at four sites of the HCV polyprotein. The NS3-4A protease activity involves a catalytic triad of three motifs including Ser-139, His-57, and Asp-81, and an oxy-anion hole comprising backbone amides of Gly-137 and Ser-139. In addition to that, NS3-4A acts as a helicase to unwind viral RNA by integrating into the HCV replication complex, although not fully understood [47]. It is an essential protease for viral replication in cell culture as well as in chimpanzees and has been considered one of the most pioneering, attractive, and well-studied drug targets for the design and development of anti-HCV therapies (*e.g.*, oral IFN-free DAAs, siRNAs, *etc.*). However, its shallow substrate-binding groove and lack of an efficient *in vitro* viral replication model hampered the researchers and investigators for decades to discover, design, and developing small and selective inhibitors against HCV NS3-4A protease as oral drug candidates. However, during the last decade, rapid advancement in molecular biology techniques, the introduction of novel technologies in molecular medicine, and drug designing strategies made it possible to overcome these two obstacles and provided a full understanding of this protease's biological functions, biochemistry, and three-dimensional structures. It culminates the efforts to demonstrate proof-of-concept anti-HCV activities of newly developed IFN-free DAAs against NS3/4A protease in treated patients. Some studies explicitly the role of NS3 in the progression of persistent HCV infection by inhibiting the host's innate immune defense mechanisms by blocking retinoic acid-inducible gene I (RIG-I) and toll-like cell signaling receptors (TLRs). It suggests that NS3-4A protease inhibition may restore the host's innate immune mechanism against viral infection in the host cells [47]. NS4A is the smallest known non-structural protein of the HCV genome and is essential as a co-factor for serine protease activity of the NS3-4A complex. It has been shown that in its absence only one cleavage site (*i.e.* NS5A/NS5B) is partially processed by NS3 protease alone. The central region of the protein (*i.e.* from residue 21 to 34) is important and sufficient for the enzymatic co-factor function [47].

NS4B

NS4B for many years was characterized mainly as a protein of unknown function [48]. However; the latest studies predict NS4B's potential role in the modulation of RdRp enzyme activity and regulation of many host signal transduction pathways leading to HCV carcinogenesis, impairment of ER function, and regulation of both viral and host mRNA translation [14]. The most significant role found recently to be involved in the formation of a novel intracellular membrane structure, known as membranous web or membrane spherules (*i.e.* a platform upon which viral replication occurs). Furthermore, specific domains within NS4B including an amphipathic helix and nucleotide-binding motif also act as attractive targets for the design and development of novel IFN-free DAAs nowadays [48].

NS5A: An Interferon Resistance Protein

NS5A is a phosphoprotein that acts as a multifunctional regulator of cellular pathways and virus replication as well as is involved in conferring resistance against IFN therapy [48]. The protein first time grabbed the attention due to its role in modulating the host cell IFN response. A domain within the protein known as the interferon-α sensitivity determining region (ISDR) was found to confer resistance against IFN treatment in HCV-infected patients [49]. It is also an essential component of the HCV replicase enzyme and exerts its wide range of effects on host cell processes including innate immunity, host cell growth, and cell proliferation [50]. In the last decade, the protein has been widely searched, investigated, and targeted to design and develop IFN-free DAAs, some of which have been approved by the US FDA to use in real-world clinical settings with promising SVR rates in treated individuals.

NS5B: RNA Dependent RNA Polymerase (RdRp)

NS5B protein also known as the RdRp enzyme, is a catalytic subunit of the replicase enzyme complex consisting of virally encoded and host proteins, which is responsible for viral RNA replication [14]. The NS5B protein sequence motifs are highly conserved among all the known RdRps and contain discrete fingers, palm, and thumb subdomains [14]. A unique feature of RdRp is an enriched active site developed due to extensive interactions between the finger and thumb subdomains. Sequence motif residues D220, D319, and D318, are actively involved in transferring nucleotide to an active catalytic subunit of the NS5B protein [14]. Being the viral RNA replication enzyme, NS5B is a potential target to develop novel nucleoside and non-nucleoside NS5B inhibitors (NIs and NNIs respectively) among which the sofosbuvir (SOF) and dasabuvir (DSV) are clinically used to treat different HCV GTs and subtypes infected individuals with promising SVR rates [14]. Nowadays some other NNIs (*e.g.*, radalbuvir) are also in the pipeline and clinical trials as an emerging regimen with increased anti-hepatitis C clinical efficacy.

3' UTR

The 3' UTR of the HCV genome is a tripartite structure located at the 3' end of the viral genome and is predominantly involved in HCV replication [6]. This region is vital for viral RNA replication, either in an *in vitro* cell culture system transfected with HCV replicon or *in vivo* chimpanzee model inoculated with full-length HCV infectious clone [51]. The 3'UTR genome contains a variable region of 26-70 nucleotides in length, a poly U/UC tract of variable length and sequence, and the X-tail of 98-100 nucleotides which is conserved among various HCV GTs [51]. The 3'UTR indispensable signals for viral RNA replication and translation while interacting with other viral genome regions in a highly orchestrated manner [14]. The sequence and secondary structure of 3'UTR are somehow conserved among different HCV GTs and subtypes. The interaction among 5'UTR, 3'UTR, and NS5B is mandatory for viral replication, particularly in the initiation of minus-strand RNA [51]. In addition to that, 3'UTR binding with NS5A is assumed to mediate genome circularization and switch on the viral translation. Recent studies predict that the viral translation and replication signals overlap among 5' UTR, 3' UTR, and other viral proteins, and studies are in progress to fully elucidate these mechanisms. Furthermore, some studies suggest that sequence and structural variability of the 3' UTR regulatory elements (*e.g.* variable region and poly U/UC tail) found in inter-genotypic and intra-genotypic isolates could be associated with the differential prevalence of HCV across the world and variable treatment responses of HCV subtypes to the same therapy [51].

CONCLUSIONS

The intricate interplay of HCV pathogenesis, epidemiology, and therapeutics is always remaining a big challenge to investigators, researchers, and physicians. Despite the revolutionary advancement in molecular biology techniques, as well as the introduction of state-of-the-art diagnostic procedures, and imperative development in current molecular medicine, the public healthcare burden of hepatitis C and associated hepatic comorbidities are still significant around the world. The multifaceted, perplexing, and intermingled interplay between hepatitis C and host cellular factors provides the survival advantage to the virus as well as progress from acute hepatitis C disease to CHC infection and subsequent other hepatic comorbidities. HCV structural and nonstructural proteins, as well as host cell regulatory factors, cell signaling, and metabolic networks assist, modulate, or impede the natural physiological role of liver cells to lead to hepatosteatosis, hepatic fibrosis, cirrhosis, and hepatocarcinogenesis in infected patients. A better understanding of all these regulatory pathways involved in the molecular pathogenesis of HCV infection could be useful to cure harder-to-treat hepatitis C-infected specific populations. The advent and approval of IFN-free DAAs to treat CHC infection has provided clinical promise in real-world clinical settings, however; their therapeutic benefits in complicated hepatitis C-induced co-morbidities (*e.g.*, decompensated cirrhotic patients, HCC, HCV/HIV, or HCV/HBV co-infected patients) and in heart, kidney, and liver transplant donors and recipients infected with HCV are remained to investigate. All these demands refocus the search for novel roles of hepatitis C-host interactions, the meaningful and smart dissection of regulatory pathways, and cell signaling networks to identify new drug targets ligands and prognosis biomarkers for the clinical diagnosis of these comorbidities. Furthermore, pharmacogenomics studies and pre-clinical trials of the new regimens in the pipeline should be considered to prevent any hepatic or systemic toxicity which may further exacerbate hepatitis C-induced extrahepatic manifestations in infected patients as well as in pre-and post-treated individuals with IFN-free DAAs.

REFERENCES

[1] Naeemi H, Aslam R, Raza SM, *et al.* Distribution of IL28B and IL10 polymorphisms as genetic predictors of treatment response in Pakistani HCV genotype 3 patients. Arch Virol 2018; 163(4): 997-1008.
[http://dx.doi.org/10.1007/s00705-018-3711-3] [PMID: 29340806]

[2] Ahmad W, Shabbiri K, Ijaz B, *et al.* Serine 204 phosphorylation and O-β-GlcNAC interplay of IGFBP-6 as therapeutic indicator to regulate IGF-II functions in viral mediated hepatocellular carcinoma. Virol J 2011; 8(1): 208.
[http://dx.doi.org/10.1186/1743-422X-8-208] [PMID: 21548981]

[3] Ahmad W, Shabbiri K, Ijaz B, *et al.* Claudin-1 required for HCV virus entry has high potential for phosphorylation and O-glycosylation. Virol J 2011; 8(1): 229.
[http://dx.doi.org/10.1186/1743-422X-8-229] [PMID: 21569618]

[4] Shahid I, Alzahrani AR, Al-Ghamdi SS, Alanazi IM, Rehman S, Hassan S. Hepatitis C diagnosis: Simplified solutions, predictive barriers, and future promises. Diagnostics (Basel) 2021; 11(7): 1253.
[http://dx.doi.org/10.3390/diagnostics11071253] [PMID: 34359335]

[5] AlMalki WH, Shahid I, Abdalla AN, Johargy AK, Ahmed M, Hassan S. Consensus small interfering RNA targeted to stem-loops II and III of IRES structure of 5′ UTR effectively inhibits virus replication and translation of HCV sub-genotype 4a isolates from Saudi Arabia. Saudi J Biol Sci 2021; 28(1): 1109-22.
[http://dx.doi.org/10.1016/j.sjbs.2020.11.041] [PMID: 33424405]

[6] AlMalki WH, Shahid I, Abdalla AN, Johargy AK, Ahmed M, Hassan S. Virological surveillance, molecular phylogeny, and evolutionary dynamics of hepatitis C virus subtypes 1a and 4a isolates in patients from Saudi Arabia. Saudi J Biol Sci 2021; 28(3): 1664-77.
[http://dx.doi.org/10.1016/j.sjbs.2020.11.089] [PMID: 33732052]

[7] Shahid I, Gull S, Ijaz B, *et al.* Stable Huh-7 cell lines expressing non-structural proteins of genotype 1a of hepatitis C virus. J Virol Methods 2013; 189(1): 65-9.
[http://dx.doi.org/10.1016/j.jviromet.2013.01.005] [PMID: 23352716]

[8] Ahmad W, Ijaz B, Gull S, *et al.* A brief review on molecular, genetic and imaging techniques for HCV fibrosis evaluation. Virol J 2011; 8(1): 53.

[http://dx.doi.org/10.1186/1743-422X-8-53] [PMID: 21299910]

[9] Houldsworth A. Exploring the possibility of arthropod transmission of HCV. J Med Virol 2017; 89(2): 187-94.
[http://dx.doi.org/10.1002/jmv.24638] [PMID: 27447819]

[10] Bolzoni L, Rosà R, Cagnacci F, Rizzoli A. Effect of deer density on tick infestation of rodents and the hazard of tick-borne encephalitis. II: Population and infection models. Int J Parasitol 2012; 42(4): 373-81.
[http://dx.doi.org/10.1016/j.ijpara.2012.02.006] [PMID: 22429768]

[11] Ijaz B, Ahmad W, Javed FT, *et al.* Association of laboratory parameters with viral factors in patients with hepatitis C. Virol J 2011; 8(1): 361.
[http://dx.doi.org/10.1186/1743-422X-8-361] [PMID: 21777434]

[12] Ansar M, Ashfaq UA, shahid I, *et al.* Inhibition of full length Hepatitis C Virus particles of 1a genotype through small interference RNA. Virol J 2011; 8(1): 203.
[http://dx.doi.org/10.1186/1743-422X-8-203] [PMID: 21535893]

[13] Shahid I, ALMalki WH, Hafeez MH, Hassan S. Hepatitis C virus infection treatment: An era of game changer direct acting antivirals and novel treatment strategies. Crit Rev Microbiol 2016; 42(4): 535-47.
[http://dx.doi.org/10.3109/1040841X.2014.970123] [PMID: 25373616]

[14] Shahid I, Almalki WH, Ibrahim MM, *et al.* Characterization of *in vitro* inhibitory effects of consensus short interference RNAs against non-structural 5B gene of hepatitis C virus 1a genotype. Indian J Med Microbiol 2018; 36(4): 494-503.
[http://dx.doi.org/10.4103/ijmm.IJMM_17_146] [PMID: 30880695]

[15] Shahid I, Ibrahim MM. All oral interferon-free direct-acting antivirals as combination therapies to cure hepatitis C. Curr Mol Med 2019; 18(7): 409-35.
[http://dx.doi.org/10.2174/1566524019666190104110439] [PMID: 30608042]

[16] Asad S, Ijaz B, Ahmad W, *et al.* Development of persistent HCV genotype 3a infection cell culture model in huh-7 cell. Virol J 2012; 9(1): 11.
[http://dx.doi.org/10.1186/1743-422X-9-11] [PMID: 22234052]

[17] Wang Y. Scotomas in molecular virology and epidemiology of hepatitis C virus. World J Gastroenterol 2013; 19(44): 7910-21.
[http://dx.doi.org/10.3748/wjg.v19.i44.7910] [PMID: 24307785]

[18] Lapa D, Garbuglia A, Capobianchi M, Del Porto P, Hepatitis C. Hepatitis C virus genetic variability, human immune response, and genome polymorphisms: which is the interplay? Cells 2019; 8(4): 305.
[http://dx.doi.org/10.3390/cells8040305] [PMID: 30987134]

[19] Webster DP, Klenerman P, Dusheiko GM, Hepatitis C. Hepatitis C. Lancet 2015; 385(9973): 1124-35.
[http://dx.doi.org/10.1016/S0140-6736(14)62401-6] [PMID: 25687730]

[20] Echeverría N, Moratorio G, Cristina J, Moreno P. Hepatitis C virus genetic variability and evolution. World J Hepatol 2015; 7(6): 831-45.
[http://dx.doi.org/10.4254/wjh.v7.i6.831] [PMID: 25937861]

[21] Matsuura K, Tanaka Y. Host genetic variants influencing the clinical course of hepatitis C virus infection. J Med Virol 2016; 88(2): 185-95.
[http://dx.doi.org/10.1002/jmv.24334] [PMID: 26211651]

[22] Bartenschlager R, Hepatitis C. Virus: From Molecular Virology to Antiviral Therapy Preface. Curr Top Microbiol Immunol 2013; 369: V-VI.
[http://dx.doi.org/10.1007/978-3-642-27340-7]

[23] Khaliq S, Khaliq SA, Zahur M, *et al.* RNAi as a new therapeutic strategy against HCV. Biotechnol Adv 2010; 28(1): 27-34.
[http://dx.doi.org/10.1016/j.biotechadv.2009.08.004] [PMID: 19729057]

[24] Khan M, Jahan S, Khaliq S, *et al.* Interaction of the hepatitis C virus (HCV) core with cellular genes in the development of HCV-induced steatosis. Arch Virol 2010; 155(11): 1735-53.
[http://dx.doi.org/10.1007/s00705-010-0797-7] [PMID: 20842391]

[25] Gawlik K, Gallay PA. HCV core protein and virus assembly: what we know without structures. Immunol Res 2014; 60(1): 1-10.
[http://dx.doi.org/10.1007/s12026-014-8494-3] [PMID: 24557493]

[26] Galli C, Julicher P, Plebani M. HCV core antigen comes of age: a new opportunity for the diagnosis of hepatitis C virus infection. Clinical Chemistry and Laboratory Medicine (CCLM) 2018; 56(6): 880-8.
[http://dx.doi.org/10.1515/cclm-2017-0754] [PMID: 29702484]

[27] Jahan S, Ashfaq UA, Khaliq S, Samreen B, Afzal N. Dual behavior of HCV Core gene in regulation of apoptosis is important in progression of HCC. Infect Genet Evol 2012; 12(2): 236-9.
[http://dx.doi.org/10.1016/j.meegid.2012.01.006] [PMID: 22266242]

[28] Moriishi K, Mori Y, Matsuura Y. Processing and pathogenicity of HCV core protein. Uirusu 2008; 58(2): 183-90.
[http://dx.doi.org/10.2222/jsv.58.183] [PMID: 19374196]

[29] Khaliq S, Jahan S, Pervaiz A. Sequence variability of HCV Core region: Important predictors of HCV induced pathogenesis and viral production. Infect Genet Evol 2011; 11(3): 543-56.
[http://dx.doi.org/10.1016/j.meegid.2011.01.017] [PMID: 21292033]

[30] Goossens N, Hoshida Y. Hepatitis C virus-induced hepatocellular carcinoma. Clin Mol Hepatol 2015; 21(2): 105-14.
[http://dx.doi.org/10.3350/cmh.2015.21.2.105] [PMID: 26157746]

[31] Jahan S, Khaliq S, Ijaz B, Ahmad W, Hassan S. Role of HCV Core gene of genotype 1a and 3a and host gene Cox-2 in HCV-induced pathogenesis. Virol J 2011; 8(1): 155.
[http://dx.doi.org/10.1186/1743-422X-8-155] [PMID: 21457561]

[32] Tanaka N, Moriya K, Kiyosawa K, Koike K, Gonzalez FJ, Aoyama T. PPARalpha activation is essential for HCV core protein-induced hepatic steatosis and hepatocellular carcinoma in mice. J Clin Invest 2008; 118(2): 683-94.
[PMID: 18188449]

[33] Moriya K, Nakagawa K, Santa T, *et al.* Oxidative stress in the absence of inflammation in a mouse model for hepatitis C virus-associated hepatocarcinogenesis. Cancer Res 2001; 61(11): 4365-70.
[PMID: 11389061]

[34] Sekine S, Ito K, Watanabe H, *et al.* Mitochondrial iron accumulation exacerbates hepatic toxicity caused by hepatitis C virus core protein. Toxicol Appl Pharmacol 2015; 282(3): 237-43.
[http://dx.doi.org/10.1016/j.taap.2014.12.004] [PMID: 25545986]

[35] Irshad M, Gupta P, Irshad K. Molecular basis of hepatocellular carcinoma induced by hepatitis C virus infection. World J Hepatol 2017; 9(36): 1305-14.
[http://dx.doi.org/10.4254/wjh.v9.i36.1305] [PMID: 29359013]

[36] Suhail M, Sohrab SS, Qureshi A, *et al.* Association of HCV mutated proteins and host SNPs in the development of hepatocellular carcinoma. Infect Genet Evol 2018; 60: 160-72.
[http://dx.doi.org/10.1016/j.meegid.2018.02.034] [PMID: 29501636]

[37] Alberstein M, Zornitzki T, Zick Y, Knobler H. Hepatitis C core protein impairs insulin downstream signalling and regulatory role of IGFBP-1 expression. J Viral Hepat 2012; 19(1): 65-71.
[http://dx.doi.org/10.1111/j.1365-2893.2011.01447.x] [PMID: 22187946]

[38] Khan AG, Miller MT, Marcotrigiano J. HCV glycoprotein structures: what to expect from the unexpected. Curr Opin Virol 2015; 12: 53-8.
[http://dx.doi.org/10.1016/j.coviro.2015.02.004] [PMID: 25790756]

[39] Law JLM, Logan M, Wong J, *et al.* Role of the E2 Hypervariable Region (HVR1) in the

Immunogenicity of a Recombinant Hepatitis C Virus Vaccine. J Virol 2018; 92(11): e02141-17. [http://dx.doi.org/10.1128/JVI.02141-17] [PMID: 29540595]

[40] Khera T, Behrendt P, Bankwitz D, *et al.* Functional and immunogenic characterization of diverse HCV glycoprotein E2 variants. J Hepatol 2019; 70(4): 593-602. [http://dx.doi.org/10.1016/j.jhep.2018.11.003] [PMID: 30439392]

[41] Alhammad Y, Gu J, Boo I, *et al.* Monoclonal Antibodies Directed toward the Hepatitis C Virus Glycoprotein E2 Detect Antigenic Differences Modulated by the N-Terminal Hypervariable Region 1 (HVR1), HVR2, and Intergenotypic Variable Region. J Virol 2015; 89(24): 12245-61. [http://dx.doi.org/10.1128/JVI.02070-15] [PMID: 26378182]

[42] Vieyres G, Dubuisson J, Patel AH. Characterization of antibody-mediated neutralization directed against the hypervariable region 1 of hepatitis C virus E2 glycoprotein. J Gen Virol 2011; 92(3): 494-506. [http://dx.doi.org/10.1099/vir.0.028092-0] [PMID: 21084495]

[43] Basu A, Beyene A, Meyer K, Ray R. The hypervariable region 1 of the E2 glycoprotein of hepatitis C virus binds to glycosaminoglycans, but this binding does not lead to infection in a pseudotype system. J Virol 2004; 78(9): 4478-86. [http://dx.doi.org/10.1128/JVI.78.9.4478-4486.2004] [PMID: 15078928]

[44] Johnson J, Freedman H, Logan M, *et al.* A Recombinant Hepatitis C Virus Genotype 1a E1/E2 Envelope Glycoprotein Vaccine Elicits Antibodies That Differentially Neutralize Closely Related 2a Strains through Interactions of the N-Terminal Hypervariable Region 1 of E2 with Scavenger Receptor B1. J Virol 2019; 93(22): e00810-19. [http://dx.doi.org/10.1128/JVI.00810-19] [PMID: 31462563]

[45] Welbourn S, Pause A. HCV NS2/3 Protease. In: Tan SL, Ed. Hepatitis C Viruses: Genomes and Molecular Biology. Norfolk (UK): Horizon Bioscience Copyright ũ 2006, Horizon Bioscience 2006.

[46] Suzuki R, Suzuki T, Ishii K, Matsuura Y, Miyamura T. Processing and functions of Hepatitis C virus proteins. Intervirology 1999; 42(2-3): 145-52. [http://dx.doi.org/10.1159/000024973] [PMID: 10516468]

[47] Lin C. HCV NS3-4A Serine Protease. In: Tan SL, Ed. Hepatitis C Viruses: Genomes and Molecular Biology. Norfolk (UK): Horizon Bioscience Copyright ũ 2006, Horizon Bioscience 2006.

[48] Sklan EH, Glenn JS. HCV NS4B: From Obscurity to Central Stage. In: Tan SL, Ed. Hepatitis C Viruses: Genomes and Molecular Biology. Norfolk (UK): Horizon Bioscience Copyright ũ 2006, Horizon Bioscience 2006.

[49] Kandangwa M, Liu Q. HCV-2a NS5A downregulates viral translation predominantly through domain I. Biochem Biophys Res Commun 2020; 529(1): 77-84. [http://dx.doi.org/10.1016/j.bbrc.2020.05.177] [PMID: 32560823]

[50] He Y, Staschke KA, Tan SL. HCV NS5A: A multifunctional regulator of cellular pathways and virus replication. In: Tan SL, Ed. Hepatitis C Viruses: Genomes and Molecular Biology. Norfolk (UK): Horizon Bioscience Copyright ũ 2006, Horizon Bioscience 2006.

[51] Shi ST, Lai MMC. HCV 5′ and 3′UTR: When Translation Meets Replication. In: Tan SL, Ed. Hepatitis C Viruses: Genomes and Molecular Biology. Norfolk (UK): Horizon Bioscience Copyright ũ 2006, Horizon Bioscience 2006.

[52] Boulant S, Montserret R, Hope RG, *et al.* Structural determinants that target the hepatitis C virus core protein to lipid droplets. J Biol Chem 2006; 281(31): 22236-47. [http://dx.doi.org/10.1074/jbc.M601031200] [PMID: 16704979]

[53] Oehler V, Filipe A, Montserret R, *et al.* Structural analysis of hepatitis C virus core-E1 signal peptide and requirements for cleavage of the genotype 3a signal sequence by signal peptide peptidase. J Virol 2012; 86(15): 7818-28. [http://dx.doi.org/10.1128/JVI.00457-12] [PMID: 22593157]

[54] Montserret R, Saint N, Vanbelle C, *et al.* NMR structure and ion channel activity of the p7 protein from hepatitis C virus. J Biol Chem 2010; 285(41): 31446-61.
[http://dx.doi.org/10.1074/jbc.M110.122895] [PMID: 20667830]

[55] Chandler DE, Penin F, Schulten K, Chipot C. The p7 protein of hepatitis C virus forms structurally plastic, minimalist ion channels. PLOS Comput Biol 2012; 8(9): e1002702.
[http://dx.doi.org/10.1371/journal.pcbi.1002702] [PMID: 23028296]

[56] Lorenz IC, Marcotrigiano J, Dentzer TG, Rice CM. Structure of the catalytic domain of the hepatitis C virus NS2-3 protease. Nature 2006; 442(7104): 831-5.
[http://dx.doi.org/10.1038/nature04975] [PMID: 16862121]

[57] Jirasko V, Montserret R, Appel N, *et al.* Structural and functional characterization of nonstructural protein 2 for its role in hepatitis C virus assembly. J Biol Chem 2008; 283(42): 28546-62.
[http://dx.doi.org/10.1074/jbc.M803981200] [PMID: 18644781]

[58] Jirasko V, Montserret R, Lee JY, *et al.* Structural and functional studies of nonstructural protein 2 of the hepatitis C virus reveal its key role as organizer of virion assembly. PLoS Pathog 2010; 6(12): e1001233.
[http://dx.doi.org/10.1371/journal.ppat.1001233] [PMID: 21187906]

[59] Yao N, Reichert P, Taremi SS, Prosise WW, Weber PC. Molecular views of viral polyprotein processing revealed by the crystal structure of the hepatitis C virus bifunctional protease helicase. Structure 1999; 7(11): 1353-63.
[http://dx.doi.org/10.1016/S0969-2126(00)80025-8] [PMID: 10574797]

[60] Brass V, Berke JM, Montserret R, Blum HE, Penin F, Moradpour D. Structural determinants for membrane association and dynamic organization of the hepatitis C virus NS3-4A complex. Proc Natl Acad Sci USA 2008; 105(38): 14545-50.
[http://dx.doi.org/10.1073/pnas.0807298105] [PMID: 18799730]

[61] Gouttenoire J, Castet V, Montserret R, *et al.* Identification of a novel determinant for membrane association in hepatitis C virus nonstructural protein 4B. J Virol 2009; 83(12): 6257-68.
[http://dx.doi.org/10.1128/JVI.02663-08] [PMID: 19357161]

[62] Gouttenoire J, Montserret R, Kennel A, Penin F, Moradpour D. An amphipathic α-helix at the C terminus of NS4B mediates membrane association. J Virol 2009; 51: 11378-84.
[http://dx.doi.org/10.1128/JVI.01122-09] [PMID: 19692468]

[63] Tellinghuisen TL, Marcotrigiano J, Rice CM. Structure of the zinc-binding domain of an essential replicase component of hepatitis C virus reveals a novel fold. Nature 2005; 435: 375-9.
[http://dx.doi.org/10.1038/nature03580]

[64] Liang Y, Ye H, Kang CB, Yoon HS. Domain 2 of nonstructural protein 5A (NS5A) of hepatitis C virus is natively unfolded. Biochemistry 2007; 46(41): 11550-8.
[http://dx.doi.org/10.1021/bi700776e] [PMID: 17880107]

[65] Hanoulle X, Badillo A, Wieruszeski JM, *et al.* Hepatitis C virus NS5A protein is a substrate for the peptidyl-prolyl cis/trans isomerase activity of cyclophilins A and B. J Biol Chem 2009; 284(20): 13589-601.
[http://dx.doi.org/10.1074/jbc.M809244200] [PMID: 19297321]

[66] Verdegem D, Badillo A, Wieruszeski JM, *et al.* Domain 3 of NS5A protein from the hepatitis C virus has intrinsic alpha-helical propensity and is a substrate of cyclophilin A. J Biol Chem 2011; 286(23): 20441-54.
[http://dx.doi.org/10.1074/jbc.M110.182436] [PMID: 21489988]

[67] Penin F, Brass V, Appel N, *et al.* Structure and function of the membrane anchor domain of hepatitis C virus nonstructural protein 5A. J Biol Chem 2004; 279(39): 40835-43. [http://dx.doi.org/10.1074/jbc.M404761200] [PMID: 15247283]

[68] Bressanelli S, Tomei L, Rey FA, De Francesco R. Structural analysis of the hepatitis C virus RNA polymerase in complex with ribonucleotides. J Virol 2002; 76(7): 3482-92. [http://dx.doi.org/10.1128/JVI.76.7.3482-3492.2002] [PMID: 11884572]

CHAPTER 2

HCV-Host Interactions: Interplay Part 2: Host Related Determinants and Intracellular Signaling

Abstract: The progression of acute HCV infection to chronic disease and subsequent extrahepatic comorbidities involve both viruses and host cellular proteins interactions as well as insurrection or subjection of cell signaling and metabolic pathways in infected cells. This interaction between host-specific factors and the hepatitis C genome also weakens or impairs other physiological or metabolic regulatory roles of the hepatocytes. Several host cell proteins promote hepatitis C infection through binding to HCV nonstructural proteins (*e.g.*, PPP2R5D). Some studies also found cytokine (*e.g.*, IL-10, IL-6, TNF-α, and TGF-β1) gene polymorphisms to be highly associated with chronic hepatitis C (CHC) infection progression, whereas, polymorphism in some host genes (*e.g.*, PNPLA3, ADAR-1, and IFIH1) are found to be actively involved in the induction of advanced liver fibrosis in patients co-infected with HIV-1/HCV. Host lipid metabolism reprogramming through host lipid regulators (*e.g.*, ANGPTL-3 and 4) is also considered essential for CHC progression to severe liver disease (*e.g.*, cirrhosis and HCC). Several microRNAs (*e.g.*, miR-122, miR135a) are supposed to be key mediators of HCV infection progression and development of HCC in infected individuals and associated hepatic comorbidities. In chapter 1, we have illustrated the potential roles of virus-specific proteins in HCV molecular pathogenesis. Herein, we will elucidate the host-specific culprits that subvert, impede or disrupt host cells' communications, cell signaling, and metabolic pathways to propagate HCV infection. We will also elaborate that how the subversion of infected host-cell signaling and metabolic pathways disrupt cellular networks to evolve advanced fibrosis and hepatocarcinogenesis in HCV-infected individuals.

Keywords: ANGPTL-3, ANGPTL-4, Cytokines, Cell signaling, FAS ligand, Gene polymorphism, Hepatocellular carcinoma, Host factors, Interferon lambda 4, Lipid metabolism, Liver cancer risk, Liver fibrosis, MicroRNA, MiR-122, MiR-135a, Metabolic pathways, Nuclear factor-ƙB, PPP2R5D, Toll-like receptors, Tumor necrosis factor-α.

INTRODUCTION

Hepatitis C infection causes the inflammation of the liver and subsequently progresses hepatic injury into severe comorbidities like fibrosis, cirrhosis, and hepatocarcinogenesis [1]. Chronic HCV infection is associated with rapid disrup-

Imran Shahid and Qaiser Jabeen

tion of normal physiological and regulatory roles of hepatocytes while eliciting or suppressing the expression of certain host factors, by modulating cell signaling and impeding metabolic networks [2]. Different HCV genome regions interact with hepatic cellular factors, cell signaling molecules, and metabolic pathways to weaken or impair the normal function of the liver in infected individuals [2]. Many host-specific factors have been identified to be involved in and regulate HCV RNA replication by different mechanisms including the disruption of viral proteins, RNA, or the viral replication complex. Indeed, the hepatitis C infection progression in hepatocytes displays a landscape of complex virus-host interactions, and unleashing those host factors is very critical to fully elucidate the mechanism of HCV RNA replication and viral pathogenesis [3]. Furthermore, genetic polymorphisms of pro- and anti-inflammatory mediators can also modulate the susceptibility of hepatitis C infection in certain populations [4]. In addition to that, differential expression of some host lipid regulators in HCV infection may contribute to post-treatment deregulation of lipid metabolism that could predispose certain individuals to HCC development [5]. In this book chapter, we discuss how host cellular factors deregulate, disrupt, or impede normal hepatic cells mechanisms upon interaction with different viral proteins which subsequently are associated with or correlate to propagate hepatitis C infection into severe hepatic diseases like hepatic fibrosis, cirrhosis, and HCC.

CERTAIN HOST SPECIFIC FACTORS ARE VITAL FOR HCV REPLICATION

PPP2R5D (Protein Phosphatase 2 Regulatory Subunit B'Delta) Protein

NS5B protein is essential for HCV replication either *in vitro* or *in vivo* and certain host factors have been reported to interact with NS5B to augment virus replication or production by different mechanisms [6]. Multiple studies report the identification and demonstration of many cell culture adaptive mutations in NS5B protein to initiate or enhance the viral RNA replication or virus production during the development of infectious HCV recombinants and full-length clones. These mutations were also proposed to confer resistance or reduce the efficacy of HCV antivirals in bioinformatics studies. Three key mutations, F1464L/A1672S/D2979G (LSG) in NS5B protein, permitted the replication of full-length HCV clones of GT-2a and 2b isolates, and the infectious clones of GT-1a, 2c, 3a, and 6a are reported in the literature [7]. However, the full mechanistic role of LSG mutations to accelerate HCV replication is still elusive [7]. Recent studies predict that HCV NS5B interacts with cellular PPP2R5D (protein phosphatase 2 regulatory subunit B'Delta) protein while initiating HCV replication and infection. PPP2R5D is a subunit of PP2A (protein phosphatase 2A) enzymes, which are involved in many regulating pathways and turn on or off gene expression by removing the phosphate group from proteins [8]. PP2A is a major and multifunctional serine/threonine-specific phosphatase consisting of a structural subunit A, a regulatory subunit B, and a catalytic subunit C [8]. PPP2R5D plays a major role in negative regulation of the PI3K/AKT signaling pathway, autism, or other brain-related disorders [9]. PP2A has been evaluated in cancer progression and this group of proteins has shown interaction with different HCV proteins [10, 11].

Micro RNAs (miRNA)

Conventionally, miRNAs (small non-coding RNAs of approximately 22 nucleotides in length) are considered important regulators of gene expression by suppressing mRNA translation and promoting mRNA decay [11]. However, contrary to their conventional suppressive role, certain liver-specific miRNAs anneal to HCV genome replication machinery and play an essential role in viral infection progression. A liver-specific microRNA (*i.e.* miR-122; which accounts for 70% of all hepatocytes miRNAs), affects both the initiation and maintenance of HCV infection [12]. Regulation of HCV liver tropism is almost dependent on miR-122 because of its liver-specific expression and is the most abundant miRNA in the hepatic cells [12]. It anneals to the HCV genomic 5' UTR and is vital for virus replication; albeit, the mechanism by which miR-122 promotes virus replication and genome amplification is not well understood and is still debated [12]. However, recent studies show that miR-122 increases the rate of viral RNA accumulation and promotes the establishment of hepatitis C infection in a greater number of hepatic cells than in the absence of miR-122 [12]. For this purpose, it associates with human Argonaute proteins (Ago 1-4; hAgo:miR-122 complex), which further binds to two sites on the upstream nucleotides of 5' UTR of the viral genome and promotes viral RNA accumulation [12]. Some other roles of miR-122 have also been identified, including viral translation stimulation, genome stabilization, and a direct role in genome amplification. Recent studies suggest that miR-122 is involved in the formation of an active or a translation-favorable viral IRES structure by modulating the 5' UTR shapes during its annealing with 5' UTR nucleotides; however, biophysical analyses are extensively required to support this hypothesis [12]. Furthermore, wild-type HCV genome replication cannot be detected in the absence of miR-122. However, certain studies document extrahepatic HCV RNA existence and replication in other tissues of the body where CHC propagates to a broad range of comorbidities including cryoglobulinemic vasculitis, diabetes Mellitus, and B-cell lymphoma. It suggests a possible role of miR-122-independent HCV replication and virus accumulation in these clinical manifestations [12].

miR-122: A Key Regulator of HCV Replication in Hepatocytes

As miR-122 is an important host factor for HCV replication and infection initiation, its antagonists have been shown to have both preclinical and clinical promises as effective anti-HCV treatment strategies resulting in a prolonged reduction of viral load [13]. However, multiple studies illustrate that HCV has been adopted to replicate in the absence of miR-122 because of selection pressure and the emergence of resistance-associated substitutions (RASs) [13]. Likewise, some studies show that the capability of HCV replication independent of miR-122 activity may completely rescue HCV replication in the absence of miR-122 by enhanced viral translation and genome stability which possibly suggest miR-122's role in the early stages of viral infection [14]. The initiation of HCV infection in the liver is more dependent on the miR-122 abundance in hepatocytes because it enhances the virus replication in hepatic cells [14]. As infection with a single or a low viral copy number genomes may require multiple rounds of replication to establish an infection, it signifies the importance of miR-122 in both the establishment and ongoing HCV replication in the liver [14]. Some other viruses like enterovirus, norovirus and rotavirus transmit among hosts in vesicle-cloaked viral clusters that are found to be more infectious than the single-free viral particles [14]. Likewise, miR-122 may also enhance HCV genome quantity by slowing its mRNA degradation. Still, there are no reports of HCV virion clusters; however, exosomes containing replication-competent HCV RNAs in complex with miR-122, Ago-2, and HSP90 can transmit HCV infection which could increase the viral copy number and stability of infecting HCV genomes [14].

miR-135a Drives Chronic Hepatitis C Infection to HCC

Another miRNA (*i.e.*miR-135a) has been documented with elevated expression in many cancers and is thought to be a candidate driver of HCV-associated HCC [15]. Although its roles in HCV infection-associated comorbidities are still investigative, it is thought that it modulates hepatitis C infection to HCC by affecting the virus core protein expression and RNA replication [15]. HCV infection upregulates miR-135a expression in infected hepatic cells that elicit viral replication as well as impede cellular networks to contribute to HCV-associated HCC [15]. Several studies point out a significant correlation between miR-135a levels and malignant behaviors in HCC patients, thus miR-135a could be a potential target for prognostic and therapeutic anti-HCV regimens [15]. Moreover, miR-135a plays an essential role to propagate portal vein tumor thrombus (PVTT) by promoting metastasis in HCC [15]. However, *in vitro* inhibition of miR-135a significantly reduces PVTT incidences, thus anti-miR135a inhibitors could be also useful in PVTT therapy [15]. In HCV patients with recurrence of HCC also expresses high levels of miR-135a within 12 months after resection. Thus, quantitative analysis of high intratumoral miR-135a expression could be a potential indicator for adjuvant therapy post-resection [15].

Cytokines Gene Polymorphisms in Chronic Hepatitis C Patients

The Importance of Cytokines against Viral Infections

Cytokines are glycoproteins of humoral immunomodulatory characteristics that are secreted by multiple cells of the human immune system like macrophages, T or B lymphocytes, mast cells, endothelial cells, fibroblasts, and stromal cells [16]. These proteins are broadly classified either based on their secretory cells like monokines (produced by monocytes cell lineage) or lymphokines (produced by lymphocytes lineage) as well as based on their functions [16]. For example, type 1 cytokines are pro-inflammatory (tumor necrosis factor (TNF)-α, interferon-γ, interleukin-2, and interleukin-12) and type 2 are by large the anti-inflammatory cytokines (*e.g.*, tumor growth factor (TGF)-β1, interleukin (IL)-4, -5, -6, -10, and IL-13) [16]. Type 1 cytokines are potentially involved to enhance cellular immune responses while type 2 supports antibody-mediated immune responses. Certain cytokines have dual characteristics like both pro-and anti-inflammatory effects (*e.g.*, IL-6) [16].

Cytokine regulation from innate immune cells is a fundamental phenomenon to control inflammation and infection dynamics in the human body. The impediment of pro- and anti-inflammatory cytokine profiles potentially impacts the pathogenesis and influences the clinical outcomes of many infections, autoimmune disorders, and malignant diseases [17]. This imbalance of equilibrium between the interactions of these two types of cytokines in host cells disrupts the normal feedback mechanisms and threatens normal tissue integrity [17]. As documented and well-studied the overexpression of type 1 cytokines results in widespread inflammatory responses and significant adverse effects in injured or damaged host cells or tissue [17].

Multiple studies augment a very close and firm correlation between the genetic polymorphism within a particular gene and its implications as individual variations in clinical features of a particular infection (either to enhance the susceptibility of infection or the progression of persistent infection to severe disease) [17]. Cytokine genetic polymorphism also implicates its harmful effects by a certain infection proliferation or progression into a severe disease among individuals [17]. The predisposing factor for this difference in cytokine profile is due to allelic polymorphism that occurs within regulatory or coding regions of the cytokines gene [17]. Non-conservative mutations in the coding genome region of cytokines may lose, abrogate, or alter the function of the expressed proteins, whereas polymorphism within the 5' and 3' regulatory elements or intron sequences of the genome may affect transcription [17].

Cytokine Gene Polymorphism for IL-10

Cytokine gene polymorphism for IL-10 (rs1800896 and rs1800871), IL-6 (rs1800795), TNF- α (rs1800629), and TGF-β1 (rs1800471) have been demonstrated with a strong association to the susceptibility of HCV infection in individuals with drug abuse [16]. In particular, IL-10 gene polymorphism rs1800871 is found to play a significant role in a patient's response toward antiviral therapy as well as susceptibility to HCV infection in drug abusers [16]. A recent meta-analysis establishes a strong correlation between IL-6 rs1800795 single nucleotide polymorphism and susceptibility to hepatic disease. An association between IL-6 rs1800871SNP and the outcome of HCV infection is also reported [16].

Cytokine Gene Polymorphism for IL-13

IL-13 is a glycosylated polypeptide of the family of IL-13/IL-4. It has an anti-inflammatory effect on cytokines and chemokines and also suppresses macrophage activity [16]. Proteins and antibodies of IL-13 polypeptide are important mediators of immunoregulatory processes in various cell types [16]. Multiple studies demonstrate elevated expression of IL-13 protein in hepatic tissues of CHC-infected patients while some others also unveil enhanced serum concentration of IL-13 in CHC-infected patients as compared to healthy controls [16]. IL-13 protein is also linked with the fibrotic stage of hepatitis C infection and is also supportive to propagate steatosis/steatohepatitis. The most important role of IL-13 is confined to tumor tissues where the protein is overexpressed and inhibition of IL-13 in cancer could have a potential therapeutic benefit as cancer immunotherapy. Interestingly, some previous studies point out that IL-13 levels were significantly higher prior to DAA treatment in HCV patients who later developed HCC and it remained higher at each subsequent time point. The studies also show that IL-13 levels were significantly higher at initial viremia and during persistent infection in HCV patients, who did not achieve SVR rates and/or acquired HCC. However, IL-13 levels were recorded lower in the patients who achieved higher SVR rates and cleared the virus [16].

Gene Polymorphisms of Tumor Necrosis Factor-alpha (TNF-α)

Tumor Necrosis Factor-alpha (TNF-α) is a pro-inflammatory cytokine released by the activation of macrophages in response to bacterial endotoxins [16]. However, various studies allude to the association of gene polymorphism of TNF- α rs1800629 with susceptibility to hepatitis C infection [16]. TNF- α SNP of A→G has been significantly associated with susceptibility to HCV infection [16].

Furthermore, TNF- α SNP of G→A at position 308 was also reported to have a link to HCV pathogenesis and advancement of CHC infection. TGF-β1 is a multifunctional protein responsible for cell differentiation and apoptosis as well as exerts strong anti-inflammatory effects. Gene polymorphism of the TGF-β1 genotype (*i.e.* rs1800471) also indicates an association with HCV infection outcome. However, some other studies from Asia, Brazil, and Caucasian populations could not find any significant relationship between TGF-β1 polymorphism and CHC infection [16].

Role of Cytokine Storm in HBV Reactivation in HBV/HCV Coinfections

HBV/HCV co-infection may exacerbate the progression of end-stage liver disease in infected individuals more rapidly than either mono-HBV or HCV infection [17]. Furthermore, HBV reactivation in HBV/HCV co-infected patients while taking DAAs to cure HCV may further devastate the infection outcomes as severe disease and in many cases death. Hence, the early prediction of HBV reactivation in HBV/HCV co-infected patients, or at the time of initiating DAA treatment for HCV cure is crucial [17]. Mechanistically, patients infected with HBV/HCV co-infection are more prone to be dominantly affected by HCV infection, and HBV viral activity, infection chronicity, and disease severity are relatively low [17]. Successful HCV cures with DAAs may inversely trigger HBV replication in HCV/HBV co-infections as previous literature reported 24% HBV reactivation after DAAs post-treatment completion [17]. During the interferon treatment era, It was supposed that diminished IFN response marked by circulating CXCL10 protein (an inflammatory chemokine that binds to CXCR3 to stimulate immune response through the activation and recruitment of leukocytes such as T cells, eosinophils, monocytes, and natural killer cells) following HCV clearance is associated with HBV reactivation in HBV/HCV co-infection [17]. However, the molecular pathogenesis of HBV reactivation after DAAs therapy is still elusive and warrants large investigations [17].

Notably, data are scarcely discussing the reactivation of HBV in HBV/HCV co-infection patients receiving DAAs therapy to treat HCV [17]. As DAAs show no significant therapeutic activity against HBV infection, it is important to unleash immunopathogenesis of HBV reactivation in CHC patients receiving DAAs. It is also of paramount interest to design effective prophylactic or therapeutic strategies to coup HBV reactivation in such patient populations. For this purpose, serum biomarkers for early prediction of HBV reactivation could be a pragmatic clinical approach in HBV/HCV co-infected patients. Some recent studies postulate that HBV-specific or -nonspecific host immune responses may be modulated during treatment of HCV with DAAs in HBV/HCV co-infection patients and propagate to HBV reactivation when HCV is cleared with DAA treatment. A recent study conducted in Taiwan analyzed serum samples for virologic and cytokine/chemokine analysis of a clinical cohort of patients infected with HBV/HCV co-infection and who received DAA-based therapy for CHC [17]. The study findings illustrate that DAAs administration for HCV treatment in HBV/HCV co-infected patients may break/disrupt the balance of certain chemokines/cytokines expression and facilitate HBV reactivation. For example, a chemokine CCL2 (also known as MCP-1), attracts monocytes, T cells, and dendritic cells during infection and provides sustained inflammatory bridges between innate and acquired immunity. It is found that higher levels of CCL2 are associated with lower viral activity implying its possible role in host immune responses against HBV replication. However, the decreasing level of CCL2 after DAAs administration for HCV treatment in HBV/HCV coinfected patients may facilitate HBV reactivation, especially for those with higher baseline CCL2 levels [17]. Further studies are still needed to clarify this underlying mechanism.

The advancement of HCV treatment with pan-genotypic DAAs in the current era for harder-to-treat populations including HCV/HBV coinfections has decreased the new incidences of HBV reactivation, but the risks are still prevailing with a growing number of novel treatments strategies [17]. The cytokine/chemokine dynamics and their fluctuating levels could be explored as the intricate mechanisms of HBV reactivation and could become the early potential predictors for the different infected populations at risk for HBV reactivation caused by different antivirals in future studies [17].

Genetic Polymorphism in Host Genetic Factors of HIV-1/HCV Coinfected Patients Progress Toward Advanced Hepatic Fibrosis

SNPs or mutations in other host genetic factors related to immune activation for HIV-1 and/or HCV infection have been reported to progress hepatic inflammation and advanced liver fibrosis in patients co-infected with HIV-1/HCV coinfection [18]. For example, SNPs in adenosine deaminase acting on RNA-1 (ADAR-1), interferon-induced helicase C domain-containing 1 (IFIH1), IFN, and mitochondrial antiviral-signaling gene (MAVS) have been potentially associated with liver fibrosis and cirrhosis [18]. ADAR-1 is considered one of the important regulators of innate immune response by the activation of TLR3/TLR4 mediated type-I IFN induction pathway (discussed below) and its silencing induces a potent IFN response that results in hepatic damage and fibrosis. IFIH1 is a viral sensor to elicit strong IFN responses and risk alleles in IFIH1 are strongly correlated to hepatic inflammation and autoimmune diseases. A recent study's findings are the first to associate IFIH1 SNP rs1990760 with advanced hepatic fibrosis regardless of patient body mass index (BMI) and peripheral visceral fat accumulation (PVFA) [18]. Previously, this SNP (IFIH1/rs1990760) was linked to inflammatory bowel disease (IBD), type 1 diabetes mellitus (DM), and vitiligo [19]. IFN lambda (IFNL) is implicated in the innate antiviral response against many RNA viruses including hepatitis C. IFNL3/4 variants have been reported as favorable predictors of spontaneous HCV clearance and response to IFN-based therapies. Similarly, SNPs in IFN lambda (IFNL) 3/4 have also been documented to link liver inflammation in CHC-infected patients (discussed below) although the data are contrary and intermingled to extrapolate a clear correlation of advanced hepatic fibrosis with the IFNL3/4 genes [20]. One study assessed 16 host genetic SNPs in 10 genes involved in innate immune response and liver metabolism and their strong correlation with hepatic steatosis and liver injury in HCV/HIV co-infected patients [18]. Another study deciphers the potential association between visceral fat accumulation (VFA) and advanced hepatic fibrosis in HIV-1/HCV coinfected patients. Instead of the availability of liver fibrosis staging methods in HCV patients, a major challenge confronted by the clinics is the lack of available biomarkers for predicting different stages of hepatic disease in individuals with HIV-1/HCV co-infection [18].

SNP or genetic variations in patatin-like phosphatase domain-containing protein 3 (PNPLA3) and transmembrane 6 superfamily member 2 (TM6SF2) genes have been documented to develop HCV-induced HCC in infected individuals [21]. Genome-wide studies predict that PNPLA3/rs738409 polymorphism is strongly correlated to an increased risk of HCC development with the PNPLA3 GG genotype (3-fold increased risk) compared to PNPLA3 CC genotype in patients with mild CHC infection. Similarly, few studies favor that TM6SF2 gene polymorphism rs58542926 is strongly correlated to increased HCC risk in HCV-infected patients; however, many deny this hypothesis and correlate it with nonalcoholic fatty liver disease (NAFLD), nonalcoholic steatohepatitis (NASH), or other non-hepatitis B non-hepatitis C (NBNC) induced HCC [21].

Genetic Polymorphisms of Interferon Lambda (IFNL 3/4) Genes in HCV Patients and its Clinical Significance

Being the most prevalent HCV GT in the world, in particular in Western countries and the USA, 50% of patients infected with HCV GT-1 failed to achieve SVRs with PEG-IFN/RBV combination therapies in the IFN treatment era [22]. It was discovered in 2009 that SNPs located near the IFNL3 locus (encoding IFNλ3; also known as IL-28B) were strongly associated with the treatment response to PEG-IFN/RBV therapy and with the spontaneous clearance of HCV infection. The patients with the rs12979860-T allele (C/T or T/T) respond poorly to PEG-IFN/RBV treatment, whereas patients with two copies of the rs12979860-C allele (C/C) respond well to this treatment [22].

The IFNL4 gene encoding IFNλ4 located near the IFNL3 locus was discovered in 2013 and interestingly found to be influenced by a germline dinucleotide frameshift variant that is located in exon 1 of the IFNL4 gene (*i.e.* rs368234815) [22]. The rs368234815-ΔG allele generates the full-length IFNλ4 protein, whereas the rs368234815-TT allele does not generate IFNλ4 because of a premature stop codon. It was also found that rs368234815-ΔG allele is strongly associated with the previously known rs12979860-T allele of the IFNL3 locus by linkage disequilibrium. CHC patients with rs368234815-ΔG allele (ΔG/TT or ΔG/ΔG) have high baseline IFN-stimulated gene (ISG) levels in the liver; however, respond poorly to PEG-IFN/RBV treatment. A recent study also emphasizes that IFNL4-ΔG/TT is the primary IFNL gene polymorphism that determines the treatment response to PEG-IFN/RBV therapy. A defective form of IFNλ4 protein is associated with a weaker induction of ISGs in the liver of CHC-infected patients, which indicates that it is the main driver of hepatic ISGs induction in CHC infection. IFNλ4 protein activates the JAK-STAT (Janus kinase-signature of transducer and activator of transcription 3) pathway to induce the expression of ISGs by binding to the IFNλ receptor. However, it remains to be elucidated why IFNλ4 protein with the rs368234815-ΔG allele (ΔG/TT or ΔG/ΔG) respond poorly to PEG-IFN/RBV treatment [22].

Multiple recent studies reveal that genetic polymorphism of the IFNL gene strongly correlates with spontaneous and IFN treatment-induced clearance of HCV infection [22]. HCV-infected individuals with the ancestral lack of IFNL4-dG allele are not capable to clear HCV in the acute phase and have a probability of more than 90% developing CHC infection. On contrary, the IFNL-dG allele encodes a fully functional IFNL4 protein with potent antiviral activity against HCV. However, a minor amount of IFNL4 protein is secreted because largely it is retained in ER where it induces ER stress. Stressed cells are significantly weaker activators of HCV-specific CD8+ T cell activation than unstressed ones. Hence, IFNL4-induced ER stress interferes with HCV antigen presentation by MHC-I complexes on CD8+ T cells. Subsequently, T-immune cell responses are attenuated in CHC patients which favors the viral escape from immune responses that are considered to be crucial for viral clearance [22].

DIFFERENTIAL EXPRESSION OF HOST CELLS LIPID METABOLISM REGULATORS IMPACT HEPATITIS C INFECTION PROGRESSION

As previously mentioned host lipid metabolism modulation is crucial for CHC progression into severe hepatic comorbidities (*e.g.*, HCC) where differential expression of certain lipid metabolism regulators (*e.g.*, angiopoietin-like protein-3/4 (ANGPTL-3/4)) regulate the clearance of plasma lipids by inhibiting cellular lipase activity and contribute their roles in tumorigenesis [23]. It is important to mention here that DAAs administration achieved higher SVR rates in HCV-treated patients, but the viral infection cure does not always protect against the HCC occurrence or recurrence in those individuals [24]. HCV antigenic protein core, and nonstructural 5A, orchestrate de novo lipogenesis and enhance hepatic lipid uptake by attenuating fatty acid catabolism through modulation of lipid-related transcription factors, thereby promoting hepatic steatosis [23]. A hallmark of HCV infection, -hepatic fibrosis- which drives and propagates CHC to HCC and also occurs roughly at the same time [23]. Hepatic stellate cells (HSCs) produce excessive extracellular matrix (ECM) proteins because of the HCV-mediated induction of fibrinogenic signaling and the secretion of profibrotic cytokines like TGF-β [23]. Although the mechanisms involved in the crosstalk of steatosis with hepatic fibrosis in HCV infection are poorly understood, it is believed that hepatic lipid accumulation independently causes elevated production of TGF-β by HSCs [23]. Mechanistically, continuous disruption of beneficial wound healing processes that are part of the standard response-to-injury regeneration programs leads from set-in fibrosis to cirrhosis in HCV-infected patients [23].

HCV patients with a cirrhotic background are always at risk to develop HCC at any timeline of their infection [23]. Hepatitis C infection transforms infected hepatocytes' malignancies by deregulating cell proliferation, differentiation, and apoptosis. Further activation of oncogenic protein signaling, chromatin remodeling, rogue epigenetic modification, production of oxidative stress, and escalation of immunotolerance all drive HCV-mediated tumorigenesis. A fundamental realization that cancer cells mainly rely on de novo lipid biosynthesis for their morphological, metabolic, and signaling needs also signify the key role of lipid metabolism in HCC development and progression. Recent studies also speculate the enormous impact of HCV on lipid metabolism reprogramming by impacting major lipid metabolism-related enzymes and specific lipid classes involved in hepatocarcinogenesis [23].

Pan-genotypic DAAs achieve more than 95% SVR rates for all HCV GTs except HCV GT-3a patients, which is still proven more resistant to this type of treatment [24]. However, HCV patients with advanced hepatic fibrosis before initiating DAAs treatment, patients with non-regressing cirrhosis, treatment failure in achieving SVR rates post-treatment, or patients with co-infections are still at risk for HCC development despite the intention to treat with DAAs [24]. Indeed scientifically evident and supported by multiple studies, HCV-induced reprogramming of host lipid metabolism, epigenetic alterations, immunotolerance, continuous deregulation of cellular signaling, and abrupt modulation of hepatic gene expression may constitute or build a viral fingerprint that persistently remains after viral eradication with DAAs [24]. Subsequently, these HCV-induced alterations are supposed to collectively promote HCC development and progression depending on the extent of the existing liver damage in some HCV-cured patients [24].

ANGPTL-3 and -4: Potent Regulators of Lipid Metabolism in Hepatocytes

ANGPTL-3 and -4 are considered two potent regulators of host cell lipid metabolism as they both increase plasma triglycerides through post-translational inhibition of lipoprotein lipase (LPL) and hepatic lipase (HL) enzymatic activity [23]. LPL metabolizes very-low-density lipoproteins (VLDL) and chylomicrons into non-esterified fatty acids and monoacylglycerol, which are then absorbed into peripheral tissues for energy utilization. HL acts in the same manner as LPL but mainly in the liver, where it utilizes intermediate-density lipoproteins (IDL) and high-density lipoproteins (HDL) as substrates. Both lipid metabolism regulators (*i.e.* ANGPTL-3 and ANGPTL-4) differ in their functional mechanisms and physiological roles according to their tissue specificity as ANGPTL-3 alone regulates low-density lipoprotein (LDL) levels *via* inhibition of endothelial lipase (*i.e.* LIPG) activity. ANGPTL-3 is more hepatic specific in its activity, acts in an endocrine manner, and remains largely irrelevant by the dietary state. However, ANGPTL-4 is mainly expressed in the liver, macrophages, adipose tissue, heart, and small intestine where it plays its part as a local regulator of LPL-dependent lipid uptake and is strongly up-regulated by fasting [23]. Previous studies demonstrate that HCV antigenic protein (*i.e.* Core (C)) down-regulates ANGPTL-3 through cancer-related kinase minibrain-related kinase/dual-specificity tyrosine-regulated kinase 1B (Mirk/Dyrk 1B)-dependent loss of hepatic nuclear factor-1α (HNF-1α) binding activity and inhibition of liver-X/retinoid-X receptor (LXR/RXR) transactivation [25].

ANGPTLs Linked to HCV Induced Hepatic Fibrosis and Tumorigenesis

Irrespective of their independent role in lipid metabolism, both ANGPTLs have also been considered to play their part in tumorigenesis [23]. Although the exact role of ANGPTL-3 in tumor development and progression is still obscure, it is assumed that it mediates both pro-survival and antimetastatic mechanisms [23]. On contrary, ANGPTL-4 levels are raised under hypoxic and inflammatory cell conditions where it upholds multiple roles as a positive regulator of angiogenesis, tumor survival, and tissue invasiveness. Some studies reported only higher levels of ANGPTL-3 in liver biopsy specimens of HCV-and HBV-associated HCC, compared to non-cancerous tissue. However, some studies illustrate elevated serum levels of both ANGPTL-3 and -4 in HCV-induced HCC. Genetic manipulation of key lipid metabolism regulators is not only required for HCV-induced hepatic disease and the initiation of hepatocarcinogenesis but also deemed important for the creation of lipid-rich cellular surroundings needed for the successful completion of viral life cycle as well as to maintain infection chronicity and severity in infected individuals. It is strongly presumed that host lipid metabolism reprogramming not only elicits hepatocarcinogenesis in HCV cirrhotic patients with active infection but also pose a high risk of HCC recurrence in genetically susceptible HCV patients even cured with DAA therapy [23].

ANGPTL Expression in Various Stages of Hepatic Fibrosis

CHC patients are grouped into three clinically relevant categories based on their fibrosis score (*i.e.* METAVIR fibrosis score) as determined by Fibroscan® measurement (discussed in chapter 4). According to this score, CHC-infected patients are mainly grouped into mild fibrosis (F0, F1, and F2), advanced fibrosis (F3), and cirrhosis (F4). Fibrosis stage 'F3' is considered as a "bridging" step between complication-free hepatic disease and cirrhosis (*i.e.*, either HCV patients with fibrosis in F0, F1, or F2 stage) whereas F3 patients are characterized by a deformed liver architecture (*i.e.* mainly liver stiffness), increased chances for HCC development, and severe systemic pathologies although patients in F3 fibrosis stage tend to have better clinical outcomes and overall survival [23]. However, some clinicians recommend patients in the F3 stage should also be monitored for HCC development even post-DAA treatment cure. Moreover, scientific clues are still not providing sufficient information to infer that HCV-mediated molecular mechanisms are involved in tumorigenesis at the F3 fibrosis stage. A recent study shows that ANGPTL-3 is least expressed in HCV treatment-naïve patients' serum samples in the F3 fibrosis state as compared to all other fibrosis stages. In contrast, ANGPTL-4 serum level was found relatively higher from the early acute HCV infection (*i.e.* mild fibrosis; F0, F1, and F2) to late cirrhosis/HCC stages (*i.e.* fibrosis state F3 and cirrhosis F4); however, expressed in a non-linear way since it peaked in HCV patients with advanced fibrosis (*i.e.* fibrosis stage F4). Surprisingly, some studies predict that both ANGPTL-3 and -4 serum levels do not statistically differ between the early stages of acute HCV infection and mild fibrosis or late-stage cirrhosis and HCC. Hence, ANGPTL-3 and -4 serum levels at the F3 stage represent an important threshold for the initiation of tumorigenesis and could be accentuated predictors of the differential regulation of ANGPTLs in HCV infection [23].

Some studies also report serum levels of ANGPTL-3 and -4 in HCV patients after a 12-week treatment period with DAAs [26, 27]. In comparison to pre-treatment levels, ANGPTL-4 levels were noticed to be altered independently of the fibrosis stage in DAA treatment-experienced patients and were subjected to a "corrective" adjustment. However, ANGPTL-3 levels did not modulate in patients with advanced fibrosis and cirrhosis even when administered to DAAs treatment. It may evident that retention of ANGPTL-3 baseline values after treatment could be linked to more severe hepatic disease. Hence, ANGPTL-3 could be one of many genes belonging to the host transcriptome, secretome, epigenome, and immunome that retain its expression levels after a successful HCV cure with DAA in patients with advanced hepatic damage. Therefore, it represents an important part of a residual HCV fingerprint that is most probably involved to promote hepatocarcinogenesis in some cured HCV patients [26]. It is obvious by the detection of similar persistently expressed immunoregulatory signatures in acute hepatitis C-infected patients who received early DAA treatment in some studies.

Several studies predict the recovery from HCV-induced hypolipidemia after DAAs therapy [28, 29]. In contrast, most studies explored that ANGPTL-targeted lipid moieties (*e.g.*, triglycerides, VLDL) did not significantly differ after post-DAA treatment, even at 24-week follow-ups [30, 31]. By analogy, a slight post-cure increase in lipids was noticed in HCV patients with mild fibrosis. However, the underlying mechanism for this partial recovery of circulating lipids remains unclear and can be attributed to increased steatosis in HCV patients with or without co-existing predisposing factors [31]. HCV-dictated remaining levels of ANGPTL-3 after viral clearance could also be involved in shaping lipid species and steatosis after treatment [30]. Ultimately, these remaining ANGPTL-3 levels after HCV clearance could promote lipotoxicity-related hepatocarcinogenesis that strengthens the emerging role of ANGPTL-3 in cancer initiation [28]. In contrast, ANGPTL-4 does not play any part in the 'corrective adjustment' of lipids in host cells after DAA treatment. Furthermore, its levels are decreased both *in vitro* and *in vivo* after DAA therapy involving other factors in the host environment like residual inflammatory activity recorded in the serum of DAA-treated patients [29].

ANGPTL-3/4 Interacts With TGF-β to Promote Hepatic Fibrosis and Cirrhosis

ANGPTL-3 and ANGPTL-4 expressions are also associated with hepatic fibrosis during hepatitis C infection. The transforming growth factor (TGF-β) protein is known as the master regulator of fibrosis and strongly implicates its involvement in the reduction of inflammation, promotion of fibrinogenesis, hepatic cancer development, and facilitation of metastasis depending on the cellular milieu [32]. TGF-β involvement in hepatic fibrosis and hepatitis C-mediated disease progression has also been validated by most studies [32, 33]. Cellular functions of TGF-β are entirely dependent on its structural configuration which is strictly regulated and dictates its active role in HCV patients with mild/advanced fibrosis and cirrhosis progression [33]. A recent study also links the TGF-β association between fibrosis and the expression pattern of ANGPTL-3 and -4 [34]. TGF-β expression was found significantly elevated in the serum samples of HCV patients with F3 fibrosis state as compared to other fibrosis stages [34]. TGF-β is also overexpressed in regenerating liver nodules enough found in advanced fibrosis (F3 stage) as promoters of wound healing [34]. Interestingly, ANGPTLs expression is inversely associated with TGF-β levels before initiation of HCV treatment by DAAs. ANGPTL-3 levels are negatively correlated with TGF-β, while ANGPTL-4 levels are positively associated with TGF-β [34]. However, the data are scarce to hypothesize any correlation between the TGF-β and both host lipid metabolism regulators (both ANGPTL-3 and -4) after post-treatment completion. Previous studies have shown that TGF-β upregulates ANGPTL-4 expression in breast and bone cancer; however, the correlation between TGF-β and ANGPTL-3 is not so far clear, although some unpublished data postulate that TGF-β influences a decrease in ANGPTL-3 mRNA in hepatoma cells [32, 33]. Hence, it can be concluded that a causal relationship exists between TGF-β and these proteins of host lipid metabolism regulators as well as other cytokines that are potentially involved to elicit hepatocarcinogenesis. Furthermore, this partial explanation of a possible correlation between ANGPTLs and fibrosis throughout the natural history of hepatitis C infection warrants further investigation in every individual fibrosis stage of the disease. It may help to use as prognostic biomarkers of fibrosis and hepatocarcinogenesis before initiating DAAs treatment in HCV patients as well as to monitor a likelihood of a future HCC recurrence or progression in cured individuals after pan-genotypic DAAs therapy.

VITAMIN D AND HCV INDUCED HEPATOCELLULAR CARCINOMA

Vitamin D (Vit. D) contains both anti-inflammatory and anti-fibrotic characteristics that may impact HCV treatment outcomes and can minimize HCV-induced hepatic comorbidities [15]. Previous studies show that vitamin D and its active metabolites can synergize interferon treatment as well as inhibit viral genome replication *in vitro* [35, 36]. Some studies indicate the positive roles of vitamin D supplements to attain virological responses to HCV therapy and its sustained serum levels significantly correlate with achieving SVR rates [37]. For example, vitamin D deficiency was documented to be a cause of poor response to PEGIFN/RBV therapy in HCV GT-1 infection [37]. However, the data are scarce, murky, and inconclusive with intermingled interpretations about vitamin D's synergistic role in HCV therapy outcomes. Vitamin D also correlates with CHC infection as its progression may lead to low serum levels of vitamin D [37]. A recent study conducted in Egypt showed that a lower serum level of vitamin D in CHC-infected patients was associated with treatment failure and the development of HCC [38]. Similarly, another study describes that CHC infection is associated with vitamin D but also due to iron overload which results in a reduced level of hepcidin [38]. HCV treatment with sofosbuvir/daclatasvir increases hepcidin, thereby reducing iron levels and increasing vitamin D. An in vitro study shows that vitamin D in combination with IFN-α synergistically reduces HCV protein production in cell culture [39]. Furthermore, *in vivo* studies postulate the role of vitamin D in HCV clearance along with IFN-α by enhancing certain gene expressions [15]. In contrast, some studies reveal that pretreatment vitamin D levels do not affect HCV treatment outcomes with DAAs. The studies also predict that higher serum vitamin D levels do not beneficially associate with response to DAA therapy and even in certain cases HCV patients with higher serum vitamin D levels were less likely to achieve SVR rates [15]. Hence vitamin D supplementation as an adjuvant therapy with DAAs has no impactful role to achieve SVR rates in HCV-infected patients [15]. Although HCV patients who achieve SVR rates with DAAs do not regress after SVR, some even worsened with an increased risk for HCC [15]. The deficiency of vitamin D is also reported to be linked with advanced stages of HCC progression and poor treatment outcomes in most studies [15]. One study explored that vitamin D deficiency was higher in hepatitis-C-related cirrhotic patients as compared to the non-cirrhotic cohort and correlated with components of hepatic function [37]. However, neither the pretreatment with vitamin D supplements nor higher serum vitamin D levels lead to increased SVR rates in HCV patients with DAAs [37].

INTRACELLULAR SIGNALING MODULATION IN HEPATITIS C INFECTION

TLR Activation and their Implications in HCV Molecular Pathogenesis

Toll-like receptors (TLR) are evolutionarily preserved receptors that have the unique capability to sense microbial pathogen-associated molecular patterns (PAMPs) and activate the expression of genes involved in inflammatory and immune responses (Fig. **1**) [40]. To date 11 humans and 13 mice, TLRs have been identified, and 3 of them are involved in the recognition of viral infections. TLR activation by viral infections is recognized in varying capacities of pathogen sensors, modifiers of the immune responses, and potential targets for therapeutic modifications [40]. These are transmembrane glycoproteins which upon ligand binding oligomerize to induce downstream cell signaling. Recent studies demonstrate that HCV has adopted strategies to interfere with IFN pathways through pattern recognition signals. HCV NS3 protein alone or NS3/4A serine protease/helicase complex down-regulate interferon regulatory factor-3 (IRF-3) activity and impedes IRF-3 mediated type 1 IFN induction (Table **1**). It indicates that HCV subverts TLR signaling pathways to escape from clearance in hepatic cells. Furthermore, the IFN-α production induced by both TLR9- and TLR7/8 also diminish in peripheral plasmacytoid dendritic cells of HCV-infected patients. Immune responses are also dysregulated in CHC-infected patients by modulating the activity of TLR2 and TLR4. HCV 'antigenic protein Core' and NS3 protein activate monocytes by binding to TLR2 receptors to produce IL-8, IL- 6, and tumor necrosis factor (TNF-α), and inhibit differentiation and antigen-presenting functions of myeloid dendritic cells. Marked up-regulation of TLR2 and TLR4 was reported in CHC patients irrespective of HCV GTs and viral load in hepatocytes, kupffer cells, and peripheral blood monocytes. HCV Core is also linked to a loss of TLR tolerance due to excessive TLR2 and TLR4 stimulation with increased cytokine activation in monocytes of HCV patients permitting ongoing pro-inflammatory cell activation [40].

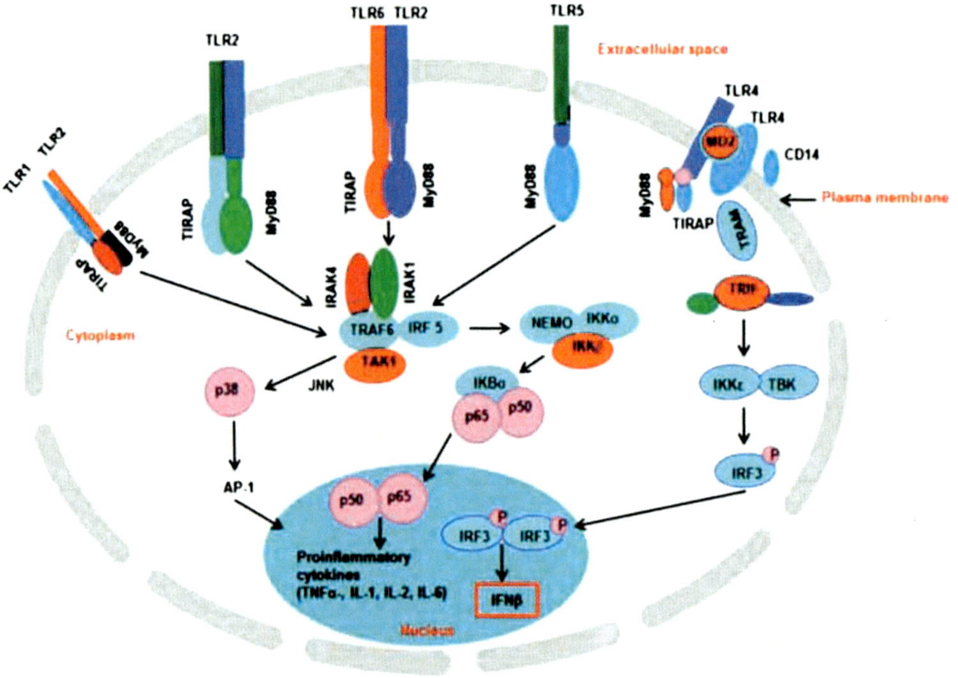

Fig. (1). Membrane-associated toll-like receptors (TLRs) and their signaling adapters. TLR; tool-like receptors, MD2; Myeloid Differentiation factor 2, CD14; Cluster of differentiation 14, TIRAP; Toll-interleukin-1 Receptor (TIR) domain-containing adaptor protein, TRAM; TRIF-related adapter molecule, MyD; Myeloid differentiation, TRIF; TIR-domain-containing adapter-inducing interferon-β, IRAK; Interleukin-1 receptor-associated kinases, IRF; Interferon regulatory factors, TRAF; tumor necrosis factor (TNF) receptor-associated factors, TAK1; Transforming growth factor β-activated kinase 1, JNK; c-Jun N-terminal kinases, NEMO; Nuclear factor-kappa B essential modulator, IKK; IκB kinase, IKB; IkappaB kinase, IKKβ; IkappaB kinase beta, NF-κB; nuclear factor kappa-light-chain-enhancer of activated B cells, AP-1; Activator protein 1, TNFα; Tumour necrosis factor α, TBK; TANK binding kinase, IFNβ; Interferon-beta..

TNF/TNF Receptor Activation in CHC Patients

Tumor necrosis factor-α (TNF-α) is a pleiotropic cytokine that regulates many cellular responses of injury and repair, inflammation and immunity, and cell proliferation [46]. It is a central regulator of hepatic physiology with perplexing signaling pathways that mediates intermingled effects of this cytokine in the liver. In particular, the researchers have been tempted to understand how it could promote either cell proliferation or death in hepatocytes under different physiologic circumstances. TNF exerts both autocrine and paracrine effects in the liver which may elicit a variety of pathophysiological states including hepatic injury, cell death, and/or hepatocellular proliferation (Fig. **2**). From a viral infection point of view, TNF cell signaling is not well understood, and established a link between CHC infection and further hepatic cell damage. However; viral proteins may promote a proinflammatory and proliferative response through increased secretion of TNF from inflammatory cells. In one study, HCV nonstructural protein NS3 expression in permissive hepatoma cell lines resulted in an increased NF-ĸB binding activity and JNK activation, suggesting that NS3 protein may augment hepatocyte signaling in response to TNF [47]. Furthermore, one study suggests that increased NF-ĸB activation in HCV core transgenic hepatocytes inhibits TNF-mediated cell death. In contrast, another study explicated increased sensitivity towards TNF-induced cell death in HCV-core transgenic hepatoma cell lines resulting from the direct interaction of core antigen with the cytoplasmic domain of TNF receptor 1 (TNF-R1). These conflicting reports on the roles of TNF and NF-ĸB signaling in CHC infection must be clarified by further studies [46].

Table 1. HCV proteins induced activation of TLRs and their signaling adaptors in hepatitis C infection and associated comorbidities.

The potential roles of TLRs in HCV pathogenesis by upregulation/downregulation of genes expression			
Hepatic Disease	**Abnormalities in Expression/dysfunctional TLRs**	**The Probable Mechanism of TLRs Dysfunction and Consequences**	**References**
HCV	TLR 1,2,3,4,6	TLR3-recognition of HCV; Hijacked by NS3/4A serine protease	[41, 42]
	TLR 7,8,9	TLR2- dendritic cells, monocyte recognition of NS3 and HCV core	[43]
		TLR4- hyperresponsive monocytes to LPS: Loss of TLR tolerance against HCV particles	[44]
		TLR7,9- decreased IFNα by plasmacytoid dendritic cells	[44]
		TLR 2,3,6,7,8,9- upregulation of mRNA in monocytes and T cells	[43]
Hepatic fibrosis	TLR 2, 4	TLR 2, 4 stellate cell activation	[45]

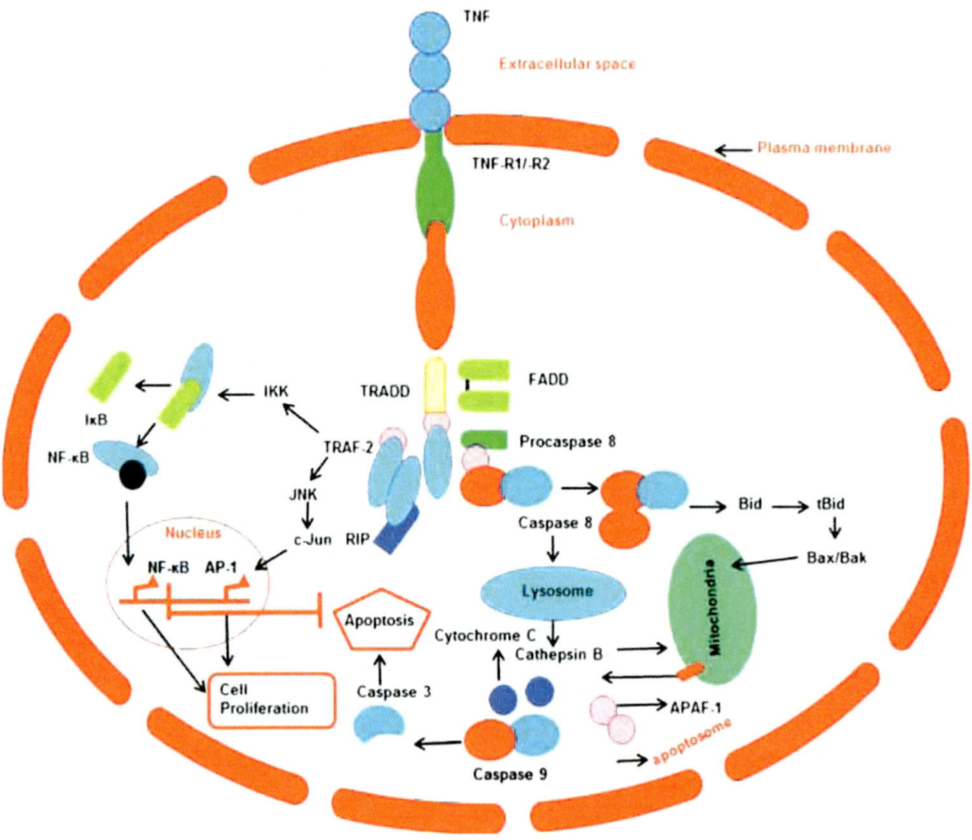

Fig. (2). TNF-induced proliferation and cell death signaling pathways. TNF- α either membrane-bound or soluble form binds to the TNF-R1/R2 and elicits the recruitment of intracellular proteins that modulate the NF-ƙB and JNK cellular signaling pathways. The responses of these signaling molecules derive cell proliferation or apoptosis in the hepatocytes. TNF; Tumor necrosis factor, TNF-R1/R2; Tumor necrosis factor receptor, FADD; FAS-Associated *via* Death Domain; TRADD; TNFR1-associated death domain protein, TRAF; tumor necrosis factor (TNF) receptor-associated factors, IKK; IκB kinase, JNK; c-Jun N-terminal kinases, IKK; IκB kinase, RIP; Receptor-interacting protein, AP-1; Activator protein 1, NF-ƙB; Nuclear factor-kappa B, Bid; BH3-interacting domain, tBid; truncated Bid, BAX; BCL2 Associated X, Bak; BCL2 Associated kinase.

An essential role of TNF-α for HBV reactivation in HCV/HBV coinfected patients has also been demonstrated [17]. Interestingly, one meta-analysis predicts this risk up to 15.6% in patients receiving TNF- α inhibitors and those with inflammatory arthritis [17]. Some animal studies show that TNF-α mediates the immune responses for HBV clearance, and its blockade could impair viral clearance and enhance viral load, demonstrating the possible mechanism of HBV reactivation. Taking these findings together, a recent study figure out that HBV/HCV coinfected patients with higher baseline TNF-α may tend to have more hepatic injury induced by HBV reactivation. However, The causal relationship between TNF-α and HBV reactivation in HBV/HCV co-infection is not fully elusive and further mechanistic studies are required [17].

FAS/FASL Activation in CHC Patients

Apoptosis is an essential phenomenon to preserve liver function and health, as it ensures the efficient removal of unwanted cells (*i.e.*, aged or virus-infected cells) through regulation of cell death and survival [48]. Apoptotic cells are ultimately fragmented into membrane-bound, organelle-containing corpses (*i.e.* apoptotic bodies) which are readily engulfed by neighboring phagocytes, mainly Kupffer cells in the liver [48]. However; this engulfment process may, under several hepatic pathological conditions, promote liver inflammation and damage by amplifying Fas-mediated hepatocyte apoptosis through FasL production by the Kupffer cells themselves. Hepatocyte apoptosis often represents an early sign of many hepatic illnesses, independent of their etiology, and it occurs mainly through the engagement of death receptors on the plasma membrane, especially Fas. For this reason, Fas is constitutively expressed by every cell type in the liver due to which several hepatic illnesses are associated with either Fas over-expression or down-regulation [48]. This equilibrium between new cell regeneration by hepatic cell division and cells dying by Fas-mediated apoptosis is disturbed during uncontrolled hepatocyte apoptosis which can progress into liver injury [48]. Tumor cells often acquire resistance to Fas-mediated apoptosis (Fig. **3**). In these cells stimulation of Fas does not result in apoptosis but triggers activation of prosurvival and pro-oncogenic signaling pathways, which promote cancer growth [48].

Interestingly, being a non-cytopathic virus, HCV itself has very mild cytopathic effects on the infected hepatic cells, and the extensive hepatic damage associated with CHC infection is generally the result of host immune responses to viral antigens [49]. During CHC infection, specific classes of cytotoxic T lymphocytes (CTL) recognize and kill viral antigen-expressing HCV-infected hepatocytes to clear the virus from the liver. However, the presence of excessive apoptotic bodies (once known as councilman bodies) overwhelms the clearance capacity of CTL that causes the initial liver damage, which is subsequently exacerbated by the influx of antigen-non-specific inflammatory cells (Fig. **3**) [49]. This killing of hepatitis C antigen-positive hepatocytes by CTL occurs *via* apoptosis pathways modulated by Fas/FasL binding, in the liver of patients infected with CHC infection, although it does not seem necessary that the Fas pathway only plays a key role in this process [49]. However; it has been unveiled that fas expression is increased in the liver of patients infected with CHC infection, and directly correlates with disease severity such as periportal and intralobular inflammation [50].

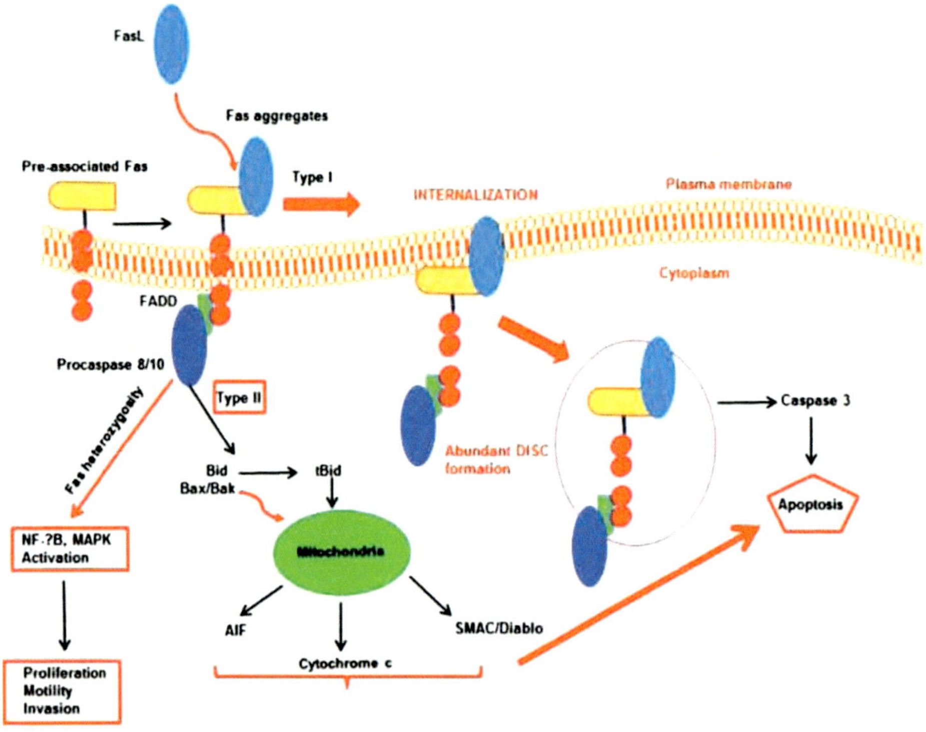

Fig. (3). Fas signaling pathways illustrating Fas-mediated apoptotic and nonapoptotic signaling pathways. FAS; (also known as APO-1 or CD95), FasL; Fas ligand, FADD; FAS-Associated *via* Death Domain; TRADD; TNFR1-associated death domain protein, TRAF; tumor necrosis factor (TNF) receptor-associated factors, Bid; BH3-interacting domain, tBid; truncated Bid, BAX; BCL2 Associated X, Bak; BCL2 Associated kinase, SMAC; supramolecular activation cluster, DISC; death-inducing signaling complex, AIF; apoptosis-inducing factor; MAPK; mitogen-activated protein kinase..

Similarly, the role of HCV proteins in Fas-mediated apoptosis is still controversial and ambiguous in that either Fas expression is mainly regulated by virus-specific proteins or by inflammatory cytokines (*e.g.*, the generation of IL-1, after the first immune response) [49]. In clinical epidemiology, FasL-positive infiltrating mononuclear cells are found very commonly in the liver of CHC-infected patients, improvising the importance of the Fas/FasL pathways in the removal of infected hepatocytes by CTL during hepatitis C infection [49]. Similarly, in another study, HCV proteins exhibited the inhibition of Fas-mediated apoptosis and death in transgenic mice by preventing the release of cytochrome c from the mitochondria [51].

All this reflects that hepatitis C proteins may either stimulate hepatocytes to Fas-induced apoptosis or inhibit apoptosis to maintain persistent hepatitis C infection. Therefore, therapeutic interventions aimed to modulate Fas-mediated apoptosis could be advantageous to reduce hepatic damage in CHC infection and subsequent progression to hepatitis C-induced HCC.

NF-ƙB Cell Signaling and HCV Progression

Nuclear factor-ƙB is essential for immunoglobulin ƙ light chain (an immunoglobulin (Ig) is constituted by two identical heavy chains and two identical light chains either kappa (ƙ) or lambda (ƛ) joined by disulfide bonds so that each heavy chain is linked to a light chain and two heavy chains are linked together) transcription, due to which it is virtually present in all known cell types and mitochondria [52]. It exceptionally regulates the transcription of a large number of genes involved in the immune and inflammatory responses, cell death, and proliferation. In the last decade, tremendous progress has been made in conditional gene knockout technology in mice to advance our understanding of the complex functions of this cell signaling pathway *in vivo* [52]. In particular, inactivating this pathway in certain tissues has highlighted its crucial functions in linking immune responses and cytokine signaling to all kinds of pathological states that had not initially been associated with inflammation (Fig. **4**) [52].

NF-ƙB cell signaling pathway influences almost every physiological process in the liver as liver cells are the preferred source of and target for cytokines, which means that modulation of NF-ƙB cell signaling in the liver plays an important role in hepatic diseases like acute liver failure, hepatic fibrogenesis, and hepatocarcinogenesis. During hepatitis C infection, both hepatitis C structural (*e.g.*, core protein) and nonstructural proteins influence NF-ƙB cell signaling pathways [53]. Hepatitis C infection may stimulate anti-apoptotic genes by activating the NF-ƙB cell signaling pathway which may lead to persistent CHC infection and ultimately hepatocarcinogenesis [54]. Furthermore, hepatitis C core protein can promote human hepatoma cell line proliferation by activating NF-ƙB thereby leading to transforming growth factor (TGF-α) induction and activation of the extracellular-signal-regulated kinase/mitogen-activated protein kinase (ERK/MAPK) pathway [55]. However; the molecular pathogenesis of NF-ƙB induced hepatocarcinogenesis differs between hepatic cell types and the early and late stages of tumor development. Like in the case of inflammatory hepatocarcinogenesis, NF-ƙB promotes tumor development in the later stages of inflammation in hepatocytes as well as the activation of IL-6 in hepatic kupffer cells, whereas NF-ƙB is a tumor suppressor in hepatocytes during the early stages of HCC development [55].

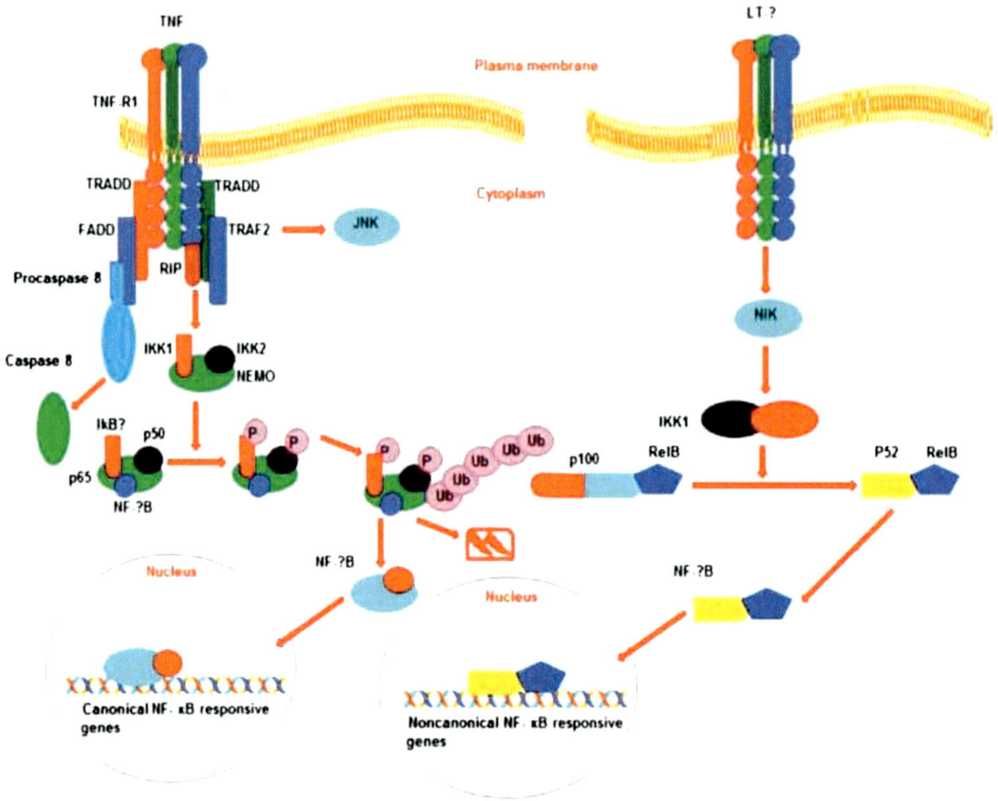

Fig. (4). Canonical and noncanonical NF- kB activation pathways and responsive genes. Canonical activation of NF- kB pathways (left): Upon binding to its receptor (*i.e.* TNF-R1; tumor necrosis factor), the IKK (IκB kinase) family adopters including IKK1, IKK2, and NEMO (Nuclear factor-kappa B essential modulator) gets activated and mediate phosphorylation and ubiquitination of the inhibitory protein IkBα, thereby releasing the p50/p65 NF-kB dimer and unmasking its nuclear localization site. NF-kB translocates to the nucleus and induces transcription of antiapoptotic and inflammatory genes. Noncanonical activation of NF-kB pathways (right): Lymphotoxin-β (LT- β) binds to its receptor leading to NF-κB inducing kinase (NIK) -dependent activation of IKK1 homodimers. The IκB kinase (IKK1) cleaves the inactive precursor protein p100 to the active NF-kB protein p52, which associates with RelB (*i.e.* Transcription factor) and other factors)) and translocates to the nucleus. FADD; FAS-Associated *via* Death Domain; TRADD; TNFR1-associated death domain protein, TRAF; tumor necrosis factor (TNF) receptor-associated factors, *JNK,* c-Ju--(N)-terminal kinase; *LT*-b lymphotoxin-b, NIK; NF-κB inducing kinase..

To summarize, NF-ƙB can perpetuate liver inflammation and block hepatocyte apoptosis in hepatitis C infection which might indicate that HCV has acquired the ability to subvert NF-ƙB regulatory roles to its advantage [56]. The prominent involvement of NF-ƙB cell signaling in almost every physiological role of the liver and its influence on hepatic disease progression signifies its importance as an attractive candidate for the development of innovative therapies based on molecular drugs by targeting this pathway [54, 55]. However; as some generalized inflammatory responses have been noticed with NF-κB inhibitors (*e.g.* molecular inhibitors of kappaB kinase (IKK)), further genetic and pre-clinical studies are urgently needed to explore the better role of NF-κB in hepatic disorders (Fig. **4**), to further dissect the pathway, and to discover novel mediators of NF-κB dependent cell signals to allow sophisticated modulation of this pathway without any hepatic or systemic toxicity in certain hepatic diseases.

CONCLUSIONS

Virus-host dependencies are vital for the production of new viral progeny and the infectiousness of a certain virus in host cells. Regardless of the viral determinants, host factors also play an integral role in the replication, translation, and transmission of HCV from an infected hepatocyte to healthy hepatic cells. Furthermore, the propagation of acute HCV infection to CHC and subsequently toward end-stage liver diseases (hepatic cirrhosis, HCC, *etc.*) also rely on various host factors to exacerbate viral proteins to take the charge of host cell machinery to disrupt normal cellular processes leading to extrahepatic manifestations of HCV. Host cell factors involved in regular functions of the cells crosstalk HCV proteins to support the virus replication and translation inside the host cells. Certain host DNA transcription and replication proteins modulation, cytokine gene polymorphism, and alteration of lipid metabolism are key host mechanisms responsible for HCV infection progression, chronicity, and transmission. Furthermore, Intracellular signaling plays a vital role in worsening the pathological states of the infected hepatocytes by activating cell proliferation, prohibiting apoptosis of damaged cells, and up or down-regulating host genes or protein functions to develop hepatocarcinogenesis. Toll-like receptors and their intricate interplay with HCV proteins, tumor necrosis factor, and FAS/FAS ligand activation are vital to leading acute HCV infection to chronic hepatitis C. Furthermore, the activation of nuclear factor-κB cell signaling by HCV augments the expression of anti-apoptotic genes to convert CHC into hepatocarcinogenesis. The thorough studies of all these pivotal host cell mechanisms would be useful to understand the etiology of the conversion of acute hepatitis C to CHC and followed by hepatocarcinogenesis. It will also help us to find indigenous anti-HCV drug targets to design and develop novel agents to be used as an adjuvant with oral interferon-free direct-acting antivirals (DAAs) to safeguard HCV-infected host cells and maintain their cellular integrity.

REFERENCES

[1] Lapa D, Garbuglia A, Capobianchi M, Del Porto P, Hepatitis C. Hepatitis C virus genetic variability, human immune response, and genome polymorphisms: which is the interplay? Cells 2019; 8(4): 305. [http://dx.doi.org/10.3390/cells8040305] [PMID: 30987134]

[2] Matsuura K, Tanaka Y. Host genetic variants influencing the clinical course of hepatitis C virus infection. J Med Virol 2016; 88(2): 185-95.

[http://dx.doi.org/10.1002/jmv.24334] [PMID: 26211651]

[3] Chigbu D, Loonawat R, Sehgal M, Patel D, Jain P, Hepatitis C. Hepatitis C Virus Infection: Host Virus Interaction and Mechanisms of Viral Persistence. Cells 2019; 8(4): 376. [http://dx.doi.org/10.3390/cells8040376] [PMID: 31027278]

[4] Buchanan R, Hydes T, Khakoo SI. Innate and adaptive genetic pathways in HCV infection. Tissue Antigens 2015; 85(4): 231-40. [http://dx.doi.org/10.1111/tan.12540] [PMID: 25708172]

[5] Bassendine MF, Sheridan DA, Bridge SH, Felmlee DJ, Neely RDG. Lipids and HCV. Semin Immunopathol 2013; 35(1): 87-100. [http://dx.doi.org/10.1007/s00281-012-0356-2] [PMID: 23111699]

[6] Shahid I, Almalki WH, Ibrahim MM, *et al.* Characterization of *In vitro* inhibitory effects of consensus short interference RNAs against non-structural 5B gene of hepatitis C virus 1a genotype. Indian J Med Microbiol 2018; 36(4): 494-503. [http://dx.doi.org/10.4103/ijmm.IJMM_17_146] [PMID: 30880695]

[7] Li YP, Ramirez S, Jensen SB, Purcell RH, Gottwein JM, Bukh J. Highly efficient full-length hepatitis C virus genotype 1 (strain TN) infectious culture system. Proc Natl Acad Sci USA 2012; 109(48): 19757-62. [http://dx.doi.org/10.1073/pnas.1218260109] [PMID: 23151512]

[8] Barski MS, Minnell JJ, Maertens GN. PP2A Phosphatase as an Emerging Viral Host Factor. Front Cell Infect Microbiol 2021; 11: 725615. [http://dx.doi.org/10.3389/fcimb.2021.725615] [PMID: 34422684]

[9] Biswas D, Cary W, Nolta JA. PPP2R5D-Related Intellectual Disability and Neurodevelopmental Delay: A Review of the Current Understanding of the Genetics and Biochemical Basis of the Disorder. Int J Mol Sci 2020; 21(4): 1286. [http://dx.doi.org/10.3390/ijms21041286] [PMID: 32074998]

[10] Loveday C, Tatton-Brown K, Clarke M, *et al.* Mutations in the PP2A regulatory subunit B family genes *PPP2R5B*, *PPP2R5C* and *PPP2R5D* cause human overgrowth. Hum Mol Genet 2015; 24(17): 4775-9. [http://dx.doi.org/10.1093/hmg/ddv182] [PMID: 25972378]

[11] Loureiro D, Tout I, Narguet S, Benazzouz SM, Mansouri A, Asselah T. miRNAs as Potential Biomarkers for Viral Hepatitis B and C. Viruses 2020; 12(12): 1440. [http://dx.doi.org/10.3390/v12121440] [PMID: 33327640]

[12] Kunden RD, Khan JQ, Ghezelbash S, Wilson JA. The Role of the Liver-Specific microRNA, miRNA-122 in the HCV Replication Cycle. Int J Mol Sci 2020; 21(16): 5677. [http://dx.doi.org/10.3390/ijms21165677] [PMID: 32784807]

[13] Thomas M, Deiters A. MicroRNA miR-122 as a therapeutic target for oligonucleotides and small molecules. Curr Med Chem 2013; 20(29): 3629-40. [http://dx.doi.org/10.2174/0929867311320290009] [PMID: 23745562]

[14] Panigrahi M, Thibault PA, Wilson JA. miR-122 affects both the initiation and maintenance of Hepatitis C Virus infections. J Virol 2021; Jvi0190321. [PMID: 34908444]

[15] Ali ME, Halby HM, Ali MY, *et al.* Role of Serum Vitamin D, Interleukin 13, and microRNA-135a in Hepatocellular Carcinoma and Treatment Failure in Egyptian HCV-Infected Patients Receiving Direct Antiviral Agents. Viruses 2021; 13(10): 2008. [http://dx.doi.org/10.3390/v13102008] [PMID: 34696438]

[16] Noh IC, Ahmad I, Suraiya S, Musa NF, Nurul AA, Ruzilawati AB. Cytokine (IL-10, IL-6, TNF-α and TGF-β1) Gene Polymorphisms in Chronic Hepatitis C Virus Infection among Malay Male Drug Abusers. Biomedicines 2021; 9(9): 1115.

[http://dx.doi.org/10.3390/biomedicines9091115] [PMID: 34572300]

[17] Huang SC, Cheng PN, Liu CH, Yang HC, Su TH, Tseng TC. Serum cytokine/chemokine profiles predict hepatitis B reactivation in HBV/HCV co-infected subjects receiving direct-acting antiviral agents. Journal of the Formosan Medical Association 2021.

[18] Franco S, Horneros J, Soldevila L, *et al.* Single nucleotide polymorphisms in PNPLA3, ADAR-1 and IFIH1 are associated with advanced liver fibrosis in patients co-infected with HIV-1//hepatitis C virus. AIDS 2021; 35(15): 2497-502.
[http://dx.doi.org/10.1097/QAD.0000000000003066] [PMID: 34482352]

[19] Della Mina E, Rodero MP, Crow YJ. Polymorphisms in IFIH1: the good and the bad. Nat Immunol 2017; 18(7): 708-9.
[http://dx.doi.org/10.1038/ni.3765] [PMID: 28632717]

[20] Eslam M, Hashem AM, Leung R, *et al.* Interferon-λ rs12979860 genotype and liver fibrosis in viral and non-viral chronic liver disease. Nat Commun 2015; 6(1): 6422.
[http://dx.doi.org/10.1038/ncomms7422] [PMID: 25740255]

[21] Longo M, Meroni M, Paolini E, *et al.* TM6SF2/PNPLA3/MBOAT7 Loss-of-Function Genetic Variants Impact on NAFLD Development and Progression Both in Patients and in In Vitro Models. Cell Mol Gastroenterol Hepatol 2022; 13(3): 759-88.
[http://dx.doi.org/10.1016/j.jcmgh.2021.11.007] [PMID: 34823063]

[22] Chen Q, Coto-Llerena M, Suslov A, *et al.* Interferon lambda 4 impairs hepatitis C viral antigen presentation and attenuates T cell responses. Nat Commun 2021; 12(1): 4882.
[http://dx.doi.org/10.1038/s41467-021-25218-x] [PMID: 34385466]

[23] Valiakou V, Eliadis P, Karamichali E, *et al.* Differential Expression of the Host Lipid Regulators ANGPTL-3 and ANGPTL-4 in HCV Infection and Treatment. Int J Mol Sci 2021; 22(15): 7961.
[http://dx.doi.org/10.3390/ijms22157961] [PMID: 34360721]

[24] Shahid I, AlMalki WH, Hassan S, Hafeez MH. Real-world challenges for hepatitis C virus medications: a critical overview. Crit Rev Microbiol 2018; 44(2): 143-60.
[http://dx.doi.org/10.1080/1040841X.2017.1329277] [PMID: 28539069]

[25] Foka P, Karamichali E, Dalagiorgou G, *et al.* Hepatitis C virus modulates lipid regulatory factor Angiopoietin-like 3 gene expression by repressing HNF-1α activity. J Hepatol 2014; 60(1): 30-8.
[http://dx.doi.org/10.1016/j.jhep.2013.08.016] [PMID: 23978712]

[26] Faillaci F, Marzi L, Critelli R, *et al.* Liver Angiopoietin-2 Is a Key Predictor of *D e N ovo* or Recurrent Hepatocellular Cancer After Hepatitis CVirus Direct-Acting Antivirals. Hepatology 2018; 68(3): 1010-24.
[http://dx.doi.org/10.1002/hep.29911] [PMID: 29604220]

[27] Khera T, Du Y, Todt D, Deterding K, Strunz B, Hardtke S, *et al.* Long-lasting Imprint in the Soluble Inflammatory Milieu despite Early Treatment of Acute Symptomatic Hepatitis C. J Infect Dis 2021. [PMID: 33517457]

[28] Graf C, Welzel T, Bogdanou D, *et al.* Hepatitis C clearance by direct-acting antivirals impacts glucose and lipid homeostasis. J Clin Med 2020; 9(9): 2702.
[http://dx.doi.org/10.3390/jcm9092702] [PMID: 32825571]

[29] Huang CF, Dai CY, Yeh ML, *et al.* Cure or curd: Modification of lipid profiles and cardio-cerebrovascular events after hepatitis C virus eradication. Kaohsiung J Med Sci 2020; 36(11): 920-8.
[http://dx.doi.org/10.1002/kjm2.12275] [PMID: 32643842]

[30] Iossa D, Vitrone M, Gagliardi M, *et al.* Anthropometric parameters and liver histology influence lipid metabolic changes in HCV chronic hepatitis on direct-acting antiviral treatment. Ann Transl Med 2021; 9(1): 35.
[http://dx.doi.org/10.21037/atm-20-669] [PMID: 33553328]

[31] Chang SW, Cheng ML, Shiao MS, *et al.* Recovery of lipid metabolic alterations in hepatitis C patients

after viral clearance: Incomplete restoration with accelerated ω-oxidation. J Clin Lipidol 2018; 12(3): 756-66.
[http://dx.doi.org/10.1016/j.jacl.2018.02.011] [PMID: 29574072]

[32] Fabregat I, Caballero-Díaz D. Transforming Growth Factor-β-Induced Cell Plasticity in Liver Fibrosis and Hepatocarcinogenesis. Front Oncol 2018; 8: 357.
[http://dx.doi.org/10.3389/fonc.2018.00357] [PMID: 30250825]

[33] Ray S, Broor SL, Vaishnav Y, *et al.* Transforming growth factor beta in hepatitis C virus infection: In vivo and in vitro findings. J Gastroenterol Hepatol 2003; 18(4): 393-403.
[http://dx.doi.org/10.1046/j.1440-1746.2003.02985.x] [PMID: 12653887]

[34] Abd El-Meguid M, Dawood RM, Mokhles MA, El Awady MK. Extrahepatic Upregulation of Transforming Growth Factor Beta 2 in HCV Genotype 4-Induced Liver Fibrosis. Journal of interferon & cytokine research : the official journal of the International Society for Interferon and Cytokine Research 2018; 38(8): 341-7.

[35] Gal-Tanamy M, Bachmetov L, Ravid A, *et al.* Vitamin D: An innate antiviral agent suppressing hepatitis C virus in human hepatocytes. Hepatology 2011; 54(5): 1570-9.
[http://dx.doi.org/10.1002/hep.24575] [PMID: 21793032]

[36] Gutierrez JA, Jones KA, Flores R, *et al.* Vitamin D Metabolites Inhibit Hepatitis C Virus and Modulate Cellular Gene Expression. J Virol Antivir Res 2014; 3(3)
[http://dx.doi.org/10.4172/2324-8955.1000129] [PMID: 26594646]

[37] Esmat G, El Raziky M, Elsharkawy A, Sabry D, Hassany M, Ahmed A. Impact of vitamin D supplementation on sustained virological response in chronic hepatitis C genotype 4 patients treated by pegylated interferon/ribavirin. Journal of interferon & cytokine research : the official journal of the International Society for Interferon and Cytokine Research 2015; 35(1): 49-54.

[38] Petta S, Ferraro D, Cammà C, *et al.* Vitamin D levels and IL28B polymorphisms are related to rapid virological response to standard of care in genotype 1 chronic hepatitis C. Antivir Ther 2012; 17(5): 823-31.
[http://dx.doi.org/10.3851/IMP2100] [PMID: 22505587]

[39] Petta S, Cammà C, Scazzone C, *et al.* Low vitamin D serum level is related to severe fibrosis and low responsiveness to interferon-based therapy in genotype 1 chronic hepatitis C. Hepatology 2010; 51(4): 1158-67.
[http://dx.doi.org/10.1002/hep.23489] [PMID: 20162613]

[40] Howell J, Angus P, Gow P, Visvanathan K. Toll-like receptors in hepatitis C infection: Implications for pathogenesis and treatment. J Gastroenterol Hepatol 2013; 28(5): 766-76.
[http://dx.doi.org/10.1111/jgh.12170] [PMID: 23432473]

[41] Otsuka M, Kato N, Moriyama M, *et al.* Interaction between the HCV NS3 protein and the host TBK1 protein leads to inhibition of cellular antiviral responses. Hepatology 2005; 41(5): 1004-12.
[http://dx.doi.org/10.1002/hep.20666] [PMID: 15841462]

[42] Li K, Foy E, Ferreon JC, *et al.* Immune evasion by hepatitis C virus NS3/4A protease-mediated cleavage of the Toll-like receptor 3 adaptor protein TRIF. Proc Natl Acad Sci USA 2005; 102(8): 2992-7.
[http://dx.doi.org/10.1073/pnas.0408824102] [PMID: 15710891]

[43] Dolganiuc A, Oak S, Kodys K, *et al.* Hepatitis C core and nonstructural 3 proteins trigger toll-like receptor 2-mediated pathways and inflammatory activation. Gastroenterology 2004; 127(5): 1513-24.
[http://dx.doi.org/10.1053/j.gastro.2004.08.067] [PMID: 15521019]

[44] Dolganiuc A, Norkina O, Kodys K, *et al.* Viral and host factors induce macrophage activation and loss of toll-like receptor tolerance in chronic HCV infection. Gastroenterology 2007; 133(5): 1627-36.
[http://dx.doi.org/10.1053/j.gastro.2007.08.003] [PMID: 17916356]

[45] Kisseleva T, Brenner DA. Role of hepatic stellate cells in fibrogenesis and the reversal of fibrosis. J

Gastroenterol Hepatol 2007; 22(s1) (Suppl. 1): S73-8.
[http://dx.doi.org/10.1111/j.1440-1746.2006.04658.x] [PMID: 17567473]

[46] Peña-Asensio J, Sanz-de-Villalobos E, Miquel J, Larrubia JR. Tumor necrosis family receptor superfamily member 9/tumor necrosis factor receptor-associated factor 1 pathway on hepatitis C viral persistence and natural history. World J Hepatol 2020; 12(10): 754-65.
[http://dx.doi.org/10.4254/wjh.v12.i10.754] [PMID: 33200014]

[47] Hassan M, Selimovic D, Ghozlan H, Abdel-Kader O. Induction of high-molecular-weight (HMW) tumor necrosis factor(TNF) alpha by hepatitis C virus (HCV) non-structural protein 3 (NS3) in liver cells is AP-1 and NF-κB-dependent activation. Cell Signal 2007; 19(2): 301-11.
[http://dx.doi.org/10.1016/j.cellsig.2006.07.002] [PMID: 16916598]

[48] Bortolami M, Kotsafti A, Cardin R, Farinati F. Fas / FasL system, IL-1β expression and apoptosis in chronic HBV and HCV liver disease. J Viral Hepat 2008; 15(7): 515-22.
[http://dx.doi.org/10.1111/j.1365-2893.2008.00974.x] [PMID: 18331250]

[49] Amoras ESG, Gomes STM, Freitas FB, *et al.* Intrahepatic mRNA Expression of FAS, FASL, and FOXP3 Genes Is Associated with the Pathophysiology of Chronic HCV Infection. PLoS One 2016; 11(5): e0156604.
[http://dx.doi.org/10.1371/journal.pone.0156604] [PMID: 27243827]

[50] Harper N, Hughes M, MacFarlane M, Cohen GM. Fas-associated death domain protein and caspase-8 are not recruited to the tumor necrosis factor receptor 1 signaling complex during tumor necrosis factor-induced apoptosis. J Biol Chem 2003; 278(28): 25534-41.
[http://dx.doi.org/10.1074/jbc.M303399200] [PMID: 12721308]

[51] Scaffidi C, Fulda S, Srinivasan A, *et al.* Two CD95 (APO-1/Fas) signaling pathways. EMBO J 1998; 17(6): 1675-87.
[http://dx.doi.org/10.1093/emboj/17.6.1675] [PMID: 9501089]

[52] Arsura M, Cavin LG. Nuclear factor-κB and liver carcinogenesis. Cancer Lett 2005; 229(2): 157-69.
[http://dx.doi.org/10.1016/j.canlet.2005.07.008] [PMID: 16125305]

[53] Boya P, Larrea E, Sola I, *et al.* Nuclear factor-κB in the liver of patients with chronic hepatitis C: Decreased RelA expression is associated with enhanced fibrosis progression. Hepatology 2001; 34(5): 1041-8.
[http://dx.doi.org/10.1053/jhep.2001.29002] [PMID: 11679977]

[54] Song X, Gao X, Wang Y, *et al.* HCV Core Protein Induces Chemokine CCL2 and CXCL10 Expression Through NF-κB Signaling Pathway in Macrophages. Front Immunol 2021; 12: 654998.
[http://dx.doi.org/10.3389/fimmu.2021.654998] [PMID: 34531848]

[55] Song X, Yao Z, Yang J, *et al.* HCV core protein binds to gC1qR to induce A20 expression and inhibit cytokine production through MAPKs and NF-κB signaling pathways. Oncotarget 2016; 7(23): 33796-808.
[http://dx.doi.org/10.18632/oncotarget.9304] [PMID: 27183919]

[56] Sato Y, Kato J, Takimoto R, *et al.* Hepatitis C virus core protein promotes proliferation of human hepatoma cells through enhancement of transforming growth factor expression *via* activation of nuclear factor- B. Gut 2006; 55(12): 1801-8.
[http://dx.doi.org/10.1136/gut.2005.070417] [PMID: 16581947]

CHAPTER 3

Immune Responses and Immunopathology of Acute and Chronic Hepatitis C Virus Infection

Abstract: An ample understanding of the HCV life cycle and infection biology has also significantly increased our knowledge of hepatitis C immune responses against acute infection to the progression of chronic hepatitis C and associated comorbidities. As expected in chimpanzees (the best *in vivo* model so far to study hepatitis C infection kinetics, molecular pathogenesis, and immunopathology) and humans, several arms of the immune responses are activated following HCV infection. Some of the underlying mechanisms both for innate immune responses and adaptive immune responses to viral clearance and persistent HCV infection are fully understood, however; some fundamental questions in hepatitis C immunopathology remain to be answered and some immune responses hypothesis demands further studies to validate. Some mechanistic issues of viral evasion strategies during infection progression and the future development of prophylactic and protective anti-HCV vaccines will be largely dependent on the full understanding of the kinetics of adaptive immune responses against HCV infection. As generally presumed the inefficient role of innate immunity in self-resolving HCV infection, the potent immune responses of CD8+ T and CD4+ T cells are critically important after the acute phase of the infection. In particular, the plausible understanding of CD4+ T cells responses against persistent infection will certainly be central to the development of future HCV vaccines. In this chapter, we overview the host immune responses against hepatitis C acute infection and subsequent CHC infection, their regulation by viral and cellular proteins, and the virus purging strategies while impairing host defense system mechanisms.

Keywords: Adaptive immune response, Anergy, Anti-HCV vaccines, Cross-reactive neutralizing antibodies, CD+ 4 T cells, CD+ 8 T cells, Dendritic cells, Cytotoxic T lymphocyte, Hepatitis C virus, Host-immune response, Immunoregulatory cells, Immunopathogenesis, Innate immune response, Natural killer cells, Priming, Protective vaccines, Prophylactic vaccines, T-cell exhaustion, Viral escape.

INTRODUCTION

Currently, all oral IFN-free DAAs are the treatment of choice for HCV infection, where the proportion of cured patients with high SVR rates has markedly increased in real-world clinical settings [1]. However, therapy costs, treatment

Imran Shahid and Qaiser Jabeen

access to poor nations, chances of re-infection after post-completion therapy, and the occurrence of some severe adverse events (SAEs) are big challenges to surmount the public healthcare burden of HCV [2]. There will be always a need for prophylactic or protective HCV vaccines to control the further dissemination of infection in populations and to reduce new HCV incidences. For this purpose, extensive knowledge and a comprehensive understanding of anti-HCV immune responses against acute and chronic hepatitis C infection, viral clearance, and viral reinfection would be required and pragmatic research approaches must be implemented in various disciplines of HCV immunopathology [3]. In addition to that, the current literature is unlikely and largely decipher the HCV immune responses in disease progression phenomena rather than in host protection [3]. Second, HCV immunology research is hampered by several difficulties. First, as mentioned in Chapter 1, acute hepatitis C infections are often asymptomatic, and therefore difficult to follow the evolution of the disease before it becomes chronic. Second, most HCV immunopathological studies and their conclusions have been based on the analysis of hepatitis C immune responses in peripheral blood, which might not be representative of the anti-HCV immune responses in the liver and secondary lymphoid organs. Finally, the lack of an efficient animal model for HCV infection studies also hampers the efforts to fully understand the host's innate and adaptive immune responses against the virus. In this chapter, we briefly overview the host's innate and adaptive immune responses against HCV and its impact on preventing disease severity and chronicity. We will also elaborate on HCV evasion strategies against host immune responses during the progression of acute hepatitis C to CHC infection. In the end, we will demonstrate the importance of anti-HCV immune responses in the development of a prophylactic or protective hep C vaccine.

THE TYPICAL TIMELINE OF HEPATITIS C VIRUS INFECTION

HCV is a blood-borne virus, so the major infection route is via the blood. Some patients who are exposed to the virus develop overt liver disease, but most of them remain in a latent state [4]. Within six months of being infected, 30% of the patients expel the virus naturally while the remaining 70% enter a phase of persistent infection [4]. Once patients enter this later phase, it is very rare for the virus to be expelled naturally, with the estimated annual rate being less than 0.2% at most. Many of the patients with persistent infection show the medical conditions of CHC and develop cirrhosis in 20 to 30 years [5]. Patients with cirrhosis develop HCC at a very high annual rate of 8%, while patients with early CHC do so at an annual rate of only 0.5% (Fig. **1**) [5]. In the absence of high levels of immunosuppression, HCV is a non-cytopathic virus. In the absence of an ongoing immune response, it infects and persists in target cells, predominantly hepatocytes, without inducing inflammation and damage [3]. This has been demonstrated in both experimental chimpanzee models and drug users or humans who were accidentally infected with contaminated needles during healthcare practice [3]. In these studies, increases in viremia were not associated with parallel increases in serum transaminase levels, thus reflecting an absence of hepatocyte damage [6]. Furthermore, following liver transplantation, the infection does not lead to liver damage for 3 weeks despite high levels of the virus [7]. The only cytopathic lesion that has been directly ascribed to HCV is the association of GT-3 infection with steatosis, the accumulation of lipids in hepatocytes [8]. Although non-cytopathic, gene microarray analysis of infected chimpanzee liver has revealed that the virus induces the expression of a large number of cellular genes as soon as a few days after HCV infection [3]. These genes include those involved in lipid metabolism and several genes associated with innate and adaptive immune responses [3].

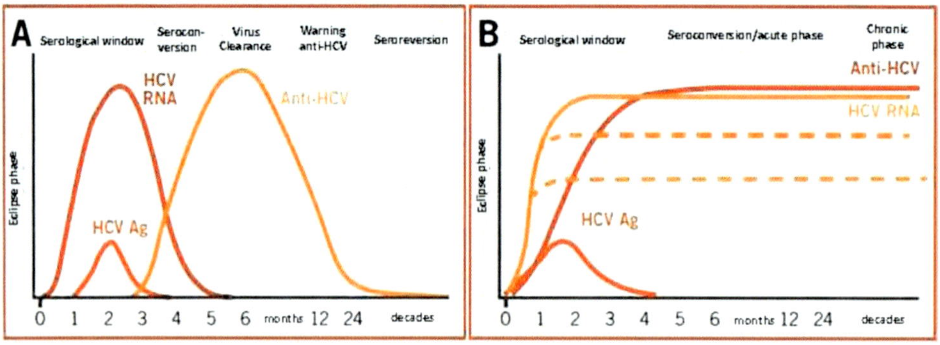

Fig. (1). Approximate time course of virological and immunological markers of hepatitis C infection [35]. **(A)** deciphers the modulation of virological and immunological markers during acute HCV infection whereas **(B)** explains the persistence of immunological markers during chronic infection. Ag; antigen.

INNATE AND ADAPTIVE IMMUNE RESPONSES AGAINST HEPATITIS C

Both the innate and adaptive immune systems appear to play an important role in the immune response to HCV [3]. The biological defense mechanism of higher organisms, including humans, is generally divided into innate immunity and adaptive immunity [3]. In the adaptive immune response, gene rearrangement by T cells and B cells enables the establishment of a defense mechanism of high specification against "the molecular microstructure of a foreign substance," and this mechanism is immunologically memorized [3]. However, as it takes a few days to induce adaptive immune responses, innate immunity works as an early defense mechanism [3]. Cells involved in innate immunity include macrophages, neutrophils, natural killer (NK), natural killer T (NKT) cells, and gamma delta ($\gamma\delta$T) cells. Important humoral factors include complements, lectins, and interferons (IFNs) [3].

Activation of Innate Immune Responses and their Implications Against HCV Replication

In Vitro Innate Immune Responses Against Hepatitis C

The innate immune response represents the first line of defense against pathogens and is maintained by complement, NK, NKT, and macrophage cells [3]. It is widely accepted that this arm of the immune system is effective in removing most pathogens that infect the body [3]. The innate immune responses also play important roles in activating and amplifying the adaptive immune system [9]. Viruses produce viral pathogen-associated molecular patterns (PAMPs) that can initiate a cascade of events leading to innate intracellular immunity [3]. In the case of HCV, the double-stranded RNA initiates two major pathways of host defense by binding to TLR-3 and retinoic-acid inducible gene I (RIG-1) [3]. Type I interferons (*i.e.*, IFNα and IFNβ proteins) and type III IFNs (*i.e.*, IFNλ proteins) are the major components of the antiviral innate immune system [3]. These proteins bind to the IFNα/β receptors (*i.e.*, IFNAR1-IFNAR2) and the IFNλ receptor (*i.e.*, IFNLR1-IL10R2), respectively [3]. Both proteins induce the expression of IFN-stimulated genes (ISGs) mediated by an IFN-stimulated gene factor 3 (ISGF3) complex formed by phosphorylated STAT1, phosphorylated STAT2, and IFN regulatory factor 9 (IRF9) [3]. HCV infection increases the expression of many ISGs which has three major roles: First to induce ISGs that have an antiviral action; second to induce the maturation of immune effector cells, and third to create a pro-inflammatory environment following upregulation of cytokine expression by hepatic cells [3]. An ongoing type I IFN response appears to be important to limit hepatitis C replication and spread until the adaptive immune responses play their roles [3]. It was noticed during *in vitro* studies that HCV replicons are extremely sensitive to IFN-α, by the high rate of viral clearance when IFN-α is administered during the acute phase of infection (*i.e.*, an approximate reduction to a 10% chronicity of infection) and by the effectiveness of IFN-α and RBV treatment in chronically infected individuals [3]. However, it was postulated that the natural induction of type I IFNs alone is unable to control hepatitis C replication [3]. It is therefore likely that the virus inhibits the downstream antiviral effects of IFNs.

In Vivo Activation of Innate Immune Responses Against Hepatitis C

Cytosolic hepatitis C RNA is sequentially sensed by RIG-I (also known as DDX58) and melanoma differentiation-associated protein 5 (MDA5; also known as IFIH1) [3]. The RIG-I-mediated IFN response dominates at the early stages of infection, whereas the MDA5-mediated IFN response occurs later. Protein kinase

R (PKR; also known as EIF2AK2) also participates in the early sensing of Hepatitis C. After binding to hepatitis C dsRNA, PKR interacts with mitochondrial antiviral signaling (MAVS) protein and induces ISGs. TLR-3 is also involved in IFN production and ISG expression by sensing hepatitis C dsRNA in endosomes. Once IFN type I and IFN type III are produced, they can suppress hepatitis C replication through the antiviral action of ISGs. That's why PEG-IFNα) has been used as a gold standard of care for hepatitis C treatment before the advent and approval of DAAs. However; hepatitis C infection can result in divergent outcomes either self-limited infection or progression to chronic infection [3]. As mentioned earlier the hepatic expression of ISGs is increased during acute hepatitis C infection, whereas virus-specific T-cell responses are induced in a delayed manner despite the early increase in virus loads. Due to this, T-cell responses coincide with liver injury (*i.e.*, increased serum levels of ALT) and virus control, even if the virus is not completely cleared [3, 6].

Antibodies Against HCV Infection

The role of hepatitis C-specific antibodies in the control of acute infection is not explained fully and it remains to be elucidated. Hepatitis C seroconversion occurs approximately from 7 to 31 weeks after primary infection, and some hepatitis C-specific antibodies are effective in blocking *in vitro* infection of target cells by HCV [10]. However, in both chimpanzees and humans, naturally acquired anti-HCV antibodies generated during this infection do not seem to be protective against secondary infection with hepatitis C [10]. It indicates that these molecules play a limited role in preventing the progression of HCV. Antibodies specific for E1 and E2 envelope glycoproteins have hepatitis C neutralizing activity [3]. However, hepatitis C-specific E1 or E2 antibodies tend to easily lose their neutralizing activity as a result of virus escape mutations [3]. Furthermore, some studies in chimpanzees indicate that resolution of infection can occur without the development of detectable antibody responses [10].

Cell-to-cell direct transmission of hepatitis C can also help the virus to escape detection by neutralizing antibodies [11]. In early studies, it was also found that hepatitis C-specific antibodies have a limited role to control the infection as those were often detected in patients or chimpanzees with persistent CHC infection rather than in hosts with spontaneous resolution of infection [11, 12]. However; the conclusions of those studies were based on the use of only a limited set of HCV pseudo-particles. Recent studies have documented that antibodies might be essential for the control of non-cytopathic viruses and to maintain protective memory [13, 14]. In a study using the hepatitis C pseudoparticle library, cross-reactive neutralizing antibodies were induced in early acute hepatitis C infection patients with spontaneous recovery, whereas neutralizing antibodies were developed in a delayed manner in patients with CHC infection [15]. Interestingly, the appearance of neutralizing antibodies was also noticed in a CHC-infected patient with spontaneous clearance of the infection that rarely occurs [15]. Similarly, a crystal structure of E2 envelope glycoprotein has been reported and broadly neutralizing antibodies with protective or therapeutic activity have been developed [16]. It is, therefore, possible that antibodies may play other unexpected roles during hepatitis C infections and must be further clarified in future studies. Furthermore, it remains to be elucidated how broadly neutralizing antibodies can be induced during CHC infection which may provide fruitful information for the development of a prophylactic or protective anti-hepatitis C vaccine. Although the recent advent of hepatitis C replicon models is likely to enhance our understanding of the role of neutralizing antibodies in hepatitis C infection, the role of T cells in viral control is better understood than the role of B cells [3].

IFN Responses in CHC Infection

As described above, ISG stimulation and IFN production are continued during hepatitis C infection despite the interference mechanisms of the virus, and many ISGs are upregulated during CHC infection [3]. However; unlike acute hepatitis C, phosphorylated STAT1 is scarcely detected in CHC-infected livers (Table **1**) [3]. Instead of that, an unphosphorylated transcription factor complex known as U-ISGF3- formed by high protein levels of STAT1, STAT2, and IRF9 without tyrosine phosphorylation of the STATs- having a role in the induction of a set of ISGs was noticed in one study [17]. Furthermore, this complex maintains the sustained expression of ISGs in hepatitis C-infected cells for a prolonged time and ultimately confers extended antiviral effects [17]. Interestingly, sustained expression of ISGs has been noticed with an adverse impact on spontaneous virus clearance and IFNα-based treatment [17]. HCV-infected patients with high levels of ISGs in their livers at baseline have been observed with worse rates of spontaneous virus clearance and poor response to PEG-IFN/RBV combination therapy [18]. The underlying mechanism for poor response to IFNα-based therapy was emphasized by the negative regulation of a ubiquitin-specific peptidase 18 (USP 18) that is responsible for unresponsiveness to IFNα [19]. USP18 is itself an ISG; however, its interaction with IFNAR2 inhibits the downregulation signals for IFNα stimulation [19]. A recent study demonstrates that prolonged exposure to endogenously produced IFNλs during HCV infection induces the sustained upregulation of ISG15 by U-ISGF3 [17]. ISG15 stabilizes the USP18 protein and causes unresponsiveness to exogenous IFNα treatment [17]. It is one of the most abundant and highly expressed ISGs in HCV-infected livers, and this unique function of ISG15 helps to explain why even the presence of high baseline levels of ISGs in HCV-infected livers are associated with poor response to PEG-IFN therapy [17]. A recently identified IFNL4 genotype is also found to strongly influence IFNα-based therapy (discussed in chapter 2).

How HCV Evades Innate Immune Responses

HCV interferes with the stimulation of ISGs and the production of IFNs. Various HCV proteins have been shown to inhibit IFN-related genes *in vitro*. Hepatitis C NS3-NS4A serine protease cleave MAVS independently of its subcellular location (*i.e*., in mitochondria, in mitochondria-associated endoplasmic reticulum membranes (MAMs)) and in peroxisomes [20]. This cleavage by NS3-NS4A serine protease was confirmed in HCV-infected liver tissue [21]. NS3–NS4A also blocks the induction of type I IFNs by functioning as an antagonist of IRF-3 [21]. Furthermore, it can cleave Toll/IL-1 receptor domain-containing adaptor inducing IFN-β (TRIF; also known as TICAM1), which is a downstream mediator of TLR-3-induced signal transduction [21]. *In vitro* studies demonstrate that HCV glycoprotein E2 and NS5A nonstructural phosphoprotein interact and can repress the double-stranded RNA-dependent protein kinase (PKR) (Table **1**) [3]. HCV has also been shown to affect the JAK-STAT pathway [3]. It should be noted that activation of the innate immune responses promulgates a cascade that is critical to the initiation and maturation of the adaptive immune responses. Thus, defects in the innate immune response induced by HCV might have crucial downstream effects on the development of adaptive immune responses capable of mediating viral clearance [3]. Interestingly, hepatitis C interferes with IFN induction to some extent, however; IFN types I and III are still produced during hepatitis C infection. It has been reported that ISGs are continuously upregulated in the hepatitis C-infected liver of chimpanzees, and ISG mRNA is simultaneously detected with hepatitis C RNA in the hepatic cells of patients infected with hepatitis c [3]. On the contrary, in cell culture models, the production of IFNλs rather than IFN-β has been demonstrated in response to hepatitis C infection. A recent study using laser-capture micro-dissection showed that IFNλs are induced only in hepatitis C-infected cells and not in neighboring uninfected cells [22]. Furthermore, plasmacytoid dendritic (pDCs; a rare type of immune cells that secrete type I IFN in response to a viral infection) cells also produce type I IFN during hepatitis C infection through TLR7-mediated recognition of hepatitis C RNA loaded in exosomes that are released from infected hepatocytes [22]. The key features of immune cell responses in acute HCV infection are demonstrated in Table **1**.

Table 1. Summary of immune responses in acute HCV infection [3]. RIG-1; retinoic acid-inducible gene I, MDA5; melanoma differentiation-associated protein 5), TLR3; Toll-like receptor 3, MAVs; Mitochondrial antiviral-signaling protein, TRIF; TIR-domain-containing adapter-inducing interferon-β, ISGs; Interferon stimulating genes, $CD4^+$ $CD25^+$ $FOXP3^+$ Treg cells; Induced regulatory T (iT_{reg}) cells. *Based on data from chimpanzee studies.

Summary of immune responses in acute HCV infections	
Immune Responses	**Acute HCV Infection**
IFN Responses (Both I and III IFNs)	
Virus-sensing receptors	RIG-I, MDA5, PKR and TLR3
Interference mechanisms	1. NS3 NS4A cleaves MAVS 2. NS3 NS4A cleaves TRIF
ISG induction in the infected liver	Increased expression of many ISGs
Antibodies	
Neutralizing antibodies	HCV easily escapes from the neutralizing activity of E1- and E2-specific antibodies
Vaccines inducing neutralizing antibodies	No approved vaccine
T cells	
Timing*	8 12 weeks after infection
Relation to the outcome of infection	Vigorous and broad (multiple epitope-specific) T-cell responses lead to spontaneous resolution of infection
$CD4^+$ $CD25^+$ $FOXP3^+$ Treg cells	Increase transiently

Adaptive Immune Responses in Hepatitis C Infection

Activation of T-helper and T-cytotoxic Immune Cells

HCV infection control and viral clearance are largely mediated by adaptive immune responses in both humans and chimpanzees where CD4+ and CD8+ cells respond and increased expression of IFN-γ expression in hepatocytes maintains the sustained viral clearance (Fig. **2**) [22]. A recent study demonstrates the critical role of memory CD4+ and CD8+ T-cells in controlling hepatitis C infection as compared to depleting those cells in experimental animals [23]. The key cells involved to mediate adaptive immune responses in HCV-infected subjects are T and B lymphocytes which express antigen-specific receptors. B cells secrete Igs to capture viral pathogens by macrophages (*i.e.* opsonization) and block viral antigenic sites critical for the life cycle of the pathogen [3]. Contrary to B cells which recognize and degrade soluble viral antigens, T lymphocytes express T cell-specific receptors to recognize the degraded form of the viral antigen associated with a molecule encoded by the major histocompatibility complex (MHC) [23]. This viral antigen-MHC complex is established, processed, and presented on the surface of APCs (*e.g.*, T-cell APCs; Dendritic cells, macrophages, and B cells). There are two distinct types of T lymphocytes based on the expression of two types of molecules that exert different functions [23]. CD4+ T-lymphocyte expresses CD4 molecules which recognize MHC class II molecules, secrete cytokines, and are commonly known as T helper cells (Th cells), whereas; CD8+ T-lymphocyte expresses CD8 molecules which recognize MHC Class I molecules, secrete cytokines with antiviral properties, kill target cells, and are known as cytotoxic T cells (CTL) or effector cells (Fig. **2**) [23].

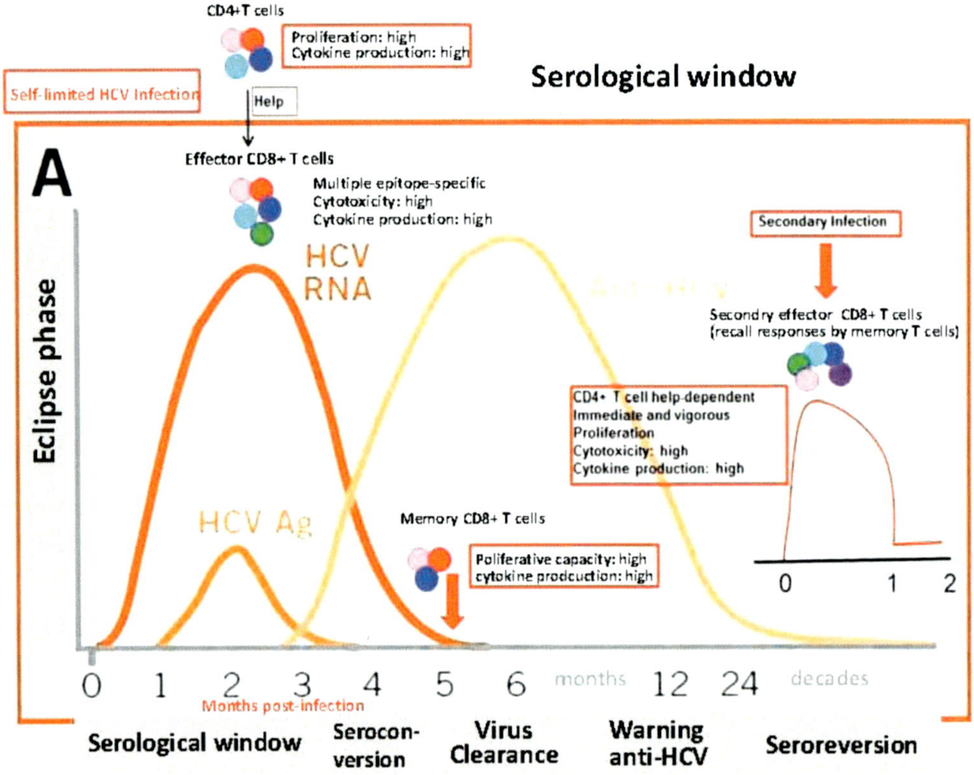

Fig. (2). T cell responses in acute self-limited hepatitis C virus (HCV) infection [35]. Acute HCV infection is associated with strong, broad, and polyfunctional $CD8^+$ T-cells. $CD4^+$ T cells are essential for help during the acute resolution of infection and the induction and maintenance of effector and memory $CD8^+$ T cells. After the natural resolution of acute HCV infection, HCV-specific memory $CD8^+$ T cells persist for decades or a lifetime and can respond immediately after secondary infection. The $CD8^+$ T cells recall their responses with the help of $CD4^+$ T cells, resulting in lower HCV viremia and more rapid HCV clearance compared with primary infection.

Immunopathology of HCV Infection and T-cell Immune Responses

To chronologically elucidate T cell immune responses during persistent HCV infection and virus clearance, the classical time course of HCV infection can be divided into three phases [3]. The first-week primary infection corresponds to an increased viral load which becomes very high during this phase irrespective of future virus clearance or persistence. CD8+ T cells specific for HCV antigens become very active with the help of CD4+ T cells (Fig. **3**). However; interestingly the responses to these cells are not detected in the blood before 1–3 months after the initial infection. The median time for the development of an IFN-γ response is 33 days. The exact reasons behind this failure to detect CD4+ and CD8+ T-cells are not fully elucidated in the initial infection. The second phase of the disease is an acute transient hepatitis C that persists for a few weeks and may progress to acute hepatitis C in infected individuals irrespective of the infection outcome. Serum ALT levels are increased indicating hepatocyte damage and are associated with detectable CD4+ and CD8+ T cell immune responses, and a drop in viral titers. These responses peak between 180–360 days after initial infection and are largely responsible for a drop in viral loads, virus clearance, and infection resolution in almost 30% of acutely HCV-infected individuals depending on the outcome of the disease. After spontaneous clearance of the virus in acute HCV-infected individuals, HCV-antigen-specific memory CD8+ T cells persist for many years and can respond immediately after secondary infection. CD8+ T cells may recall response, which depends on Th cells' help that results in normal ALT levels, lower viral load, and more rapid virus clearance compared with primary infection (Fig. **3**) [3].

Around 70% of acute HCV infections may lead to CHC infection where weak and narrow CD8+ T cell responses without CD4+ T cell help result in persistent CHC infection [3]. CD4+ T cell loss seems to be very critical for the development of persistent viral infections [24] and might be responsible for the impaired function of CD8+ T cells during CHC infection [25]. HCV genome mutations (also called resistance-associated substitutions (RAS)/or virus escape mutations)) elicit narrow specificity to CD8+ T cells recognition of virus antigen and cause CD8+ T cells exhaustion (Fig. **3**). It has been possible now to derive some CD4+ T cell lines from the blood of CHC-infected patients by repeated stimulation with recombinant proteins, confirming the presence of such T cells [25].

CD4+ T cells specific for HCV core antigen are more easily detected than those specific for HCV nonstructural proteins, which indicates that the loss of CD4+ T cells in CHC might depend on the nature of the epitope (discussed in the section, 'T cell exhaustion) [25]. As a result of virus escape mutations, CD8+ T cells of narrow specificity can easily lose their antiviral activity and prolonged exposure to virus antigens causes the functional exhaustion of CD8+ T cells, which is characterized by the upregulation of various inhibitory receptors such as PD1 (programmed cell death protein 1) [3]. Blockade of the PD1-PDL1 pathway restores the function of exhausted T cells and combinatorial blockade of the inhibitory receptors (PD1, TIM3, and/or CTLA4; please see the T-cell exhaustion for more details) further invigorates the exhausted CD8+ T cells *ex vivo* function (Fig. **3**) [26]. A recent study reported that IFN-free DAAs partially rescue the exhausted T cells, although this needs to be further confirmed by additional studies [27]. Interestingly, the key features of T lymphocyte cells in CHC infection are also observed in chronic HBV infection [27]. Some studies have shown that more CD4+ T cell lines can be derived from the liver than the blood, which indicates that HCV-specific CD4+ T cells might be sequestered in the liver [3, 26, 27]. HCV-specific T cells are enriched within the liver up to 10- to 30-fold for CD8+ T cells and 2-fold for CD4+ T cells [3].

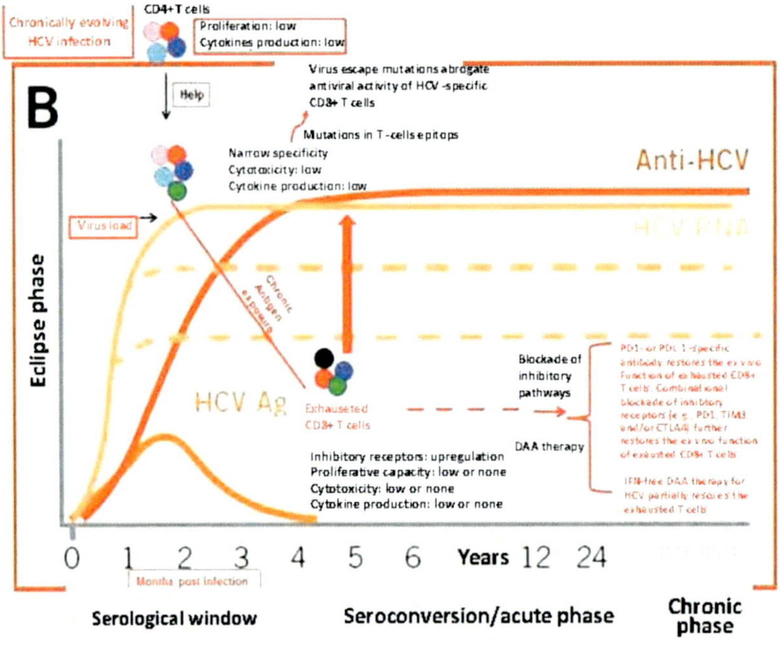

Fig. (3). T cell responses in chronic hepatitis C virus (HCV) infection [35]. The immunopathology of chronic HCV infection demonstrates weak and narrow CD8⁺ T cell immune responses without CD⁺ T cell help. CD8⁺ T cells of narrow specificity can easily lose their antiviral potential as a result of the emergence of the virus escape mutations (also known as resistance-associated substitutions; RASs). During chronic HCV infection, CD8⁺ T cells also functionally exhaust due to continuous exposure to HCV antigens characterized by the upregulation of various inhibitory receptors (*e.g.*, PD1). However, blockade of the PD1-PDL1 pathway may restore the function of exhausted T cells, and the combinatorial blockade of inhibitory receptors further reinvigorates the exhausted CD8⁺ T cells. A recent study points out that direct-acting antivirals (DAAs) partially rescue the functionality of exhausted CD8⁺ T cells; albeit, it requires further studies to be confirmed. CTLA4; cytotoxic T lymphocytes antigen 4, IFN; interferon, PD1; Programmed cell death protein 1.

THE ROLE OF VIRAL PROTEINS IN HCV IMMUNOPATHOLOGY

HCV directly affects the recognition of MHC/peptide complexes by cytotoxic T lymphocytes (CTL; *i.e.* CD8+ T cells), thus preventing the killing of infected cells and favoring viral persistence very early after viral infection (Table **1**) [3]. Albeit the development of *in vitro* HCV replication systems 20 years ago, functional evidence for this mechanism is lacking. However, while using subgenomic replicons expressing all hepatitis C structural proteins, the investigators have demonstrated that HCV structural protein expression affects the glycosylation and cell surface expression of MHC class I molecules [28]. Similarly, some researchers by using transfected cell lines have shown that HCV core protein (nucleocapsid) interact with TNF-related molecules involved in CTL activity, such as Lymphotoxin-β receptor (LT-βR) or Tumor necrosis factor receptor I (TNF-R1) and modulate NFκB activity mediated by TNF-α and LT-α1 β2 (Table **1**) [29]. However, as mentioned earlier, the relevance of these findings cannot be established to natural HCV infection and remains to investigate. It is also possible that HCV structural and non-structural proteins might be used in different alternative mechanisms to protect the infected cells from being recognized and killed, thus favoring the establishment of the viral infection in the host [3]. One plausible example is the core protein that has been shown to bind to the complement receptor gC1qR expressed by T cells and inhibits their proliferation by inducing the expression of suppressors of cytokine signaling (SOCS) molecules [29]. Similarly, it has been unveiled that antigen-presenting cells (APC; *e.g.* dendritic cells (DCs)) isolated from CHC patients are impaired in their ability to present antigen and secrete IL-12, suggesting that the virus targets the antigen presentation ability of DCs [3]. However, the question still arises that how non-HCV-specific T cells would be protected against the inhibitory effect of free core antigen particles circulating within the bloodstream of HCV-infected individuals. The experimental evidence is still inconclusive and murky and requires further research work to prove it.

T-cell Exhaustion

T- cell exhaustion is the primary explanation for T-cell dysfunction in CHC infection and has been extensively studied. HCV-specific T cells might be present in the hepatocytes, however; the virus may escape from the T cells' responses through mutations [30]. If T cell epitopes are present without mutations, T cells become exhausted and functionally impaired during CHC infection because of the sustained antigenic stimulation (*i.e.* HCV core antigen) [30]. Prolonged exposure to HCV antigens is the main reason for T cell exhaustion during which the inhibitory receptors on T cells are upregulated [31]. These receptors include PD1 (programmed cell death protein 1), CTLA4 (cytotoxic T lymphocyte antigen 4),

TIM3, KLRG1 (Killer cell lectin-like receptor G1), CD160, 2B4 (also known as CD244), and elevated expression of CD39 [31]. However, intrahepatic CD8+ T cells in CHC patients have been characterized by the co-expression of multiple inhibitory receptors. The *in-vitro* blockade of the PD1-PDL1 pathway has been shown to rescue T cell exhaustion in CHC-infected patients and restore the effector functions of CD8+ T cells [32]. However, its alone blockade is not sufficient to reinvigorate exhausted HCV-specific CD8+ T cells and to fully restore T cell functions in CHC-infected patients and seems to be required the combinatorial blockade of other inhibitory receptors (*i.e.* CTLA4, TIM3, and/or 2B4) [31]. In contrast, a limited therapeutic effect of PD1-specific antibody administration by the blockade of the PD1-PDL1 pathway alone has been demonstrated in CHC-infected patients and chimpanzees [3].

T cell functions are also suppressed by an increased number of CD4+CD25+FOXP3+ T_{reg} cells in CHC-infected persons [33]. It has been demonstrated that the number of these cells tends to increase in the blood and liver during CHC infection and their frequency is positively correlated with virus load. It means that T_{reg} cells contribute to virus persistence by suppressing HCV-specific effector T cells. The suppression of effector T cell functions by T_{reg} cells occurs through a direct cell-to-cell contact mechanism during CHC infection and is independent of the secretion of IL-10 and TGF-β [33]. In contrast, intrahepatic T_{reg} cells express increased levels of PD1 in patients with CHC infection. The proliferation and suppressive functions of these T_{reg} cells are inhibited by PDL1 through the attenuation of STAT5 phosphorylation [26].

SOME PRETTY MIND-BOGGLING ASPECTS OF HCV IMMUNOLOGY

The inability of immune responses (either innate or adaptive) to mediate virus clearance in the majority of hepatitis C-infected individuals thus enabling viral persistence and ensuing chronic necroinflammatory liver diseases (*e.g.*, fibrosis, cirrhosis, hepatocellular carcinoma) has raised some fundamental, outstanding, and mind-boggling questions about the current knowledge of immune responses against HCV that could be summarized as mentioned below:

1- Why does hepatitis C infection persists in the majority of infected individuals despite a detectable immune response in many, while some patients control viral load and resolve the infection?

2- No general immunosuppression is associated with HCV, Why?

3- Lack of any proposed model to explain why HCV infection with the same hepatitis C strain can lead to two different outcomes.

4- Why T cells isolated from the blood of HCV-infected patients are not representative of intrahepatic lymphocytes?

5- Why the immune system is under the continuous attack of virus antigens in HCV-infected patients?

Although the recent advancements *in vitro* HCV replication models help to understand the answers to some of these perplexing aspects of HCV immune responses, the relevance of these findings cannot be implied to *in vivo* HCV infections and remains unclear as these mechanisms do not explain fully the *in vivo* aspects of HCV immunology [3]. Subsequently, these are the hot-spot issues in HCV immunology and vaccinology research and should be comprehensively answered along with the progress in the development of a prophylactic or protective HCV vaccine.

PROPHYLACTIC HCV VACCINES

Some prophylactic HCV vaccine candidates are in different phases of their clinical trials to elicit HCV-specific memory T cells and/or broadly neutralizing antibodies (Discussed in detail in chapter 10) [34]. Neutralizing antibodies can only protect hosts from the infection itself. However, HCV-specific memory T cells may prevent the progression of acute hepatitis C to chronic persistent infection [3]. The crucial and productive role of T cell responses in protective immunity to HCV infection and reinfection has been evident from studies in infected patients and virus-inoculated chimpanzees [3]. Virus-specific memory T cells protect HCV-rechallenged chimpanzees and naturally reinfected patients, as shown by low viral load and a shorter duration of viremia. It also provides a rationale for the development of T cell-based vaccines. Viral vectors including adenovirus, modified vaccinia virus Ankara (MVA), vaccinia virus and others, virus-like particles, recombinant DNA plasmids, and yeast vectors that express HCV proteins have been shown to induce HCV-specific T cell responses that mediate protective immunity in chimpanzees [34]. The early proliferation of polyfunctional CD8+ T cells upon HCV infection and high levels of expression of the memory precursor marker CD127 is considered the key immunological factors for successful vaccine-induced protective immunity [34]. A simian adenoviral vector expressing HCV non-structural proteins primed HCV-specific CD4+ and CD8+ T cells, and a boost immunization with MVA expressing the same HCV proteins elicited sustained memory and effector T cell responses with enhanced functionality and proliferative capacity in a phase I trial in healthy human volunteers [34]. This vaccine candidate is currently proceeding to a phase II trial.

Most studies support the evidence that broadly neutralizing antibodies has also roles in the control of HCV infection [3, 34]. Furthermore, neutralizing antibodies have been shown to protect against a heterologous HCV challenge or abolished established HCV infection in a chimeric mouse model. In addition to that, cross-reactive neutralizing antibodies are also assumed to be associated with protection against chronic HCV infection in the setting of reinfection of injection drug users (IDUs) [13]. A recombinant E1-E2 vaccine successfully induced broadly neutralizing antibodies in chimpanzees challenged with homologous or heterologous HCV strains providing the base for an antibody-based prophylactic vaccine [34]. Similarly, the generation of cross-genotype neutralizing antibodies was also reported in healthy volunteers in clinical trials using recombinant E1-E2 proteins plus adjuvant [34, 35].

CONCLUSIONS

Despite significant achievements in HCV diagnostic and treatment algorithms in the last two decades, some fundamental aspects of HCV immunopathology and immune system responses upon persistent infection are still answerable. In parallel to that, HCV immunology research was not modulated toward the cellular aspects of the immune system responses against hepatitis C infection and most conclusions were drawn based on the findings of the immune system interplay with the virus in circulatory blood. Consequently, a dream for the development of an effective prophylactic or protective HCV vaccine is still far away. Even the vaccine models in the pipeline or preclinical stage are not given the preference to be evaluated in phase III clinical trials. Furthermore, variable immune responses with different outcomes even with the homologous viral strains infection during *in vitro* and *in vivo* studies also raise the concern to design an appropriate effective vaccine against hepatitis C. No doubt adaptive immune responses are much crucial to tackle persistent HCV infection in the infected hosts and well studied for HCV immunopathology; however, a complete understanding of innate immune responses are also integral to curb the infection at the acute stage and for the development of prophylactic HCV vaccines. T-cell exhaustion may drive persistent HCV infection for a long time and further progression to severe hepatic diseases. Hence, thorough mechanistic studies to reinstate T-cell functions could be helpful to reinvigorate host cell immune responses to clear the virus and would be helpful to design adjuvant therapies that can synergize DAAs attaining SVR rates in treated patients. Overall, HCV immunopathology and immune response studies/research should be integrated just like HCV diagnostics and therapeutics in the last decade to design and develop the first effective vaccine to eliminate HCV by 2030 as an ambitious goal of the World Health Organization (WHO).

REFERENCES

[1] Shahid I, AlMalki WH, AlRabia MW, *et al. In vitro* inhibitory analysis of consensus siRNAs against NS3 gene of hepatitis C virus 1a genotype. Asian Pac J Trop Med 2017; 10(7): 701-9. [http://dx.doi.org/10.1016/j.apjtm.2017.07.011] [PMID: 28870347]

[2] Shahid I, AlMalki WH, Hassan S, Hafeez MH. Real-world challenges for hepatitis C virus medications: a critical overview. Crit Rev Microbiol 2018; 44(2): 143-60.

[http://dx.doi.org/10.1080/1040841X.2017.1329277] [PMID: 28539069]

[3] Shin EC, Sung PS, Park SH. Immune responses and immunopathology in acute and chronic viral hepatitis. Nat Rev Immunol 2016; 16(8): 509-23. [http://dx.doi.org/10.1038/nri.2016.69] [PMID: 27374637]

[4] Ahmad W, Ijaz B, Javed FT, *et al.* HCV genotype distribution and possible transmission risks in Lahore, Pakistan. World J Gastroenterol 2010; 16(34): 4321-8. [http://dx.doi.org/10.3748/wjg.v16.i34.4321] [PMID: 20818816]

[5] Ahmad W, Ijaz B, Javed FT, *et al.* A comparison of four fibrosis indexes in chronic HCV: Development of new fibrosis-cirrhosis index (FCI). BMC Gastroenterol 2011; 11(1): 44. [http://dx.doi.org/10.1186/1471-230X-11-44] [PMID: 21507271]

[6] Ahmad W, Ijaz B, Javed FT, *et al.* HCV genotype-specific correlation with serum markers: Higher predictability for genotype 4a. Virol J 2011; 8(1): 293. [http://dx.doi.org/10.1186/1743-422X-8-293] [PMID: 21663629]

[7] Hiet MS, Bauhofer O, Zayas M, *et al.* Control of temporal activation of hepatitis C virus-induced interferon response by domain 2 of nonstructural protein 5A. J Hepatol 2015; 63(4): 829-37. [http://dx.doi.org/10.1016/j.jhep.2015.04.015] [PMID: 25908268]

[8] Arnaud N, Dabo S, Akazawa D, *et al.* Hepatitis C virus reveals a novel early control in acute immune response. PLoS Pathog 2011; 7(10): e1002289. [http://dx.doi.org/10.1371/journal.ppat.1002289] [PMID: 22022264]

[9] Dustin LB, Rice CM. Flying under the radar: the immunobiology of hepatitis C. Annu Rev Immunol 2007; 25(1): 71-99. [http://dx.doi.org/10.1146/annurev.immunol.25.022106.141602] [PMID: 17067278]

[10] Werner JM, Heller T, Gordon AM, *et al.* Innate immune responses in hepatitis C virus-exposed healthcare workers who do not develop acute infection. Hepatology 2013; 58(5): 1621-31. [http://dx.doi.org/10.1002/hep.26353] [PMID: 23463364]

[11] Timpe JM, Stamataki Z, Jennings A, *et al.* Hepatitis C virus cell-cell transmission in hepatoma cells in the presence of neutralizing antibodies. Hepatology 2008; 47(1): 17-24. [http://dx.doi.org/10.1002/hep.21959] [PMID: 17941058]

[12] Logvinoff C, Major ME, Oldach D, *et al.* Neutralizing antibody response during acute and chronic hepatitis C virus infection. Proc Natl Acad Sci USA 2004; 101(27): 10149-54. [http://dx.doi.org/10.1073/pnas.0403519101] [PMID: 15220475]

[13] Cashman SB, Marsden BD, Dustin LB. The Humoral Immune Response to HCV: Understanding is Key to Vaccine Development. Front Immunol 2014; 5: 550. [http://dx.doi.org/10.3389/fimmu.2014.00550] [PMID: 25426115]

[14] Esteban-Riesco L, Depaulis F, Moreau A, *et al.* Rapid and sustained autologous neutralizing response leading to early spontaneous recovery after HCV infection. Virology 2013; 444(1-2): 90-9. [http://dx.doi.org/10.1016/j.virol.2013.05.037] [PMID: 23890816]

[15] Osburn WO, Snider AE, Wells BL, *et al.* Clearance of hepatitis C infection is associated with the early appearance of broad neutralizing antibody responses. Hepatology 2014; 59(6): 2140-51. [http://dx.doi.org/10.1002/hep.27013] [PMID: 24425349]

[16] Raghuraman S, Park H, Osburn WO, Winkelstein E, Edlin BR, Rehermann B. Spontaneous clearance of chronic hepatitis C virus infection is associated with appearance of neutralizing antibodies and reversal of T-cell exhaustion. J Infect Dis 2012; 205(5): 763-71. [http://dx.doi.org/10.1093/infdis/jir835] [PMID: 22293431]

[17] Sung PS, Cheon H, Cho CH, *et al.* Roles of unphosphorylated ISGF3 in HCV infection and interferon responsiveness. Proc Natl Acad Sci USA 2015; 112(33): 10443-8. [http://dx.doi.org/10.1073/pnas.1513341112] [PMID: 26216956]

[18] Cheon H, Holvey-Bates EG, Schoggins JW, *et al.* IFNβ-dependent increases in STAT1, STAT2, and IRF9 mediate resistance to viruses and DNA damage. EMBO J 2013; 32(20): 2751-63. [http://dx.doi.org/10.1038/emboj.2013.203] [PMID: 24065129]

[19] Randall G, Chen L, Panis M, *et al.* Silencing of USP18 potentiates the antiviral activity of interferon against hepatitis C virus infection. Gastroenterology 2006; 131(5): 1584-91. [http://dx.doi.org/10.1053/j.gastro.2006.08.043] [PMID: 17101330]

[20] Bender S, Reuter A, Eberle F, Einhorn E, Binder M, Bartenschlager R. Activation of Type I and III Interferon Response by Mitochondrial and Peroxisomal MAVS and Inhibition by Hepatitis C Virus. PLoS Pathog 2015; 11(11): e1005264. [http://dx.doi.org/10.1371/journal.ppat.1005264] [PMID: 26588843]

[21] Li K, Foy E, Ferreon JC, *et al.* Immune evasion by hepatitis C virus NS3/4A protease-mediated cleavage of the Toll-like receptor 3 adaptor protein TRIF. Proc Natl Acad Sci USA 2005; 102(8): 2992-7. [http://dx.doi.org/10.1073/pnas.0408824102] [PMID: 15710891]

[22] Wang Y, Li J, Wang X, Ye L, Zhou Y, Ho W. Induction of interferon-λ contributes to Toll-like receptor-3-activated hepatic stellate cell-mediated hepatitis C virus inhibition in hepatocytes. J Viral Hepat 2013; 20(6): 385-94. [http://dx.doi.org/10.1111/jvh.12040] [PMID: 23647955]

[23] Semmo N, Day CL, Ward SM, *et al.* Preferential loss of IL-2-secreting CD4+ T helper cells in chronic HCV infection. Hepatology 2005; 41(5): 1019-28. [http://dx.doi.org/10.1002/hep.20669] [PMID: 15841456]

[24] Zhou Y, Callendret B, Xu D, *et al.* Dominance of the CD4+ T helper cell response during acute resolving hepatitis A virus infection. J Exp Med 2012; 209(8): 1481-92. [http://dx.doi.org/10.1084/jem.20111906] [PMID: 22753925]

[25] Zhao J, Zhang Z, Luan Y, *et al.* Pathological functions of interleukin-22 in chronic liver inflammation and fibrosis with hepatitis B virus infection by promoting T helper 17 cell recruitment. Hepatology 2014; 59(4): 1331-42. [http://dx.doi.org/10.1002/hep.26916] [PMID: 24677193]

[26] Franceschini D, Paroli M, Francavilla V, *et al.* PD-L1 negatively regulates CD4+CD25+Foxp3+ Tregs by limiting STAT-5 phosphorylation in patients chronically infected with HCV. J Clin Invest 2009; 119(3): 551-64. [http://dx.doi.org/10.1172/JCI36604] [PMID: 19229109]

[27] Martin B, Hennecke N, Lohmann V, *et al.* Restoration of HCV-specific CD8+ T cell function by interferon-free therapy. J Hepatol 2014; 61(3): 538-43. [http://dx.doi.org/10.1016/j.jhep.2014.05.043] [PMID: 24905492]

[28] Sevvana M, Keck Z, Foung SKH, Kuhn RJ. Structural perspectives on HCV humoral immune evasion mechanisms. Curr Opin Virol 2021; 49: 92-101. [http://dx.doi.org/10.1016/j.coviro.2021.05.002] [PMID: 34091143]

[29] Hajikhezri Z, Roohvand F, Maleki M, *et al.* HCV Core/NS3 Protein Immunization with "N-Terminal Heat Shock gp96 Protein (rNT (gp96))" Induced Strong and Sustained Th1-Type Cytokines in Immunized Mice. Vaccines (Basel) 2021; 9(3): 215. [http://dx.doi.org/10.3390/vaccines9030215] [PMID: 33802466]

[30] Lee J, Suh WI, Shin EC. T-cell dysfunction and inhibitory receptors in hepatitis C virus infection. Immune Netw 2010; 10(4): 120-5. [http://dx.doi.org/10.4110/in.2010.10.4.120] [PMID: 20844736]

[31] Nakamoto N, Cho H, Shaked A, *et al.* Synergistic reversal of intrahepatic HCV-specific CD8 T cell exhaustion by combined PD-1/CTLA-4 blockade. PLoS Pathog 2009; 5(2): e1000313. [http://dx.doi.org/10.1371/journal.ppat.1000313] [PMID: 19247441]

[32] Golden-Mason L, Palmer B, Klarquist J, Mengshol JA, Castelblanco N, Rosen HR. Upregulation of PD-1 expression on circulating and intrahepatic hepatitis C virus-specific CD8+ T cells associated with reversible immune dysfunction. J Virol 2007; 81(17): 9249-58. [http://dx.doi.org/10.1128/JVI.00409-07] [PMID: 17567698]

[33] Cabrera R, Tu Z, Xu Y, *et al.* An immunomodulatory role for CD4+CD25+ regulatory T lymphocytes in hepatitis C virus infection. Hepatology 2004; 40(5): 1062-71. [http://dx.doi.org/10.1002/hep.20454] [PMID: 15486925]

[34] Hartlage AS, Kapoor A, Hepatitis C. Hepatitis C Virus Vaccine Research: Time to Put Up or Shut Up. Viruses 2021; 13(8): 1596. [http://dx.doi.org/10.3390/v13081596] [PMID: 34452460]

[35] WHO guidelines on hepatitis B and C testing. Geneva: World Health Organization. 2017. Available from: https://www.who.int (Accessed on: 3rd December 2021).

CHAPTER 4

Consensus-based Approaches for Hepatitis C Screening and Diagnosis in General and Vulnerable Populations

Abstract: Hepatitis C screening and diagnosis are both pre-requisite to predicting infection endemicity, transmission risks and identifying vulnerable hepatitis C infected populations in highly endemic areas of the infection prevalence. It is also pivotal to select optimal treatment choices and their impact, including cost and access to care, especially in resource-constrained areas in an era of all oral interferon-free direct-acting antivirals. Furthermore, hepatitis C screening is also very crucial to "find the missing millions" to achieve the hepatitis C elimination goal by 2030. It seems only possible by implementing new screening and diagnostic approaches like RNA point-of-care (RNA-POC) testing, rapid diagnostic tests (RDTs), and dried blood spot (DBS) sample testing, especially in remote communities having poor health infrastructure and where phlebotomies are a major concern for samples collection from patients who inject drugs (PWIDs). In addition to that, it is also very much required to bring HCV diagnostic facilities to decentralized healthcare centers which provide care for people at high risk or opportunistic infection of hepatitis C transmission by sexual contacts (*e.g.*, men who have sex with men (MSM), sex workers, current or former IDUs, people who are incarcerated, and people in drug harm reduction centers). In this book chapter, we will discuss consensus-based recommendations and approaches for hepatitis C screening and diagnosis in general and vulnerable populations with their potential significance for the identification and diagnosis of high-risk individuals of hepatitis C transmission. We will also emphasize the importance of initial HCV screening before the start of HCV treatment.

Keywords: Baby Boomers, Centralized HCV Testing, Disease Assessment, Decentralized HCV Testing, Dried Blood Spot, ELISA, Fibroscan, HCV Core Antigen Detection, Hepatitis C Virus, Hepatitis C Screening, High-risk Individuals, MSM, Nanoparticle-based Diagnostics, Patients who Inject Drugs, Point of Care Testing, Qualitative RNA, Quantitative RNA, Rapid Diagnostic Tests,task-shifting, Vulnerable Populations.

INTRODUCTION

Since the hepatitis C virus discovery in 1989, remarkable progress has been made in hepatitis C diagnosis from the traditional methods of anti-HCV antibodies det-

Imran Shahid and Qaiser Jabeen

ection (anti-HCV Abs) in plasma samples by enzyme-linked immunosorbent assay (ELISA) to the emerging state-of-the-art diagnostic tests including RNA-POCT and novel diagnostic strategies like rapid RDTs and DBS sampling used in both clinical and community settings [1]. Furthermore, qualitative and quantitative RNA viral load assessment before therapy, during therapy, and post-treatment completion by some sophisticated polymerase chain reaction (PCR) machines and real-time PCR analysis are also valuable, reliable, and authentic predictors of DAA choice for treatment initiation, to select dosage algorithms, and treatment outcomes in infected individuals [1]. These state-of-the-art screening methods and diagnostic procedures are also helpful to identify the recurrence of viral breakthroughs, reinfections, and viral relapse in treatment-failure patients [2]. In addition to that, hepatitis C RNA sequencing by traditional methods like Sanger sequencing, as well as innovative current ones by next-generation sequencing (NGS), are also very pragmatic to detect the emergence of resistance-associated substitutions (RAS) in treated patients or treatment failure patients with IFN plus ribavirin (RBV), and treatment-experienced patients without any virologic responses or virologic failure with IFN-free DAAs [1]. Besides that, hepatitis C screening and diagnosis are very useful to find many hepatitis C-infected anonymous individuals in hard-hit communities as well as in vulnerable populations who do not know their infection status and cannot afford high-cost screening in governmental and private clinical settings [1]. In this chapter, we overview the current status of hepatitis C screening and diagnostic algorithms in general and vulnerable infected populations, why we need large-scale hepatitis C screening in highly endemic areas, recommendations, and strategies to screen everyone for hepatitis C to prevent further transmission, and to decide treatment choices for those who need on prioritizing basis.

GRADING OF EVIDENCE AND RECOMMENDATION

International health organizations, policy-making committees, and research organizations provide evidence-based clinical recommendations for the physicians, clinicians, health care providers (HCPs), infectious disease experts, and primary care providers (PCPs) who refer to screening, diagnosis, and treat patients with acute and CHC infection (Table **1**). These recommendations are entirely based on comprehensive medical literature reviews and demonstrate consensus among panels of HCV experts. Each recommendation is weighed out for the strength and quality of the evidence (Table **1**) [3]. However; for the recommendations based on an expert opinion, the rationale for the opinion is included.

Table 1. Grading of evidence and recommendations for HCV screening and diagnostics [4].

Strength of Recommendation	Quality of Supporting Evidence
A = Strong	1 = ≥ 1 randomized trial with clinical outcomes and/or validated laboratory endpoints.
B = Moderate	2 = < 1 or more well-designed, nonrandomized trial or observational cohort studies with long-term clinical outcomes.
C = Optional	3 = Expert opinion

RECOMMENDATIONS BEFORE SCREENING AND DIAGNOSIS OF HEPATITIS C VIRUS

The core principles prior to screening and diagnosing an HCV-infected individual are based on who to test, where to test, and how to test. By in large, worldwide, HCV screening and diagnosis are provided in centralized lab settings, decentralized testing premises, POCT, and integrated testing approaches/ facilitation (Fig. **1**) [5].

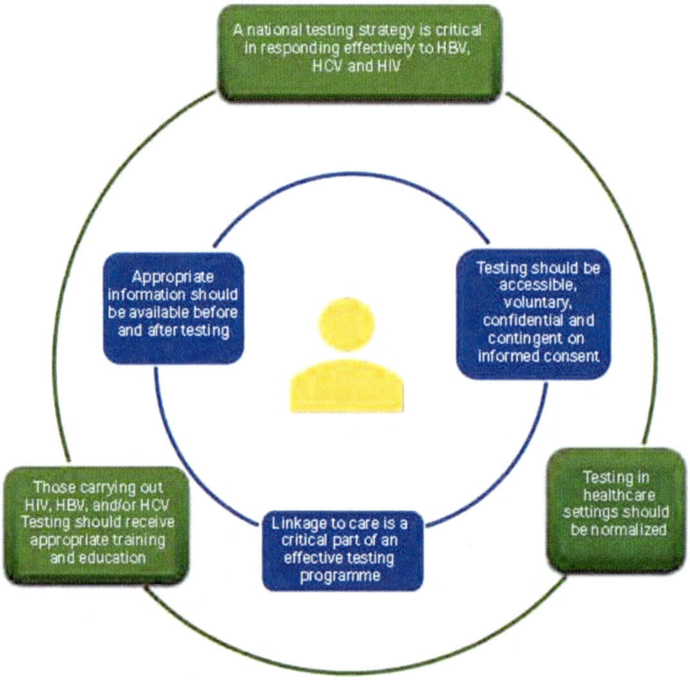

Fig. (1). Key components of integrated testing of HBV, HCV, and HIV [5].

The bottom line message from all these hepatitis C screening and diagnostic models must be a single sentence, "test and treat everyone who is in need" (Fig. **3**). However, universal hepatitis C screening/diagnosis and treatment seems an ambitious and uphill task that demands excessive resources in terms of finance, research and development, healthcare infrastructure, manpower, and testing/diagnostic supplies [1]. Because of this, international health organizations, policy-making committees, and research organizations add recommendation guidelines to support universal screening for HCV in vulnerable populations as well as in individuals who need it the most (Fig. **1**) [1]. Herein we briefly overview the guidelines which are followed by the physicians, clinicians, HCPs, and infectious disease experts prior to recommending someone for HCV screening, infection diagnosis, and, ultimately linkage to care (Fig. **2**). Being not exhaustive and considering page limit constraints, only key points are considered with a plausible explanation.

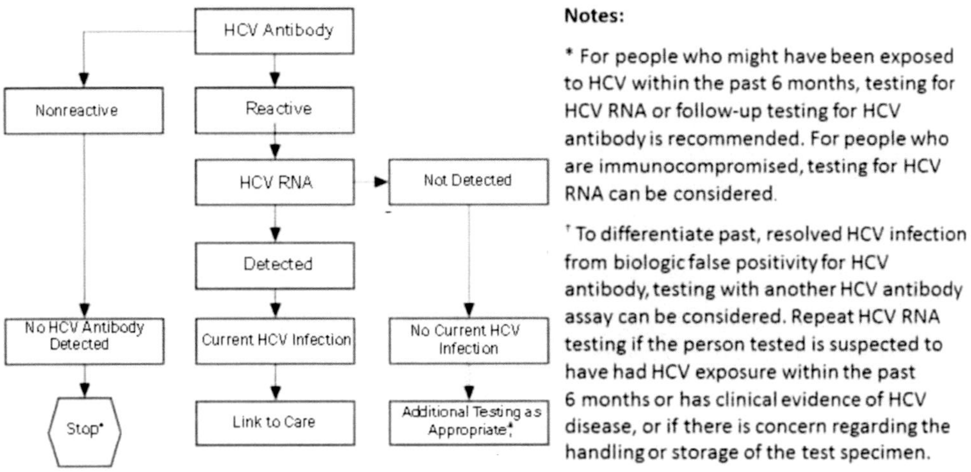

Fig. (2). An overlay summary of HCV diagnostic algorithms and link to care [6].

Key Points

1. According to WHO, 50% of hepatitis C-affected individuals are not aware of their current HCV infection status.
2. 75% of the cases belong to baby boomers (*i.e.*, born between 1945 to 1965) with no infection symptoms (asymptomatic) and no recognized risk factors.
3. HCV screening in specific birth cohorts may increase treatment for baby boomers.
4. Universal HCV screening for pregnant or who are planning to get pregnant will be helpful to prevent vertical transmission of HCV infection.
5. HCPs should perform risk-based screening for HCV infection to evaluate other risk factors for infection transmission.

6. Cohort studies, as well as risk-based HCV screening, both are vital to identifying adults with hepatitis C infection.
7. HCV screening should be performed on all individuals in highly prevalent HCV endemic areas where communities might have been exposed to hepatitis C through any mode of transmission.
8. HCPs should refer chronic HCV-infected individuals, as well as patients with decompensated liver disease, and who are pre-or post-transplant to a liver disease specialist [3, 7].

WHO TO TEST FOR CHRONIC HCV INFECTION

Testing approach And population	Recommendations*
Focused testing in most affected populations	1. In all settings (and regardless of whether delivered through facility- or community-based testing), it is recommended that serological testing for HCV antibody (anti-HCV)[1] be offered with linkage to prevention, care and treatment services to the following individuals: • **Adults and adolescents from populations most affected by HCV infection**[2] (i.e. who are either part of a population with high HCV seroprevalence or who have a history of exposure and/or high-risk behaviours for HCV infection); • **Adults, adolescents and children with a clinical suspicion of chronic viral hepatitis**[3] (i.e. symptoms, signs, laboratory markers). *Strong recommendation, low quality of evidence* *Note: Periodic re-testing using HCV NAT should be considered for those with ongoing risk of acquisition or reinfection.*
General population testing	2. In settings with a ≥2% or ≥5%[4] HCV antibody seroprevalence in the general population, it is recommended that all adults have access to and be offered HCV serological testing with linkage to prevention, care and treatment services. General population testing approaches should make use of existing community- or facility-based testing opportunities or programmes such as HIV or TB clinics, drug treatment services and antenatal clinics[5]. *Conditional recommendation, low quality of evidence*
Birth cohort testing	3. This approach may be applied to specific identified birth cohorts of older persons at higher risk of infection[6] and morbidity within populations that have an overall lower general prevalence. *Conditional recommendation, low quality of evidence*

Abbreviations: NAT: nucleic acid test; anti-HCV: HCV antibody; PWID: people who inject drugs; MSM: men who have sex with men
*The GRADE system (Grading of Recommendations, Assessment, Development and Evaluation) was used to categorize the strength of recommendations as strong or conditional (based on consideration of the quality of evidence, balance of benefits and harms, acceptability, resource use and programmatic feasibility) and the quality of evidence as high, moderate, low or very low.

[1] This may include fourth-generation combined antibody/antigen assays
[2] Includes those who are either part of a population with higher seroprevalence (e.g. some mobile/migrant populations from high/intermediate endemic countries, and certain indigenous populations) or who have a history of exposure or high-risk behaviours for HCV infection (e.g. PWID, people in prisons and other closed settings, MSM and sex workers, and HIV-infected persons, children of mothers with chronic HCV infection especially if HIV-coinfected).
[3] Features that may indicate underlying chronic HCV infection include clinical evidence of existing liver disease, such as cirrhosis or hepatocellular carcinoma (HCC), or where there is unexplained liver disease, including abnormal liver function tests or liver ultrasound.
[4] A threshold of ≥2% or ≥5% seroprevalence was based on several published thresholds of intermediate and high seroprevalence. The threshold used will depend on other country considerations and epidemiological context.
[5] Routine testing of pregnant women for HCV infection is currently not recommended.
[6] Because of historical exposure to unscreened or inadequately screened blood products and/or poor injection safety.

Fig. (3). WHO recommendations for HCV screening and diagnosis [3].

Cohort-Based Screening

Recommendations [4]:
• "HCV-Abs screening be offered to every individual born between 1945 and 1965 (*i.e.*, baby boomers) who receives healthcare services from a physician, physician assistant, or nurse practitioner in a primary care or inpatient hospital setting." • Hepatitis C screening is required unless the HCP believes that: 1) the individual is being treated for a life-threatening emergency; 2) the individual has previously been offered or has received a hepatitis screening test; or 3) the individual lacks the capacity to consent to a hepatitis C screening test.

Risk-Based Screening

Recommendations [4]:
• "Clinicians should perform hepatitis C screening *at least once* for all patients aged 18 years and older who are not known to have hepatitis C infection." (A2) • "Clinicians should repeat hepatitis C screening in all patients who are planning to get pregnant (A2) or are currently pregnant (B3), and screening should be repeated with each pregnancy." (B3) • Clinicians should perform hepatitis C screening *at least once* for patients of any age who are not known to have hepatitis C infection and currently have, or have a history that includes, any of the following hepatitis C transmission risk factors: 1. Injection drug use (IDU) (A1), 2. Intranasal drug use (A2), 3. Sex partner(s) with hepatitis C infection (A2), 4. Incarceration (A2), 5. Long-term hemodialysis (A1), 6. A mother with a positive HCV-Abs test result (A1), 7. HIV infection (A2), 8. Receipt of blood transfusion or organs before 1992, or of clotting factor concentrates from human plasma before 1987 (A1), 9. Tattoo, piercing, or acupuncture in a nonsterile environment (A2), 10. Unexplained hepatic disease or abnormal liver transaminase levels (A1). • "Clinicians should offer repeat hepatitis C screening based on individual exposure to the following risk factors, at least once if risk exposure is episodic and annually if it is ongoing. 1. Injection (A1) or intranasal (A2) drug use. 2. Hemodialysis. (A1), 3. HIV diagnosis. (A1), 4. Sex partner(s) with hepatitis C infection, (A2) 4. Tattoo, piercing, or acupuncture obtained in a non-sterile environment. (A2), 5. Incarceration. (A2), 6. Unexplained hepatic disease or abnormal hepatic transaminase levels." (A1)

Pregnancy and Hepatitis C Screening

Recommendations [4]:
• Clinicians should perform hepatitis C screening on all patients who are pregnant or planning to get pregnant. (B3) • Clinicians should advise pregnant patients with hepatitis C infection to reschedule treatment with DAAs until they are no longer pregnant or breastfeeding. (A2) • If an individual with hepatitis C virus infection becomes pregnant during DAA treatment, clinicians should (A3): 1. "Advise that the use of DAAs is not currently recommended during pregnancy because no data are currently available on the effects of medications on the fetus." 2. "Discuss the risks and benefits of continuing DAAs treatment. " • "Clinicians should refer pregnant patients who are diagnosed with hepatitis C infection (HCV-Abs positive and HCV RNA detectable), or who are known to have hepatitis C infection and become pregnant before or during DAA treatment, to a specialist experienced in counseling about hepatitis C infection in pregnancy.

(A3) Specialists may include but are not limited to, hepatologists, gastroenterologists, ID specialists, or high-risk OBs."
• "If a pregnant patient with hepatitis C infection has a substance use disorder, the clinician should provide its treatment, including harm reduction services, or refer the patient for these services." (A3)
• "It is imperative to recognize and acknowledge the influence of stigma toward pregnant individuals with hepatitis C infection."
• "The possible effects of stigma cannot be underestimated."
• "One cannot assume that hepatitis C infection is associated with current or past IDUs. Such assumptions can result in personal, family, and legal consequences for the patient, particularly among pregnant patients."

Post-partum Patient and Hepatitis C Screening

Recommendations [4]:
• "Clinicians should advise pregnant and postpartum individuals with hepatitis C mono-infection that breastfeeding is considered safe, and hepatitis C is not transmitted through breastmilk." (B3)
• "Clinicians should advise patients that if they have or develop cracked or bleeding nipples, breastfeeding should be discontinued and milk should be expressed and discarded until the bleeding has resolved." (B3)
• "Clinicians should refer infants born to individuals with hepatitis C to clinicians with experience in hepatitis C care for further counseling and testing and notify the clinician of the mother's hepatitis C status." (A3)

Annual HCV Screening

Recommendations [4]:
• "Clinicians should offer hepatitis C screening *at least annually* to individuals who are not known to have hepatitis C infection and;"
1. Use injection drugs (A2), 2. Use intranasal drugs (A2), 3. Receive current long-term hemodialysis (A2).
• "Clinicians should offer repeat hepatitis C screening *at least annually* to MSM and to others who are not known to have HCV infection and:"
1. "Engage in receptive anal sex and other behaviors that may tear mucous membranes." (A2), 2. Have multiple sex partners. (A2), 3. Are taking pre-exposure prophylaxis (PrEP) to prevent HIV acquisition? (A3), 4. Are transgender women? (B3), 5. Engage in sex while using recreational mind-altering drugs, *e.g.*, methamphetamine (A2), 6. Have been diagnosed with another sexually transmitted infection (STI) within the previous 12 months. (A2)

Screening for Occupational or Other HCV Exposure

Recommendations [4]:
• "Clinicians should perform repeat HCV screening for individuals who are not known to have hepatitis C infection and have a possible exposure in a healthcare setting (Figs. **4** and **5**), including those who:"
1. "Have a break in the skin caused by a sharp object that is contaminated with blood, visibly bloody fluid, or other potentially infectious material or that has been in the source patient's blood vessel." (A2)
2. "Have been bitten by an individual with visible bleeding in the mouth that causes bleeding in the exposed worker." (A2)
3. "Have been splashed on a mucosal surface with blood, visibly bloody fluid, or other potentially infectious material." (A2)
4. "Have non-intact skin (*e.g.*, dermatitis, chapped skin, abrasion, or open wound) that has been exposed to blood, visibly bloody fluid, or other potentially infectious material." (A2)

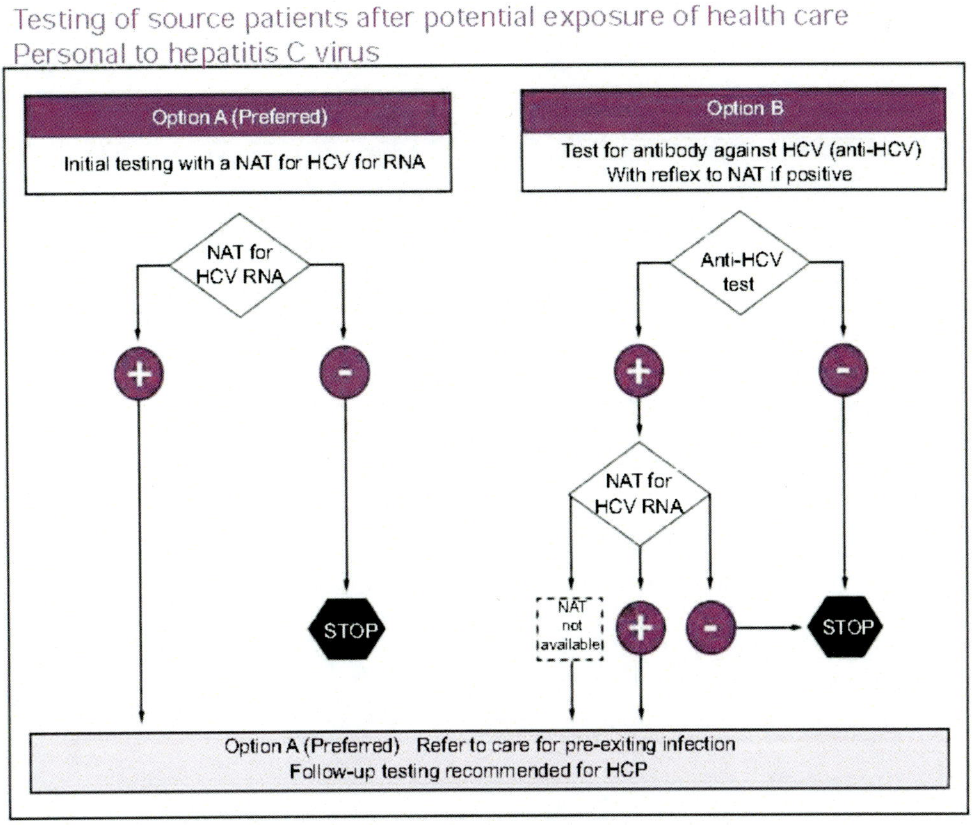

- *Testing of the source patient should be performed as soon as possible (preferably within 48 hours) after exposure.*
- Testing may follow option A (preferred), which is testing with a NAT for HCV RNA, or option B, which is testing for anti-HCV with reflex to NAT for HCV RNA if positive. If the source patient is known or suspected to have recent behaviors that increase the risk for HCV acquisition (e.g., injection drug use within the previous 4 months) or if risk cannot be reliably assessed, initial testing of the source patient should include a NAT for HCV RNA.
- A source patient found to be positive for HCV RNA should be referred to care.
- Follow-up testing of HCP is recommended if the source patient is HCV RNA positive, anti-HCV positive with HCV RNA status unknown, or cannot be tested.
- *Persons with detectable HCV RNA at any point* should be referred to care consistent with current AASLD-IDSA guidelines for evaluation and treatment of all persons with acute or chronic HCV infection. Guidance for hepatitis C treatment (https://www.hcvguidelines.org) is evolving with emerging data on treatment with direct-acting antivirals.

Abbreviations: AASLD-IDSA = American Association for the Study of Liver Diseases and the Infectious Diseases Society of America; HCP = health care personnel; HCV = hepatitis C virus; NAT = nucleic acid test.

Fig. (4). Summary of HCV screening and diagnostics for source individuals after potential exposure of HCPs to HCV [8].

Testing of health care personnel after potential exposure to hepatitis C virus

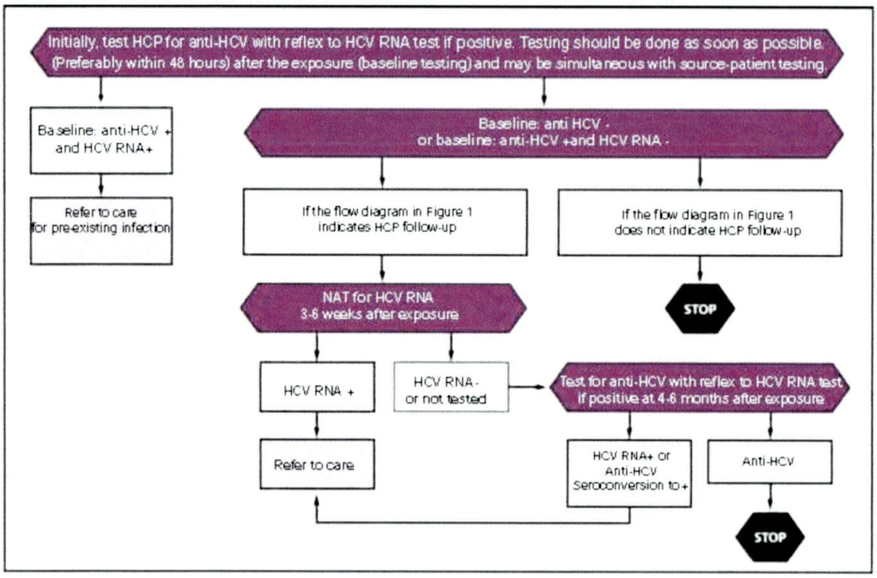

- ***Baseline testing of HCP for anti-HCV with reflex to a NAT for HCV RNA if positive should be done as soon as possible*** (preferably within 48 hours) after the exposure and may be simultaneous with source-patient testing.
- ***If follow-up testing is recommended based on the source-patient's status, test for HCV RNA at 3–6 weeks postexposure.*** Testing for HCV RNA performed at 6 weeks postexposure has the advantage of coinciding with human immunodeficiency virus (HIV) postexposure testing schedules if HIV surveillance is recommended.
- ***If HCV RNA is negative at 3–6 weeks postexposure, a final test for anti-HCV at 4–6 months postexposure is recommended due to the possibility of intermittent periods of aviremia in acute HCV infection. If the HCP was anti-HCV positive and HCV RNA negative at baseline, testing at this time should be conducted for HCV RNA detection, as persons successfully treated for HCV infection will remain anti-HCV positive and HCV RNA negative unless reinfected.*** Testing performed at 6 months postexposure has the advantage of coinciding with hepatitis B virus (HBV) postexposure testing schedules if HBV testing is recommended.
- ***HCP with anti-HCV seroconversion and negative HCV RNA should be referred for further evaluation.*** False-positive anti-HCV results are known to occur among low-risk populations.
- Anti-HCV seroconversion occurs on average 8–11 weeks after exposure, although cases of delayed seroconversion have been documented among persons with immunosuppression such as in HIV infection. ***For persons who had a negative anti-HCV result and are immunocompromised, testing for HCV RNA can be considered.***
- Also, for persons with a positive anti-HCV and negative HCV RNA result, HCV RNA testing should be repeated if an additional potential HCV exposure occurred within the past 6 months, clinical evidence of HCV infection is present, or concerns exist about specimen integrity, including handling and storage conditions that might have compromised test results. ***Exposed persons who develop viral syndromes suggestive of acute HCV infection at any point should be retested for HCV RNA.***
- ***Persons with detectable HCV RNA at any point should be referred to care consistent with current AASLD-IDSA guidelines for evaluation and treatment of all persons with acute or chronic HCV infection.*** Guidance for hepatitis C treatment (https://www.hcvguidelines.org) is evolving with emerging data on treatment with direct-acting antivirals.

Fig. (5). Summary of HCV screening and diagnostic testing for health care personnel after potential exposure to HCV [8].

Screening for at-risk Adolescents and Young Adults

Recommendations [4]:
• Hepatitis C screening in all patients aged 18 years and older is an essential first step in identifying and treating adults with hepatitis C infection. • Hepatitis C testing should be performed in individuals younger than 18 years of age who are at risk for infection. • Hepatitis C screening in young male and female IDUs primarily in suburban and rural areas where epidemics of hepatitis C infection have been observed parallel to opioid-use epidemics.

Screening for Acute HCV Infection

Recommendations [4]:
• "Clinicians should suspect acute hepatitis C infection if a patient who had a negative anti-HCV Abs test documented within the previous 6 months has a new positive anti-HCV Abs or has detectable HCV RNA in the absence of a positive anti-HCV Abs test." (A3) • "Clinicians should not prescribe pre- or post-exposure prophylaxis to prevent hepatitis C infection." (A1) • "If chronic hepatitis C infection is established, clinicians should evaluate patients for treatment." (A1) • "Clinicians should screen all patients with possible acute hepatitis C infection for HIV, hepatitis A virus (HAV), and hepatitis B virus (HBV) infections, given the similar risk factors for acquisition." (A3)

Diagnosing HCV Infection

Recommendations [4]:
1. Screening Tests • Clinicians should perform hepatitis C screening using either a laboratory-based anti-HCV Abs test or a point-of-care (POC) rapid antibody (Ab) test (Fig. **6**). (A1) **2. Confirmatory Testing** • If the anti-HCV Abs test result is positive, clinicians should obtain confirmatory HCV RNA testing from a laboratory that uses an HCV-RNA nucleic acid test (HCV-RNA-NAT) approved by the U.S. FDA. (A1) • If HCV RNA is detected after a positive anti-HCV Abs result, the patient has confirmed hepatitis C infection and clinicians should evaluate for treatment of chronic or acute hepatitis C infection. (A2) • If the anti-HCV Abs result is negative: 1. Clinicians should perform subsequent hepatitis C screening based on individual patient risk factors (A3) 2. *And* if acute hepatitis C infection is suspected, clinicians should perform a diagnostic HCV-RNA test using an FDA-approved NAT (Fig. **7**). (A1) • In patients with a history of a positive anti-HCV Abs test, clinicians should use an HCV-RNA test (not an anti-HCV Abs test) for subsequent screening. (A1)

Vulnerable Population Groups to be Considered for Targeted Hepatitis C Screening with Suggested Diagnostic Algorithms

Population group [5]	**Who to test**	**How often to test (HCV testing frequency)**
MSM	• Individuals with aggressive sexual behavior • Sexualized drug use • PrEP or PEP use	Up to every 6-12 months depending on ongoing risk, sexual behavior, HIV PrEP use, history of STIs, IDUs, and local hepatitis C prevalence/incidence

	• HIV infection • History of rectal bacterial STI	
Transgender people	All-trans gender individuals	Up to every 6-12 months depending on ongoing risk, sexual behavior, HIV PrEP use, history of STIs, injecting drug use, and local hepatitis C prevalence/incidence
Sex workers	All sex workers	Up to every 6-12 months depending on ongoing risk, sexual behavior, history of STIs, HIV PrEP use, injecting drug use and local hepatitis C prevalence/incidence
People who inject drugs (PWIDs)	All PWIDs	Up to every 6 months for those at ongoing risk or more frequently depending on local hepatitis C prevalence/ incidence
People in prison	Everyone in prison	Up to every year depending on individual risk assessment
Migrants including from a country of intermediate or high endemicity for hepatitis C virus or local migrants belonging to communities with high prevalence/incidences of hepatitis C infection	All migrants	Once; However; retesting can be performed based on individual risk assessment and local HCV epidemiology
Homeless people	Individual risk assessment	Once; However, can be repeated based on individual risk assessment and local HCV epidemiology
Pregnant women	To be considered based on individual risk assessment	With each pregnancy
Haemodialysis recipients	All individuals in this group	Once; however, retesting can be performed every 6 months or more often in case of an HCV outbreak, or if hemodialysis is performed in a substandard infection control setting
People who received blood products, organs, or surgical interventions before 1992 or in settings with suboptimal infection control standards	All individuals in this group	Once
Sexual partners and injecting partners of people diagnosed with hepatitis C and household contacts of people diagnosed with hepatitis C infection	All sexual and injecting partners of people diagnosed with hepatitis C	Once. Retesting is dependent upon the window period and type of HCV screening test used

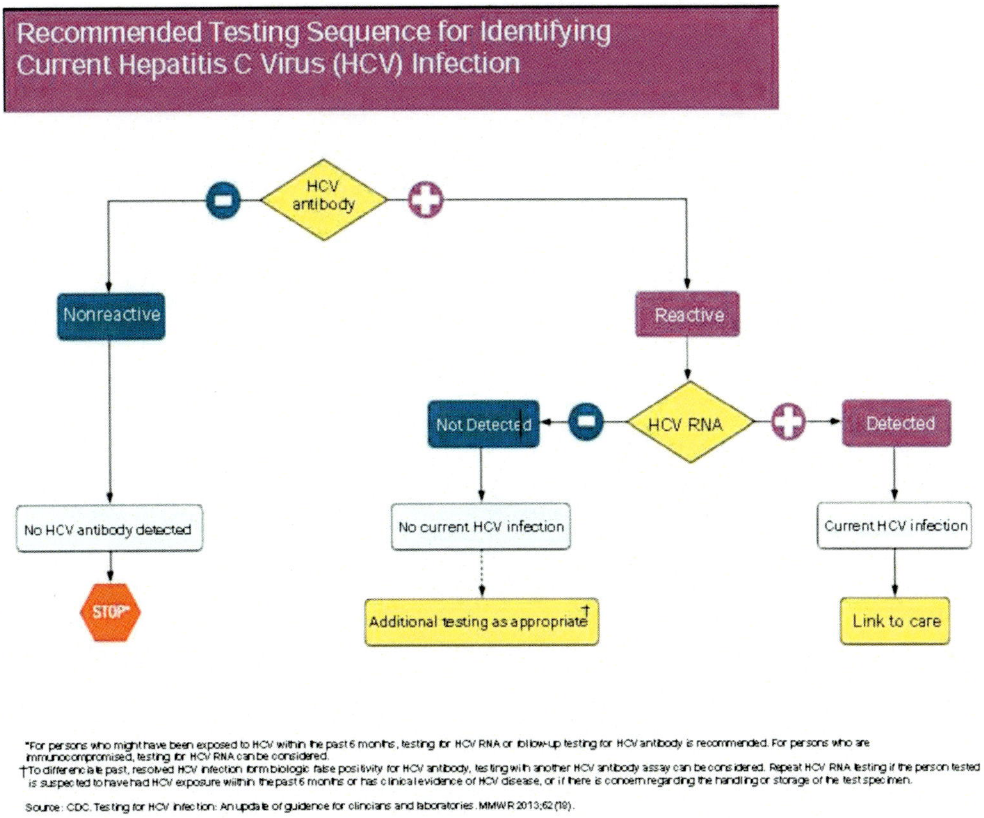

Fig. (6). Recommended testing scheme for identifying current HCV infection [9].

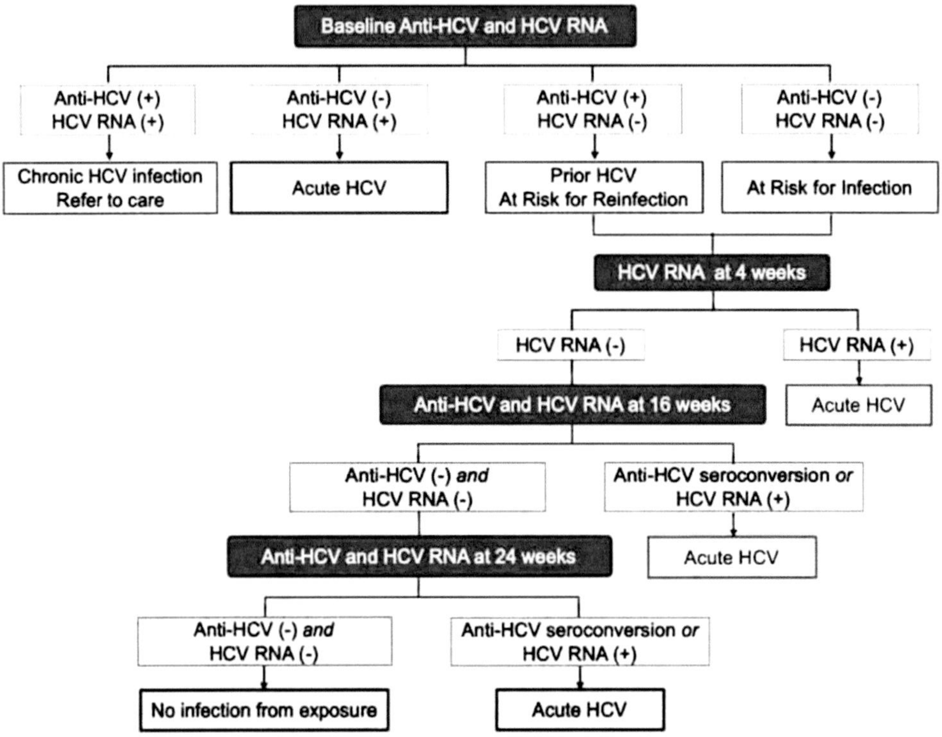

Fig. (7). Recommended testing scheme for identifying acute HCV infection at baseline before initiating HCV treatment, during the treatment, and post-DAA treatment [6].

CURRENT PARADIGMS OF HEPATITIS C SCREENING AND DIAGNOSIS

The WHO guidelines as well as world-renowned healthcare committees, institutes, and organizations working on hepatitis elimination provide time-to-time guidelines and algorithms for screening, diagnosis, treatment, and monitoring of hepatitis C infection. Furthermore published literature and expert opinion/consensus also provide simplified hepatitis C screening and diagnostic algorithms (Table **2**). Herein we comprehensively overview the screening and diagnostic parameters of hepatitis C in general as well as in vulnerable populations by using existing technologies and briefly highlight the innovative diagnostic solutions in the pipeline or late-stage of their development.

Table 2. Overview of existing technologies for HCV screening and diagnostic testing with their advantages and disadvantages [5].

Technology	Description
Laboratory-based immunoassay	A serological assay that detects anti-HCV Abs, HCV core antigen, or a combination of both. Typically used as the front line in HCV testing. These tests are relatively low cost compared to HCV-RNA NATs.
Alternative to laboratory-based immunoassays	
Rapid diagnostic test (RDT)	HCV-RDTs using serum, plasma, finger stick (FS) whole blood, or oral (crevicular) fluid can be used instead of classical immunoassays. A single-use immunoassay that detects Abs or antigens can give same-day results (<30 minutes). Most RDTs can be performed with blood collected by FS sampling. RDTs are robust and simple to perform. They can be useful in settings where access to laboratory infrastructure is limited and with populations for which access to RDTs can facilitate linkage to care, *e.g.* in outreach remote settings. Disadvantages include lower assay sensitivity/specificity and more subjective interpretation of results compared to other HCV diagnostics. For anti-HCV Abs testing, whole blood sampled from dried blood spots (DBS) can be used as an alternative to serum or plasma obtained by venipuncture.
Nucleic acid test (NAT)	Test using molecular techniques, *e.g.*, polymerase chain reaction (PCR), to detect viral RNA or DNA, either qualitatively or quantitatively. An HCV-RNA test is typically used to detect the presence of HCV RNA, active HCV infection, whether treatment is required, and monitor the course of the infection. However; laboratory-based HCV NATs are expensive and require highly trained staff to perform.
Alternative to laboratory-based NAT	
Point-of-care (POC) NAT	Anti-HCV Abs screening can be replaced by a point-of-care (POC) HCV RNA assay with a lower limit of detection (LLoD; <1000 IU/mL) or HCV core Ag assay if available. Consideration is given to cost-effectiveness and affordability.

BASICS OF HEPATITIS C SCREENING AND DIAGNOSIS

Hepatitis C diagnosis is a two-step process including:

1. Screening (*i.e.*, Anti-hepatitis C antibody (Ab) tests; and
2. Diagnostic HCV testing (also known as confirmatory tests) includes;
    a. A viral load test (also known as HCV RNA or nucleic acid testing (NAT; both qualitative and quantitative NAT); and
    b. An HCV core antigen (HCV cAg) test to detect viral/antigenic protein of hepatitis C [10].

Step 1: Hepatitis C Screening

Anti-HCV Antibody Screening

Hepatitis C screening involves determining whether an asymptomatic healthy individual has the infection. Hepatitis C screening detects antibodies (Abs) that the body makes against HCV, instead of looking for the virus itself (Fig. **8**). Anti-hepatitis C Abs are produced when HCV as an antigen (Ag) elicits an immune response in the human immune system [10]. The approximate window period to produce Abs against hepatitis C Ag in the human body may remain from 6 to 24 weeks. However; anti-HCV Abs stay for long (even for the rest of an individual's life) in a person's body even if the triggering antigen disappears or clears from the affected organs (this is commonly called immunological memory). If similar HCV Ag enters an individual again, even months or years later, the immunological memory of the immune system remembers the HCV Ag and produces Abs to target it for destruction [10].

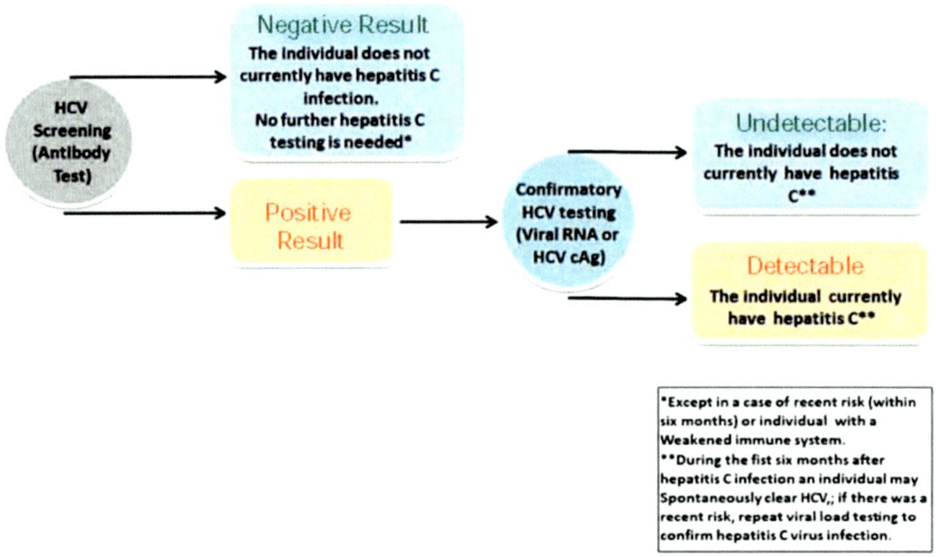

Fig. (8). Flow-chart of HCV screening and confirmatory tests with their interpretations [10].

What it means is that he/she will always test positive for anti-HCV Abs, even if the virus does not exist in their blood and they are not at risk for getting sick [10]. Furthermore, anti-HCV Abs screening confirms a past/previous hepatitis C infection (Fig. **8** and Table **3**). The immune system of some acutely infected hepatitis C patients clears the virus by itself (*i.e.* spontaneous viral clearance; as discussed in chapter 3) and generally one in four individuals may spontaneously clear HCV within 6 months of becoming infected [43]. Interestingly, the WHO estimates that around 30% (CI; 15 to 45%) of suspected hepatitis C infected persons will spontaneously clear HCV provided that those are young women, individuals not infected with other co-infections (*e.g.*, HIV and HBV), and persons with genetic variations that might strengthen their immune system [10].

Table 3. Overview of anti-HCV Abs test and their result interpretation [10].

Step 1: Anti-HCV Antobody (Ab) Test	
Anti-HCV Ab Positive	**Anti-HCV Ab Negative**
Three potential meanings: 1) The individual was recently infected with hepatitis C; or 2) The individual may have CHC; or 3) The individual was infected with hepatitis C in the past, but cleared the virus and is no longer infected. **Final Interpretation:** The individual needs a quantitative RNA (*i.e.*, viral load) test to confirm hepatitis C infection (Fig. 9).	**Three potential meanings:** 1) The individual has never been infected with the hepatitis C virus. **Final Interpretation:** The individual does not need a quantitative RNA (*i.e.*, viral load) test to confirm hepatitis C infection. 2) The individual may have been recently exposed to hepatitis C within the last 2 weeks; or 3) The individual is HIV positive, with a CD4 count <200 cells/mm^3, or has a weakened immune system. This individual may have a chronic hepatitis C infection. **Final Interpretation:** The individual needs a quantitative RNA (*i.e.*, viral load) test to confirm hepatitis C infection (Fig. **10**).

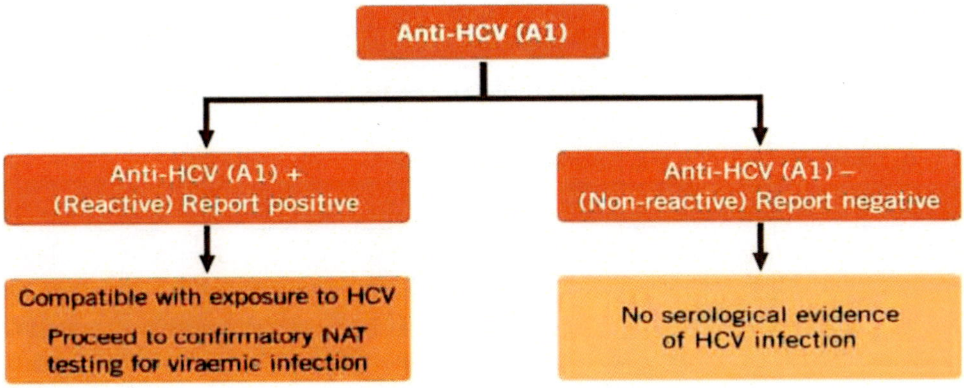

Fig. (9). Interpretation of one-assay serological (anti-HCV Abs) testing strategy for HCV testing [3].

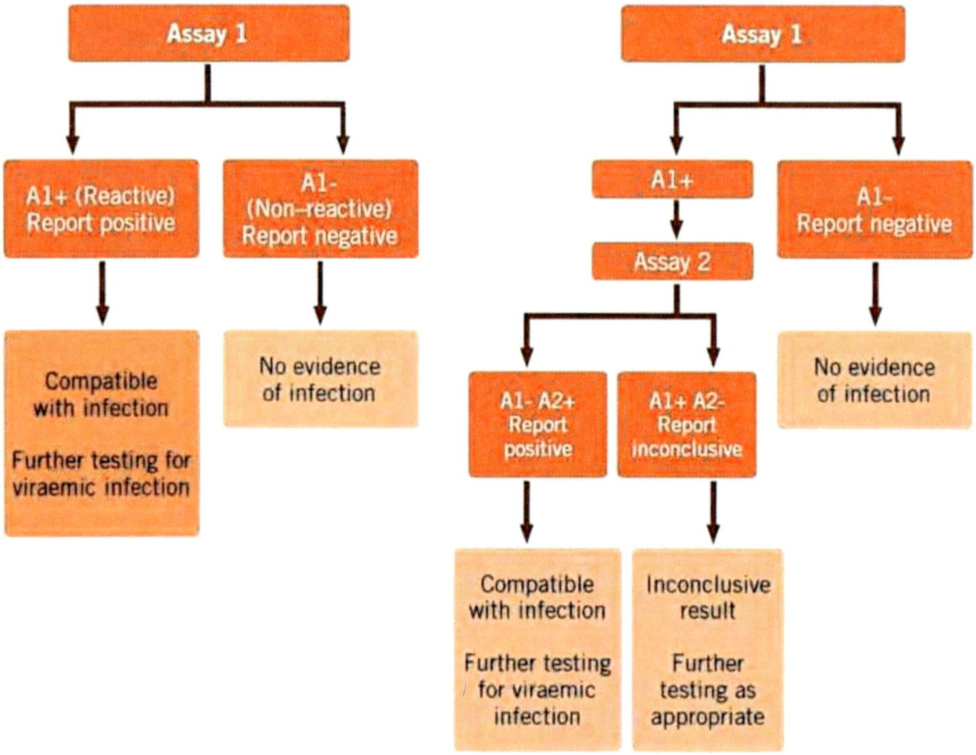

Fig. (10). Interpretation of two-assay serological (*i.e.* anti-HCV Abs) testing strategy for HCV testing [3].

Step 2: Hepatitis C Diagnosis Confirmation Tests

HCV RNA or HCV Core Ag (cAg) Confirmation

Hepatitis C virological/confirmatory testing rule out hepatitis C disease in a suspected individual or confirm current hepatitis C infection and directly relates to the virus itself [43]. Hepatitis C confirmation tests are categorized into two types including HCV NAT which are used to detect the virus in the blood and hepatitis C core antigen (HCV cAg) tests to detect hepatitis C cAg in the blood usually found within two weeks. However; the HCV cAg facility is available in central lab settings in big hospitals (Figs. **11** and **12**). Currently, HCV RNA load tests are preferable to cAg tests and are divided into two types:

1. HCV RNA Qualitative tests: Qualitative RNA tests are used to check HCV RNA in the bloodstream. The test results are either the virus is detectable (positive RNA test) in the bloodstream or nondetectable (negative RNA test).

2. HCV RNA Quantitative test: Quantitative RNA analysis measures the amount

of HCV RNA in the bloodstream (Usually expressed in IU/mL). As not widely accessible and affordable in many low-to-middle-income countries (LMICs), so specifically used before pretreatment assessment, prognosis, and post-HCV treatment [10].

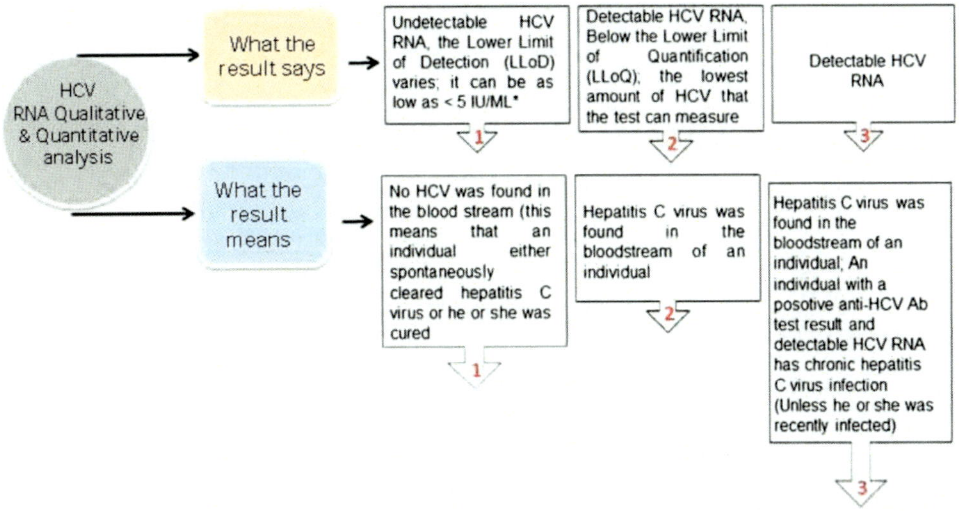

Fig. (11). HCV RNA confirmatory tests (RNA qualitative and quantitative) with their interpretations [10].

Step 2: Confirm Hepatitis C Diagnosis	
Detectable HCV RNA or cAg	**Undetectable HCV RNA or cAg**
Two potential meanings: 1) The individual may be recently infected with hepatitis C; or 2) The individual may have chronic hepatitis C; **Final Interpretation:** This individual should be pre-assessed for hepatitis C treatment.	**Two potential meanings:** 1) The individual has never been infected with hepatitis C. 2) The individual was once infected with hepatitis C in the past but has now cleared the virus. **Final Interpretation:** This individual should be assessed for follow-up testing.

HCV GENOTYPING/SUBTYPING

Currently, there are 6 known and WHO-classified HCV genotypes (GTs) and more than 70 subtypes [12]. An individual infected with one GT in the past or with a current infection may be reinfected with the same or different GTs in the future [13]. Mixed hepatitis C GTs infections have also been reported widely where the HCV genome exhibits different genotypic kinetics of one or different HCV GTs or subtypes in an affected person (commonly known as quasispecies HCV infections) [13]. HCV GTs identification and further subtyping are pivotal for the treatment choice, treatment duration, prognosis, therapeutic outcome, and

HCV cure [13]. By advantage, of the recommendations of pangenotypic oral direct-acting antivirals to treat all HCV GTs infected individuals, HCV genotype identification is becoming less relevant and unnecessary. The WHO guidelines 2018 recommend the skipping of HCV GTs identification if pangenotypic DAAs are used to treat hepatitis C infections [14].

Interpretation of Results of Tests for Hepatitis C Virus (HCV) Infection and Further Actions

TEST OUTCOME	INTERPRETATION	FURTHER ACTION
HCV antibody non reactive	No HCV antibody detected	Sample can be reported as nonreactive for add HCV antibody. No further action required. If recent exposure in person tested is suspected, test for HCV RNA. *
HCV antibody reactive	Presumptive HCV infection	Repeatedly reactive result with current HCV infection, all past at CV infection that has resolved, are biologic false positivity for HCV antibody. Test for HCV or RNA to identify current infection
HCV antibody reactive HCV RNA detected	Current HCV infection	Provide person tested with appropriate counseling and Link person tested to care and treatment.
HCV antibody reactive HCV RNA not detected	No current HCV infection	No further action required in most cases. If distinction between true positivity and biologic false positivity for HCV antibody is desired, and if sample is repeatedly reactive in the initial test, best with another at HCV antibody essay. In certain situations, follow-up with HCV RNA testing and appropriate counseling.

*If HCV RNA is not feasible and person tested is not immunocompromised, do not follow-up for testing for HCV antibody to demonstrate seoconversion. If the person tested is immunocompromised, consider testing for HCV RNA.

It is recommended before initiating antiviral therapy to retest for HCV RNA in a subsequent blood sample to confirm HCV RNA positivity.

§ If the person tested is suspected of having HCV exposure within the past 6 months, or has clinical evidence of HCV disease, or if there is concern regarding the handling or storage of the test specimen

Fig. (12). Interpretation of HCV testing outcomes and further actions [11].

HCV LIVER DISEASE STAGING ASSESSMENT

The detection of HCV disease staging in the liver is also vital as targeting the virus early stage of the infection is more fruitful before the hepatocytes or liver becomes more damaged [15]. It may help to choose the right treatment and to determine the length of treatment, and treatment outcomes. IFN-free DAAs are promising to cure CHC-infected individuals without cirrhosis by achieving 95%

SVR rates; however, the patients affected with compensated cirrhosis are more difficult to manage, treat, and cure. The inclusion of other regimens to treat cirrhosis or a long duration of treatment is generally recommended in those patients. Even if not managed timely, compensated cirrhosis may ultimately progress to decompensated cirrhosis, and further leads to HCC and end-stage liver disease (*i.e.* liver failure). Similarly, HCV GT-3 infections with cirrhosis are known as a harder-to-treat even with the administration of some pan-genotypic IFN-free DAAs. Additional factors that make HCV GT-3 treatment difficult by oral IFN-free DAAs are more likely for the patient to develop steatosis along with cirrhosis [15]. To what extent the liver has been damaged before initiating treatment in hepatitis C-infected individuals is measured by two types of approaches including;

1. Invasive tests (*e.g.*, liver biopsy: a small piece of a hepatic tissue sample with a needle for the assessment of prognostic biomarkers of hepatic damage), and;
2. Noninvasive tests (*e.g.*, ultrasound imaging or direct blood biomarkers);
3. Liver function tests (LFTs) can also be considered to check hepatic enzyme levels in individuals who are HCV/HBV or HCV/HIV co-infected and taking HBV or HIV antiretrovirals (ARTs) as well as who are on tuberculosis (TB) treatment. Furthermore, their hepatic enzymes profile should be monitored regularly as these antiviral regimens are not easily metabolized and biotransformed into the liver. For liver health and monitoring of hepatitis C infection progression, the hepatic levels of Alanine aminotransferase (ALT; also known as serum glutamic pyruvic transaminase [SGPT] that is made in the liver) and Aspartate aminotransferase (AST; also known as serum glutamic-oxaloacetic transaminase [SGOT] that is mainly made in heart, intestines, and muscles) are routinely measured (Table **4**). An increased level of ALT indicates the sign of HCV infection progression; however, cannot predict how much the liver has been damaged and may not infer to what extent hepatitis C infection has progressed [10]. Alkaline Phosphatase (ALP), gamma-glutamyl transferase (GGT), bilirubin, albumin, prothrombin (PT), and other important liver biomarkers can also be measured to assess liver health in hepatitis C infected individuals (Table **4**) [10].

Table 4. Overview of methods for liver disease staging technologies with potential advantages and disadvantages [5].

Methods for Liver Disease Staging (Fibrosis)	
Technology	**Applications/Advantages**
Indirect serum markers	APRI (AST to Platelet Ratio Index), FIB-4 (Fibrosis-4 score; calculators are available online), noninvasive; inexpensive, Limited ability to differentiate intermediate stages of fibrosis

(Table 4) cont.....

Direct markers	FibroSure, FibroTest, FibroMeter, FIBROSpect II, and HepaScore, Noninvasive; easily accessible, Limited ability to differentiate intermediate stages of fibrosis
Vibration Control Transient Elastography (VCTE)	Mechanically generated shear wave across the liver to derive a liver stiffness, noninvasive; assesses the large volume of liver parenchyma, May be difficult to interpret in F2 and F3 liver disease; limited availability
Liver biopsy	Pathologic examination, diagnostic standard; diagnoses a concurrent liver disease, invasive procedure; costly; sampling error

Liver Fibrosis Detection

Recommendations

• Clinicians should assess the degree of hepatic fibrosis in patients with chronic hepatitis C infection to aid in determining the following (A1):
1. Need for pretreatment screening for varices and HCC.
2. Duration of DAAs treatment.
3. Need to include ribavirin (RBV) in the treatment regimen.
4. Need for post-treatment follow-up.
• Clinicians should assess patients with CHC infection for decompensated liver disease. (A1)
• Clinicians should refer patients with decompensated cirrhosis to a liver disease specialist. (A3)

Liver Fibrosis Evaluation Tests

Liver fibrosis can be accessed with liver biopsy, Fibroscan or FibroTest/ActiTest, APRI, and FIB-4 tests. However, liver biopsy is becoming obsolete after the development of sophisticated and robust noninvasive technologies/procedures to assess liver cirrhosis [10]. Ultrasound imaging tests (*i.e.* FibroScan or FibroTest/ActiTest) that use sound waves are operated by liver specialists to look at liver stiffness. The FibroScan test can be used to ascertain the level of hepatic damage as well as the degeneration of hepatic cells. However; the results of FibroTest/ActiTest are shipped to a Biopredictive company to interpret by specific software which takes additional time (Table **5**). FibroScan is recommended in WHO guidelines, but FibroTest is not included yet. Furthermore, these tests are very expensive and not easily accessible/affordable in most LMICs (Table **5**). However, in Georgia, interestingly portable FibroScan devices were used in harm reduction clinics with appropriate training of paramedics under the supervision of medical specialists to assess liver fibrosis and hepatitis C progression in PWIDs as the country launched HCV elimination campaigns in 2017. The ultimate advantage of this approach was to examine liver disease staging within five minutes and the patient received results immediately. Fibroscan is used as a prevention and noninvasive assessment tool to educate people about their liver health in settings where mass HCV screening and diagnostic campaigns are launched and for patients who have no insurance reimbursements from healthcare services providers. In addition to that, it is also useful in drug harm reduction centers/services and in mobile clinics to monitor hepatitis C risk factors, and disease progression, and ultimately link them with HCV care cascade and social services (Table **5**). The WHO recommends APRI or FIB-4 in LMICs to assess liver function tests as well as hepatic fibrosis as those are comparatively less expensive than noninvasive procedures. However; the test turnaround time is long and patients may wait for pretreatment assessment which may delay hepatitis C treatment and cure. Furthermore, it will add more steps to the HCV cascade of care which leads to more costs in overall hepatitis C diagnosis, treatment, and care. The former is an AST to platelet ratio index, which is a formula used to determine the level of hepatic cirrhosis, while the latter is an inexpensive and noninvasive test to determine the amount of hepatic scarring by using a patient's age, platelet count, AST, and ALT [10].

$$\text{APRI} = \frac{\dfrac{\text{AST level (IU/L)}}{\text{AST (Upper limit of Normal) (IU/L)}} \times 100}{\text{Platelet count } (10^9/\text{L})}$$

$$\text{FIB-4} = \frac{\text{Age (years)} \times \text{AST (U/L)}}{\text{Platelet count } (10^9/\text{L}) \times \sqrt{\text{ALT (U/L)}}}$$

Table 5. A comparison of potential advantages and disadvantages of FibroScan and FibroTest used for liver fibrosis evaluation [10].

Comparison of FibroScan and FibroTest		
Features	**FibroScan**	**FibroTest**
Platform Cost	Fibroscan platforms are very expensive ranging from a minimum price of US$70,000 to US$300,000	Cost varies depending on the country's procurement policy and the analysis of the results with Biopredictive's software technology
Test Cost	Per test is expensive starting from US$50, (generally ranging from US$60 to 80 per test)	Starting from US$59 to over US$100 per test
Testing Accessibility	Suitable for clinics or POC settings; however, for a large number of individuals, multiple devices would be required	Hospital laboratory settings
Resource Settings	Preferably in urban and resource-rich settings; however, can be considered for rural patients, and community settings to engage patients and peers linked to healthcare services and HCVcascade of care	Patients in both urban and rural areas can be evaluated; however, the test facility is more easily accessible in urban areas than in rural areas because of specimens/results shipping or transport problems. Available in both resource-rich and resource constraint nations.

(Table 5) cont.....

Result findings and interpretations	Detailed imaging of hepatic fibrosis	Not a hepatic imaging platform. It is an integrated work of blood tests to evaluate direct liver fibrosis biomarkers with specific software analysis
Advantages over other fibrosis evaluation technologies	Superior to FibroTest, APRI, or FIB-4 analysis while considering the accuracy, sensitivity, and specificity of the findings	Superior to FIB-4 or APRI for accuracy/interpretation of the results in particular for patients with hepatic cirrhosis or advanced hepatic disease.
Transportation of specimen/results	No specific requirement	Reliable specimens/results shipping or transport infrastructure
Linkage to care	Patient referral is required or follow-up for advanced hepatic disease (*e.g.*, HCC) diagnosis	Patient referral or follow-up is required
Equipment maintenance	No reagent is required; however, maintenance is recommended after every 6 months	Manufacturers or companies bargain or express monopolies on required reagents/kits and instrument maintenance

Liver Cirrhosis Evaluation

Recommendations [4] :
• Clinicians should refer all patients with hepatitis C-related cirrhosis for an upper endoscopy to screen for the presence of esophageal varices. (A3) • Clinicians should screen for HCC with ultrasound, computerized axial tomography (CT), or magnetic resonance imaging (MRI) every 6 months in patients with hepatitis C-related bridging fibrosis or cirrhosis. (A3)

Liver Cirrhosis Evaluation Tests

Hepatitis C treatment with pangenotypic IFN-free DAAs in hepatitis C-affected patients with compensated cirrhosis dramatically decreases the advanced infection events like hepatic decompensation, HCC, and end-stage liver disease mortalities [12]. To link HCV-infected patients with an appropriate care cascade, hepatic cirrhosis is evaluated and classified by the clinicians, hepatologists, and infectious disease experts by calculating the Model for End-Stage Liver Disease score (MELD calculator) or the Child-Turcotte-Pugh (CTP) score as mentioned in Table **6**.

Table 6. Calculating the CTP score for severity of cirrhosis in hepatitis C infected patients [4].

Evaluation of Liver cirrhosis severity (Based on Child-Turcotte-Pugh [CTP] score]) [16]			
	1 point*	2 points*	3 points*
Encephalopathy	None	Stages 1 to 2 (or precipitant induced)	Stage 3 or 4 (or chronic)

(Table 6) cont.....

Ascities	None	Mild/moderate (diuretic-responsive	Severe (diuretic-refractory)
Bilirubin (mg/dL)	<2.0	2.0 to 3.0	>3.0
Albumin (g/dL)	>3.5	2.8 to 3.5	<2.8
Prothrombin time (sec prolonged) or INR	<4.0	4.0 to 6.0	>6.0
	<1.7	1.7 to 2.3	>2.3
*CTP score is obtained by adding the score for each parameter. CTP class: A= 5 to 6 points (compensated cirrhosis, least severe hepatic disease) B= 7 to 9 points (decompensated cirrhosis, moderately severe hepatic disease) C= 10 to 15 points (decompensated, most severe liver disease) [16]			

WHY ARE WE IN NEED OF SCREENING MORE PATIENTS FOR HEPATITIS C?

Current CDC Guidelines Miss 25% of Hepatitis C Infections

Current CDC recommendations and guidelines for hepatitis C screening are inadequate and miss 25% of infections according to the findings of a study conducted in an urban emergency department (ED) in the U.S [6]. A review of blood specimens for nearly 5000 individuals who were seen in the Johns Hopkins Hospital Emergency Department, Baltimore City, Maryland, during 8 weeks demonstrated that the CDC recommendations for hepatitis C screening miss up to a quarter of all cases. Hence one-time universal HCV screening is needed [17]. Furthermore, high prevalence rates of hepatitis C in young adult patients, advocating the expansion of HCV testing beyond the baby boomer cohort [18]. EDs of urban health care systems should consider expanding CDC recommendations to facilitate more robust identification of unknown hepatitis C status of suspected individuals [19]. The transmission of hepatitis C infection in EDs patients could be high because EDs serve as a medical safety net for many citizens who are also at high risk for hepatitis C [19]. Seroprevalence of hepatitis C antibodies has been demonstrated very high in some urban ED populations in the U.S., (*i.e.*, approximately from 13% to 18%) [19]. Few EDs have weighed out the underlying burden of hepatitis C infection in their populations, Yet EDs are integral venues for hepatitis C testing because of the population served and their rationale for successful HIV screening [20]. Furthermore, it would help to establish the overall burden of undocumented hepatitis C infection in EDs to guide the implementation of ED-based hepatitis C testing recommendations. In addition to that testing, all ED patients born after 1945 might efficiently reduce HCV-associated comorbidities burden on the elderly [17]. High hepatitis C seroprevalence in young adolescent and adult patients is also linked with injection drug users (IDUs) of oxymorphone, methadone, and amphetamine [8]. Broad HCV screening instead of risk-based screening and the CDC-established birth cohort screening for baby boomers highlight an integral role for EDs to identify hepatitis C in the communities they serve [15]. However; many individuals with a high risk of hepatitis C prevalence (*e.g.*, MSM, sex workers, IDUs, incarcerated, *etc.*) do not share their risk information with ED staff, so universal hepatitis C screening, besides the CDC recommendations, could be a feasible way to identify as many hepatitis C missing individuals as possible [21].

Hepatitis C Prevalence in Women of Reproductive Age (WORA)

Anti-HCV Abs prevail in pregnant females around 0.1 to 3.6% with potential adverse neonatal outcomes worldwide [17]. It represents an enhanced risk of vertical transmission of hepatitis C infection (*i.e.* maternal hepatitis C infection that is passed to the infant) at a rate of 5% in children and is presumed to be the further key transmission source of infection in adults and child-contacted people [22]. Current and past IDUs represent the most common risk factor for hepatitis C, although effective treatment in the form of IFN-free DAAs is available, albeit; expensive, and not easily accessible in many low-to-middle-income countries (LMICs) [17]. In addition to that, ongoing high-risk behavior can result in repeat HCV infection. The CDC data demonstrate that the increased use of the opioid substance by parenteral route among young adults might be the sole reason for the higher prevalence of hepatitis C among WORA, and the number of infants born to HCV-infected mothers is increasing dramatically [23]. Vertical transmission of hepatitis C infection is demonstrated by almost 6% of children born to infected mothers [17] and more likely with high hepatitis C viral loads or concomitant HIV infection [24]. No therapeutic intervention is currently recommended to prevent vertical hepatitis C transmission [17]. HCV screening involves anti-HCV Abs tests, along with HCV-RNA tests to confirm active infection when Abs screens are positive. However; clinicians should bear in mind that Anti-HCV Abs screening is substantially associated with false-positive outcomes. Currently, the American Congress of Obstetricians and Gynecologists (ACOG) recommends that pregnant females with risk factors should be screened for hepatitis C [17].

Furthermore, The American Association for the Studies of Liver Diseases (AASLD) and the Infectious Diseases Society of America (IDSA) updated guidelines in 2018 that recommended universal hepatitis C screening with each pregnancy, except in premises where prevalence is less than 0.1% [19]. Besides that, CDC demonstrates that HCPs should also assess nonpregnant females of childbearing age for hepatitis C risk factors and screen accordingly [19]. What could be the health benefits of this strategy are not ascertained? However, the use of highly effective contraceptives such as an intrauterine device (IUD) or implant, referral for rehabilitative treatment to eliminate high-risk behavior, and referral for treatment of hepatitis C can be encouraged for those who harbor infection [25]. Once the infection is treated/cured, the females could pursue pregnancy if they intend to do so. Accordingly, many barriers have to be overcome for screening nonpregnant females in preventing subsequent vertical hepatitis C transmission [25].

Low HCV Screening Rates Among Children Exposed to Pregnancy

Hepatitis C infection is soaring among pregnant females due to the opioid epidemic in developed nations as well as unsafe sex practices in LMICs [19]. Hence, the percentage of most perinatally infected children is on the rise due to insufficient hepatitis C screening. Current guidelines suggest the screening of all infants perinatally exposed to hepatitis C infection to evaluate the risk of perinatal HCV transmission [26]. Currently, the rate of HCV screening is lower for perinatally exposed infants and warrants novel strategies to improve and escalate screening [19]. With a rise in hepatitis C prevalence among pregnant females and the difficulties of obtaining demographics with current or remote histories of substance abuse, universal hepatitis C screening, and diagnostic strategies are eagerly awaited for all pregnant females [19]. A U.S based study estimates that among 88,000 pregnant females who gave birth between 2006 and 2014, 1.2% had hepatitis C infection [27]. Most of them were younger than 30, white, and covered by Medicaid insurance as compared with hepatitis C-uninfected females [27]. During the study period of nine-years, the investigators demonstrated a high rate of hepatitis C infection among females giving birth at the hospital (*i.e.* 60% high; from 1,026 to 1,637/100,000 females) [27]. Interestingly, from 1,025 infants born to HCV-infected mothers, only 323 (32%) received well-child services, only 96 were screened for hepatitis C, and only about three-quarters received an optimal initial hepatitis C screening test [27]. Seven infants (8.4%) were documented with evidence of perinatal hepatitis C transmission [27].

As the treatment options for hepatitis C-infected children are well documented and better-tolerated, much-focused HCV screening programs for pregnant females are vital to vanquishing the long-term sequelae of HCV infection [28, 29] (see chapter 7). Furthermore, undiagnosed infants with potential perinatal HCV transmission risk when growing may become symptomatic or have abnormal hepatic enzyme levels [29]. Similarly, delays in HCV screening could lead to delays in linkage to care, and curative treatment or may transform into irreversible hepatic diseases (*e.g.*, cirrhosis or HCC) [29]. Another study conducted between 2009 to 2014 found an 89% increase in hepatitis C cases among pregnant females in the U.S [23]. Further investigations are needed on interventions to escalate screening in perinatal hepatitis C infection-risk infants, like using digital healthcare to improve the transfer of maternal hepatitis C status to the pediatric medical record and enhancing pediatricians' awareness regarding hepatitis C screening guidelines [29].

HCV Infections Among Infants are Vastly Underreported

HCV infection among infants is vastly underreported, suggesting the need for routine testing in pregnant women, as most studies found [17, 30]. These studies provide data that signifies the importance of hepatitis C screening in all pregnant women to safeguard their health and protect their offspring from hepatitis C transmission [17, 19, 24]. These studies analyzed data from two of the largest population data sets available in the United States: the National Notifiable Diseases Surveillance System (NNDSS) from 2006 to 2014 and the Quest Diagnostics Health Trends national database from 2011 to 2014. The studies included 171,801 WORA (15 - 44 years) and 1859 children (aged 2 - 13 years) with HCV infection reported to the NNDSS and 2.1 million reproductive-aged women and 56,684 children who underwent hepatitis C testing by Quest Diagnostics® [17, 19, 31]. Between 2006 and 2014, the number of reproductive-aged women with acute hepatitis C infection reported to the NNDSS rose 3.4-fold, from 249 per year to 848. Similarly, the number of past or present cases reported doubled, from 15,301 to 30,191. From 2011 to 2014, Quest Diagnostics® tested 581,255 pregnant women; of those, 4232 (0.73%; 95% CI, 0.71% - to 0.75%) had hepatitis C infection [17, 19, 31]. Until now, no Hepatitis C treatments are approved by the U.S. FDA for use in pregnant women (albeit; the clinical trials of some promising oral interferon-free pangenotypic DAAs are in the pipeline) and clinical pregnancy may be the only time a young woman is seen by a clinician, so some clinicians already are screening pregnant women known or suspected to be at risk for HCV infection according to current WHO guidelines [31]. During the same period, Quest Diagnostics® tested 57,136 children (86,783 tests) aged 2 to 13 years. Of those, 882 (1.54%; CI, 1.44% -1.65%) had past or present HCV infection, 432 (0.76%; CI, 0.69% - 0.83%) had a current infection, and 56,252 (98.45%; CI, 98.35% -98.55%) were not currently infected [17, 19, 31]. The studies predicted that the rate of infection was 3.2-fold higher among those aged 2 to 3 years (1.62%; CI, 1.34% - 1.96%) compared with those aged 12 to 13 years (0.50%; CI, 0.41% - 0.62%) [17, 19, 31]. When the hepatitis C infection rate was applied to annual live births from 2011 to 2014, it was estimated an average of 29,000 women (CI, 27 400 - 30 900 women) infected with HCV gave birth to 1700 infants (CI, 1200 - 2200 infants) with the infection annually [31].

On the flip side of the coin, only about 200 childhood hepatitis C cases per year are reported to the NNDSS, which may suggest a need for wider screening for hepatitis C in pregnant women and their infants, as is recommended for HIV and HBV [31]. However, recommendations for screening in pregnant women and clear testing guidelines for infants born to HCV-infected mothers are needed to be improved [17]. The recognition of hepatitis C infection in pregnant women and neonates is possible by using some emerging diagnostic tests and clinical trials of DAAs may show safety and efficacy in pregnant women and children [8]. At least screening pregnant women for hepatitis C infection risk factors, as well as risk-based testing, requires more emphasis [31]. Similarly, the lack of authoritative, consensus-based recommendations for the identification, testing, and case management of newborns of infected mothers is also a big challenge to coup in this scenario [31].

Hepatitis C And Drug Abuse Often Go Hand in Hand, but HCV Screening Lags

Hepatitis C is a virus that causes inflammation to the liver, in some cases leading to scarring, liver cancer, and death [1]. It is transmitted through blood, including contaminated needles that people share when they inject drugs. The initial test for hepatitis C is an inexpensive blood test to check for Abs in the blood that indicates exposure to the virus [1]. If that Abs test is positive, a second test is necessary to find out if the virus is circulating in the bloodstream, which would mean someone is infected with the virus [1]. As the number of people who inject drugs has soared, the rate of hepatitis C infection, frequently tied to sharing needles, has climbed steeply, too [1, 17]. When peoples seek help at a drug treatment center for opioid addiction, concerns about having contracted hepatitis C are generally low on their list [1]. They've often reached a crisis point in their lives but they just want to handle their drug problem and sometimes they don't have the bandwidth to take on too many other things. Even though health care facilities that serve people who use drugs are well-positioned to initiate screening, too often that is not happening, recent studies have shown [1, 17, 19, 32]. Not testing these patients for hepatitis C is an enormous missed opportunity as many public health experts agree [32]. As early hepatitis C infection is identified, it can be cured at that moment; However, in hepatitis C patients who inject drugs, no testing is incomprehensible when you look at what hepatitis C does to their bodies and their livers [32]. People who are infected with hepatitis C can go for years without symptoms, so they may not have any inkling that they're sick. That delayed onset makes screening important, advocates say, since people may unwittingly infect others [32].

Screening people who misuse drugs for the deadly virus is a commonsense strategy to get people cured and break the cycle of transmission [1]. But there are obstacles - sometimes a lack of money, staff, or other resources [32]. Reimbursement rates for hepatitis C testing often don't match the cost and if patients test positive, they need to be linked to treatment, and financial support for staffing to do that is often limited [1]. In the USA, only 27.5 percent of 12,166 substance abuse facilities reported offering testing for hepatitis C in 2017 [17]. In primary care settings, the situation sometimes isn't much better, even when patients have a diagnosed "opioid-use disorder [8]. An analysis by Boston Medical Center researchers of nearly 270,000 medical records of people aged 13 to 21 who visited federally qualified health centers from 2012 to 2017 found that 36 percent of the 875 patients with that diagnosis were tested for hepatitis C [31]. The same situation was noticed even in a setting with an identified risk factor in opioid-use disorder, where too few youths are being screened for hepatitis C [32].

To be sure, primary health care centers worldwide, and in particular in LMICs must be made testing for hepatitis C a priority particularly to test many of their patients who are at high risk because of injection drug use or unsafe sexual practices, such as having sex with an infected partner [1, 32]. The screenings can often be done on an annual basis, with a reminder to the medical personnel in the patient's electronic or manual medical record.

HCV Diagnostic and Treatment Costs Would Always be a Crosscutting Barrier for HCV Affected IDUs

In recent years, as the drug epidemic has taken hold worldwide, new infections have been concentrated among young people who inject drugs, in particular those between ages 18 and 29, according to the CDC report [31]. Complicating the effort to get people screened is the fact that many of the people who enroll in drug treatment programs are uninsured or cannot afford the expenditure of HCV infection diagnosis and treatment (Table **7**) [1]. Insurance coverage isn't the only challenge. If people have to come back to a clinic for the second test, chances are they may fall through the cracks and not get that follow-up [1]. When a patient tests positive, a nurse or counselor at the drug treatment center, who is likely overbooked working with patients to address their addiction, must carve out time to explain this new diagnosis and talk through treatment options [33]. Unlike for HIV, such a health care system does not exist for hepatitis C at this time even in resource-rich nations [33]. Finding resources to pay for treatment is also difficult. The high costs of the new drugs when they were introduced led some public and private insurers to strictly limit access [1]. But, in recent years, drug prices have come down as more drugs hit the market.

Occurrence of New Hepatitis C Incidences in Public Services Screening

HCV infection frequently occurs in populations that do not have regular contact with healthcare workers [34]. Most health departments have not yet initiated widespread screening services for a couple of reasons. First, it was not until 2013 that the CDC recommended screening for everyone born from 1945 to 1965 [31]. Second, DAAs that can effectively cure hepatitis C have only become available in recent years, and initially cost as much as $80,000 a year [12]. To identify infected patients and link them to healthcare providers (HCPs), in public venues one study targeted hepatitis C screening for baby boomers, people with a long-term partner infected with hepatitis C, people with tattoos or ear piercings done by unregulated providers, and people with a history of (IDUs), other illegal drug use, HIV infection, incarceration, or exchanging sex for drugs [35].

Table 7. Prices of HCV diagnostics [36]. Ab; antibody, HCV; Hepatitis C virus, NAT; nucleic acid test, POC; point of care, RDT; rapid diagnostic test.

-	Product	Manufacturer	Technology	Min (Price US$)	Max Price (US$)
HCV testing	**SD Bioline**	Standard Diagnostics Korea	RDT (Ab)	1	
	OraQuick	OraSure	RDT (Ab)	7	
Confirmatory testing	GeneXpert	Cepheid	near-POC	13	18
	Genedrive	Genedrive	near-POC	25	30
	Truelab/Truenat	Molbio Diagnostics	POC	20	
	Architect	Abbott	NAT	25	50
	Generic	Biocentric	NAT	23	
	Aptima	Hologic	NAT	10	25
	CAP/CTM HCV	Roche	NAT	35	45
	Versant HCV	Siemens	NAT	72	100
Test-of-cure	Truelab/Truenat	Molbio Diagnostics	POC	20	
	RealTime	Abbott	NAT	11	23
	Generic	Biocentric	NAT	23	
	Aptima	Hologic	NAT	10	25
	Artus HCV	Qiagen	NAT	16	45
	Versant HCV	Siemens	NAT	72	100
				Min price (US$)	**Max price (US$)**
Price per patient (HCV testing + confirmatory testing + test-of-cure)				22	207

The screening was also targeted at people who had more than five sexual partners in the previous 12 months and at men who had sex with men (MSM) in the previous 12 months [35]. Hepatitis C Ab and reflex RNA testing were used for hepatitis C infection identification [35]. Of the 4558 people screened from March 2016 to April 2017, 230 (5.0%) were positive for both Abs and RNA. Most of the positive tests - 41.7% - came from people in jail. The majority of people identified as having CHC were male, nearly half were black, 39% were baby boomers, 55% were previous or current IDUs, 23% were or had been incarcerated, and 4% were infected with HIV [35].

The prevalence of chronic infection was highest in the jail population, where 96 of 1246 (7.7%) people screened tested positive. It was least prevalent in women tested at maternal health clinics, where only two of the 489 (0.4%) people screened tested positive [35]. Of the 230 people with positive tests, 147 (64%) were linked to healthcare through the program. Of those, 27% were seen in primary care, 41% by a specialist, and 16% by a healthcare provider in prison. Another 17% met only with a bridge counselor. Of the 36% not linked to healthcare, 42% were lost to follow-up, 27% were homeless, 19% moved out of the area, and 12% could not be contacted for other reasons [35]. Working with inmates is particularly challenging because they probably have "a lot of other social issues, whether it's substance abuse, mental health, housing, or transportation [37]. More work needs to be done to screen and treat people in jail, as it seems a very natural place to find individuals with hepatitis C and concentration on this population is important.

Liver Cancer on the Rise in Backdrop of Undiagnosed Hepatitis C

Liver cancer is one of the greatest challenges to hepatologists today and it will become an even greater challenge in the near future [38]. It is increasing in most Western countries, partly because of the hepatitis C epidemic that occurred in the 1950s and 1960s and those people are now 60 to 70 years old and have had their disease for a very long time [38]. Now they are starting to come down with end-stage liver cancer. With ascertain, in the U.S., Canada, and most probably in LMICs, the majority of patients with hepatitis C have not yet been diagnosed [1]. Similarly, there is a handful of existing and emerging treatments for advanced hepatocellular carcinoma, but they are not highly effective [12]. Transplanting everybody with end-stage liver disease is not possible, so we need to be able to manage the end-stage liver disease better than we currently do [12]. Similarly, there is currently a shortage of centers equipped to manage what is expected to be the burgeoning number of patients with end-stage liver cancer.

Birth Cohort Screening for Hepatitis C

A study based on three independent trials determine the relative probability of identifying hepatitis C infections using birth cohort testing [39]. Hepatitis C testing of persons in the 1945-1965 birth cohort without previous ascertainment of hepatitis C risk was five times more effective in identifying persons with previous or current hepatitis C infection compared with standard of care [40]. The study strongly supports the effectiveness of the recommendations that baby boomers must be screened for HCV infection [39].

Following the CDC recommendations, in 2013, New York State mandated that primary care providers (PCP) offer hepatitis C Ab testing to all persons born between 1945 and 1965 [41]. In New York City, as many as 146,500 residents (2.4% of the adult population) have chronic hepatitis C infection; it is estimated that one-half of these people are unaware of their infection [30]. Therefore, a strategy called the 'Check Hep C campaign' was designed to integrate hepatitis C testing and linkage to care into community-based organizations to improve hepatitis C testing rates [41]. The testing method involved targeted outreach and point-of-care (POC) rapid antibody testing. After a positive Ab test, an immediate blood draw was obtained to assess hepatitis C RNA status [41]. From May 2012 to April 2013, a total of 4751 individuals were tested; 19% were hepatitis C Ab positive, and 76% of those were documented by hepatitis C RNA testing to have a current infection [41]. Of those, 85% attended their first medical appointment and 50% remained in care to receive treatment. The high overall prevalence (15%) of current infection among baby boomers supports the New York State Testing Law and CDC recommendations [41]. Expanding this model to more settings with high-risk populations in LMICs will aid in successfully identifying and linking HCV-positive individuals into care.

To Increase Quality-adjusted Life Years (QALY) in Hepatitis C Infected Individuals

At present, less than 10% of patients with CHC have been treated successfully because of the failure of risk-based screening to identify all infected patients and the low efficacy and high rate of side effects from regimens based on IFN and RBV [1]. One study explored the health and economic impact of the recommended one-time birth cohort screening for hepatitis C in the era of highly effective DAAs regimens [42]. A decision-analytic Markov model that used computer-simulated patients was used to compare four strategies for screening individuals born from 1945-to 1965 without known HCV infection [42].

1- Risk-based screening with treatment based on the stage of liver disease (RBS)
2- Risk-based screening and treat all without staging (RBA)
3- Birth cohort screening with treatment based on the stage of liver disease (BCSS)
4- Birth cohort screening and treatment all without staging (BCSA)

Treatment based on staging was applied for fibrosis stages F2-F4, with subsequent staging every 5 years for F0-F2. IFN-free DAA therapy was assumed to achieve a 98% SVR rate at US$1000/day for 12 weeks, with no disutility of treatment, because the quality of life is better on treatment [42]. The effectiveness was measured in quality-adjusted life-years (QALYs) and disease progression. The study findings estimated that about 100 million people would be screened and that 1.4 million would be found to have (unknown) HCV infection [31]. BCSA was the most cost-effective strategy ($32,263/QALY) compared with the RBS strategy. The BCSA strategy would cost an extra $123 billion but produce an additional 22.9 million QALYs [42]. The study concluded that the availability of highly efficacious IFN-free DAA regimens, with excellent tolerability, makes screening of baby boomers extremely cost-effective, with great health and economic benefits at the population level. The bottom line message is to screen and then treat all who needed the treatment without prioritizing based on liver fibrosis stages [42].

Screen All New Cancer Patients for Hepatitis C

Multiple studies have found "a large reservoir of patients with cancer and undiagnosed hepatitis virus infections" and have reignited the question of whether all newly diagnosed cancer patients should be screened for hepatitis [43]. One study named 'Screening in Newly Diagnosed Cancer Patients' (S1204) involved 3051 patients and found that 6.5% had previously been infected with HBV, 0.6% had chronic HBV infection, 2.4% had HCV infection, 1.1% were infected with HIV [43]. At enrollment, 87.3% of patients did not know that they had previously been infected with HBV. Similarly, 42.1% of the cases of chronic HBV infection, 31.0% of the cases of HCV infection, and 5.9% of the cases of HIV infection were undiagnosed [43]. Cancer patients with HBV or HCV infection are at risk for viral reactivation and potentially life-threatening clinical outcomes. Many patients had no known risk factors for infection, suggesting that current risk-based models for screening may be insufficient. Universal screening for HBV and HCV before cancer therapy "may be warranted. The investigators mentioned, however, that "the low rate of undiagnosed HIV infection may not support universal screening of newly diagnosed cancer patients for HIV [43].

Hepatitis C Screening Could Prevent Complications in Cancer patients

Universal screening for HBV, HCV, and HIV infection is not routinely performed in patients diagnosed with cancer. What's more, the use of such screening remains controversial among oncologists [44]. The findings of multiple studies provide new evidence to inform a discussion in the oncology community about whether cancer patients should require hepatitis C screening [32 - 34]. Universal screening could prevent complications from hepatitis, such as liver failure and kidney disease. Immunosuppressive cancer drugs such as rituximab (*Rituxan*®, Genentech, Biogen Idec) - used to treat CD20+ T-cell lymphomas and leukemias - can cause some viruses to reactivate and multiply [45]. Because the true risk of severe adverse events associated with most cancer treatments in persons with latent infections is unknown, the putative benefits of delaying or modifying cancer treatment remain speculative; however, the risk that these changes pose to outcomes for patients with newly diagnosed cancer is real [45]. One study conducted in 2018, reported that 15% of HCV-infected patients who had different primary cancers developed HCV-associated HCC as a second primary malignancy [45]. This is an often-overlooked presentation of liver cancer. Similarly, most studies suggest that universal HBV testing is more efficient than risk-based screening and selective screening practices for HCV are not optimal for identifying all infected cancer patients [46]. Although, with the availability of nucleos(t)ide analogs to treat HBV and oral IFN-free DAAs to treat HCV, infected cancer patients can be treated to prevent viral reactivation, progression of liver disease, and allow access to cancer treatment, including clinical trials [35]. There is evidence of the impact of reactivation of HBV and HCV infection in patients undergoing immunosuppressive chemotherapy [44]. In two separate studies, the researchers concluded that greater surveillance for HBV and safer hematologic-sparing treatments for HCV are required to surmount the burden of these two infections in cancer patients [33, 34]. In 2015, the American Gastroenterological Association issued a guideline for the prevention and treatment of HBV reactivation during immunosuppressive drug therapy [47]. Until more data are available, the US Centers for Disease Control and Prevention (CDC) and the US Preventive Services Task Force (USPSTF) recommend that universal one-time HIV screening be conducted in patients aged 13 to 65 years and in women who are pregnant [31]. One-time screening for HCV is also recommended for individuals born between 1945 and 1965 [21]. However; universal screening for three infectious diseases (*i.e.* HIV, HBV, and HCV) would increase the cost of cancer care [31]. The studies are needed in this direction to determine the cost-effectiveness of universal hepatitis B, C, and HIV screening in cancer patients. Three multiple studies present cost analyses in the United States and Europe and show that universal HCV screening in the community is cost-effective [43]. Similar results are expected in cancer patients, given the significant morbidity and mortality of HCV in this patient population.

To Minimize the Steps to Hepatitis C Cascade of Care

The Global Health Sector Strategies (GHSS) in 2016 set an ambitious goal of HCV elimination by 2030 considering it a major public health threat [1]. Achieving this ambitious goal requires a 90% decrease in the new incidence of hepatitis C infection, 90% of hepatitis C-infected patients to be diagnosed, and 80% of those to be treated. Furthermore, a 65% reduction in hepatitis C-associated mortalities is to be achieved [1]. However, the current cascade of hepatitis C care in many parts of the world in particular for LMICs represents a different scenario which requires 10 single visits from hepatitis C screening to cure, 9 phlebotomies, HCV genotyping assessment, and liver disease staging for disease assessment (Fig. **13**) [1]. Anti-hepatitis C Abs rapid diagnostic testing (RDTs) from infection screening to treatment requires 4 single visits, 1 phlebotomy for active infection confirmation, and skipping hepatitis C genotype assessment provided that prescribed to pan-genotypic DAAs regimens for treatment; however, liver disease staging for disease assessment may require for determining cirrhosis status of the patient (*i.e.*, present or absent; compensated or decompensated cirrhosis), for treatment initiation, treatment type, and length of hepatitis C treatment for HCV GT-3 infected patients [1]. The patients on dried blood spot (DBS) sample testing by anti-hepatitis C Abs RDTs receives diagnosis report within two visits [1]. While, the individuals adopting anti-HCV Abs RDT and HCV RNA-POCT for active viremic infection may confirm, diagnose, and receive DAAs treatment in a single visit [1]. It reflects the importance of a simplified HCV diagnostic pathway to overcoming the obstacles of multiple visits, phlebotomies, and increased time that potentially may lose many patients from HCV screening to diagnosis, treatment monitoring, and cure follow-ups in real-world clinical settings. Adoption and implementation of those simplified diagnostic algorithms are also helpful to remove the hurdles to scale-up hepatitis C diagnosis in vulnerable HCV populations (*i.e.* sex workers, MSM, PWIDs, IDUs, incarcerated people, *etc.*) where social stigma and poor venous access are always major challenges for the patient adherence to diagnostic algorithms and draw a venous blood sample respectively in many LMICs.

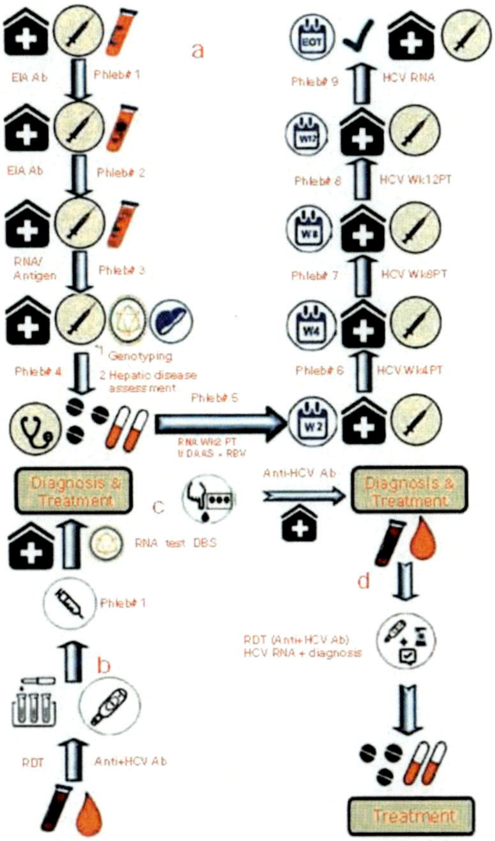

Fig. (13). A schematic diagram demonstrating the advantages of rapid HCV diagnostic tests, dried blood spot sample tests, and HCV RNA reflex testing over traditional HCV screening and diagnostic algorithms. **a)** The existing HCV screening and diagnostic approaches used in many parts of the world and in particular in many LMICs require 10 single visits from hepatitis C screening to cure, 9 phlebotomies, and one test for HCV genotyping assessment, and one procedure for liver disease staging for disease assessment. **b)** anti-hepatitis C Abs rapid diagnostic testing (RDTs) from infection screening to treatment requires 4 single visits, 1 phlebotomy for active infection confirmation, and skipping hepatitis C genotype assessment provided that prescribed to pan-genotypic DAAs regimens for treatment; however, liver disease staging for disease assessment may require for determining cirrhosis status of the patient. **c)** Dried blood spot (DBS) sample testing by anti-hepatitis C Abs RDTs receives diagnosis report in two visits. **d)** The patients adopting HCV RNA reflex testing options including anti-HCV Abs RDT and HCV RNA-POCT for active viremic infection may confirm, diagnose, and receive DAAs treatment in a single visit. EIA; enzyme immunoassay, Ab; antibody, Phleb; phlebotomy, DBS; dried blood spot, RDT; rapid diagnostic test, wk; week.

CONCLUSIONS

To eradicate HCV worldwide by 2030, HCV screening and diagnosis will play an essential role to link infected individuals to the cascade of care. Despite the advent and approvals of highly efficacious treatment regimens (*i.e.* IFN-free DAAs), HCV diagnostic algorithms are not fully implemented in many LMICs where the infection is almost endemic and even in resource-replete nations where social determinants of health (*e.g.*, stigma, criminalization, and marginalization) pose a big hurdle to reach vulnerable HCV populations (MSM, sex workers, IDUs, PWIDs, and inmates). The implementation of consensus guidelines on who to test for CHC infection in general and in vulnerable populations will help to reduce the transmission of HCV from high-risk individuals to healthy communities as well as link identified ones to care cascade. It will also determine which types of testing and diagnostic approaches would be required for different patient cohorts. HCV RDTs and POC testing may play an essential role to screen HCV-infected individuals in remote areas having poor health infrastructure as well as harder-to-reach populations. PWIDs and vertical transmission of HCV infection are two big concerns to achieve WHO HCV elimination goals by 2030; hence, universal HCV screening for pregnant females and identifying PWIDs and IDUs are pre-requisite in certain guidelines and must be a part of the national hepatitis C plan of the countries who are off-track to achieve WHO HCV elimination goals by 2030. Furthermore, HCV data surveillance along with accurate HCV diagnosis will help to treat everyone who is in need and the implementation of novel HCV diagnostic algorithms will support reducing patient visit numbers, as well as cutting the testing and treatment costs, and patient loss during follow-ups. It will also minimize the steps for a patient's 'test to treat' or 'test to care' cascade in particular for HCV-infected individuals in LMICs where most of the patients are reluctant, non-responsive, and non-adherent to conventional HCV testing and treatment approaches involving multiple visits.

REFERENCES

[1] Martinez MA, Franco S. Impact of COVID-19 in Liver Disease Progression. Hepatol Commun 2021; 5(7): 1138-50.
[http://dx.doi.org/10.1002/hep4.1745] [PMID: 34533001]

[2] Shahid I, Alzahrani AR, Al-Ghamdi SS, Alanazi IM, Rehman S, Hassan S. Hepatitis C diagnosis: simplified solutions, predictive barriers, and future promises. Diagnostics (Basel, Switzerland). 2021; 11(7).

[3] Sidharthan S, Kohli A, Sims Z, *et al.* Utility of hepatitis C viral load monitoring on direct-acting antiviral therapy. Clin Infect Dis 2015; 60(12): 1743-51.
[http://dx.doi.org/10.1093/cid/civ170] [PMID: 25733369]

[4] Guideline HCV. 2020.https://www.ncbi.nlm.nih.gov/books/NBK559965/

[5] Childs-Kean LM, Hong J. Detectable viremia at the end of treatment with direct-acting antivirals can be associated with subsequent clinical cure in patients with chronic hepatitis C: A case series. Gastroenterology 2017; 153(4): 1165-6.
[http://dx.doi.org/10.1053/j.gastro.2017.06.062] [PMID: 28881195]

[6] Steinebrunner N, Sprinzl MF, Zimmermann T, *et al.* Early virological response may predict treatment response in sofosbuvir-based combination therapy of chronic hepatitis c in a multi-center "real-life" cohort. BMC Gastroenterol 2015; 15(1): 97.
[http://dx.doi.org/10.1186/s12876-015-0328-9] [PMID: 26239732]

[7] Backus LI, Belperio PS, Shahoumian TA, Loomis TP, Mole LA. Real-world effectiveness of ledipasvir/sofosbuvir in 4,365 treatment-naive, genotype 1 hepatitis C-infected patients. Hepatology

2016; 64(2): 405-14.
[http://dx.doi.org/10.1002/hep.28625] [PMID: 27115523]

[8] Recommendations for Hepatitis C Screening. Washington University; 2022 Jan. Available from: https://www.hepatitisc.uw.edu/go/screening-diagnosis/recommendations-screening/core-concept/all.

[9] AASLD-IDSA. HCV Guidance: Recommendations for testing, management, and treating hepatitis C. Monitoring patients who are starting HCV treatment, are on treatment, or have completed therapy. [AASLD-IDSA Hepatitis C Guidance].

[10] U.S. Food and Drug Administration. FDA Drug Safety Communication: FDA warns about the risk of hepatitis B reactivating in some patients treated with direct-acting antivirals for hepatitis C. [U.S. Food and Drug Administration].

[11] Yoshida EM, Sulkowski MS, Gane EJ, *et al.* Concordance of sustained virological response 4, 12, and 24 weeks post-treatment with sofosbuvir-containing regimens for hepatitis C virus. Hepatology 2015; 61(1): 41-5.
[http://dx.doi.org/10.1002/hep.27366] [PMID: 25314116]

[12] Boettler T, Newsome PN, Mondelli MU, *et al.* Care of patients with liver disease during the COVID-19 pandemic: EASL-ESCMID position paper. JHEP Reports 2020; 2(3)100113
[http://dx.doi.org/10.1016/j.jhepr.2020.100113] [PMID: 32289115]

[13] Yu ML, Chen PJ, Dai CY, *et al.* Taiwan consensus statement on the management of hepatitis C: Part (II) special populations. Journal of the Formosan Medical Association 2020; 119(7): 1135-57.

[14] Yeon JE. Recent update of the 2017 Korean Association for the Study of the Liver (KASL) treatment guidelines of chronic hepatitis C: Comparison of guidelines from other continents, 2017 AASLD/IDSA and 2016 EASL. Clin Mol Hepatol 2018; 24(3): 278-93.
[http://dx.doi.org/10.3350/cmh.2018.1002] [PMID: 29716179]

[15] Tada T, Kumada T, Toyoda H, *et al.* Viral eradication reduces all-cause mortality, including non-live--related disease, in patients with progressive hepatitis C virus-related fibrosis. J Gastroenterol Hepatol 2017; 32(3): 687-94.
[http://dx.doi.org/10.1111/jgh.13589] [PMID: 27577675]

[16] Pisaturo M, Macera M, Alessio L, Calò F, Coppola N, Hepatitis B. Hepatitis B Virus (HBV) Reactivation Following Pharmacological Eradication of Hepatitis C Virus (HCV). Viruses 2019; 11(9): 850.
[http://dx.doi.org/10.3390/v11090850] [PMID: 31540223]

[17] Asselah T, Marcellin P, Schinazi RF. Treatment of hepatitis C virus infection with direct-acting antiviral agents: 100% cure? Journal of the International Association for the Study of the Liver. 2018; 38 Suppl 1(Suppl 1): 7-13.

[18] Marcellin F, Roux P, Protopopescu C, Duracinsky M, Spire B, Carrieri MP. Patient-reported outcomes with direct-acting antivirals for the treatment of chronic hepatitis C: current knowledge and outstanding issues. Expert Rev Gastroenterol Hepatol 2017; 11(3): 1-10.
[http://dx.doi.org/10.1080/17474124.2017.1285227] [PMID: 28116926]

[19] Cacoub P, Desbois AC, Comarmond C, Saadoun D. Impact of sustained virological response on the extrahepatic manifestations of chronic hepatitis C: a meta-analysis. Gut 2018; 67(11): 2025-34.
[http://dx.doi.org/10.1136/gutjnl-2018-316234] [PMID: 29703790]

[20] Morgan RL, Baack B, Smith BD, Yartel A, Pitasi M, Falck-Ytter Y. Eradication of hepatitis C virus infection and the development of hepatocellular carcinoma: a meta-analysis of observational studies. Ann Intern Med 2013; 158: 329-37.
[http://dx.doi.org/10.7326/0003-4819-158-5-201303050-00005] [PMID: 23460056]

[21] van der Meer AJ, Veldt BJ, Feld JJ, *et al.* Association between sustained virological response and all-cause mortality among patients with chronic hepatitis C and advanced hepatic fibrosis. JAMA 2012; 308(24): 2584-93.

[http://dx.doi.org/10.1001/jama.2012.144878] [PMID: 23268517]

[22] Maylin S, Martinot-Peignoux M, Moucari R, *et al.* Eradication of hepatitis C virus in patients successfully treated for chronic hepatitis C. Gastroenterology 2008; 135(3): 821-9. [http://dx.doi.org/10.1053/j.gastro.2008.05.044] [PMID: 18593587]

[23] Ferm VH, Willhite C, Kilham L. Teratogenic effects of ribavirin on hamster and rat embryos. Teratology 1978; 17(1): 93-101. [http://dx.doi.org/10.1002/tera.1420170117] [PMID: 415379]

[24] Feld JJ, Jacobson IM, Sulkowski MS, Poordad F, Tatsch F, Pawlotsky JM. Ribavirin revisited in the era of direct-acting antiviral therapy for hepatitis C virus infection 2017. [http://dx.doi.org/10.1111/liv.13212]

[25] Grebely J, Oser M, Taylor LE, Dore GJ. Breaking down the barriers to hepatitis C virus (HCV) treatment among individuals with HCV/HIV coinfection: action required at the system, provider, and patient levels. The Journal of infectious diseases. 2013;207 Suppl 1(Suppl 1):S19-25.

[26] Meyer JP, Moghimi Y, Marcus R, Lim JK, Litwin AH, Altice FL. Evidence-based interventions to enhance assessment, treatment, and adherence in the chronic Hepatitis C care continuum. Int J Drug Policy 2015; 26(10): 922-35. [http://dx.doi.org/10.1016/j.drugpo.2015.05.002] [PMID: 26077144]

[27] Roberts SS, Miller RK, Jones JK, *et al.* The Ribavirin Pregnancy Registry: Findings after 5 years of enrollment, 2003-2009. Birth Defects Res A Clin Mol Teratol 2010; 88(7): 551-9. [http://dx.doi.org/10.1002/bdra.20682] [PMID: 20564430]

[28] Ward RP, Kugelmas M. Using pegylated interferon and ribavirin to treat patients with chronic hepatitis C. Am Fam Physician 2005; 72(4): 655-62. [PMID: 16127955]

[29] Cacoub P, Desbois AC, Isnard-Bagnis C, Rocatello D, Ferri C. Hepatitis C virus infection and chronic kidney disease: Time for reappraisal. J Hepatol 2016; 65(1) (Suppl.): S82-94. [http://dx.doi.org/10.1016/j.jhep.2016.06.011] [PMID: 27641990]

[30] Dore GJ, Altice F, Litwin AH, *et al.* Elbasvir Grazoprevir to Treat Hepatitis C Virus Infection in Persons Receiving Opioid Agonist Therapy. Ann Intern Med 2016; 165(9): 625-34. [http://dx.doi.org/10.7326/M16-0816] [PMID: 27537841]

[31] Hoofnagle JH. Course and outcome of hepatitis C. Hepatology 2002; 36(5) (Suppl. 1): S21-9. [PMID: 12407573]

[32] Maheshwari A, Ray S, Thuluvath PJ. Acute hepatitis C. Lancet 2008; 372(9635): 321-32. [http://dx.doi.org/10.1016/S0140-6736(08)61116-2] [PMID: 18657711]

[33] Micallef JM, Kaldor JM, Dore GJ. Spontaneous viral clearance following acute hepatitis C infection: a systematic review of longitudinal studies. J Viral Hepat 2006; 13(1): 34-41. [http://dx.doi.org/10.1111/j.1365-2893.2005.00651.x] [PMID: 16364080]

[34] Kamal SM. Acute hepatitis C: a systematic review. Am J Gastroenterol 2008; 103(5): 1283-97. [http://dx.doi.org/10.1111/j.1572-0241.2008.01825.x] [PMID: 18477352]

[35] Grebely J, Page K, Sacks-Davis R, *et al.* The effects of female sex, viral genotype, and *IL28B* genotype on spontaneous clearance of acute hepatitis C virus infection. Hepatology 2014; 59(1): 109-20. [http://dx.doi.org/10.1002/hep.26639] [PMID: 23908124]

[36] WHO guidelines on hepatitis B and C testing. Geneva: World Health Organization; 2017. Available from: https://www.who.int.

[37] Blackard JT, Shata MT, Shire NJ, Sherman KE. Acute hepatitis C virus infection: A chronic problem. Hepatology 2008; 47(1): 321-31. [http://dx.doi.org/10.1002/hep.21902] [PMID: 18161707]

[38] Newsum AM, Schinkel J, van de Laar TJW, van der Meer JTM, Prins M. Spontaneous clearance of hepatitis C virus infection among human immunodeficiency virus infected men who have sex with men. Open Forum Infect Dis 2017; 4(2)ofx090
[http://dx.doi.org/10.1093/ofid/ofx090] [PMID: 28638847]

[39] Nguyen GC, Sam J, Thuluvath PJ. Hepatitis C is a predictor of acute liver injury among hospitalizations for acetaminophen overdose in the United States: A nationwide analysis. Hepatology 2008; 48(4): 1336-41.
[http://dx.doi.org/10.1002/hep.22536] [PMID: 18821593]

[40] Chou R, Wasson N. Blood tests to diagnose fibrosis or cirrhosis in patients with chronic hepatitis C virus infection: a systematic review. Ann Intern Med 2013; 158(11): 807-20.
[http://dx.doi.org/10.7326/0003-4819-158-11-201306040-00005] [PMID: 23732714]

[41] Boursier J, de Ledinghen V, Zarski JP, *et al.* Comparison of eight diagnostic algorithms for liver fibrosis in hepatitis C: new algorithms are more precise and entirely noninvasive. Hepatology 2012; 55(1): 58-67.
[http://dx.doi.org/10.1002/hep.24654] [PMID: 21898504]

[42] Duarte-Rojo A, Altamirano JT, Feld JJ. Noninvasive markers of fibrosis: key concepts for improving accuracy in daily clinical practice. Ann Hepatol 2012; 11(4): 426-39.
[http://dx.doi.org/10.1016/S1665-2681(19)31456-5] [PMID: 22700624]

[43] Gara N, Zhao X, Kleiner DE, Liang TJ, Hoofnagle JH, Ghany MG. Discordance among transient elastography, aspartate aminotransferase to platelet ratio index, and histologic assessments of liver fibrosis in patients with chronic hepatitis C. Journal of the American Gastroenterological Association. 2013; 11(3): 303-8.

[44] Cloherty G, Cohen D, Sarrazin C, *et al.* HCV RNA assay sensitivity impacts the management of patients treated with direct-acting antivirals. Antivir Ther 2015; 20(2): 177-83.
[http://dx.doi.org/10.3851/IMP2810] [PMID: 24941124]

[45] Cobb B, Pockros PJ, Vilchez RA, Vierling JM. HCV RNA viral load assessments in the era of direct-acting antivirals. Am J Gastroenterol 2013; 108(4): 471-5.
[http://dx.doi.org/10.1038/ajg.2012.248] [PMID: 23552304]

[46] Vermehren J, Kau A, Gärtner BC, Göbel R, Zeuzem S, Sarrazin C. Differences between two real-time PCR-based hepatitis C virus (HCV) assays (RealTime HCV and Cobas AmpliPrep/Cobas TaqMan) and one signal amplification assay (Versant HCV RNA 3.0) for RNA detection and quantification. J Clin Microbiol 2008; 46(12): 3880-91.
[http://dx.doi.org/10.1128/JCM.00755-08] [PMID: 18799708]

[47] Strassl R, Rutter K, Stättermayer AF, *et al.* Real-Time PCR Assays for the Quantification of HCV RNA: Concordance, Discrepancies and Implications for Response Guided Therapy. PLoS One 2015; 10(8): e0135963.
[http://dx.doi.org/10.1371/journal.pone.0135963] [PMID: 26274922]

CHAPTER 5

The Current Paradigms of Hepatitis C Diagnosis and Innovations in the Pipeline

Abstract: Considering advances in hepatitis C therapy, global management of HCV infection becomes practicable, but some influential factors, like the capacity of countries to identify and proper diagnosis of infected individuals with immense HCV genotypic variations among different global regions and at-risk populations, cannot be passed over. Approximately, 71 million people are infected with chronic HCV infection and about 80% of them remain undiagnosed. Standard protocol for HCV diagnosis includes a preliminary serological (HCV antibody) test accompanied by an expensive confirmatory test for HCV RNA detection in serum samples of patients. However, gaps remain in the accessibility, affordability, and availability of gold-standard HCV diagnostic strategies. In pursuance of achieving the goals of the World Health Organization (WHO) for HCV elimination as a public health threat by 2030, efficient, reliable, and simplified diagnostic pathways are needed to unveil. As such, simplified sensitive strategies that can enhance the single-test diagnostic approach might assist linkage to care and direct-acting antivirals (DAAs) treatment uptake. Herein, we will discuss a few advanced diagnostic approaches to subdue some of these constraints. HCV self-testing and digital devices for the detection of HCV infection would be of prime importance in the near future. Furthermore, the availability of smart, robust, and mobile diagnostic platforms to find the missing millions in harder-to-reach populations and vulnerable individuals would also be required to link every diagnosed one with cascades of care. We will briefly cover all aspects of HCV screening and diagnostic algorithms in this book chapter along with potential advantages and disadvantages.

Keywords: Core Antigen Assay, Dried Blood Spot, HCV RNA Detection, HCV EIA Assays, Multi-disease Analyzers, Nanocomposites, Point-of-care Testing, Quick portable Tests, Rapid diagnostic Tests, Real-world Challenges, RNA POC Accuracy, Scale-up HCV Screening.

Imran Shahid and Qaiser Jabeen

INTRODUCTION

HCV Serology and RNA Detection

The gold standard diagnostic pathway for screening and detection of active HCV infection is based on three techniques that might be used alone or in combination [1]. These techniques include; 1) IgG antibody detection by ELISA 2) HCVcAg detection 3) and HCV RNA detection *via* PCR. HCVcAg and HCV RNA detection techniques are used to confirm viral active infection (Table **1**) [1]. HCV antibody detection approach includes the false-positive results and the diagnosis of individuals who have cleared the active infection either automatically or through antiviral treatment. Therefore, HCVcAg and viral RNA detection techniques are used for the confirmation of active infection [2, 3]. Though the specificity and sensitivity of HCVcAg testing depict remarkable performance when compared with PCR assays; however, there are still some uncertainties over whether the antigen detection test is adequately accurate to be broadly executed as a central diagnostic tool [2 - 4]. Therefore, recent WHO guidance rules recommend the utilization of HCV antibody tests as a preliminary screening process [5]. A cautious balance between cost management and specificity optimization with high sensitivity must be made [6, 7]. In a study performed by Adland *et al.*, gold standard algorithm techniques were compared among infected patients. HCV antibody testing got 87% PPV when compared to repeat antibody testing in a reference laboratory. Thereby emphasizing the increased potency for false-positive results. HCVcAg testing depicted 100% PPV in correlation with HCV RNA detection assay in multiple recent studies. Similarly, a significant correlation ($P < 0.0001$) was found between quantitative HCVcAg and viral RNA load [8]. Briefly, HCVcAg testing performs well as a diagnostic tool in comparison to RNA PCR for the identification of HCV replication.

Numerous diagnostic techniques are being evaluated regarding their multiple parameters to develop potent, rapid, and simplified HCV testing techniques. Being not exhaustive and avoiding iteration, we are discussing here novel HCV diagnostic platforms with their sensitivity, specificity, and efficacy in real-world clinical practices as well as their potential advantages and disadvantages (Table **2**). However, advanced research is further required in the field of multiple testing techniques, diagnostic platforms, and assay validation to accurately test for different simples, the diagnostic platforms which are robust, and assays that could be pragmatic in real-life HCV diagnostics.

Table 1. A summary of HCV serological and confirmatory tests with their interpretation for acute or recent infection, confirmed but unspecified resolved or chronic infection, and confirmed infant infection [10, 44].

Confirmed Case: Acute or Recent Infection	Detection of hepatitis C virus antibodies (anti-HCV) or hepatitis C virus RNA (HCV RNA) in a person with discrete onset of any symptom or sign of acute viral hepatitis within 6 months preceding the first positive HCV test **AND** • negative anti-HAV IgM, and negative anti-HBc IgM or HBsAg tests **AND** • serum alanine aminotransferase (ALT) greater than 2.5 times the upper normal limit **OR** • detection of hepatitis C virus antibodies (anti-HCV) in a person with a documented anti-HCV negative test within the preceding 12 months **OR** • detection of hepatitis C virus RNA (HCV RNA) in a person with a documented HCV RNA negative test within the preceding 12 months.
Confirmed Case: Unspecified (including chronic and resolved infections)	Detection of hepatitis C virus antibodies (anti-HCV Abs) **OR** detection of hepatitis C virus RNA (HCV RNA).
Confirmed Case: Infants < 18 months**	PCR positive for HCV-RNA^.
HCV PCR is important as viremic individuals will be considered for antiviral treatment and is a useful diagnostic tool in immuno-compromised individuals who might not mount an antibody response.	
**In infants < 18 months of age, anti-HCV testing should not be performed as the presence of anti-HCV may represent a passive maternal antibody. The cord blood should not be used because of potential cross-contamination with maternal antibodies. ^ If testing for HCV-RNA is done, it should be delayed beyond 4-12 weeks in order to avoid false-negative HCV-RNA test results.	

Table 2. The WHO essential diagnostic list of current and emerging HCV diagnostic platforms and tests with WHO prequalification, CE marked, and those which are in late-stage development [10, 42]. ND = not defined, PQ = prequalification, CE = Conformitè Europëenne, LMICs = low-to-midd-e-income countries, CE-IVD = Conformitè Europëenne in vitro diagnostics, POC = point of care, NAT = nucleic acid testing, HAV = hepatitis A virus, IVD= in vitro diagnostics, TB = tuberculosis, GTs = genotyping, TK = to come.

HCV Enzyme Immunoassay (HCV EIA)							
Test Name	**Sample Type/Setting**	**Turnaround Time**	**Multiplexing**	**Price**	**Regulatory Status**	**WHO PQ Review**	**Suitability**
INNOTEST HCV Ab IV	Serum, plasma	179 min	Yes (HIV & other markers)	ND	WHO PQ	-	Central labs
INNO-LIA HCV Score	Serum, plasma	1 day	No	ND	WHO PQ CE-marked	-	Strip-based method but requires cold chain and other small equipment

(Table 2) cont.....

Test Name	Sample Type/Setting	Turnaround Time	Multiplexing	Price	Regulatory Status	WHO PQ Review	Suitability
HCV Enzyme Immunoassay (HCV EIA)							
Bioelisa HCV 4.0	Serum, plasma	150 min	Yes (HIV, HBV, HEV, among others)	ND	WHO PQ, CE-marked	-	Central labs
Murex Anti-HCV 4.0	Serum, plasma	120 min	Yes (HIV, HBV, HEV, among others)	ND	WHO PQ, CE-marked	-	Central labs
Enzygnost Anti-HCV 4.0	Serum, plasma	120 min	Yes (HBV, HAV)	ND	Did not receive WHO PQ approval	-	Central labs
HCV Core Antigen (HCV cAg Assay)							
Abbott ARCHITECT HCV Ag assay	Serum, plasma	ND	Yes (HIV, HBV, HAV, among others)	US$8-23 (€7–20) per test; US$100,000 per instrument	CE-marked, WHO PQ	-	Central labs
Monolisa HCV Ag-Ab ULTRA V2	Serum, plasma	150-180 minutes	Yes (HIV, HBV, HAV, among others)	ND	CE-marked,	WHO PQ (Jan 2020)	Central labs
HCV Rapid Diagnostic Tests (HCV-RDTs)							
OraQuick HCV RDT	Oral, fingerstick, venous blood	20 min	No	US$8 (MSF price); US$12 per test	FDA Approved CE-marked WHO PQ	-	Price remains too expensive for LMICs
SD Bioline	10 µL whole blood, serum, plasma	5-20 min	HIV	US$1-2.40 per test	WHO PQ	-	-
Intec Rapid anti-HCV	10 µL, whole blood, serum, plasma	15-20 min	No	<US$1-2.40 per test	WHO PQ, CE-marked	-	-
Standard Q HCV Ab Test	Whole blood, serum, plasma	10-15 min	No	ND	CE-IVD	WHO PQ March 2020	POC
Premier Medical Corporation First Response® HCV Card Test	Whole blood, serum, plasma	ND	No	US$0.60-1 per test	CE-marked	WHO PQ under review	-
ABON HCV Rapid Test Device	Whole blood, serum, plasma	ND	No	ND		WHO PQ under review	-
HCV RNA/nucleic acid tests (HCV-RNA/NAT)							
Cepheid Xpert VL Assay (use with Cepheid GeneXpert)	Plasma samples, can be PoC	Same-day results in 108-110 min	HIV, TB	US$17,000 per instrument; US$14.90 per test (for all virological tests in LMICs)	WHO PQ, CE-marked, not approved in United States	-	Can be used for all genotypes; need WHO recommendations for use in all genotypes

(Table 2) cont.....

HCV Enzyme Immunoassay (HCV EIA)							
Test Name	**Sample Type/Setting**	**Turnaround Time**	**Multiplexing**	**Price**	**Regulatory Status**	**WHO PQ Review**	**Suitability**
Cepheid Xpert VL Fingerstick	100 μL, capillary blood, Fingerstick Tertiary PoC: harm reduction settings, maybe easier to give for some PWID with poor vein access	Within 60 min	HIV	ND	CE-IVD; Not FDA-approved	Modified version of the VL assay; CE-marked, not approved in United States	Tertiary PoC, harm reduction settings
Genedrive HCV RNA	30 μL plasma, serum	90 min	No	US$5000 per device; US$25-35 per test US$30-40/test in India US$14-18/test for Africa	CE-IVD	WHO PQ (May 2020)	PoC; Decentralized diagnosis
RealTime HCV Viral Load	0.5 mL plasma, 0.2 mL serum, DBS (FS)	ND	HIV	US$11–23 per test; Global Fund price varies according to test volume/term commitment	CE-IVD (for HIV DBS and HCV RNA)	WHO PQ	Lab HCV viral load, All six GTs detected
Abbott Alinity m HCV assay RNA	Plasma, serum	135 minutes	No	US$50 per test	FDA-approved in March 2020	CE-IVD, WHO PQ (March 2020)	Lab, clinical. All HCV GTs detected
Hologic Aptima HCV Quant	Serum, plasma	ND	HIV	US$10–15 per test; US$12 (€12–15) all-inclusive price for HCV VL	FDA- approved	-	CE-marked; Lab-based
Biocentric Generic HCV PCR assay	Serum, plasma	ND	HIV	US$23 per test, US$13.50-17 per test	-	-	CE-marked
Roche Cobas 6800/8800 systems (HCV RNA)	Lab-based, High volume clinical settings	First 96 results <3.5 hours, every 90 min for 96 more results (Cobas 6800 System); first 96 results <3.5 hours, every 30 min for 96 more results (Cobas 8800 System)	HIV	US$35–45 per test; US$340,000-US$475,000 per instrument (depending on instrument and volume)	-	-	CE-marked, FDA approved
HCV diagnostics in the pipeline							
ARCHITECT HCV cAg assay	Serum, DBS	ND		US$8-23	CE-IVD	WHO PQ	Lab
HCV Self-Test	Oral fluid, capillary blood	-	-	<US$4 per test	TK	-	PoC; sexual health clinics, harm reduction centers, at home
Well anti-HCV RDT; Self-Test	Oral	15-20 minutes		TK	TK	-	POC; primary care, at-home settings

(Table 2) cont.....

HCV Enzyme Immunoassay (HCV EIA)							
Test Name	**Sample Type/Setting**	**Turnaround Time**	**Multiplexing**	**Price**	**Regulatory Status**	**WHO PQ Review**	**Suitability**
TrueNAT HCV PCR	250 µL whole blood, 500 µL plasma	40 minutes	polyvalent	US$10,000 (small); US$14,000-18,000 (large) US$18 per test, depending on the volume	CDSCO-India approval in 2019;	CE-IVD and WHO PQ (Estimated in 2020)	POC; primary healthcare
COBAS® Plasma Separation Card	Whole blood, plasma, dried plasma spots	-	-	TK, GPRO range: US$10-15 per test Egypt (high-volume): US$7 per test	Not FDA approved	CE-IVD (for HIV only, in development for HCV in 2020/2021)	lab
DBS on various PCR platforms	0.2 mL serum DBS (finger stick)	-	-	TK	Real*Time* HCV Viral load, CE-IVD (for HIV DBS and HCV RNA); WHO PQ (Dec 2019) COBAS® AmpliPrep/COBAS TaqMan HCV Test CE-IVD (for HIV only) Aptima® HCV Quant Dx Assay (TK)	-	Lab

Hepatitis C Virus Rapid Diagnostics Tests (HCV-RDTs)

WHO guidance rules propose single, sensitive, and quality-based *in vitro* serological diagnostic tests including rapid diagnostic tests (RDTs) and immunoassays. RDTs serve as an alternative for scaling up HCV screening because they utilize numerous matrices like plasma, serum, finger sticks whole blood, or oral fluid (Tables **3** and **4**) [1, 5]. Advantages of RDTs include robust performance, simplicity, minimal training, and the least requirement of equipment. For various low- and middle-income countries (LMICs) where HCV diagnostic facilities are limited, RDTs may prove very effectual, as they are robust and easy to conduct without sophisticated laboratory equipment [1]. RDTs already have affirmed their efficiency in other disease areas like the detection of the human immunodeficiency virus (HIV) (Table **3**). The broad accessibility of low-cost RDTs for HIV has considerably improved access to diagnostic tests succeeding in > 600 million individuals being diagnosed with HIV in LMICs from the year 2010 to 2014 [4]. The unavailability of quality-based RDTs for HCV serology assays is an important limitation to large-scale accessibility to HCV detection [4]. Currently, multiple studies are being conducted for the evaluation of assorted HCV RDTs concerning percentage performance using clinical samples collected from a wide range of geographic regions. One of these studies included retrospective, observational and multicenter laboratory assessment of 13 HCV RDTs (Table **5**).

Table 3. Potential advantages and disadvantages of current HCV diagnostics [10, 43].

HCV screening/diagnostic Assay	Advantages	Disadvantages
Laboratory-based immunoassays (EIA, CLIA, ECL)	1. Currently superior clinical/diagnostic and analytical sensitivity/specificity for HCV Ags 2. High throughput possible (>40 per day operator) 3. High throughput is greater when used automated immunoanalysers 4. Objective, automated reading of results, but not for line blots or simple assays 5. Within-assay procedural quality control	1. Requires laboratory facilities, equipment, *e.g.*, EIA plate, washers, readers, incubators or immunoanalysers, or random-access analyzers 2. Requires trained laboratory technician 3. Reagents require refrigeration 4. Requires venepuncture to obtain a specimen 5. Time to result around 3 hrs and generally batched as one run if manual EIA
Rapid diagnostic tests (RDTs)	1. Accessible at the lowest level of the healthcare system (including community settings) 2. Does not specifically require laboratory facilities 3. May be carried out by trained lab providers and healthcare workers, as well as laboratory technicians. 4. Can be used with less invasive specimens that do not require venepuncture such as capillary whole blood or oral fluid 5. If testing at or near to point of care, same-day results are possible, which may reduce the number of individuals that are lost to follow-up and therefore do not receive their test results 6. Devices can be stored at 2-30 °C	1. Lower clinical and analytical sensitivity/specificity for HBsAg 2. Less sensitive in certain populations such as immunosuppressed, including HIV-positive individuals 3. Ineffective within-assay quality control, i.e. most RDTs do not control for specimen addition 4. Lack of test kit external control reagents for quality control with most RDTs, but some exceptions, *e.g.* Oraquick 5. Stability at room temperature is impacted by environmental factors, *e.g.* heat, humidity, storage conditions 6. Subjective reading and interpretation of results 7. Requires the manual transcription of testing results into laboratory logbook/testing register, partially mitigated by automated RDT readers
Nucleic acid testing (NAT) technologies	1. May be used at or near the point of care 2. May be carried out by trained lay providers and healthcare workers, as well as laboratory technicians 3. Can be used with less invasive specimens that do not require venepuncture such as capillary whole blood 4. Devices can be stored at 2 30 °C	1. Currently requires laboratory facilities and equipment, but this may not apply to future point-of-care options 2. Requires trained laboratory technician 3. Reagents require refrigeration 4. Requires venepuncture to obtain a specimen 5. Time to result in ~3 hours and generally batched as one

Table 4. An overview of populations most affected by HCV infection with a summary of risk factors, primary routes of transmission, and seroprevalence rates[10, 43].

Key and priority populations	Risk factors, primary routes of transmission, and seroprevalence rates of Hepatitis C
People who inject drugs (PWID)	1- High risk of infection through parenteral exposure, most commonly from sharing of needles and other injecting equipment. 2- Global prevalence estimated to be 67% among PWID in 77 countries and over 80% in 12 countries). Prevalence is particularly high in settings where PWID are criminalized and lack access to harm reduction services. 3- Non-injecting drug use, *e.g.* through intranasal drug use, has been associated with a small but increased risk of HCV infection.
People in prisons and closed settings	1- High risk of infection through parenteral exposure, most commonly from sharing of needles and razor blades, and other injecting equipment, particularly when safe injecting equipment is not available. 2- Potential for increased risk of sexual transmission due to unsafe sex behaviors, lack of availability of prevention hardware such as condoms, and higher risk of experiencing men-on-men sexual violence. 3- Estimated global prevalence ranges from 23% to 29%, with rates as high as 40% reported from some regions, including Australia, North America, Western Europe, Central Asia, and East and South-East Asia.
Mobile or migrant populations	1- Migrant populations represent a heterogeneous group and HCV seroprevalence estimates vary widely. 2- Some marginalized mobile populations may be more likely to belong to other populations at high risk for HBV and HCV transmissions, such as PWID or sex workers.
Indigenous populations	Some indigenous populations may be more likely to belong to other high-risk populations, such as PWID.
Sex workers	1- Overall, the risk of sexual transmission of HCV is low. There may be a small, increased risk of transmission among persons with multiple sex partners. 2- Sex workers may be more likely to belong to other high-risk populations, such as PWID and persons in prisons or closed settings.
Transgender people	Transgender people may be at increased risk for viral hepatitis through using unsafe injecting equipment for the administration of hormones or through sexual transmission.
Men who have sex with men (MSM)	1- The risk of sexual transmission of HCV is low among HIV-negative MSM. HIV-positive MSM is at significantly increased risk of sexual transmission of HCV, particularly those who engage in high-risk sex behaviors such as unprotected anal sex. 2- In several outbreaks of HCV infection among MSM in Europe, Australia, and the US, transmission has been linked to sexual exposure as well as potentially to underreported use of injecting and non-injecting recreational drugs.

(Table 4) cont.....

Health-care workers	1- The greatest proportion of occupational transmission of viral hepatitis is due to percutaneous injury via needles during vascular access. 2- Transmission may also occur through exposure to blood and body fluids on skin lesions and mucous membranes. 3- Multiple factors contribute to a higher risk of occupational acquisition in LMICs. These include: working among populations with a higher prevalence of infection, higher rates of unnecessary injections in healthcare settings, use of unsterilized needles and equipment lacking a needle-stick safety mechanism, lack of implementation of standard precautions, and inadequate coverage of HBV vaccination. 4- The risk of HCV infection after percutaneous exposure is estimated to be 1.8%.
Persons exposed to healthcare settings	1- High risk of parenteral transmission in settings with a higher background seroprevalence of HBV and HCV and where infection control practices are inadequate (*e.g.* diagnostic and therapeutic procedures), and blood transfusions and other tissue donations are not screened for viral hepatitis. 2- Persons who may have multiple exposures, such as patients with thalassemia or hemophilia who receive multiple transfusions, and patients on hemodialysis, are at higher risk.
Persons exposed via other invasive procedures	There is a small but increased risk of HBV and HCV transmission with other procedures where there is a risk of blood-to-blood transmission via contaminated equipment, including cosmetic procedures (such as tattooing and body piercing), and traditional medical procedures such as scarification and circumcision.
Persons living with HIV and those living with other sexually transmitted infections (STIs)	1- Particularly in high HBV and HCV-prevalence settings, children who have been exposed to HIV through mother-to-child transmission (MTCT) are at increased risk of HBV and HCV infection. 2- There is an increased risk of HCV infection among persons living with HIV.
Infants born to infected mothers	1- MTCT is the most common cause of HCV infection in young children. 2- The risk of HCV transmission is 4 8% in the perinatal period, and 10% 25% among children born to mothers coinfected with HIV.
Children	1- Based on limited data, horizontal transmission does not appear to be a significant contributor to HCV transmission in children. 2- High prevalence in some settings such as in children treated in hospital for malignancy, renal failure requiring hemodialysis, and those who have undergone surgical procedures likely reflects iatrogenic transmission.
Adolescents	1- Overall, the risk of sexual transmission of HCV is low. However, there is a small increased risk among persons with multiple sex partners. 2- Vulnerable adolescents may be more likely to belong to other high-risk key populations, including PWID and sex workers, for example.
Couples, partners, and household contacts	1- Overall, the risk of sexual transmission of HCV is low. However, the risk is increased among persons with multiple sex partners. 2- There is no evidence to support transmission among household contacts who are not sexual partners.

Table 5. Summary of diagnostic accuracy of different anti-HCV Abs RDTs with different assay formats and comparators, populations, specimen types, and oral kit brands[10, 43].

Comparison	Pooled Sensitivity (95% CI)	Pooled Specificity (95% CI)
Assay format and comparators		
RDT versus EIA only (N=5)	99 (98 100)	100 (100 100)
RDT versus NAT or immunoblot (N=13)	93 (91 95)	98 (97 99)
RDT versus EIA, NAT, or immunoblot (N=14)	97 (96 98)	100 (100 100)
Antibody and antigen combo testing (N=6)	86 (79 94)	99 (98 100)
Populations (RDT versus EIA, NAT, or immunoblot)		
General population (N=17)	95 (94 96)	99 (98 99)
Key populations (N=19)	97 (96 98)	94 (94 95)
Hospital patients (N=16)	97 (96 98)	100 (100 100)
Specimen type (RDT vs EIA, NAT, or immunoblot)		
Blood specimens (N=45)	98 (97 98)	98 (98 99)
Oral fluid specimens (N=12)	94 (93 96)	100 (100 100)
Oral RDT versus blood reference (N=12)	94 (93 96)	99.9 (99.8 100)
Oral kit brands		
OraQuick (N=8)	98 (97 99)	100 (100 100)
Other brands (Chembio DPP, BIioeasy, ImmunoComb II (N=6)	88 (84 92)	99 (99 100)
EIA: enzyme immunoassay; NAT: nucleic acid test; RDT: rapid diagnostic test		

Vetter *et al.* evaluated two lots of 13 RDTs in three different laboratories using HIV-co-infected and uninfected clinical samples collected from four different countries (Cambodia, Georgia, Belgium, and Nigeria). For HIV-uninfected samples, sensitivity for most of the RDTs was ≥ 98% in one or both lots, and the majority of the RDTs had ≥ 99% specificity. While in HIV co-infected samples, high specificity accompanied by lower sensitivity was elucidated as compared to HIV-uninfected samples [9]. In a study performed by Mane *et al.*, five HCV RDTs (OraQuick™, Advanced Quality Flaviscreen™, Alere Truline™, and SD Bioloine™) were analyzed using two trial groups of known HCV positive and negative samples. The one-trial group included Indian patient samples and the other comprised samples obtained from the US Centers for Disease Control and Prevention (CDC), Atlanta. Overall sensitivities for both trial groups for all five RDTs were ≥ 86.2% on average. Combined specificities for both trial groups for all five RDTs were found 99.7%. Inter-observer variability for all five RDTs was ≥ 98.6% [4]. Another study done by Kabamba *et al.* evaluated the analytical performance of six RDTs for HCV detection and 100% sensitivity and negative predictive value (NPV) was achieved followed by a range of 46%-98.1% specificity and positive predictive value (PPV). Moreover, for SB BioLine HCV detection test specificity, sensitivity, NPV, and PPV parameters were found ≥ 93.9% [10]. Conclusively, RDTs could help in HCV diagnosis more expeditiously and essential to the scale-up screening of HCV.

Hepatitis C Point-of-Care Testing (HCV-POCT)

HCV Point-of-care tests (POCTs) are rapid and simple with approachable results thereby they can provide the opportunity to expand HCV screening efforts [11]. Likewise, the detection of antibodies in oral fluid is relatively a cost-effective, non-invasive, much more convenient, and safer method as compared to serum collection and diagnostic testing [12]. Accordingly, POCTs are developed for the diagnosis of antibodies in the oral fluid that includes OraQuick®, a rapid test for HCV antibody detection [4]. The high sensitivity and specificity of OraQuick® for the detection of HCV antibodies have been demonstrated after testing in the United States, Europe, South Korea, and many other countries of the world [13, 14]. Jiangsu Well Biotech Co., Ltd. has developed the Well oral anti-HCV assay® which is designed to detect HCV antibodies in oral fluids with the characteristics of low cost and simplicity [15]. Liu *et al.* evaluated the performance of a new point-of-care oral anti-HCV diagnostic test in terms of its potential utility specifically in the areas of limited resources. The Well anti-HCV assay® exhibited a specificity of 98% and sensitivity of 91.8%. The consistency between InTec® and the Well assays was found as 97% while the consistency between OraQuick and the Well assays was 97%. In addition, self-testing results were found consistent with the researcher-administered tests [15]. Recently, Kimble *et al.* analytically assessed a better efficiency of the OraQuick® HCV diagnostic test with self-collected oral fluid [16]. Research findings depict the Well oral anti-HCV assay® as user-friendly and might be used for HCV self-testing [4].

Hepatitis C Core (C) Antigen Detection Assay

The gold standard HCV diagnostic algorithm depends on preliminary antibody testing followed by an HCV RNA test for confirmation of viral replication [16]. Core antigen testing for HCV (HCVcAg), as a substitute for RNA replication test; reveals the potency in reducing HCV detection costs if it illustrates sensitivity and specificity without needing PCR testing [17]. Due to cost-effectiveness, the HCV core antigen test is recommended for employment in LMICs [18]. Currently, limited data are available regarding the efficiency of core antigen testing for its implementation in routine testing. At present, worldwide various research groups are carried out for analysis of HC core antigen performance (Table **6**). A recent study by Pollock *et al.* evaluated the use of HCV core antigen assay to detect active infection among HCV antibody-positive individuals while introducing it in the routine testing scheme. The assay sensitivity of 82.1% and specificity of 99.8% for HCV core antigen (HCVcAg) as a diagnostic tool was demonstrated by Pollock *et al.* in one study [19]. Another recent study by Catlett *et al.* evaluated the sensitivity and specificity of HCVcAg assay for the detection of active HCV infection in capillary whole blood dried blood spots (DBS) and plasma specimens in comparison to viral RNA testing in plasma samples (Abbott RealTime® HCV viral load). Sensitivity for HCVcAg detection to identify active infection in plasma was 98.1% and 100% when comparing with viral RNA thresholds of ≥12 and ≥1000 IU/mL respectively. The sensitivity for the diagnosis of active viral infection through HCVcAg assay in DBS was 90.7% and 92.5% when correlated with viral RNA thresholds of ≥12 and ≥1000 IU/mL respectively. Specificity for active infection detection through HCVcAg was 100% for all clinical samples and RNA thresholds [20]. Research data indicate that HCVcAg testing could be a useful diagnostic tool for the detection of active HCV infection as prompt extensive testing, linkage to care, and therapy management specifically when plasma samples are collected by venipuncture [20]. Daktari diagnostics (Boston, USA) developed the method for HCVcAg detection that might specifically be correlated for assay specification in many LMICs. This diagnostic system is based on microfluidic principles and would help in analyzing a drop of blood in a single cartridge within 30 minutes [21]. Patients can get their test results just in one visit thus assisting their access to HCV diagnosis. Concisely, HCVcAg detection from plasma samples employing Abbott® HCV Ag testing might be detected with high specificity and sensitivity in comparison to gold standard Abbott® HCV RNA assay.

Table 6. Summary of diagnostic accuracy of different HCV core antigen assays compared to nucleic acid tests (NATs) [10, 43].

Index test	Sample size (range)	Diagnostic accuracy (95% CI)	
		Sensitivity	Specificity
Abbott Diagnostics GmbH, ARCHITECT HCV Ag Assay	20 (11 820)	93.4% (88.7 96.2)	98.7% (96.9 99.4)
Ortho-Clinical Diagnostics, Ortho ELISA-Ag	5 (1 177)	93.2% (81.6 97.7)	99.2% (87.9 99.9)
Bio-RAD Monolisa HCV Ag-Ab ULTRA	5 (525)	28.6 95%[a]	94.9% (89.9 99.8)[b]
EIKEN Lumispot HCV Ag	2 (235)	97.5 98.1%[a]	ND
Fujirebio Lumipulse Ortho HCV Ag	1 (80)	95% (90.2 99.8)[b]	ND
Hunan Jynda HCV Core Ag ELISA	4 (524)	59.5% (46 71.7)	82.9% (58.6 94.3)

(Table 6) cont.....

DiaSorin S.A. Murex HCV Ag/Ab	4 (730)	50 100%[a]	83.8 100%[a]
CI: confidence interval; ND = no data. [a]Meta-analysis not possible. Range of results seen across studies reported. [b]Result from one study only.			

Nanocomposites as Hepatitis C Diagnostic Approach

Another important and advanced parameter for the theragnosis of HCV is nanotechnology specifically representing to POCT system due to the least requirement of sample volume and equipment besides their time-affordability, sensitivity, and cost-effectiveness. This paper-based diagnostic system does not exhibit transport and storage issues [22, 23]. In a study performed by Ghanbari *et al.*, a sensitive aptamer conjugated graphene quantum dots (GQD) nanocomposite diagnostic system was developed. The electrochemical impedance spectroscopy (EIS) scheme was used to implement GQDs as nanoconjugates for the ultrasensitive diagnosis of HCVcAg with a detection limit of 3.3 pg/mL [24]. Such aptasensor-based nanocomposites might serve as a specific, sensitive, and rapid detection system for the HCVcAg diagnosis and can provide a potent strategy in clinical diagnosis. Roh *et al.* developed a potent diagnostic approach for the detection of HCV NS3 protein using a nanocomposite-encapsulated aptamer probe. Using quantum dots with the carboxylic group as the imaging probe and 5'-amino group-modified RNA oligomer as capturing probe, HCV NS3 was detected visually on the chip. Such nanoparticle-based RNA aptamer conjugating systems possess high specificity and sensitivity with a 5 ng/mL detection limit for NS3 protein [25]. However, limited data are available regarding HCV detection through nanotheragnosis. Further research might enhance the utilization of nanotechnology tools in clinical diagnostics.

Hepatitis C Detection in Dried Blood Spot (DBS) Samples

Remarkable scaling up in HCV diagnostics is dependent upon numerous parameters including the detection process, facilitation regarding access to diagnostics specifically in remote areas with limited access, and among more susceptible populations like people who inject drugs (PWIDs) and prisoners (Table **7**) [26]. DBS sampling provides an alternative sample collection procedure through capillary finger sticks or heel pricking in infants. DBS sampling involves the embedding of blood drops upon filter paper and can further be transported to a diagnostic place or laboratory [27]. The ease of sample collection, transport, and storage devices make DBS specimens a potential alternative for gold standard diagnostic algorithms (Table **8**). In a study done by Lange *et al.*, diagnostic performance was evaluated for DBS samples versus venous blood samples for the detection of HCV RNA.

Table 7. HCV specimen collection, storage, and time to testing [10, 43].

Specimen type	Time to processing/storage/time to testing
Venous whole blood Fresh whole blood collected by venepuncture	Use the specimen immediately.
Serum Freshly collected whole blood is allowed to coagulate, and serum fraction is collected away from the clotted red blood cells.	1- Collect whole blood, mix by hand 4 5 times immediately and let stand for the clot to form. 2- Process within 30 minutes of collection. 3- Store at 2 8 °C. Test within 5 days or as specified by the instructions for the assay to be used.
Plasma Freshly collected whole blood is added to the recommended anticoagulant, such as EDTA, heparin, or citrate. After centrifugation, the plasma is separated.	1- Collect whole blood, mix by hand 8 10 times immediately and centrifuge for up to 10 minutes. 2- Process within 6 hours of collection. 3- Store at 2 8 °C. Test within 5 days or as specified by the instructions for the assay to be used.
Capillary whole blood Capillary (finger-stick) whole blood is collected using a lancet and a specimen transfer device.	1- Use the specimen immediately, with the specimen transfer device recommended by the instructions for use. 2- Note that the specimen transfer device may or may not include an anticoagulant. An anticoagulant contributes to accuracy.
Oral fluid Oral mucosal transudate (not saliva) is collected from the gums using a collection device.	Use the specimen immediately, with the specimen transfer device recommended in the instructions for use.
Dried blood spot (DBS) Venous or capillary whole blood is applied to a filter paper by hanging drop or microcapillary action. Whole blood is later eluted from the filter paper and used for the test procedure.	1- Store at 4 °C for up to 3 months, or at 20 °C for longer. 2- Use of specific assays with DBS should be validated by the manufacturer. If the manufacturer has not validated their assay for DBS, the use of DBS is considered "off-label", or unauthorized for returning medical results.

Table 8. Potential advantages and disadvantages of HCV DBS testing [10, 43].

Benefits	Challenges and Concerns
Ease of specimen collection. DBS specimen collection involves pricking a finger or a heel without the need for venepuncture, and so avoids the need for a trained health worker.	**Storage conditions.** Few studies have systematically examined the effects of storage and transport conditions on the accuracy of results from DBS specimens. However, some data suggest that there may be instability of results when stored for prolonged durations (more than 14 days) at high temperatures (room temperature and above) and humidity, particularly for serological testing.

(Table 8) cont.....

Ease of sample transport. Specimen transport and logistics are simplified as, apart from the advantage of avoiding venepuncture, DBS specimen handling does not require high skill, and the biohazard risk is thought to be less.	**Manufacturers' validation.** Most manufacturers have not validated the use of their commercial assays with DBS specimens. In particular, procedures for the pre-analytical treatment of specimens are not standardized, such as the type of filter paper, volume of capillary whole blood to be used, type of elution buffer, and elution procedure. The impact on assay performance is uncertain but may result in potentially lower sensitivity/specificity.
Minimal training required. When DBS specimens are used for serological testing, the need for training in how to use and interpret RDTs is eliminated. Lay providers can be trained to take capillary whole blood samples without having to be trained in the use and reading of RDTs.	**Lack of assays with regulatory approval.** At present, there are few if any assays that have regulatory approval for the use of DBS as a specimen type for any HBsAg, anti-HCV, HBV DNA, or HCV RNA assay.
Facility to allow multiplex testing. Multiplex testing of multiple diseases may be possible, such as HIV/HBV/HCV in combination using the same DBS specimen card. Both serological testing and NAT can be conducted from multiple spots on the same DBS card at the same laboratory, thereby avoiding the need for collecting a second sample from the patient.	**Assay cut-offs.** The use of a DBS specimen may require adjustment of the assay cut-off to determine test positivity for serological screening, as DBS specimens use a small volume of blood.
-	**Laboratory capacity.** The actual laboratory work can be more difficult with a DBS specimen compared to a serum/plasma specimen, because it involves manual specimen processing, and requires a laboratory experienced in and competent at handling and processing these specimens. It also involves the need to maintain quality assurance of testing a specimen potentially off-label from the manufacturers' validated specimen types.

The consolidated specificity and sensitivity of HCV RNA detection for DBS specimens was 98% for both [28]. However, there is a need to develop standard protocols by manufacturers for the utilization of DBS sampling with their assays. Another study performed by Lange *et al.* elucidated the diagnostic accuracy for the detection of HCV antibodies from DBS specimens in comparison to venous samples. Pooled specificity and sensitivity were 99% and 98% respectively while the overall quality and heterogeneity of the study were reported as moderate [29]. Vázquez-Morón *et al.* performed a meta-analysis study for HCV screening in DBS samples. For HCV antibodies detection consolidated diagnostic accuracy estimates were found a specificity of 99.2%, sensitivity of 96.1%, PPV of 105, and NPV of 0.04 with a diagnostic odds ratio (DOR) of 2692.9. For HCV RNA detection, pooled diagnostic accuracy measures were found a specificity of 99.2%, a sensitivity of 97.8%, a PPV of 44.8, NPV of 0.04 with a diagnostic odds ratio (DOR) of 1966.9 [30].

In short, HCV testing in DBS specimens exhibits remarkable diagnostic efficiency without detecting any difference between the techniques used for DBS and gold-standard testing (Tables **9** and **10**). However, external validity is required for their use in commercial diagnostics. In a study performed by Catlett *et al.*, aptima® HCV Quant Dx assay was evaluated for HCV RNA detection from DBS and venepuncture collected specimens. The sensitivity and specificity of the Aptima® assay for HCV RNA detection from DBS samples were 95.6% and 94.1% while RNA quantification sensitivity and specificity were 100% for both [31]. To summarize the above, Aptima® Quant assay effectively detects active viral infection from DBS that is clinically in proportionate to plasma specimens.

Table 9. WHO listed recommendations of HCV DBS testing for serological and virological screening and diagnosis of hepatitis C[10, 43].

Topic	Recommendations*
Serological testing	The use of DBS specimens for HBsAg and HCV antibody serology testing1 may be considered in settings where: - There are no facilities or expertise to take venous whole blood specimens; or - RDTs are not available or their use is not feasible; or - There are persons with poor venous access (*e.g.* in drug treatment programs, and prisons). Conditional recommendation, moderate (HBV)/low (HCV) quality of evidence
Detection of viremia (nucleic acid testing)	The use of DBS specimens to test for HBV DNA and HCV RNA for diagnosis of HBV and HCV viraemia[1], respectively, may be considered in settings where: - There is a lack of access to sites or nearby laboratory facilities for NAT, or provision for timely delivery of specimens to a laboratory; or - There are persons with poor venous access (*e.g.* in drug treatment programs, and prisons). Conditional recommendation, low (HBV)/moderate (HCV) quality of evidence

(Table 9) cont.....

Uptake of testing and linkage to care	• All facility- and community-based hepatitis testing services should adopt and implement strategies to enhance the uptake of testing and linkage to care. Strong recommendation, moderate quality of evidence • The following evidence-based interventions should be considered to promote the uptake of hepatitis testing and linkage to care and treatment initiation: (Conditional recommendations) -**Peer and lay health worker support in community-based settings** (moderate quality of evidence). -**Clinician reminders** to prompt provider-initiated, facility-based HBV and HCV testing in settings that have electronic records or analogous reminder systems (very low quality of evidence). -**Provision of hepatitis testing as part of integrated services** within mental health/substance use services (very low quality of evidence).
*The GRADE system (Grading of Recommendations, Assessment, Development, and Evaluation) was used to categorize the strength of recommendations as strong or conditional (based on consideration of the quality of evidence, the balance of benefits and harms, acceptability, resource use, and programmatic feasibility) and the quality of evidence as high, moderate, low or very low. [1]Well-functioning laboratory specimens referral network and system for the return of results should be in place to maximize the impact of DBS specimens. There are currently few assays where the manufacturer's instructions state that DBS specimens are validated for use. Therefore, currently, the use of DBS specimens would be considered "off-label".	

Table 10. Diagnostic performance of DBS specimens for serological and nucleic acid testing (NAT) of HBV and HCV [10, 43].

	DBS for HBsAg	DBS for anti-HCV	DBS for HBV DNA[1]	DBS for HCV RNA
No. of included studies	10 (SR), 9 (meta-anal)	18 (SR), 14 (meta-anal)	10 (SR), 9 (meta-anal)	9 (SR & meta-anal)
Total sample size	2481	4524	608	1250
Overall pooled sensitivity (95% CI)	92.9% [86.2 96.5]	98% [94 99]	96% [90 98]	96.0% [93.4 97.6]
Overall pooled specificity (95% CI)	99.0% [96.2 99.7]	99% [97 100]	99% [55 100]	97.7% [94.7 99.0]
Impact of storage	Cold chain: SN 78.7% [70 85] SP: 98.6% [68 100] ≥RT: SN: 96.1% [92 98] SP: 99.7% [98 100]	Storage at 20 °C associated with less variation compared to RT	Not possible to calculate because all accuracy studies conducted at 20 °C	Better result at 20 °C compared to RT; conflicting results re deterioration of sample at RT

(Table 10) cont.....

Impact of duration of storage	Accuracy not affected if RT for ≤15 days (1 study) or 63 days (another study)	Accuracy not affected if RT for ≤3 days (1 study) or ≤6 days (another study) or ≤60 days (another study)	No effect on accuracy if 4 37 °C for ≤7 days (2 studies)	Conflicting results re- deterioration over time
DBS: dried blood spot; meta-anal: meta-analysis; RT: room temperature; SN: sensitivity; SP specificity; SR: systematic review [1]HBV DNA testing is not recommended for ruling out HBV infection if HBsAg is positive. HBV DNA detection can be used to explore occult HBV infection in persons testing negative for HBsAg. A large proportion of HBV-infected persons have a low HBV replication level (inactive carriers).				

Multi-disease Analyzers

Multi-disease analyzers are used to perform integrated diagnosis of HCV along with other pathogens like syphilis and HIV. Low sample volume and efficiency for the detection of multiple pathogens at the same time make this technique favorable. Multiple RDTs are in the process of development for anti-HCV/ant--HIV, anti-HCV/HBsAg, and anti-HCV/syphilis/anti-HIV Ags detections [32]. More research data are required to depict their diagnostic sensitivity and specificity before their implementation. Generally, they are suitable for provincial and national level laboratories, as the recent multiplex analyzers require some precision steps, plasma/serum samples, proper electricity, and equipment maintenance.

REAL-WORLD CHALLENGES TO IMPLEMENT CURRENT HEPATITIS C DIAGNOSTICS AND PLAUSIBLE SOLUTIONS

Though multiple diagnostic strategies are being discovered for the detection of active HCV infection, still gaps remain in diagnostic systems specifically for LMICs. From the above discussion, it is evident that research efforts are equally contributing to developing robust, simplified, and cost-effective clinical diagnostic tools to counteract the health care and financial burden of HCV. Hereby, it is necessary to highlight those multiple factors that are causing hindrances in achieving the WHO-set goals for HCV diagnosis worldwide to eliminate the hepatitis C pandemic by 2030.

Millions of HCV Infected are Still Undiagnosed

Besides the remarkable disease burden of HCV and HIV-HCV coinfection, and the availability of advanced therapeutic options, most of the patients coinfected with HIV-HCV remain unaware and undiagnosed for their infection [5]. Data depicts that not more than 5% of HCV-infected individuals know their disease status specifically in LMICs this is much lower (*i.e.* < 1%) [1, 3]. This approximation is much lower for different populations like PWIDs, sex workers, and prisoners to whom access to diagnosis and treatment is already difficult [1]. Hence, there are several key challenges to the implementation of current HCV screening and diagnostic testing schemes (Fig. **1**). There are some major issues specific to HCV diagnosis in consideration of HIV coinfection. Coinfection leads to the rapid progression of liver disease into advanced stages like cirrhosis and liver cancer (*i.e.* HCC), especially in those who have low $CD4^+$ cell count. In HCV/HIV coinfected patients, HIV lowers the $CD4^+$ count in the body as a result, the HCV antibody screening test produces false-negative results. In the case of coinfection, earlier-generation HCV serological assays produce false positives and false negatives [1, 6]. Sufficient data regarding the performance of RDTs for HCV screening in coinfected patients are not available. Further studies are required to see the impact of multiple biological parameters of HIV positivity upon the specificity and sensitivity of HCV serological assays specifically RDTs and also to validate RDTs and EIAs with simplified and less invasive sample collection methods like DBS and oral fluid *etc.*

HOW TO TEST FOR CHRONIC HCV INFECTION AND MONITOR TREATMENT RESPONSE

Topic	Recommendations
Which serological assays to use	• To test for serological evidence of past or present infection in adults, adolescents and children (>18 months of age[1]), an HCV serological assay (antibody or antibody/antigen) using either RDT or laboratory-based immunoassay formats[2] that meet minimum safety, quality and performance standards[3] (*with regard to both analytical and clinical sensitivity and specificity*) is recommended. - In settings where there is limited access to laboratory infrastructure and testing, and/or in populations where access to rapid testing would facilitate linkage to care and treatment, RDTs are recommended. *Strong recommendation, low/moderate quality of evidence*
Serological testing strategies	In adults and children older than 18 months[1], a single serological assay for initial detection of serological evidence of past or present infection is recommended prior to supplementary nucleic acid testing (NAT) for evidence of viraemic infection. *Conditional recommendation, low quality of evidence*
Detection of viraemic infection	• Directly following a reactive HCV antibody serological test result, the use of quantitative or qualitative NAT for detection of HCV RNA is recommended as the preferred strategy to diagnose viraemic infection. *Strong recommendation, moderate/low quality of evidence* • An assay to detect HCV core (p22) antigen, which has comparable clinical sensitivity to NAT, is an alternative to NAT to diagnose viraemic infection.[4] *Conditional recommendation, moderate quality of evidence*
Assessment of HCV treatment response	• Nucleic acid testing for qualitative or quantitative detection of HCV RNA should be used as test of cure at 12 or 24 weeks (i.e. sustained virological response (SVR12 or SVR24)) after completion of antiviral treatment. *Conditional recommendation, moderate/low quality of evidence*

Abbreviations: DBS: dried blood spot; IVD: in vitro diagnostics; NAT: nucleic acid test; RDT: rapid diagnostic test

* The GRADE system (Grading of Recommendations, Assessment, Development and Evaluation) was used to categorize the strength of recommendations as strong or conditional (based on consideration of the quality of evidence, balance of benefits and harms, acceptability, resource use and programmatic feasibility) and the quality of evidence as high, moderate, low or very low.

[1] HCV infection can be confirmed in children under 18 months only by virological assays to detect HCV RNA, because transplacental maternal antibodies remain in the child's bloodstream up until 18 months of age, making test results from serology assays ambiguous.
[2] Laboratory-based immunoassays include enzyme immunoassay (EIA), chemoluminescence immunoassay (CLIA), and electrochemoluminescence assay (ECL).
[3] Assays should meet minimum acceptance criteria of either WHO prequalification of IVDs or a stringent regulatory review for IVDs. All IVDs should be used in accordance with manufacturers' instructions, and where possible at testing sites enrolled in a national or international external quality assessment scheme.
[4] A lower level of analytical sensitivity can be considered, if an assay is able to improve access (i.e. an assay that can be used at the point of care or suitable for dried blood spot (DBS) specimens) and/or affordability. An assay with a limit of detection of 3000 IU/mL or lower would be acceptable and would identify 95% of those with viraemic infection, based on available data.

Fig. (1). Screening and diagnostic approaches for current or past HCV infection (HCV exposure) identification and monitoring treatment response [43].

A Need for Short Turnaround Time Diagnostic Platforms for Mass HCV Screening Campaigns

As mentioned above, the biggest challenge for HCV diagnostics is the majority of persons remain undiagnosed. Pragmatic diagnostic strategies are required to test services specifically in countries with limited resources and high HCV prevalence. Mass Testing campaigns are required to upraise awareness of diagnosis and identify infected persons. The recently approved point-of-care Xpert HCV Viral Load® test is based on sample collection *via* venepuncture with a time of 2 hrs for results. The 2nd generation iteration of this test includes the cartridge for the sample collection *via* finger-stick and result interpretations in one hour with increased specificity and sensitivity [7]. However, this improved testing is not yet clinically approved and further studies are required to build up robust HCV RNA tests getting results in 5-10 minutes considering low-cost RNA detection strategies. Robust clinical assessment and approval for potent diagnostic tools are required to make a step forward in novel diagnostic discoveries that ultimately translate into daily clinical practice. However, this is a challenging situation for diagnostic companies with limited resources and numerous contending priorities but they need to find avenues to boost clinical trials and make efforts for diagnostic approval through collaborations with their stakeholders.

Costs of HCV Screening and Diagnostic Platforms in LMICs

For LMICs to achieve WHO targets to improve diagnosis for HCV elimination, the cost of the diagnostic tests must be dropped down. In many countries, the process of HCV testing exceeds the cost of HCV treatment [1, 7]. So, the cost and access to diagnostic facilities are major challenges in resources limited and developing countries. Numerous diagnostic companies offer discounts for diagnosis specifically in disease-burden areas. Therefore, streamlined strategies are required to provide low-cost diagnostic kits to LMICs while maintaining facilities for companies to spend on diagnostics for sale in medium- and high-income regions of the world [33]. Quality assurance of HCV RNA POCTs along with their linkage to central laboratories is another critical challenge. The availability of trained staff for the assessment of POCT quality is required (Fig. **2**). Where possible, linkage of POCTs to local centralized laboratories accompanied by existing diagnostic expertise and a long-standing history of conducting quality assurance programs may provide the solution to set out quality assurance [34].

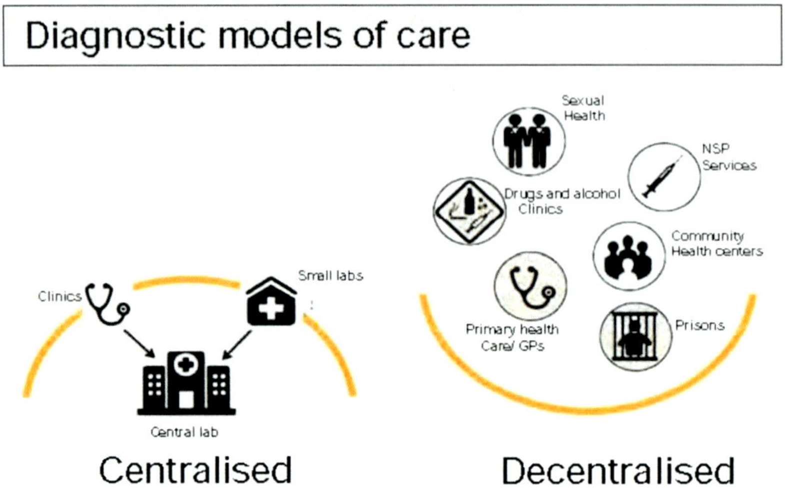

Fig. (2). A comparison of centralized and decentralized diagnostic models of care [35]. Decentralized diagnostic models of care are handier to integrate HCV diagnostics and care under one umbrella while reducing testing and treatment costs as well as decreasing multiple visits and follow-ups.

DBS testing has proved to enhance HCV diagnosis but some disadvantages make this technique less favorable. DBS diagnostic tool needs to be performed in centralized well-equipped laboratories and requires more than one visit to get results [1, 36]. This is again a major barrier in distant areas and among at-risk populations like PWIDs, MSM, sex workers, and inmates. Moreover, less specimen volumes are involved with several pricks and sometimes this may result in lower HCV RNA titre that ultimately affects the sensitivity of the assay.

HCV RNA POC Test With Good Accuracy in Real-world Clinical Practice

Hepatitis C RNA point-of-care (HCV-RNA POC) tests that can detect active hepatitis C infection from a finger-stick sample in less than two hours showed good sensitivity, accuracy, and specificity in a multicenter study [7]. The Xpert® HCV Viral Load test (Cepheid, Sunnyvale, Calif) represents an advance over current antibody-based tests, which indicate only past exposure to HCV. The test can detect HCV RNA in capillary whole blood collected by finger-stick and in plasma collected by venipuncture [7]. An open observational cohort study conducted at five sites including three drug and alcohol clinics, one homelessness service, and one needle and syringe program (NSP) revealed the efficacy of the Xpert® HCV Viral Load test in real-life experience [1]. The study recruited participants aged 18 or older and either with a history of injection drug use or recruited from the homelessness service. The final analysis population of 150 participants had a median age of 44. Most patients (87%) were male. The sensitivity of the Xpert® HCV Viral Load assay for HCV RNA detection in plasma collected by venipuncture was 100.0% and the specificity was 99.1%. The assay's sensitivity for HCV RNA detection in samples collected by finger-stick was 95.5% and specificity was 98.1%. The Abbot RealTime® HCV Viral Load RNA assay was used as the gold standard against which the Xpert HCV Viral Load was compared. A modified Xpert HCV Viral Load assay is under development with a time to result of 60 minutes [1]. The study results were encouraging, albeit; the performance of the test was noticed as poorer in clinical settings than in the laboratory. However; instead of that 25% of people will spontaneously clear their hepatitis C infection, the availability of RNA POC test to detect hepatitis C infection represents a major advance over previous hepatitis C POC tests which only test for exposure to the virus [1].

The purpose of this initiative is to move toward low-cost and rapid tests for detecting active hepatitis C infection in low-income countries where the cost of screening is a big barrier to large improvements in hepatitis C diagnosis [1]. Furthermore, the testing principle of the kit by collecting whole blood by finger-stick is particularly appropriate for populations with a high prevalence of hepatitis C infection. This on-spot testing is feasible and opportunistic to engage people in testing who are highly marginalized, as well as linkage to care, and treatment in a single visit which may reduce drop-outs along the hepatitis C cascade of care [1]. However; the test is not yet approved in many countries and further studies are needed to evaluate the assay in different settings and populations like patients given IFN-free DAAs therapy, those with SVR rates, or those with HIV/HCV co-infection. Though not ideal, a turnaround time of fewer than two hours can overcome the problem of patients not returning to the testing site for their results, and the waiting time can be used for HCV education and harm-reduction activities [1]. Furthermore, rapid testing enables immediate action for those hepatitis C patients who are often lost to follow-up or who are living with the transient nature of hepatitis C infection while the patient is temporarily engaged in the healthcare system. Another advantage of the Xpert® HCV Viral Load POC test is that it does not rely only on antibodies [1]. The sine qua non of HCV diagnosis is the detection of viremia in the form of HCV RNA, but such a POC test has been lacking until now. It is a 'potentially field-ready test' and could be especially important in LMICs. Though refinements are still needed, it would be ideal to shave the time down, so the patient could leave with a care plan in place. In addition to that, the RNA POC test can reduce the impact of some of the substantial obstacles that keep hepatitis C-infected individuals from accessing care, including the shortcomings of current diagnostic tests [1].

HCV-antigens EIA Detects Viremic Hepatitis C Virus Infection

A new one-step enzyme immunoassay (EIA) can reliably diagnose viremic hepatitis C infection [37]. The current hepatitis C screening requires a two-step testing process that is suboptimal, time-consuming, and not widely available or affordable globally. This new method is based on four HCV nonstructural protein antigens which were tested in 176 serum specimens without and 189 with viremic HCV infection [6, 37]. The test proved to have a sensitivity of 100% for detecting acute or chronic viremic hepatitis C infection, with positive test results detected 59 to 65 days before the appearance of anti-HCV antibodies [6]. Results were similar in denatured and non-denatured serum samples. Specificity was 99% using non-denatured serum specimens, but 88.6% using denatured serum specimens. The positive predictive value was 99% for the non-denaturation method and 90.4% for the denaturation method, whereas the negative predictive value was 100% for both methods [6]. Furthermore, the HCV-antigens EIA test is well correlated to hepatitis C replication as determined by serum HCV RNA RT-PCR. In addition to that, its sensitivity is superior to those reported for HCV core antigen assays. The assay also offers improved specificity by excluding sample denaturation and provides a highly specific and reliable one-step test to screen and diagnose hepatitis C infection [6].

HCV Core Antigen Could be Cost-Saving Alternative for Diagnosing Hepatitis C

HCV-core-antigen testing is a cost-saving alternative to HCV RNA testing for diagnosing hepatitis C infection, according to a retrospective study [38]. The study validates the recommendations of WHO and the European Association for the Study of the Liver (EASL) to use the core (C) antigen in place of HCV RNA, particularly in regions where cost is a major consideration. It can be reliably used to confirm the presence or absence of infection and can be used for treatment monitoring when it is required [6]. HCV core antigen is more stable at room temperature than HCV RNA, allowing for unrefrigerated transport. It can be tested on the same platform that is used for HCV antibodies [38]. HCV-RNA testing by reverse-transcription quantitative PCR is also more expensive. The researchers sought to determine if HCV core antigen could be used for confirmation of HCV infection in HCV antibody-positive samples, as well as for on-treatment monitoring and assessment of treatment response in samples from patients treated with DAAs [1]. In more than 10,000 screening samples, the HCV core antigen was 94% sensitive and 100% specific for confirming viremia [1].

The diagnostic performance of HCV core antigen among patients receiving antiviral treatment varied at different treatment time points [39]. Sensitivity ranged from 34.6% at four weeks of treatment to 50.0% at the end of treatment, 98.2% at follow-up week 12, and 100% at follow-up week 24. Specificity ranged from 86.6% at four weeks to 97.5% at the end of treatment, 97.7% at follow-up week 12, and 100% at follow-up week 24 [38, 39]. Based on these estimates, a screening program in which HCV core antigen replaced HCV-RNA testing for confirmation of viremia in patients who test positive for HCV antibodies would save 0.22 US dollars per person screened [39]. If negative HCV-core-antigen results excluded the need for HCV-RNA testing for confirmation, the savings would amount to 2.81 US dollars per patient screened [39]. The use of confirmatory HCV-RNA testing for samples that test negative for HCV core antigen would cost an estimated 19,325 US dollars per quality-adjusted life-year (QALY), still well within most willingness-to-pay thresholds [38]. However, the patients who test hepatitis C-antibody positive but hepatitis C-core-antigen negative should consider having a hepatitis C RNA RT-PCR to confirm the absence of infection [39]. This approach is important for a small percentage of people who have the infection but will test core-antigen negative. However, for widespread screening in LMICs, hepatitis C testing is reasonable to confirm infection only, with significant potential cost savings by avoiding hepatitis C RNA testing [1]. The overall performance of the hepatitis C core antigen test was found impressive in this study [38]; however, few discordant results were noted at the time of SVR12. SVR12 is a point that determines the cure of a hepatitis C patient treated with DAAs at post-completion of therapy at week 12. In almost all cases, the hepatitis C core antigen test agreed with HCV-RNA results at SVR 12; however, the risk that someone is incorrectly deemed to be cured or scheduled for unnecessary retreatment is obviously a concern [38]. For this reason, HCV RNA detection at 3 months post-treatment would still be prudent to determine whether an individual is cured. However; this testing approach would provide optimism for a major simplification and scale-up of hepatitis C screening and treatment worldwide [39]. It was also found that this approach can also be used as an alternative to HCV-RNA testing as a marker of viremia. This means that in resource-limited settings where molecular tests to detect hepatitis C virus are neither affordable nor accessible (because of a lack of laboratories that can perform such assays), more HCV-antibody-positive patients can now be tested to determine if they require treatment (Fig. **3**). It would be helpful for immediate confirmation of viremia in patients found to be positive for HCV antibodies [1].

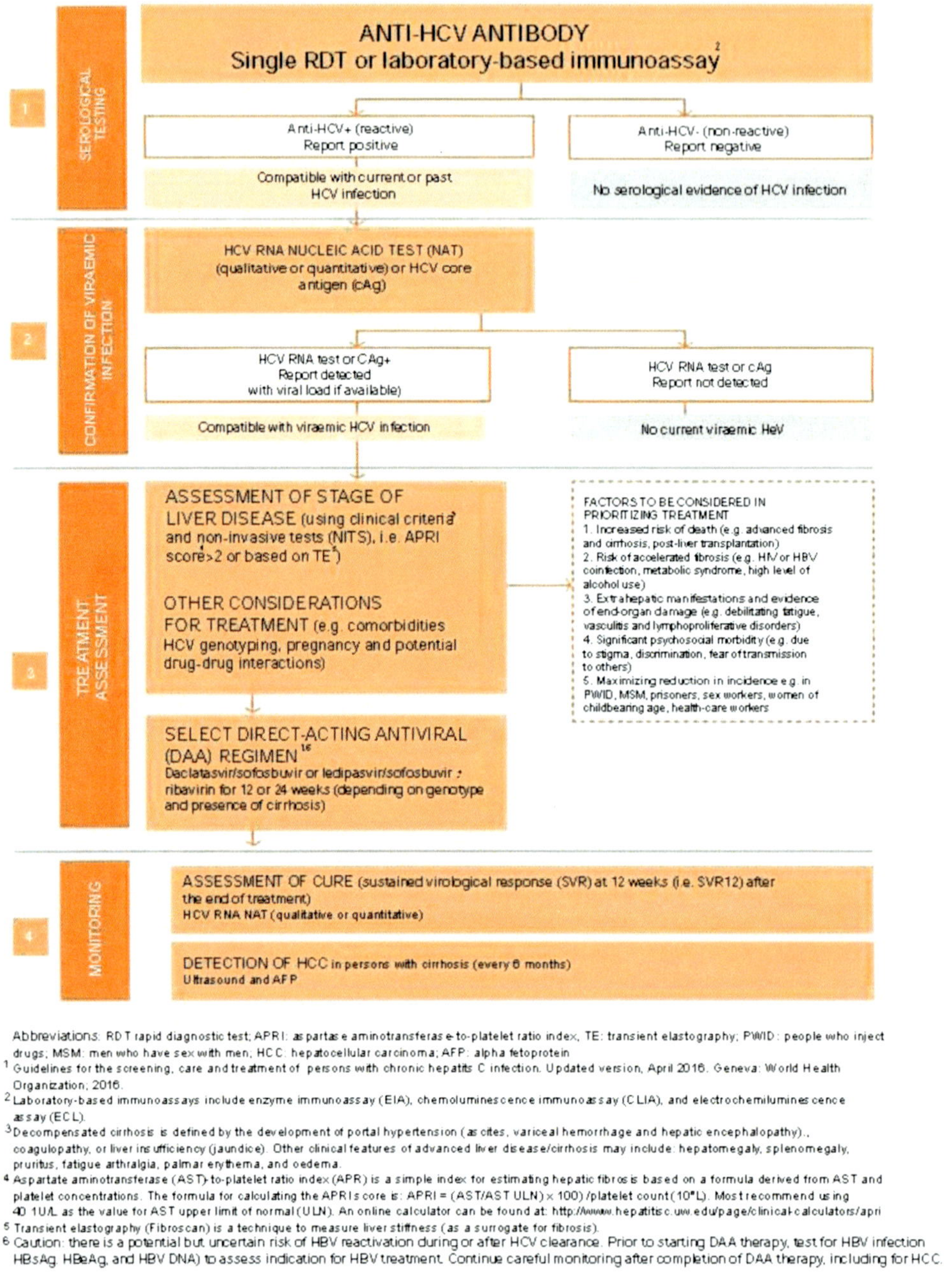

Fig. (3). A layout summary of WHO-suggested algorithms for the diagnosis, treatment, and monitoring of chronic HCV infection [43].

Quick Portable Test Could Widen Reach of HCV Diagnosis

A POC assay for HCV infection running on the portable Genedrive® molecular diagnostic platform shows high specificity and sensitivity during initial clinical testing [40]. Whilst IFN-free DAAs have revolutionized therapeutic options for treating hepatitis C patients, the challenge remains to identify people infected with the virus, many of whom are living in geographic regions that lack access to state-of-the-art diagnostics [1]. To help close that gap, the investigators developed the POC assay for the qualitative detection of HCV RNA using the 600-gram battery-operatable Genedrive® device. The assay results were compared with those obtained with the Abbott RealTime® HCV test when applied to 422 patients chronically infected with HCV and 503 controls negative for anti-HCV and HCV RNA. Samples were tested across 12 Genedrive® instruments, five operators, and three different assay batches [41].

The POC assay identified all six major HCV GTs, with 98.6% sensitivity and 100% specificity [40, 41]. A real-life clinical setting validation study of the assay was conducted in South Africa with samples obtained from various African countries and the performance of the Genedrive® HCV assay was found equally specific and sensitive [41]. It is a rapid point-of-need test that enables real-time treatment and management of chronic hepatitis C patients in decentralized settings. The team also points out that although final costs remain to be defined, the instrument is available for about US$5,000 and each Genedrive® hepatitis C test will cost around US$30 to $40 [41]. This promising entry into the POC HCV RNA testing space has high sensitivity and specificity and meets the WHO target product profile for a POC assay. It has low blood volume requirements and is a portable, low-cost instrument [41]. These features make it potentially quite attractive for deployment for field testing in LMICs and could help narrow the gap between HCV-infected patients and highly effective treatment.

CONCLUSIONS

We have IFN-free DAAs to cure hepatitis C in 8 to 12 weeks but do not have the means to test all populations at risk for hepatitis C in vulnerable and hard-hit communities. Studies on alerts in medical health records to improve screening, POC testing, systematic linkage to care, and special populations (*e.g.*, PWIDs, IDUs, sex workers, patients in prison, and patients coinfected with HIV and hepatitis C) must be addressed and managed. Most of the remote areas and places of aboriginal populations where hepatitis C may concentrate are difficult to penetrate, so novel ways will have to find to integrate screening in these communities. The key objective of hepatitis C screening should access the ways to provide treatment as it alone itself does not do anything. In this scenario, an initiative that offers rapid hepatitis C antibody screening and counseling, a syringe access program, and a drug harm reduction clinic or center should be implemented. When a test is reactive, the patient is referred to a navigation specialist who sets up RNA testing and subsequent appointments. A screening program operating in a detention center, with follow-up assistance for transportation, health insurance, and appointments, should be adopted. For patients undergoing blood tests, a pop-up alert in electronic medical records that reminds providers to screen patients whose hepatitis C status is not documented and who are born between 1945 and 1965 should be followed. Enhancing HCV testing and linkage to care and treatment services are critical to reaching the 2030 HCV elimination goal. Furthermore, robust, short turnaround time, and portable digital HCV screening and diagnostic devices are in the pipeline and will be a part of decentralized HCV testing facilities as well as in harder-to-reach HCV-affected communities very soon. Conventional, RDT algorithms include the use of immunoassays that detect antibodies or antigens and provide results within 30 minutes by using alternative sampling methods. Recent validation studies on rapid HCV RNA assays based on both standard and alternative sampling methods (finger-stick capillary whole blood) confirm the acceptable sensitivity and specificity of these assays. The main contribution of rapid molecular assays is the possibility to diagnose active infection with HCV in a single visit enabling real-time treatment decisions and potentially supporting elimination. HCV self-testing could be encouraged to raise awareness about HCV infection and to be alert about current infection status or reinfection in high-risks and occupational exposure to the virus both in centralized and decentralized testing facilities. It may also be supportive to know the current infection status in the unprecedented working environment and safety measures regulations due to the spread of a viral outbreak across the world.

REFERENCES

[1] Shahid I, Alzahrani AR, Al-Ghamdi SS, Alanazi IM, Rehman S, Hassan S. Hepatitis C Diagnosis: Simplified solutions, predictive barriers, and future promises. Diagnostics 2021; 11: 7.

[2] Easterbrook PJ, Roberts T, Sands A, Peeling R. Diagnosis of viral hepatitis. Curr Opin HIV AIDS 2017; 12(3): 302-14. [http://dx.doi.org/10.1097/COH.0000000000000370] [PMID: 28306597]

[3] Coffie PA, Egger M, Vinikoor MJ, *et al.* Trends in hepatitis B virus testing practices and management in HIV clinics across sub-Saharan Africa. BMC Infect Dis 2017; 17(S1) (Suppl. 1): 706. [http://dx.doi.org/10.1186/s12879-017-2768-z] [PMID: 29143625]

[4] WHO Guidelines Approved by the Guidelines Review Committee. Guidelines for the Screening Care and Treatment of Persons with Chronic Hepatitis C Infection: Updated Version. Geneva: World Health Organization Copyright © World Health Organization. 2016.

[5] Easterbrook PJ. Who to test and how to test for chronic hepatitis C infection 2016 WHO testing guidance for low- and middle-income countries. J Hepatol 2016; 65(1): S46-66. [http://dx.doi.org/10.1016/j.jhep.2016.08.002] [PMID: 27641988]

[6] Chevaliez S. Strategies for the improvement of HCV testing and diagnosis. Expert Rev Anti Infect Ther 2019; 17(5): 341-7.
[http://dx.doi.org/10.1080/14787210.2019.1604221] [PMID: 30950298]

[7] Saludes V, Antuori A, Lazarus JV, *et al.* Evaluation of the Xpert HCV VL Fingerstick point-of-care assay and dried blood spot HCV-RNA testing as simplified diagnostic strategies among people who inject drugs in Catalonia, Spain. Int J Drug Policy 2020; 80: 102734.
[http://dx.doi.org/10.1016/j.drugpo.2020.102734] [PMID: 32470849]

[8] Freiman JM, Wang J, Easterbrook PJ, *et al.* Deriving the optimal limit of detection for an HCV point-of-care test for viraemic infection: Analysis of a global dataset. J Hepatol 2019; 71(1): 62-70.
[http://dx.doi.org/10.1016/j.jhep.2019.02.011] [PMID: 30797050]

[9] Reipold EI, Trianni A, Krakower D, *et al.* Values, preferences and current hepatitis B and C testing practices in low- and middle-income countries: results of a survey of end users and implementers. BMC Infect Dis 2017; 17(S1) (Suppl. 1): 702.
[http://dx.doi.org/10.1186/s12879-017-2769-y] [PMID: 29143612]

[10] Vetter BN, Reipold EI, Ongarello S, *et al.* Sensitivity and specificity of rapid diagnostic tests for hepatitis C virus with or without HIV coinfection: a multicentre laboratory evaluation study. J Infect Dis 2020; jiaa389.
[PMID: 32614451]

[11] Mane A, Sacks J, Sharma S, *et al.* Evaluation of five rapid diagnostic tests for detection of antibodies to hepatitis C virus (HCV): A step towards scale-up of HCV screening efforts in India. PLoS One 2019; 14(1): e0210556.
[http://dx.doi.org/10.1371/journal.pone.0210556] [PMID: 30653562]

[12] Kabamba AT, Mwamba CM, Dessilly G, Dufrasne F, Kabamba BM, Longanga AO. Evaluation of the analytical performance of six rapid diagnostic tests for the detection of viral hepatitis B and C in Lubumbashi, Democratic Republic of Congo. J Virol Methods 2020; 285: 113961.
[http://dx.doi.org/10.1016/j.jviromet.2020.113961] [PMID: 32860797]

[13] Martinello M, Hajarizadeh B, Grebely J, Dore GJ, Matthews GV. Management of acute HCV infection in the era of direct-acting antiviral therapy. Nat Rev Gastroenterol Hepatol 2018; 15(7): 412-24.
[http://dx.doi.org/10.1038/s41575-018-0026-5] [PMID: 29773899]

[14] Khuroo MS, Khuroo NS, Khuroo MS. Diagnostic accuracy of point-of-care tests for hepatitis C virus infection: a systematic review and meta-analysis. PLoS One 2015; 10(3): e0121450.
[http://dx.doi.org/10.1371/journal.pone.0121450] [PMID: 25816332]

[15] Cameron SO, Carman WF. The use of the OraSure collection device for hepatitis virus testing in health care settings. Journal of clinical virology : the official publication of the Pan American Society for Clinical Virology 2005; 34(Suppl 1): 22-8.
[http://dx.doi.org/10.1016/S1386-6532(05)80006-X]

[16] Cha YJ, Park Q, Kang ES, *et al.* Performance evaluation of the OraQuick hepatitis C virus rapid antibody test. Ann Lab Med 2013; 33(3): 184-9.
[http://dx.doi.org/10.3343/alm.2013.33.3.184] [PMID: 23667844]

[17] Pallarés C, Carvalho-Gomes Â, Hontangas V, Conde I, Di Maira T, Aguilera V. Performance of the OraQuick Hepatitis C virus antibody test in oral fluid and fingerstick blood before and after treatment-induced viral clearance. Journal of clinical virology : the official publication of the Pan American Society for Clinical Virology 2018; 102: 77-83.

[18] Liu L, Zhang M, Hang L, *et al.* Evaluation of a new point-of-care oral anti-HCV test for screening of hepatitis C virus infection. Virol J 2020; 17(1): 14.
[http://dx.doi.org/10.1186/s12985-020-1293-7] [PMID: 32005264]

[19] Kimble MM, Stafylis C, Treut P, Saab S, Klausner JD. Clinical evaluation of a hepatitis C antibody

rapid immunoassay on self-collected oral fluid specimens. Diagn Microbiol Infect Dis 2019; 95(2): 149-51.
[http://dx.doi.org/10.1016/j.diagmicrobio.2019.05.010] [PMID: 31204109]

[20] Jülicher P, Chulanov VP, Pimenov NN, Chirkova E, Yankina A, Galli C. Streamlining the screening cascade for active Hepatitis C in Russia: A cost-effectiveness analysis. PLoS One 2019; 14(7): e0219687.
[http://dx.doi.org/10.1371/journal.pone.0219687] [PMID: 31310636]

[21] Pollock KG, McDonald SA, Gunson R, *et al.* Real-world utility of HCV core antigen as an alternative to HCV RNA testing: Implications for viral load and genotype. J Viral Hepat 2020; 27(10): 996-1002.
[http://dx.doi.org/10.1111/jvh.13337] [PMID: 32479681]

[22] Catlett B, Lamoury FMJ, Bajis S, *et al.* Evaluation of a hepatitis C virus core antigen assay from venepuncture and dried blood spot collected samples: A cohort study. J Viral Hepat 2019; 26(12): 1423-30.
[http://dx.doi.org/10.1111/jvh.13196] [PMID: 31448470]

[23] Abdollahi-Aghdam A, Majidi MR, Omidi Y. Microfluidic paper-based analytical devices (μPADs) for fast and ultrasensitive sensing of biomarkers and monitoring of diseases. Bioimpacts 2018; 8(4): 237-40.
[http://dx.doi.org/10.15171/bi.2018.26] [PMID: 30397578]

[24] Eletxigerra U, Martinez-Perdiguero J, Merino S, Villalonga R, Pingarrón JM, Campuzano S. Amperometric magnetoimmunoassay for the direct detection of tumor necrosis factor alpha biomarker in human serum. Anal Chim Acta 2014; 838: 37-44.
[http://dx.doi.org/10.1016/j.aca.2014.05.047] [PMID: 25064241]

[25] Ghanbari K, Roushani M, Azadbakht A. Ultra-sensitive aptasensor based on a GQD nanocomposite for detection of hepatitis C virus core antigen. Anal Biochem 2017; 534: 64-9.
[http://dx.doi.org/10.1016/j.ab.2017.07.016] [PMID: 28728900]

[26] Warkad SD, Song KS, Pal D, Nimse SB. Developments in the HCV Screening Technologies Based on the Detection of Antigens and Antibodies. Sensors (Basel) 2019; 19(19): 4257.
[http://dx.doi.org/10.3390/s19194257] [PMID: 31575036]

[27] Snijdewind IJM, van Kampen JJA, Fraaij PLA, van der Ende ME, Osterhaus ADME, Gruters RA. Current and future applications of dried blood spots in viral disease management. Antiviral Res 2012; 93(3): 309-21.
[http://dx.doi.org/10.1016/j.antiviral.2011.12.011] [PMID: 22244848]

[28] Komas NP, Vickos U, Hübschen JM, *et al.* Cross-sectional study of hepatitis B virus infection in rural communities, Central African Republic. BMC Infect Dis 2013; 13(1): 286.
[http://dx.doi.org/10.1186/1471-2334-13-286] [PMID: 23800310]

[29] Lange B, Roberts T, Cohn J, *et al.* Diagnostic accuracy of detection and quantification of HBV-DNA and HCV-RNA using dried blood spot (DBS) samples a systematic review and meta-analysis. BMC Infect Dis 2017; 17(S1) (Suppl. 1): 693.
[http://dx.doi.org/10.1186/s12879-017-2776-z] [PMID: 29143616]

[30] Lange B, Cohn J, Roberts T, *et al.* Diagnostic accuracy of serological diagnosis of hepatitis C and B using dried blood spot samples (DBS): two systematic reviews and meta-analyses. BMC Infect Dis 2017; 17(S1) (Suppl. 1): 700.
[http://dx.doi.org/10.1186/s12879-017-2777-y] [PMID: 29143672]

[31] Vázquez-Morón S, Ardizone Jiménez B, Jiménez-Sousa MA, Bellón JM, Ryan P, Resino S. Evaluation of the diagnostic accuracy of laboratory-based screening for hepatitis C in dried blood spot samples: A systematic review and meta-analysis. Sci Rep 2019; 9(1): 7316.
[http://dx.doi.org/10.1038/s41598-019-41139-8] [PMID: 31086259]

[32] Catlett B, Bajis S, Starr M, *et al.* Evaluation of the Aptima HCV Quant Dx Assay for Hepatitis C Virus RNA Detection from Fingerstick Capillary Dried Blood Spot and Venepuncture-Collected

Samples. J Infect Dis 2021; 223(5): 818-26.
[http://dx.doi.org/10.1093/infdis/jiaa442] [PMID: 32710758]

[33] Fourati S, Feld JJ, Chevaliez S, Luhmann N. Approaches for simplified HCV diagnostic algorithms. Journal of the International AIDS Society 2018; 21(Suppl 2): e25058.
[http://dx.doi.org/10.1002/jia2.25058]

[34] Patel AA, Bui A, Prohl E, *et al.* Innovations in Hepatitis C Screening and Treatment. Hepatol Commun 2021; 5(3): 371-86.
[http://dx.doi.org/10.1002/hep4.1646] [PMID: 33681673]

[35] Lamoury F, Hajarizadeh B, Soker A, Martinez D, Quek C, Cunningham P. Hepatitis C virus core antigen and dried blood spots as simplified hepatitis C virus diagnostic tools.

[36] Pawlotsky JM, Ramers CB, Dillon JF, Feld JJ, Lazarus JV. Simplification of Care for Chronic Hepatitis C Virus Infection. Semin Liver Dis 2020; 40(4): 392-402.
[http://dx.doi.org/10.1055/s-0040-1713657] [PMID: 32725611]

[37] Grebely J, Applegate TL, Cunningham P, Feld JJ. Hepatitis C point-of-care diagnostics: in search of a single visit diagnosis. Expert Rev Mol Diagn 2017; 17(12): 1109-15.
[http://dx.doi.org/10.1080/14737159.2017.1400385] [PMID: 29088981]

[38] Wong XZ, Amirah A, Gan CC, *et al.* Hepatitis C virus core antigen as alternative diagnostic algorithm for active hepatitis C virus infection among haemodialysis population: Cost implications. Nephrology (Carlton) 2021; 26(5): 463-70.
[http://dx.doi.org/10.1111/nep.13862] [PMID: 33580732]

[39] Wang Y, Jie W, Ling J, Yuanshuai H. HCV core antigen plays an important role in the fight against HCV as an alternative to HCV-RNA detection. J Clin Lab Anal 2021; 35(6): e23755.
[http://dx.doi.org/10.1002/jcla.23755] [PMID: 33788295]

[40] Padhi A, Gupta E, Singh G, Agarwal R, Sharma MK, Sarin SK. Evaluation of the Point of Care Molecular Diagnostic Genedrive HCV ID Kit for the detection of HCV RNA in clinical samples. Epidemiol Infect 2020; 1-23.
[http://dx.doi.org/10.1017/S0950268820002812] [PMID: 33203484]

[41] Lamoury FMJ, Njouom R, Amougou-Atsama M, Yiagnigni Mfopou E, Berishvili N, Sologashvili M. Diagnostic Performance and Usability of the Genedrive(®) HCV ID Kit in Two Decentralized Settings in Cameroon and Georgia. Diagnostics 2021; 11: 5.

[42] Activist Guide to Hepatitis C Virus Diagnostics. Available from: https://www.hepcoalition.org/advocate/advocacy-tools/article/activist-guide-to-hepatitis-c-virus-diagnostics

[43] WHO guidelines on hepatitis B and C testing. Geneva: World Health Organization. 2017. Available from: https://www.who.int

[44] HCV Guideline Committee of the New York State Department of Health AIDS Institute (NYSDOH AI). Treatment of Chronic HCV with Direct-Acting Antivirals. Baltimore (MD): Johns Hopkins University. 2020. Available from: https://www.ncbi.nlm.nih.gov/books/NBK559965/

CHAPTER 6

Current Landscape of HCV Therapeutics

Abstract: During the last decade, the advent and approval of almost a dozen all-oral interferon-free direct-acting antivirals (IFN-free DAAs) to cure hepatitis C-infected general and harder-to-treat populations have entirely changed the treatment paradigms against this "silent epidemic". The clinical trials of generic IFN-free DAAs, while achieving 95% to 100% sustained virologic response rates (SVRs) in treated individuals, have proven their worth as "magic pills" in hepatitis C therapeutics. Following their real-world clinical usage data with SVR rates, more than 95% have raised the hopes to treat everyone infected with hepatitis C in near future, albeit certain barriers still need to be broken. These regimens, in combination or as a fixed-dose combination (FDC) of a single pill, are highly efficacious against all major hepatitis C genotypes and sub-genotypes. Furthermore, the regimens are well tolerable, with fewer adverse events, and with lesser chances of post-treatment viral relapse or breakthrough in treated patients. The dose algorithms are well-defined for all adult patient groups and in different pathological states of the infection and their recommendations are according to extrahepatic manifestations of hepatitis C in infected individuals. Furthermore, the clinical trials of some DAAs are underway to approve their recommendations in HCV-infected infants, children, and pregnant female patients. In this chapter, we will illustrate the most attractive pharmaco-characteristics of these novel therapeutic regimens to be considered while treating hepatitis C-infected populations. We will also elaborate on the infected subpopulations for which such regimens are not recommended and further research is extensively needed.

Keywords: Cirrhosis, Direct-acting antivirals, Fibrosis, Hepatocellular carcinoma, HCV/HBV Co-infection, HCV/HIV Co-infection, HCV/CKD Co-infection, Harder-to-treat populations, HCV Therapeutics, Resistance-associated substitutions, Sustained virologic response, Treatment-naïve patients, Treatment-experienced patients, Treatment-associated adverse events.

INTRODUCTION

The overall cure rates to once 'gold standard of care' (*i.e.*, pegylated interferon (PEG-IFN α) and ribavirin (RBV)) have been dismally poor with dual therapy completion in chronically infected HCV patients along with the emergence of severe adverse events [1]. All oral interferon-free direct-acting antivirals (DAAs) were awaited eagerly not only to avoid the administration of PEG-IFN α to intole-

Imran Shahid and Qaiser Jabeen

rant interferon patients but also to decrease the frequency of associated adverse events and viral breakthroughs (HCV RNA remains the lower limit of quantification, but increased to ≥100 IU/ml or ≥1 $\log_{10}$ during PEG-IFNα/RBV dual therapy) in infected patients [2]. The current therapies are not only safe and highly effective, but the relative ease of administration also allows for widespread use outside of a specialist's office. These oral IFN-free antivirals are reported to achieve sustained virologic response rates (SVR; undetectable hepatitis C viral load at week 12 or 24 at the end of therapy) higher than 95% in treated individuals [3]. With the availability of these safe and highly effective (yet costly) drugs, the clinical question becomes "treat selectively or treat everyone?" Furthermore, the therapeutic regimens are well tolerated, express unrestricted genotype efficacy, and result in excellent on-treatment virologic responses [3]. However, the successful use of these therapeutic regimens would depend on various factors including; previous patient history of treatment, HCV viral load monitoring during treatment, additional adverse events, possible drug-drug interactions (DDIs), and the emergence of viral escape mutants [3]. These treatment strategies are being investigated for HCV by deriving some established findings in the treatment of HIV infection, where the combination of different drugs with different anti-viral efficacy and antiviral resistance substantially decreases the risk of viral breakthroughs [4].

Although the current status of anti-HCV drug development and therapeutics is a dense, ever-changing menu of new agents, it is beyond the scope of this book chapter to cover all relevant studies. Even then, the bottom-line message from this matter-of-fact book chapter is simple: "Agent X (fill in the blank) leads to the achievement of high SVRs and cure hepatitis C". The current DAAs are therapeutically active while working at different stages of the virus life cycle by only targeting and inhibiting hepatitis C nonstructural proteins that are potentially involved in virus replication and translation [1]. Current DAAs for the treatment of hepatitis C target 3 nonstructural proteins of HCV upon which they are classified accordingly as shown in Fig. (**1**). As of August 2020, the following DAAs are no longer used in the USA for the treatment of HCV; boceprevir, daclatasvir, dasabuvir, elbasvir, grazoprevir, ombitasvir, paritaprevir, simeprevir, and telaprevir. Similarly, telaprevir and boceprevir are obsolete and no longer recommended in the rest of the world to treat HCV, but the remaining DAAs are prescribed by clinicians to treat hepatitis C [5]. Second, DAAs are only effective to achieve high SVR rates or cure hepatitis C when administered in combinations within a similar or different class or as a fixed-dose combination (FDC) of different DAAs as a single co-formulated pill [1]. Fig. (**2**) depicts the most promising direct-acting antivirals according to their classification while Table **1** demonstrates the salient features of the FDA-approved interferon-free DAA combinations for hepatitis C treatment.

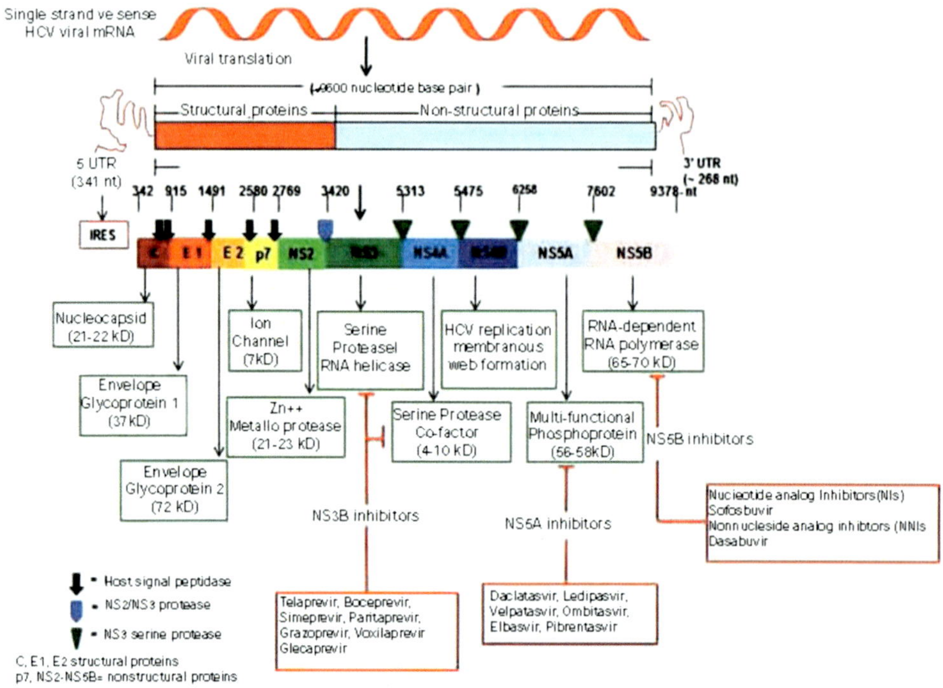

Fig. (1). Direct-acting antivirals acting on their targeted sites (highlighted in rectangular boxes) of the HCV genome UTR; untranslated region.

MECHANISM OF ACTION OF DAAS

As previously described, an ample understanding of the HCV genome and its life cycle enabled efforts to improve drug efficacy and tolerability to cure the infection [1]. The early treatment in the form of pegylated interferon (PEG-IFN) plus ribavirin (RBV) could not seem highly efficacious against HCV GTs 3 and 4 and their subtypes [2]. This led to the development of multiple direct-acting antivirals (DAAs) which target specific proteins pivotal for the HCV life cycle [1]. DAAs are drug molecules that target specific nonstructural proteins of HCV and disrupt viral replication, translation, and ultimately the infection [1]. There are four main classes of DAAs defined by their mechanism of action and therapeutic target. The four classes include;

1- Nonstructural protein 3/4A (NS3/4A) protease inhibitors (PIs)

2- NS5B nucleoside polymerase inhibitors (NPIs)

3- NS5B non-nucleoside polymerase inhibitors (NNPIs)

4- NS5A inhibitors

Here in we illustrate the mechanism of action of each DAAs class. Other important issues related to the selection of treatment choice, patient evaluation, and other management issues are discussed elsewhere in this book.

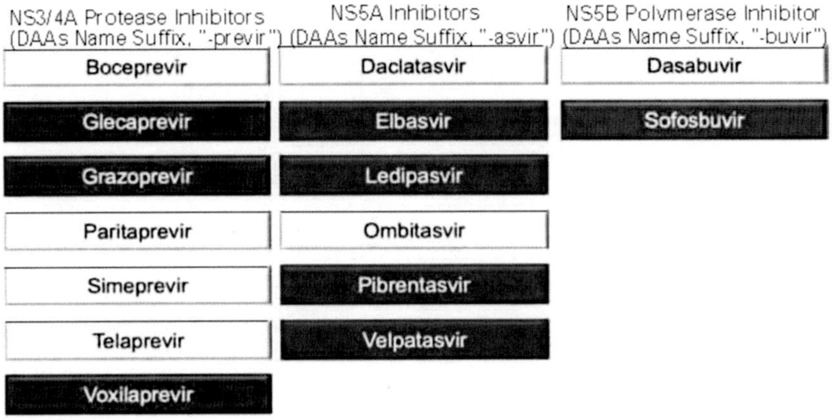

Fig. (2). Direct-acting antiviral classification according to their target sites [6].

NS3/4A Protease Inhibitors (NS3/4A PIs)

NS3/4A PIs inhibit NS3/4A serine protease, an enzyme integral for post-translational processing and replication of HCV [1]. PIs disrupt HCV genome polyprotein processing by blocking the NS3 catalytic site or interaction between NS3 and NS4A (a coenzyme for NS3 protease as well as helicase activity). Besides NS3/4A's pivotal role in viral polyprotein processing, it blocks TRIF-(TIR-domain-containing adapter-inducing interferon-β) mediated Toll-like receptor (TLR) signaling and Cardif-mediated retinoic acid-inducible gene 1 (RIG-1) signaling, resulting in impaired induction of IFN and block virion elimination. Hence, inhibition of NS3/4A protease contributes to antiviral activity by two mechanisms [1].

HCV NS3/4A protease enzyme is a serine proteinase with a catalytic site, two substrate binding sites, an NS4A-binding site and NS2/NS3 proteinase substrate-recognition site, a helicase single-strand RNA-binding site, and a zinc-binding site [2]. This multitargeted structure offers multiple potential avenues to inhibit the enzyme and block HCV-RNA translation (Fig. **3**).

Table 1. The most promising interferon-free DAA combinations approved by the US FDA for the treatment of the hepatitis C virus.

Referenced Clinical Trials[a]	Drug Efficacy[b]	Drug Resistance Barrier[c]	Pan-genotypic coverage[d]	Severe Adverse Effects[e]	Drug-drug Interactions[f]	Development Phase	Target Site
Ledipasvir (LDV/LED) and sofosbuvir (SOF) combination (Pan-genotypic regimen) [Harvoni®]							
NCT01701401 NCT01768286 NCT01851330 NCT02073656	+++	+++	+++	+	+	Approved	NS5A/NS5B active site
Sofosbuvir (SOF) and simeprevir (SMV) combination [Sovaldi®+ Olysio®]							
NCT01466790 NCT02114177 NCT02114151	+++	++	++	+	++	Approved	NS5B/NS3 serine protease active site
Daclatasvir (DCV) and sofosbuvir (SOF) combination (Pan-genotypic regimen) [Daklinza® + Sovaldi®]							
NCT02032875 NCT01359644 NCT02032888 NCT02032901	+++	+++	++	+	+	Approved	NS5A/NS5B active site + mRNA chain
Sofosbuvir (SOF) and velpatasvir (VEL) combination (Pan-genotypic regimen) [Epclusa®]							
NCT02201940 NCT02201953 NCT02220998 NCT02201901 NCT02480712	+++	+++	+++	+	+	Approved	NS5B/NS5A active site + mRNA chain
Daclatasvir (DCV), asunaprevir (ASV) and beclabuvir (BCV) combination [DCV-TRIO®]							
NCT01979939 NCT01973049	+++ +++	+++ ++	++ ++	+ ++	++ ++	Approved	NS5A/NS3-4A serine protease active site /NNIs
Paritaprevir (PTV) –ombitasvir (OBV)-ritonavir (r) and dasabuvir (DSV) combination [Viekira Pak®, PrOD®]							
NCT01716585 NCT01715415 NCT01704755 NCT01939197 NCT01674725 NCT01767116 NCT01833533	+++	+++	++	+	+	Approved	NS3-4A serine protease/NS5A active site/NNIs
Paritaprevir (PTV)-ombitasvir (OBV) and ritonavir (r) combination [Technivie®]							
NCT01685203 NCT02265237 NCT02247401	+++	++	+	+++	+	Approved	NS3-4A serine protease/NS5A active site

(Table 1) cont.....

Elbasvir (EBV) and grazoprevir (GZR) combination [Zepatier®]							
NCT02105688 NCT02105662 NCT02105701 NCT02105467 NCT02092350	+++	++	+++	++	++	Approved	NS3-4A/NS5A serine protease active site
Daclatasvir (DCV) and asunaprevir (ASV) combination [Daklinza® + Sunvepra®]							
NCT01581203 NCT01573351	+++	+++	+	+	+++	Approved in Japan	NS5A/NS3-4A serine protease active site
Sofosbuvir (SOF), velpatasvir (VEL), and voxilaprevir (VOX) combination [Vosevi®]							
NCT02607735 NCT02607800 NCT02639338 NCT02639247 NCT02745535	+++	++	+	+	+	Approved	NS3-4A/NS5A/NS5B active site
Glecaprevir (GLE) and Pibrentasvir (PIB) combination (Pan-genotypic regimen) [Mavyret®]							
NCT02604017 NCT02640482 NCT02640157 NCT02636595 NCT02966795 NCT02642432 NCT02738138 NCT02651194 NCT03069365 NCT03089944 NCT02446717 NCT02243280 NCT02243280 NCT02243293	+++	+++	+	+	+	Approved	NS3-4A/NS5A active site

[a]Only those phase II/III clinical trials were mentioned in (Table **1**) which were reported to the US FDA for the approval of interferon-free DAA combination and were registered to the clinicaltrials.gov website. [b]Drug efficacy profile was based on the overall SVR rates achieved in phase II/III clinical trials where SVRs > 95% = high profile, SVRs > 90% = average profile, and SVRs > 85-90% = low profile. [c]Drug resistance barrier was based on the clinical data registered to clinicaltrials.gov. [d]Pan-genotypic coverage was based on the fact that the DAA combination achieved SVR at the end of treatment. SVR 1 through 6 genotypes = high profile, two/three genotypes = average profile, and one genotype = low profile. [e]Severe adverse event (SAEs) profile was accomplished based on the percentage occurrence of adverse effects in phase II/III clinical trials which caused treatment discontinuation in treated individuals, where 10% SAEs > high profile, 10→5% SAEs > average profile, and 5→0% SAEs > low profile. [f]Drug-drug interaction profile was established based on the DAA's ability to induce/inhibit hepatic cytochrome P450 system, P-glycoprotein (P-gp), and organic transporting polypeptide (OATP) induction/inhibition. CYP 450, P-gp, and OATP induction/inhibition= high profile, P-gp and OATP induction/inhibition= average profile, and one or none of these CYP 450 or P-gp or OATP induction/inhibition = low profile.High profile = +++, Average profile = ++, and low profile= +

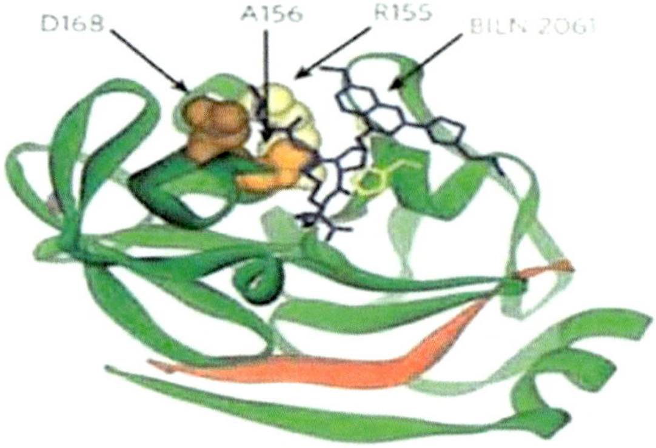

Fig. (3). Binding of protease inhibitors to NS3/4A serine protease [7]. The structure of two PIs (BILN 2061 and VX-950) and the NS3 serine protease domain (green) are complex with the central domain of NS4A (red). The amino acid residues histidine 57, aspartate 81, and serine 139 constitute the catalytic triad of the enzyme and are shown as yellow (stick representation). The structural zinc atom is indicated in purple. Protease inhibitor (BILN 2061) is modeled in the active site of the enzyme. Amino acid substitutions (D168, A156, and R155) responsible for resistance to PIs are shown in space-filling mode and color-coded [7].

Telaprevir and boceprevir belonged to first-generation NS3/4A PIs and were available as the first DAAs for the treatment of HCV [3]. Both were used in conjunction with PEG/IFN plus RBV for the treatment of HCV GT-1 infection. As the progress toward searching for other potent DAAs with better tolerability and high efficacy continued, the clinical importance of first-generation PIs substantially diminished because of their cumbersome dosage frequencies, severe adverse events, drug-drug interactions, and the emergence of drug resistance [1]. The subsequent second and next-generation NS3/4A PIs offer several clinical benefits over first-generation PIs, including improved dosage frequency, fewer adverse drug effects, and lesser drug-drug interactions [3]. Moreover, the newer PIs are highly efficacious against HCV GT-1 and its subtypes; albeit, some newer PIs have limited efficacy against other HCV GTs and subtypes. In addition to that, the resistance barrier against NS3/4A PIs was also reported relatively low. Simeprevir belonged to the second-generation NS3/4A PIs and was once infrequently used in the US; however, it obsoleted after the development of next-generation PIs but is used in other parts of the world [3]. Following are the NS3/4A PIs available in the United States and the rest of the world in combination with other DAAs targeting different HCV proteins.

1- Glecaprevir is a potent, pangenotypic PI available in combination with pibrentasvir (an NS5A inhibitor).

2- Grazoprevir is also a potent, pangenotypic PI available in combination with elbasvir.

3- Paritaprevir is a potent PI available in combination with low-dose ritonavir (not a PI with any anti-HCV activity and boosts the pharmacological effects of other DAAs). Both paritaprevir and ritonavir are available in a fixed-dose combination (FDC) with ombitasvir (an NS5A inhibitor) and dasabuvir (a non-nucleoside NS5B inhibitor (NNIs).

4- Voxilaprevir is also a potent, pangenotypic PI available in combination with sofosbuvir (an NS5B inhibitor) and velpatasvir (an NS5A inhibitor).

NS5A Inhibitors

HCV nonstructural protein NS5A plays essential roles in viral replication and the assembly of HCV [2]. However, the underlying mechanisms responsible for these vital functions accomplished by NS5A protein are still not fully elucidated. Hence, the exact molecular mechanisms of NS5A inhibitors are also still unclear [2]. However, it is hypothesized that a hierarchy of interaction establishes between HCV-encoded proteins, HCV RNA genome, and host factors (HF) that results in the formation of replication complexes (RCs) on the endoplasmic reticulum (ER) membrane [2]. Interestingly, at this time point, NS5B inhibitors inhibit the RNA-dependent RNA polymerase (RdRp; NS5B protein) activity within preformed viral RCs; however, the activity of NS5A protein sequester within preformed RCs and is refractory to inhibit by NS5A-targeting compounds [3]. Most probably viral and host proteins interaction during the formation of the RCs mask the targeted binding site of a drug molecule of NS5A in RCs; however, prior to the *de novo* RCs formation, NS5A is accessible for inhibition. An NS5A inhibitor after binding to NS5A alters or locks the NS5A protein conformational changes not permissive for incorporation into RCs. Hence, protein assemblies devoid of NS5A, and NS5A-mediated incorporation of essential HF fail to form functional RCs [3]. Subsequently, inhibited NS5A proteins shuttled to the surface of lipid droplets ("because the failure of NS5A to be sequestered into RCs results in the protein adopting a distribution reminiscent of that when expressed in the absence of other HCV-encoded proteins") (Fig. **4**).

NS5A inhibitors are generally quite potent and highly efficacious across all HCV GTs but have a low genetic barrier to resistance and variable drug toxicity profile [1]. NS5A inhibitors showed significantly reduce HCV RNA levels and excellent SVR rates when used in combination with PEG-IFN plus RBV. SVR rates were also shown to be very high when used in combination with other DAAs with or without RBV among patients with HCV GT-1 infection. Daclatasvir belonged to the first-generation NS5A inhibitor used in combination with sofosbuvir [2]. It is now infrequently used in the USA but still used in combination with other DAAs in the rest of the world. Elbasvir is another NS5A inhibitor available as an FDC with NS3/4A PI "grazoprevir". Ledipasvir is the first NS5A inhibitor available in the USA as an FDC with "sofosbuvir" (an NS5B inhibitor) [3]. An NS5A inhibitor "ombitasvir" is available as an FDC with "paritaprevir" and ritonavir which is usually administered in combination with "dasabuvir" (a non-nucleotide NS5B inhibitor) [1]. "Pibrentasvir" is a pangenotypic NS5A inhibitor and is available only as an FDC with "glecaprevir" (an NS3/4A PIs). Velpatasvir is another pangenotypic NS5A inhibitor and is available as an FDC with sofosbuvir (an NS5B inhibitor) [1].

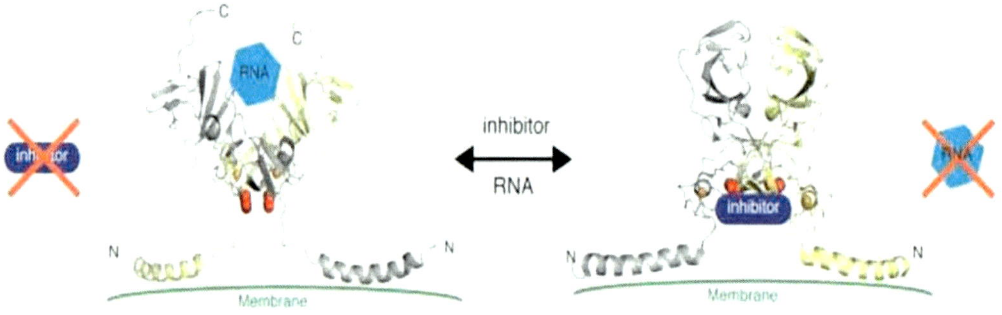

Fig. (4). Proposed mechanism of action of NS5A inhibitors. NS5A inhibitors bind to domain 1 of NS5A protein and prevent RNA binding for viral replication. Models of NS5A observed dimer conformations are displayed as cartoons and colored by monomers. The location of amino acid substitutions Y93 (responsible for antiviral resistance against NS5A inhibitors) in each monomer is indicated by red cpk and the Zn^{+2} ions are orange spheres [8].

NS5B RNA-dependent RNA Polymerase Inhibitors

HCV nonstructural protein NS5B acts as an RNA-dependent RNA polymerase (RdRp) enzyme which is involved in post-translational processing that is essential for viral replication [2]. The enzyme has a catalytic site for nucleoside analog inhibitors (NIs) and four other sites to bind non-nucleoside analog inhibitors (NNIs) (Fig. **5**).

HCV RdRp is highly conserved across all HCV GTs and compounds that inhibit or inactivate RdRp activity are efficacious against all six HCV GTs [1]. HCV NS5B protein inhibitors are classified into two types; nucleoside/nucleotide analog inhibitors (NIs) and non-nucleoside analog inhibitors (NNIs). NIs target the catalytic site of NS5B protein that is potentially involved in HCV RNA replication thus causing viral mRNA chain termination [2]. This mode of action makes the viral variants less fit and unable to replicate. Hence, NS5B NIs express a high barrier to antiviral drug resistance. On the other hand, NNIs act as allosteric inhibitors or incorporate conformational changes in four allosteric binding pockets of NS5B protein [3]. NS5B NIs are activated within hepatocytes through phosphorylation to active drug metabolites as nucleoside triphosphate which competes with nucleotides of viral mRNA chain. These nucleoside triphosphates (*i.e.* active drug metabolite) act as false nucleotide bases in the growing viral mRNA chain and result in chain termination during RNA replication of the viral genome. NS5B active site for NIs binding is relatively more intolerant to amino acid substitutions [2]. Therefore, mutations within NS5B actives sites that confer resistance against NIs are more likely to impair RdRp activity as compared to mutations emerging in NNIs allosteric binding pockets. Subsequently, the mutant virus genome renders less "fit" compared to the wild-type virus. HCV NS5B NIs contain moderate to high clinical efficacy against all HCV GTs and show equal drug efficacy against GT-1 subtypes 1a and 1b having a very high barrier to antiviral drug resistance [3]. However, as a class of drug, NS5B NIs represent a very limiting number of drugs (till now only one NIs "sofosbuvir" is approved by the US FDA to cure HCV) completing late development and is plagued with toxicity problems. Sofosbuvir is the first and sole NS5B PIs available in various combinations with other DAAs administered for different indications of HCV infections all over the world [1].

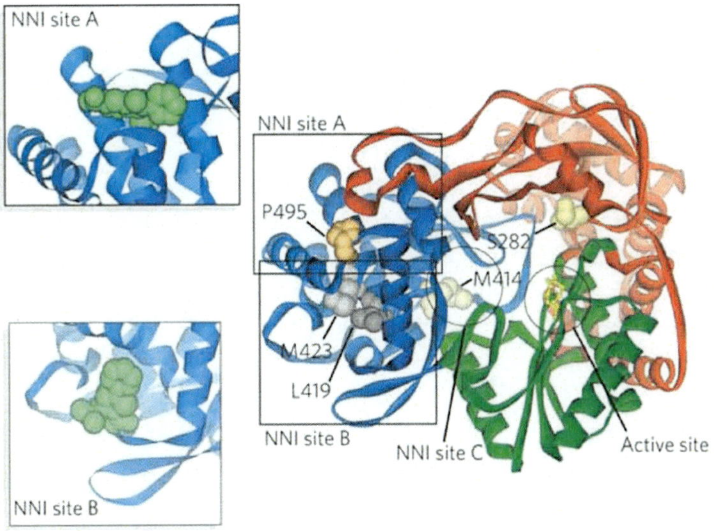

Fig. (5). Catalytic active sites for NIs and NNIs inhibitors within NS5B protein [7]. The thumb, palm, and finger domains of NS5B proteins are colored blue, green, and red, respectively. The side chains of the two catalytic aspartates are yellow in the active site. The amino acid substitutions responsible for antiviral drug resistance against NIs and NNIs like serine 282 (S282), proline 495 (P495), methionine 419 or threonine 423 (M419/T423), and methionine 414 (M414) respectively are shown in space-filling style and indicated in the fig. The two insets show the details of RdRp in binding with two different NNIs (*i.e.* NNI site A or NNI site B). For clarity on how NNIs bind to their targeted sites, those are shown in the insets in bright green. NNI site C depicts a tentative location for the NNI of a drug class thiadiazine [7].

The four allosteric sites of NS5B protein that act as targets for NNIs are thumb domains 1 and 2 and palm domains 1 and 2 [1]. As a class of drugs, NNIs are less potent than NS5B NIs; however, they are more HCV genotype-specific (*e.g.*, All NNIs in clinical development has been optimized for HCV GT-1). Furthermore, they contain a low to moderate genetic barrier to resistance and variable toxicity profiles across different HCV GTs and subtypes [1]. Because of these characteristics, NNIs were primarily studied as an adjunct regimen along with other DAAs with higher barriers to drug resistance. Dasabuvir is the sole member of the drug class approved for HCV treatment in combination with ombitasvir-paritaprevir-ritonavir [3].

PANGENOTYPIC DAA REGIMENS

With the advancement and an ample understanding of hepatitis C genome replication and polyprotein processing determinants, the design and development of pan-genotypic DAAs targeting specific hepatitis C proteins have revolutionized the treatment paradigms for HCV difficult-to-treat individuals and are being used in real-world clinical practice since 2017 (Table **1**) [9]. Now the treatments are available for all patients who are treatment-naïve or treatment-experienced (*i.e.*, previous treatment failure with PEG-IFN/RBV or DAAs failure), who contain HCV with cirrhosis (either compensated or decompensated) or not, who are concomitantly suffering from co-infections (*e.g.*, HCV/HBV, HCV/HIV, or HCV/CKD) or who are suffering from any HCV GTs/subtypes, or mixed GTs/subtypes (*i.e.* quasispecies nature of infection) or with "undetected" or "indeterminate" HCV GTs/subtypes [10]. Before the availability of these promising DAAs to attain higher SVR rates (*i.e.*, >95%) or cure of HCV-affected individuals, both the patients and clinicians were reluctant to initiate, adhere, or complete the treatment with pegylated interferon (PEG-IFN) and ribavirin (RBV) based therapies due to suboptimal SVR rates, significant rates of SAEs, potential drug toxicities, and possible DDIs with pole frequency medications [9]. However, these concerns have been significantly reduced and are no longer applicable to current pan-genotypic DAAs. Interestingly, the current pan-genotypic DAAs are therapeutically active while working at different stages of the virus life cycle by only targeting and inhibiting HCV nonstructural proteins that are potentially involved in virus replication and translation (Table **1**) [9]. Data from real-life clinical situations explore that cure rates are found to be almost similar with pangenotypic DAAs administration across all HCV GTs/subtypes with some exceptions of GT-3 infected patients either treatment naïve or who failed prior treatment with PEG-IFN/RBV or first and second-generation DAAs [9]. It seems that effective HCV treatment is now a reality provided to surmount some cross-cutting barriers to provide these regimens to everyone who is diagnosed with HCV [4]. Furthermore, the AEs associated with pan-genotypic DAAs administration are also mostly manageable. However, co-administration of RBV with these regimens may cause insomnia in treating patients, and adjustment of the timing of the dose earlier in the afternoon can avoid any sleep disruption [3].

GOALS OF HCV TREATMENT

The goals of treating hepatitis C-infected patients can be threefold including;

1. Global HCV elimination,
2. Improving HCV-related health outcomes and survival both in general populations as well as in vulnerable HCV-affected proportion of the general population, and;
3. To prevent HCV transmission to unaffected ones.

The integrated subgoals with DAAs administrations are evidenced by an SVR, to reduce hepatitis C-related morbidities (*e.g.*, HCC, end-stage liver disease) and mortalities, as well as extrahepatic manifestations of CHC infection (*e.g.*, advanced fibrosis, cirrhosis, ascites, and cryoglobulinemic vasculitis) [11]. With the advent and approval of DAAs, all HCV-infected patients regardless of the severity of disease (either acute or chronic HCV infection), fibrosis, and cirrhosis stage are considered potential candidates for anti-HCV DAAs therapies [12]. The treatment window is wider now while considering individual patient demographics and infection kinetics (*e.g.*, hepatitis C genotype, presence or absence of cirrhosis, previous treatment history, *etc*.,) [13]. Furthermore, in each category of classified DAAs, several options are available for treatment in each category, and no single DAA regimen is prioritized or recommended over another in each category. Likely, for the treatment choices, specific individual patient factors including concomitant medical conditions, potential DDIs, and cost/coverage are also considered. Herein, we discuss the recommended DAA regimens for adults aged 18 and older to guide clinicians, practitioners, and other healthcare providers (HCPs) in treating patients with HCV infection. Recommended treatment regimens for patients aged 17 years and younger would also be briefly highlighted. All DAAs about drug regimen tables for all HCV GT/subtypes refer to oral medications [13].

Evidence	**Notes**	**Symbol**
High	Further research is very unlikely to change our confidence in the estimate of effect.	A
Moderate	Further research is likely to have an important impact on our confidence in the estimate of effect and may change the estimate.	B

Evidence	Notes	Symbol
Low or very low	Further research is very likely to have an important impact on our confidence in the estimate of effect and is likely to change the estimate. Any estimate of the effect is uncertain.	C
Recommendation	**Notes**	**Symbol**
Strong	Factors influencing the strength of the recommendation included the quality of the evidence, presumed patient-important outcomes, and cost.	1
Weak	Variability in preferences and values, or more uncertainty. The recommendation is made with less certainty; higher cost or resource consumption.	2

HCV GT-1 TREATMENT

HCV GT-1 prevalence: 49.1% worldwide, 70 to 75% in the USA		
HCV GT-1, subtype 1a treatment[13]		
Initial Treatment **In Past:** From 1998-2013 • Interferon (IFN) monotherapy • Pegylated interferon (PEG-IFN) plus RBV • Pegylated interferon (PEG-IFN) plus RBV plus NS3/4A protease inhibitor (boceprevir or telaprevir)		
Present treatment **Considerations prior to choosing initial treatment regimens:** • presence or absence of cirrhosis • medication cost or insurance considerations. • Baseline resistance testing		
Recommended regimens for HCV GT-1a patients' initial treatment: • ledipasvir • sofosbuvir • elbasvir • grazoprevir • glecaprevir • pibrentasvir • velpatasvir • voxilaprevir • ribavirin		
Treatment naïve patients with no cirrhosis [5, 10, 14]	**Duration**	**Brands**
Glecaprevir 300 mg/pibrentasvir 120 mg once daily (A1); This is taken as 3 tablets once daily with each fixed-dose tablet containing glecaprevir (100 mg)/pibrentasvir (40 mg).	8 weeks	GLE/PIB; (Mavyret®)
Sofosbuvir 400 mg/velpatasvir 100 mg once daily (A1)	12 weeks	SOF/VEL; (multiple brands)

For non-black patients, HIV-uninfected, and have HCV RNA <6 million copies/mL [15-17]. **Ledipasvir 90 mg/sofosbuvir 400 mg once daily (A2)**	8 weeks	LED/SOF; (multiple brands)
Ledipasvir 90 mg/sofosbuvir 400 mg once daily (A1)	12 weeks	LED/SOF; (multiple brands)
Fixed-dose combination of elbasvir (50 mg)/grazoprevir (100 mg) one tablet once daily (A1)	12 weeks	EBR/GZR; (Zepatier®)
Treatment naïve patients with compensated cirrhosis [11, 18, 19]		
Glecaprevir 300 mg/pibrentasvir 120 mg once daily (A1)	8 weeks	GLE/PIB; (Mavyret®)
Ledipasvir 90 mg/sofosbuvir 400 mg once daily (A1)	12 weeks	LED/SOF; (multiple brands)
Sofosbuvir 400 mg/velpatasvir 100 mg once daily (A1)	12 weeks	SOF/VEL; (multiple brands)
Fixed-dose combination of elbasvir (50 mg)/grazoprevir (100 mg) one tablet once daily	12 weeks	(EBR/GZR); (Zepatier®)
Retreatment options for patients with no cirrhosis and PEG-IFN failure [11, 20, 21]		
Glecaprevir 300 mg/pibrentasvir 120 mg once daily (A1)	8 weeks	GLE/PIB; (Mavyret®)
Ledipasvir 90 mg/sofosbuvir 400 mg once daily (A1)	12 weeks	LED/SOF; (multiple brands)
Sofosbuvir 400 mg/velpatasvir 100 mg once daily (A1)	12 weeks	SOF/VEL; (multiple brands)
Retreatment options for patients with compensated cirrhosis and PEG-IFN/RBV failure [11, 18, 20]		
Glecaprevir 300 mg/pibrentasvir 120 mg once daily (A1)	12 weeks	GLE/PIB; (Mavyret®)
Ledipasvir 90 mg/sofosbuvir 400 mg once daily (A1)	24weeks	LED/SOF; (multiple brands)
Ledipasvir 90 mg/sofosbuvir 400 mg once daily plus weight-based ribavirin twice daily (A1)	12 weeks	LED/SOF; (multiple brands) plus RBV (Copegus®)
Sofosbuvir 400 mg/velpatasvir 100 mg once daily (A1)	12 weeks	SOF/VEL; (multiple brands)
Retreatment options for patients with or without compensated cirrhosis and sofosbuvir (SOF) failure [22, 23]		
Fixed-dose combination of sofosbuvir (400 mg)/velpatasvir (100 mg)/voxilaprevir (100 mg) one tablet once daily (A1)	12 weeks	SOF/VEL/VOX; (Vosevi®)
Fixed-dose combination of glecaprevir (300 mg)/pibrentasvir (120 mg) once daily (A2)	16 weeks	GLE/PIB; (Mavyret®)
Retreatment options for patients with or without compensated cirrhosis and elbasvir/grazoprevir (EBR/GZR) failure [22]		

Fixed-dose combination of sofosbuvir (400 mg)/velpatasvir (100 mg)/voxilaprevir (100 mg) one tablet once daily (A1)	12 weeks	SOF/VEL/VOX; (Vosevi®)
Retreatment options for patients with or without compensated cirrhosis and glecaprevir/pibrentasvir (GLE/PIB) failure [24]		
• Fixed-dose combination of glecaprevir (300 mg)/pibrentasvir (120 mg) once daily (B2); plus • Sofosbuvir (400 mg) one tablet once daily (B2); plus • Ribavirin 1000 mg if <75 kg or 1200 mg if ≥75 kg (the daily dose is given in two divided doses) (B2) • Fixed-dose combination of sofosbuvir (400 mg)/velpatasvir (100 mg)/voxilaprevir (100 mg) one tablet once daily (B2)	16 weeks	GLE/PIB; (Mavyret®)
	16 weeks	SOF; (multiple brands)
	16 weeks	RBV; (Copegus®)
	12 weeks	SOF/VEL/VOX; (Vosevi®)
Retreatment options for patients with decompensated cirrhosis and glecaprevir/pibrentasvir (GLE/PIB) failure [24]		
• Fixed-dose combination of sofosbuvir (400 mg)/velpatasvir (100 mg)/voxilaprevir (100 mg) one tablet once daily (B2) plus • Ribavirin 1000 mg if <75 kg or 1200 mg if ≥75 kg (the daily dose is given in two divided doses) (B2)	12 weeks	SOF/VEL/VOX; (Vosevi®)
	12 weeks	RBV; (Copegus®)
Retreatment options for patients with multiple DAA treatment failures (SOF+VEL+VOX or SOF+GLE+PIB) [25]		
• Fixed-dose combination of glecaprevir (300 mg)/pibrentasvir (120 mg) once daily (B2); plus • Sofosbuvir (400 mg) one tablet once daily (B2); plus • Ribavirin 1000 mg if <75 kg or 1200 mg if ≥75 kg (the daily dose is given in two divided doses) (B2) (Or) • Fixed-dose combination of glecaprevir (300 mg)/pibrentasvir (120 mg) once daily (B2); plus • Ribavirin 1000 mg if <75 kg or 1200 mg if ≥75 kg (the daily dose is given in two divided doses) (B2)	16 weeks	GLE/PIB; (Mavyret®)
	16 weeks	SOF; (multiple brands)
	16 weeks	RBV; (Copegus®)
	24 weeks	GLE/PIB; (Mavyret®)
	24 weeks	RBV; (Copegus®)
HCV GT-1, subtype 1b treatment [13]		
Initial Treatment **In Past:** From 1998-2013 • Interferon (IFN) monotherapy • Pegylated interferon (PEG-IFN) plus RBV • Pegylated interferon (PEG-IFN) plus RBV plus NS3/4A protease inhibitor (boceprevir or telaprevir)		
Present treatment **Considerations prior to choosing initial treatment regimens:** • presence or absence of cirrhosis • medication cost or insurance considerations. • Baseline resistance testing		

Recommended regimens for GT-1b patient's initial treatment:

- ledipasvir
- sofosbuvir
- elbasvir
- grazoprevir
- glecaprevir
- pibrentasvir
- velpatasvir
- voxilaprevir
- ribavirin

Treatment naïve patients with no cirrhosis [11, 20]	**Duration**	**Brands**
Glecaprevir 300 mg/pibrentasvir 120 mg once daily (A1); This is taken as 3 tablets once daily with each fixed-dose tablet containing glecaprevir (100 mg)/pibrentasvir (40 mg).	8 weeks	GLE/PIB; (Mavyret®)
Sofosbuvir 400 mg/velpatasvir 100 mg once daily (A1)	12 weeks	SOF/VEL; (multiple brands)
For non-black patients, HIV-uninfected, and have HCV RNA <6 million copies/mL [15-17]. Ledipasvir 90 mg/sofosbuvir 400 mg once daily (A2)	8 weeks	LED/SOF; (multiple brands)
Ledipasvir 90 mg/sofosbuvir 400 mg once daily (A1)	12 weeks	LED/SOF; (multiple brands)
Fixed-dose combination of elbasvir (50 mg)/grazoprevir (100 mg) one tablet once daily (A1)	12 weeks	EBR/GZR; (Zepatier®)
For black patients, HIV-infected, and have HCV RNA ≥6 million copies/mL [15-17] Ledipasvir 90 mg/sofosbuvir 400 mg once daily (A2)	12 weeks	LED/SOF; (multiple brands)
Treatment naïve patients with compensated cirrhosis [6, 9, 10]		
Glecaprevir 300 mg/pibrentasvir 120 mg once daily (A1)	8 weeks	GLE/PIB; (Mavyret®)
Ledipasvir 90 mg/sofosbuvir 400 mg once daily (A1)	12 weeks	LED/SOF; (multiple brands)
Sofosbuvir 400 mg/velpatasvir 100 mg once daily (A1)	12 weeks	SOF/VEL; (multiple brands)
Fixed-dose combination of elbasvir (50 mg)/grazoprevir (100 mg) one tablet once daily	12 weeks	(EBR/GZR); (Zepatier®)
Retreatment options for patients with no cirrhosis and PEG-IFN/RBV failure [11, 21, 23, 26]		
Glecaprevir 300 mg/pibrentasvir 120 mg once daily (A1)	8 weeks	GLE/PIB; (Mavyret®)
Ledipasvir 90 mg/sofosbuvir 400 mg once daily (A1)	12 weeks	LED/SOF; (multiple brands)
Sofosbuvir 400 mg/velpatasvir 100 mg once daily (A1)	12 weeks	SOF/VEL; (multiple brands)
Retreatment options for patients with compensated cirrhosis and PEG-IFN/RBV failure [11, 18]		

Glecaprevir 300 mg/pibrentasvir 120 mg once daily (A1)	12 weeks	GLE/PIB; (Mavyret®)
Ledipasvir 90 mg/sofosbuvir 400 mg once daily (A1)	24weeks	LED/SOF; (multiple brands)
Ledipasvir 90 mg/sofosbuvir 400 mg once daily plus weight-based ribavirin twice daily (A1)	12 weeks	LED/SOF; (multiple brands) plus RBV (Copegus®)
Sofosbuvir 400 mg/velpatasvir 100 mg once daily (A1)	12 weeks	SOF/VEL; (multiple brands)
Retreatment options for patients with or without compensated cirrhosis and sofosbuvir (SOF) failure [27]		
Fixed-dose combination of sofosbuvir (400 mg)/velpatasvir (100 mg)/voxilaprevir (100 mg) one tablet once daily (A1)	12 weeks	SOF/VEL/VOX; (Vosevi®)
Fixed-dose combination of glecaprevir (300 mg)/pibrentasvir (120 mg) once daily (A2)	16 weeks	GLE/PIB; (Mavyret®)
Retreatment options for patients with or without compensated cirrhosis and elbasvir/grazoprevir (EBR/GZR) failure [27]		
Fixed-dose combination of sofosbuvir (400 mg)/velpatasvir (100 mg)/voxilaprevir (100 mg) one tablet once daily (A1)	12 weeks	SOF/VEL/VOX; (Vosevi®)
Retreatment options for patients with or without compensated cirrhosis and glecaprevir/pibrentasvir (GLE/PIB) failure [24]		
• Fixed-dose combination of glecaprevir (300 mg)/pibrentasvir (120 mg) once daily (B2); plus • Sofosbuvir (400 mg) one tablet once daily (B2); plus • Ribavirin 1000 mg if <75 kg or 1200 mg if ≥75 kg (the daily dose is given in two divided doses) (B2) (Or) • Fixed-dose combination of sofosbuvir (400 mg)/velpatasvir (100 mg)/voxilaprevir (100 mg) one tablet once daily (B2) (Or) • Fixed-dose combination of sofosbuvir (400 mg)/velpatasvir (100 mg)/voxilaprevir (100 mg) one tablet once daily (C2); plus • Ribavirin 1000 mg if <75 kg or 1200 mg if ≥75 kg (the daily dose is given in two divided doses) (C2)	16 weeks	GLE/PIB; (Mavyret®)
	16 weeks	SOF; (multiple brands)
	16 weeks	RBV; (Copegus®)
	12 weeks	SOF/VEL/VOX; (Vosevi®)
	12 weeks	SOF/VEL/VOX; (Vosevi®)
	12 weeks	RBV; (Copegus®)
Retreatment options for patients with compensated cirrhosis and glecaprevir/pibrentasvir (GLE/PIB) failure [24]		
• Fixed-dose combination of sofosbuvir (400 mg)/velpatasvir (100 mg)/voxilaprevir (100 mg) one tablet once daily (C2); plus • Ribavirin 1000 mg if <75 kg or 1200 mg if ≥75 kg (the daily dose is given in two divided doses) (C2)	12 weeks	SOF/VEL/VOX; (Vosevi®)
	12 weeks	RBV; (Copegus®)
Retreatment options for patients with multiple DAA treatment failures (SOF+VEL+VOX or SOF+GLE+PIB) [25]		

<table>
<tr><td rowspan="5">• Fixed-dose combination of glecaprevir (300 mg)/pibrentasvir (120 mg) once daily (B2); plus
• Sofosbuvir (400 mg) one tablet once daily (B2); plus
• Ribavirin 1000 mg if <75 kg or 1200 mg if ≥75 kg (the daily dose is given in two divided doses) (B2)
(Or)
• Fixed-dose combination of sofosbuvir (400 mg)/velpatasvir (100 mg)/voxilaprevir (100 mg) one tablet once daily (B2); plus
• Ribavirin 1000 mg if <75 kg or 1200 mg if ≥75 kg (the daily dose is given in two divided doses) (B2)</td><td>16 weeks</td><td>GLE/PIB;
(Mavyret®)</td></tr>
<tr><td>16 weeks</td><td>SOF;
(multiple brands)</td></tr>
<tr><td>16 weeks</td><td>RBV;
(Copegus®)</td></tr>
<tr><td>24 weeks</td><td>SOF/VEL/VOX;
(Vosevi®)</td></tr>
<tr><td>24 weeks</td><td>RBV;
(Copegus®)</td></tr>
</table>

HCV GT-2 TREATMENT

<table>
<tr><td colspan="3">HCV GT-2 prevalence: 11.0% worldwide, 13 to 15% in the USA</td></tr>
<tr><td colspan="3">HCV GT-2 treatment [13]</td></tr>
<tr><td colspan="3">Initial Treatment
In Past:
• Interferon (IFN) monotherapy
• Pegylated interferon (PEG-IFN) plus RBV
• Pegylated interferon (PEG-IFN) plus RBV plus NS3/4A protease inhibitor (boceprevir or telaprevir)
• Sofosbuvir plus ribavirin
• Declatasvir plus sofosbuvir</td></tr>
<tr><td colspan="3">Present treatment
Considerations prior to choosing initial treatment regimens:
• presence or absence of cirrhosis
• medication cost or insurance considerations.
• Baseline resistance testing</td></tr>
<tr><td colspan="3">Recommended regimens for HCV GT-2 patients' initial treatment:
• ledipasvir
• sofosbuvir
• elbasvir
• grazoprevir
• glecaprevir
• pibrentasvir
• velpatasvir
• voxilaprevir
• ribavirin</td></tr>
<tr><td>Treatment naïve patients with no cirrhosis [20, 27]</td><td>Duration</td><td>Brands</td></tr>
<tr><td>Glecaprevir 300 mg/pibrentasvir 120 mg once daily (A1); This is taken as 3 tablets once daily with each fixed-dose tablet containing glecaprevir (100 mg)/pibrentasvir (40 mg).</td><td>8 weeks</td><td>GLE/PIB;
(Mavyret®)</td></tr>
<tr><td>Sofosbuvir 400 mg/velpatasvir 100 mg once daily (A1)</td><td>12 weeks</td><td>SOF/VEL;
(multiple brands)</td></tr>
</table>

Treatment naïve patients with compensated cirrhosis [5, 10, 28, 29]		
Glecaprevir 300 mg/pibrentasvir 120 mg once daily (A1)	8 weeks	GLE/PIB; (Mavyret®)
Sofosbuvir 400 mg/velpatasvir 100 mg once daily (A1)	12 weeks	SOF/VEL; (multiple brands)
Retreatment options for patients with no or compensated cirrhosis and PEG-IFN/RBV failure [20, 23]		
No cirrhosis: Glecaprevir 300 mg/pibrentasvir 120 mg once daily (A1)	8 weeks	GLE/PIB; (Mavyret®)
Compensated cirrhosis: • Glecaprevir 300 mg/pibrentasvir 120 mg once daily (A1)	12 weeks	GLE/PIB; (Mavyret®)
• Sofosbuvir 400 mg/velpatasvir 100 mg once daily (A1)	12 weeks	SOF/VEL; (multiple brands)
Retreatment options for patients with or without compensated cirrhosis and sofosbuvir (SOF) failure [27]		
Fixed-dose combination of sofosbuvir (400 mg)/velpatasvir (100 mg)/voxilaprevir (100 mg) one tablet once daily (A1)	12 weeks	SOF/VEL/VOX; (Vosevi®)
Fixed-dose combination of glecaprevir (300 mg)/pibrentasvir (120 mg) once daily (A2)	16 weeks	GLE/PIB; (Mavyret®)
Retreatment options for patients with or without compensated cirrhosis and elbasvir/grazoprevir (EBR/GZR) failure [27]		
Fixed-dose combination of sofosbuvir (400 mg)/velpatasvir (100 mg)/voxilaprevir (100 mg) one tablet once daily (A1)	12 weeks	SOF/VEL/VOX; (Vosevi®)
Retreatment options for patients with or without compensated cirrhosis and glecaprevir/pibrentasvir (GLE/PIB) failure [24]		
• Fixed-dose combination of glecaprevir (300 mg)/pibrentasvir (120 mg) once daily (B2); plus	16 weeks	GLE/PIB; (Mavyret®)
• Sofosbuvir (400 mg) one tablet once daily (B2); plus	16 weeks	SOF; (multiple brands)
• Ribavirin 1000 mg if <75 kg or 1200 mg if ≥75 kg (the daily dose is given in two divided doses) (B2)	16 weeks	RBV; (Copegus®)
• Fixed-dose combination of sofosbuvir (400 mg)/velpatasvir (100 mg)/voxilaprevir (100 mg) one tablet once daily (B2)	12 weeks	SOF/VEL/VOX; (Vosevi®)
• Fixed-dose combination of sofosbuvir (400 mg)/velpatasvir (100 mg)/voxilaprevir (100 mg) one tablet once daily (C2) plus	12 weeks	SOF/VEL/VOX; (Vosevi®)
• Ribavirin 1000 mg if <75 kg or 1200 mg if ≥75 kg (the daily dose is given in two divided doses) (C2)	12 weeks	RBV; (Copegus®)
Retreatment options for patients with multiple DAA treatment failures (SOF+VEL+VOX or SOF+GLE+PIB) [25]		

• Fixed-dose combination of glecaprevir (300 mg)/pibrentasvir (120 mg) once daily (B2); plus • Sofosbuvir (400 mg) one tablet once daily (B2); plus • Ribavirin 1000 mg if <75 kg or 1200 mg if ≥75 kg (the daily dose is given in two divided doses) (B2) (Or) • Fixed-dose combination of sofosbuvir (400 mg)/velpatasvir (100 mg)/voxilaprevir (100 mg) one tablet once daily (C2) plus • Ribavirin 1000 mg if <75 kg or 1200 mg if ≥75 kg (the daily dose is given in two divided doses) (B2)	16 weeks	GLE/PIB; (Mavyret®)
	16 weeks	SOF; (multiple brands)
	16 weeks	RBV; (Copegus®)
	24 weeks	GLE/PIB; (Mavyret®)
	24 weeks	RBV; (Copegus®)

HCV GT-3 TREATMENT

HCV GT-3 prevalence: 17.9% worldwide, 10% in the USA		
HCV GT-3 treatment [13]		
Initial Treatment **In Past:** • Sofosbuvir plus weight-based ribavirin (12 or 16 weeks; low SVR rates) • Sofosbuvir plus pegylated interferon plus weight-based ribavirin (12 weeks; low SVR rates) • Sofosbuvir plus ribavirin (24 weeks) • Sofosbuvir plus daclatasvir (16 or 24 weeks)		
Present treatment **Considerations prior to choosing initial treatment regimens:** • The presence of baseline NS5A resistance-associated substitution Y93H (screening required for patients with cirrhosis or prior treatment experience in whom sofosbuvir-velpatasvir or daclatasvir plus sofosbuvir is being considered) • Patient cirrhosis status • Prior treatment experience • Coexistent renal disease • Drug interactions • Medication cost and/or insurance considerations		
Recommended regimens for HCV GT-3 patients' initial treatment: • ledipasvir • sofosbuvir • elbasvir • grazoprevir • glecaprevir • pibrentasvir • velpatasvir • voxilaprevir • ribavirin		
Treatment naïve patients with no cirrhosis [30]	**Duration**	**Brands**

Glecaprevir 300 mg/pibrentasvir 120 mg once daily (A1); This is taken as 3 tablets once daily with each fixed-dose tablet containing glecaprevir (100 mg)/pibrentasvir (40 mg).	8 weeks	GLE/PIB; (Mavyret®)
Sofosbuvir 400 mg/velpatasvir 100 mg once daily (A1)	12 weeks	SOF/VEL; (multiple brands)
Treatment naïve patients with compensated cirrhosis [10, 28, 31]		
Glecaprevir 300 mg/pibrentasvir 120 mg once daily (A1)	8 weeks	GLE/PIB; (Mavyret®)
Sofosbuvir 400 mg/velpatasvir 100 mg once daily (A1)	12 weeks	SOF/VEL; (multiple brands)
• Sofosbuvir 400 mg/velpatasvir 100 mg once daily (A2); plus • Ribavirin 1000 mg if <75 kg or 1200 mg if ≥75 kg (the daily dose is given in two divided doses)	12 weeks	SOF/VEL; (multiple brands)
	12 weeks	RBV; (Copegus®)
Fixed-dose combination of sofosbuvir (400 mg)/velpatasvir (100 mg)/voxilaprevir (100 mg) one tablet once daily (A1); plus	12 weeks	SOF/VEL/VOX; (Vosevi®)
Retreatment options for patients with no cirrhosis and PEG-IFN/RBV failure [30]		
Glecaprevir 300 mg/pibrentasvir 120 mg once daily (A1)	16 weeks	GLE/PIB; (Mavyret®)
Sofosbuvir 400 mg/velpatasvir 100 mg once daily (A1)	12 weeks	SOF/VEL; (multiple brands)

Retreatment options for patients with compensated cirrhosis and PEG-IFN/RBV failure [28]		
Glecaprevir 300 mg/pibrentasvir 120 mg once daily (A1)	16 weeks	GLE/PIB; (Mavyret®)
Sofosbuvir 400 mg/velpatasvir 100 mg once daily (A1)	12 weeks	SOF/VEL; (multiple brands)
Retreatment options for patients with or without compensated cirrhosis and sofosbuvir (SOF) failure [27]		
Fixed-dose combination of sofosbuvir (400 mg)/velpatasvir (100 mg)/voxilaprevir (100 mg) one tablet once daily (A1)	12 weeks	SOF/VEL/VOX; (Vosevi®)
Fixed-dose combination of glecaprevir (300 mg)/pibrentasvir (120 mg) once daily (A2)	16 weeks	GLE/PIB; (Mavyret®)
Retreatment options for patients with or without compensated cirrhosis and elbasvir/grazoprevir (EBR/GZR) failure [27]		
Fixed-dose combination of sofosbuvir (400 mg)/velpatasvir (100 mg)/voxilaprevir (100 mg) one tablet once daily (A1)	12 weeks	SOF/VEL/VOX; (Vosevi®)
Retreatment options for patients with or without compensated cirrhosis and glecaprevir/pibrentasvir (GLE/PIB) failure [24]		

• Fixed-dose combination of glecaprevir (300 mg)/pibrentasvir (120 mg) once daily (B2); plus • Sofosbuvir (400 mg) one tablet once daily (B2); plus • Ribavirin 1000 mg if <75 kg or 1200 mg if ≥75 kg (the daily dose is given in two divided doses) (B2)	16 weeks	GLE/PIB; (Mavyret®)
	16 weeks	SOF; (multiple brands)
	16 weeks	RBV; (Copegus®)
• Fixed-dose combination of sofosbuvir (400 mg)/velpatasvir (100 mg)/voxilaprevir (100 mg) one tablet once daily (B2)	12 weeks	SOF/VEL/VOX; (Vosevi®)
• Fixed-dose combination of sofosbuvir (400 mg)/velpatasvir (100 mg)/voxilaprevir (100 mg) one tablet once daily (C2) plus • Ribavirin 1000 mg if <75 kg or 1200 mg if ≥75 kg (the daily dose is given in two divided doses) (C2)	12 weeks	SOF/VEL/VOX; (Vosevi®)
	12 weeks	RBV; (Copegus®)
Retreatment options for patients with multiple DAA treatment failure (SOF-VEL-VOX or SOF plus GLE-PIB) [25]		
• Fixed-dose combination of glecaprevir (300 mg)/pibrentasvir (120 mg) once daily (B2); plus • Sofosbuvir (400 mg) one tablet once daily (B2); plus • Ribavirin 1000 mg if <75 kg or 1200 mg if ≥75 kg (the daily dose is given in two divided doses) (B2) (Or) • Fixed-dose combination of sofosbuvir (400 mg)/velpatasvir (100 mg)/voxilaprevir (100 mg) one tablet once daily (C2) plus • Ribavirin 1000 mg if <75 kg or 1200 mg if ≥75 kg (the daily dose is given in two divided doses) (B2)	16 weeks	GLE/PIB; (Mavyret®)
	16 weeks	SOF; (multiple brands)
	16 weeks	RBV; (Copegus®)
	24 weeks	GLE/PIB; (Mavyret®)
	24 weeks	RBV; (Copegus®)

HCV GT-4 TREATMENT

HCV GT-4 prevalence: 8 to 20% worldwide, 1 to 2% in the USA
HCV GT-4 treatment [13]
Initial Treatment **In Past:** • Interferon • Pegylated interferon plus weight-based ribavirin (48 weeks; very low SVR rates) • Sofosbuvir plus ribavirin • Simeprevir plus sofosbuvir • Simeprevir plus peginterferon plus ribavirin • Daclatasvir plus peginterferon plus ribavirin
Present treatment **Considerations prior to choosing initial treatment regimens:** • Patient cirrhosis status • Prior treatment experience • Coexistent renal disease • Medication cost and/or insurance considerations

Recommended regimens for HCV GT-4 patients' initial treatment:

- ledipasvir
- sofosbuvir
- elbasvir
- grazoprevir
- glecaprevir
- pibrentasvir
- velpatasvir
- voxilaprevir
- ribavirin

Treatment naïve patients with no cirrhosis or compensated cirrhosis [5, 20, 29, 31, 32]	**Duration**	**Brands**
Glecaprevir 300 mg/pibrentasvir 120 mg once daily (A1); This is taken as 3 tablets once daily with each fixed-dose tablet containing glecaprevir (100 mg)/pibrentasvir (40 mg).	8 weeks	GLE/PIB; (Mavyret®)
Fixed-dose combination of elbasvir (50 mg)/grazoprevir (100 mg) one tablet once daily (A1)	12 weeks	EBR/GZR; (Zepatier®)
Sofosbuvir 400 mg/velpatasvir 100 mg once daily (A1)	12 weeks	SOF/VEL; (multiple brands)
Ledipasvir 90 mg/sofosbuvir 400 mg once daily (A1)	12 weeks	(LED/SOF; (multiple brands)
Retreatment options for patients with NO or compensated cirrhosis and PEG-IFN/RBV failure [11, 20, 31]		
No cirrhosis: Glecaprevir 300 mg/pibrentasvir 120 mg once daily (A1)	8 weeks	GLE/PIB; (Mavyret®)
Compensated cirrhosis: Glecaprevir 300 mg/pibrentasvir 120 mg once daily (A1)	12 weeks	GLE/PIB; (Mavyret®)
Sofosbuvir 400 mg/velpatasvir 100 mg once daily (A1)	12 weeks	SOF/VEL; (multiple brands)
Ledipasvir 90 mg/sofosbuvir 400 mg once daily (A1)	12 weeks	(LED/SOF; (multiple brands)
Retreatment options for patients with or without compensated cirrhosis and sofosbuvir (SOF) failure [27]		
Fixed-dose combination of sofosbuvir (400 mg)/velpatasvir (100 mg)/voxilaprevir (100 mg) one tablet once daily (A1)	12 weeks	SOF/VEL/VOX; (Vosevi®)
Fixed-dose combination of glecaprevir (300 mg)/pibrentasvir (120 mg) once daily (A2)	16 weeks	GLE/PIB; (Mavyret®)
Retreatment options for patients with or without compensated cirrhosis and elbasvir/grazoprevir (EBR/GZR) failure [27]		
Fixed-dose combination of sofosbuvir (400 mg)/velpatasvir (100 mg)/voxilaprevir (100 mg) one tablet once daily (A1)	12 weeks	SOF/VEL/VOX; (Vosevi®)
Retreatment options for patients with or without compensated cirrhosis and glecaprevir/pibrentasvir (GLE/PIB) failure [24]		

<table>
<tr><td rowspan="3">• Fixed-dose combination of glecaprevir (300 mg)/pibrentasvir (120 mg) once daily (B2); plus
• Sofosbuvir (400 mg) one tablet once daily (B2); plus
• Ribavirin 1000 mg if <75 kg or 1200 mg if ≥75 kg (the daily dose is given in two divided doses) (B2)</td><td>16 weeks</td><td>GLE/PIB; (Mavyret®)</td></tr>
<tr><td>16 weeks</td><td>SOF; (multiple brands)</td></tr>
<tr><td>16 weeks</td><td>RBV; (Copegus®)</td></tr>
<tr><td>• Fixed-dose combination of sofosbuvir (400 mg)/velpatasvir (100 mg)/voxilaprevir (100 mg) one tablet once daily (B2)</td><td>12 weeks</td><td>SOF/VEL/VOX; (Vosevi®)</td></tr>
<tr><td rowspan="2">• Fixed-dose combination of sofosbuvir (400 mg)/velpatasvir (100 mg)/voxilaprevir (100 mg) one tablet once daily (C2) plus
• Ribavirin 1000 mg if <75 kg or 1200 mg if ≥75 kg (the daily dose is given in two divided doses) (C2)</td><td>12 weeks</td><td>SOF/VEL/VOX; (Vosevi®)</td></tr>
<tr><td>12 weeks</td><td>RBV; (Copegus®)</td></tr>
<tr><td colspan="3">Retreatment options for patients with multiple DAA treatment failure (SOF-VEL-VOX or SOF plus GLE-PIB) [25]</td></tr>
<tr><td rowspan="5">• Fixed-dose combination of glecaprevir (300 mg)/pibrentasvir (120 mg) once daily (B2); plus
• Sofosbuvir (400 mg) one tablet once daily (B2); plus
• Ribavirin 1000 mg if <75 kg or 1200 mg if ≥75 kg (the daily dose is given in two divided doses) (B2)
(Or)
• Fixed-dose combination of sofosbuvir (400 mg)/velpatasvir (100 mg)/voxilaprevir (100 mg) one tablet once daily (C2) plus
• Ribavirin 1000 mg if <75 kg or 1200 mg if ≥75 kg (the daily dose is given in two divided doses) (B2)</td><td>16 weeks</td><td>GLE/PIB; (Mavyret®)</td></tr>
<tr><td>16 weeks</td><td>SOF; (multiple brands)</td></tr>
<tr><td>16 weeks</td><td>RBV; (Copegus®)</td></tr>
<tr><td>24 weeks</td><td>GLE/PIB; (Mavyret®)</td></tr>
<tr><td>24 weeks</td><td>RBV; (Copegus®)</td></tr>
</table>

HCV GT-5 TREATMENT

<table>
<tr><td>HCV GT-5 prevalence: Less than 5% worldwide, Fewer than 2% in the USA</td></tr>
<tr><td>HCV GT-5 treatment [13]</td></tr>
<tr><td>Initial Treatment
In Past:
• Interferon plus weight-based ribavirin (48 weeks)
• Pegylated interferon plus weight-based ribavirin (48 weeks)</td></tr>
<tr><td>Present treatment
Considerations prior to choosing initial treatment regimens:
• Patient cirrhosis status
• Prior treatment experience</td></tr>
</table>

Recommended regimens for HCV GT-5 patients' initial treatment: • ledipasvir • sofosbuvir • elbasvir • grazoprevir • glecaprevir • pibrentasvir • velpatasvir • voxilaprevir • ribavirin		
Treatment naïve patients with no cirrhosis OR compensated cirrhosis [5 - 11, 20, 29, 32]	**Duration**	**Brands**
Glecaprevir 300 mg/pibrentasvir 120 mg once daily (A1); This is taken as 3 tablets once daily with each fixed-dose tablet containing glecaprevir (100 mg)/pibrentasvir (40 mg).	8 weeks	GLE/PIB; (Mavyret®)
Fixed-dose combination of elbasvir (50 mg)/grazoprevir (100 mg) one tablet once daily (A1)	12 weeks	EBR/GZR; (Zepatier®)
Sofosbuvir 400 mg/velpatasvir 100 mg once daily (A1)	12 weeks	SOF/VEL; (multiple brands)
Ledipasvir 90 mg/sofosbuvir 400 mg once daily (A1)	12 weeks	(LED/SOF; (multiple brands)
Retreatment options for patients with no or compensated cirrhosis and PEG-IFN/RBV failure [11, 20, 32]		
No cirrhosis: Glecaprevir 300 mg/pibrentasvir 120 mg once daily (A1)	8 weeks	GLE/PIB; (Mavyret®)
Compensated cirrhosis: Glecaprevir 300 mg/pibrentasvir 120 mg once daily (A1)	12 weeks	GLE/PIB; (Mavyret®)
Sofosbuvir 400 mg/velpatasvir 100 mg once daily (A1)	12 weeks	SOF/VEL; (multiple brands)
Ledipasvir 90 mg/sofosbuvir 400 mg once daily (A1)	12 weeks	(LED/SOF; (multiple brands)
Retreatment options for patients with or without compensated cirrhosis and sofosbuvir (SOF) failure [27]		
Fixed-dose combination of sofosbuvir (400 mg)/velpatasvir (100 mg)/voxilaprevir (100 mg) one tablet once daily (A1)	12 weeks	SOF/VEL/VOX; (Vosevi®)
Fixed-dose combination of glecaprevir (300 mg)/pibrentasvir (120 mg) once daily (A2)	16 weeks	GLE/PIB; (Mavyret®)
Retreatment options for patients with or without compensated cirrhosis and elbasvir/grazoprevir (EBR/GZR) failure [27]		
Fixed-dose combination of sofosbuvir (400 mg)/velpatasvir (100 mg)/voxilaprevir (100 mg) one tablet once daily (A1)	12 weeks	SOF/VEL/VOX; (Vosevi®)
Retreatment options for patients with or without compensated cirrhosis and glecaprevir/pibrentasvir (GLE/PIB) failure [24]		

• Fixed-dose combination of glecaprevir (300 mg)/pibrentasvir (120 mg) once daily (B2); plus • Sofosbuvir (400 mg) one tablet once daily (B2); plus • Ribavirin 1000 mg if <75 kg or 1200 mg if ≥75 kg (the daily dose is given in two divided doses) (B2)	16 weeks	GLE/PIB; (Mavyret®)
	16 weeks	SOF; (multiple brands)
	16 weeks	RBV; (Copegus®)
• Fixed-dose combination of sofosbuvir (400 mg)/velpatasvir (100 mg)/voxilaprevir (100 mg) one tablet once daily (B2)	12 weeks	SOF/VEL/VOX; (Vosevi®)
• Fixed-dose combination of sofosbuvir (400 mg)/velpatasvir (100 mg)/voxilaprevir (100 mg) one tablet once daily (C2) plus • Ribavirin 1000 mg if <75 kg or 1200 mg if ≥75 kg (the daily dose is given in two divided doses) (C2)	12 weeks	SOF/VEL/VOX; (Vosevi®)
	12 weeks	RBV; (Copegus®)
Retreatment options for patients with multiple DAA treatment failure (SOF-VEL-VOX or SOF plus GLE-PIB) [25]		
• Fixed-dose combination of glecaprevir (300 mg)/pibrentasvir (120 mg) once daily (B2); plus • Sofosbuvir (400 mg) one tablet once daily (B2); plus • Ribavirin 1000 mg if <75 kg or 1200 mg if ≥75 kg (the daily dose is given in two divided doses) (B2) (Or) • Fixed-dose combination of sofosbuvir (400 mg)/velpatasvir (100 mg)/voxilaprevir (100 mg) one tablet once daily (C2) plus • Ribavirin 1000 mg if <75 kg or 1200 mg if ≥75 kg (the daily dose is given in two divided doses) (B2)	16 weeks	GLE/PIB; (Mavyret®)
	16 weeks	SOF; (multiple brands)
	16 weeks	RBV; (Copegus®)
	24 weeks	GLE/PIB; (Mavyret®)
	24 weeks	RBV; (Copegus®)

HCV GT-6 TREATMENT

HCV GT-6 prevalence: 5% worldwide, Fewer than 2% in the USA
HCV GT-6 treatment [13]
Initial Treatment **In Past:** • Interferon plus weight-based ribavirin (48 weeks) • Pegylated interferon plus weight-based ribavirin (48 weeks)
Present treatment **Considerations prior to choosing initial treatment regimens:** • Patient cirrhosis status • Prior treatment experience

Recommended regimens for HCV GT-6 patients' initial treatment: • ledipasvir • sofosbuvir • elbasvir • grazoprevir • glecaprevir • pibrentasvir • velpatasvir • voxilaprevir • ribavirin		
Treatment naïve patients with no cirrhosis or compensated cirrhosis [5 - 11, 22]	**Duration**	**Brands**
Glecaprevir 300 mg/pibrentasvir 120 mg once daily (A1); This is taken as 3 tablets once daily with each fixed-dose tablet containing glecaprevir (100 mg)/pibrentasvir (40 mg).	8 weeks	GLE/PIB; (Mavyret®)
Fixed-dose combination of elbasvir (50 mg)/grazoprevir (100 mg) one tablet once daily (A1)	12 weeks	EBR/GZR; (Zepatier®)
Sofosbuvir 400 mg/velpatasvir 100 mg once daily (A1)	12 weeks	SOF/VEL; (multiple brands)
Ledipasvir 90 mg/sofosbuvir 400 mg once daily (A1)	12 weeks	(LED/SOF; (multiple brands)
Retreatment options for patients with no or compensated cirrhosis and PEG-IFN/RBV failure [11, 20]		
No cirrhosis: Glecaprevir 300 mg/pibrentasvir 120 mg once daily (A1)	8 weeks	GLE/PIB; (Mavyret®)
Compensated cirrhosis: Glecaprevir 300 mg/pibrentasvir 120 mg once daily (A1)	12 weeks	GLE/PIB; (Mavyret®)
Sofosbuvir 400 mg/velpatasvir 100 mg once daily (A1)	12 weeks	SOF/VEL; (multiple brands)
Ledipasvir 90 mg/sofosbuvir 400 mg once daily (A1)	12 weeks	(LED/SOF; (multiple brands)
Retreatment options for patients with or without compensated cirrhosis and sofosbuvir (SOF) failure [27]		
Fixed-dose combination of sofosbuvir (400 mg)/velpatasvir (100 mg)/voxilaprevir (100 mg) one tablet once daily (A1)	12 weeks	SOF/VEL/VOX; (Vosevi®)
Fixed-dose combination of glecaprevir (300 mg)/pibrentasvir (120 mg) once daily (A2)	16 weeks	GLE/PIB; (Mavyret®)
Retreatment options for patients with or without compensated cirrhosis and elbasvir/grazoprevir (EBR/GZR) failure [27]		
Fixed-dose combination of sofosbuvir (400 mg)/velpatasvir (100 mg)/voxilaprevir (100 mg) one tablet once daily (A1)	12 weeks	SOF/VEL/VOX; (Vosevi®)
Retreatment options for patients with or without compensated cirrhosis and glecaprevir/pibrentasvir (GLE/PIB) failure [24]		

• Fixed-dose combination of glecaprevir (300 mg)/pibrentasvir (120 mg) once daily (B2); plus • Sofosbuvir (400 mg) one tablet once daily (B2); plus • Ribavirin 1000 mg if <75 kg or 1200 mg if ≥75 kg (the daily dose is given in two divided doses) (B2)	16 weeks	GLE/PIB; (Mavyret®)
	16 weeks	SOF; (multiple brands)
	16 weeks	RBV; (Copegus®)
• Fixed-dose combination of sofosbuvir (400 mg)/velpatasvir (100 mg)/voxilaprevir (100 mg) one tablet once daily (B2)	12 weeks	SOF/VEL/VOX; (Vosevi®)
• Fixed-dose combination of sofosbuvir (400 mg)/velpatasvir (100 mg)/voxilaprevir (100 mg) one tablet once daily (C2) plus • Ribavirin 1000 mg if <75 kg or 1200 mg if ≥75 kg (the daily dose is given in two divided doses) (C2)	12 weeks	SOF/VEL/VOX; (Vosevi®)
	12 weeks	RBV; (Copegus®)
Retreatment options for patients with multiple DAA treatment failure (SOF-VEL-VOX or SOF plus GLE-PIB) [25]		
• Fixed-dose combination of glecaprevir (300 mg)/pibrentasvir (120 mg) once daily (B2); plus • Sofosbuvir (400 mg) one tablet once daily (B2); plus • Ribavirin 1000 mg if <75 kg or 1200 mg if ≥75 kg (the daily dose is given in two divided doses) (B2) (Or) • Fixed-dose combination of sofosbuvir (400 mg)/velpatasvir (100 mg)/voxilaprevir (100 mg) one tablet once daily (C2) plus • Ribavirin 1000 mg if <75 kg or 1200 mg if ≥75 kg (the daily dose is given in two divided doses) (B2)	16 weeks	GLE/PIB; (Mavyret®)
	16 weeks	SOF; (multiple brands)
	16 weeks	RBV; (Copegus®)
	24 weeks	GLE/PIB; (Mavyret®)
	24 weeks	RBV; (Copegus®)

RECENT ADVANCES IN THE DEVELOPMENT OF NEW DAAS

The excellent improvements in the development of pan-genotypic DAAs eliminated most of the remaining challenges in anti-HCV treatment [1]. Furthermore, the advent and approval of next-wave NS3/4A PIs, NS5A, and NS5B proteins inhibitors in the last 5 years made it possible to cure most HCV-infected patients without any relevant severe adverse outcomes by using a PEG-IFN-free DAA combination [3]. These treatment approaches are sufficient for most HCV-infected patients worldwide and essential for global HCV elimination. However; some difficult-to-cure HCV patient populations (*e.g.*, decompensated liver disease, HCV GT-3 infected patients, HCV/HIV co-infected patients, and liver transplant patients) still remain to be treated and a few patient populations fail to respond to first-line DAA therapy but also even retreatment with pan-genotypic DAAs [1]. Hence, the improvements in current DAAs kinetics and the development of newer ones would be continued to enable these regimens to cure the difficult-to-treat HCV populations. A combination of ravidasvir (a pan-genotypic NS5A inhibitor) and sofosbuvir appears to be an effective treatment for chronic (HCV) infection across a diverse pool of patients without cirrhosis or with compensated cirrhosis [33]. To test this regimen, 301 HCV patients were enrolled in the first stage of STORM-C-1, a two-stage, open-label, phase-2/3 single-arm trial taking place in six centers in Malaysia and four centers in Thailand [33]. Half of the participants (52%) had genotype-3 HCV infection, 33% of patients had genotype-1a, 9% had genotype-1b, 1% had genotype 2 and 5% had genotype 6. A second stage of the trial including 300 additional patients is currently ongoing. Among the patients in stage 1 of the trial, 27% were already experiencing compensated cirrhosis, 30% had an HIV co-infection and 33% had received previous interferon-based treatment [33]. The trial assessed the efficacy, safety, tolerability, and pharmacokinetics of ravidasvir and sofosbuvir through 12-week and 24- week ribavirin-free regimens. Patients without cirrhosis were prescribed once-daily ravidasvir at 200 mg and sofosbuvir at 400 mg for 12 weeks, while patients with cirrhosis were given the same prescription for 24 weeks. The primary endpoint was an overall sustained virological response at 12 weeks after treatment (SVR12), defined as HCV RNA <12 IU/mL in Thailand and HCV RNA <15 IU/mL in Malaysia [34]. Of the 300 patients in the analysis set, 291 (97%) achieved SVR12. Among the 153 (97%) of 158 patients with genotype-3 infection, who met the SVR12 threshold, a subset of 51 (96%) of the 53 patients who also had cirrhosis within that group did so as well. No difference was found in SVR12 outcomes based on HIV co-infection or previous interferon treatment. The overall SVR rates were wonderful surprises for three difficult-to-treat HCV-infected populations (*i.e.*, HCV GT-3, cirrhotic, and HIV-coinfected patients). Despite the high number of comorbidities within the patient population, the ravidasvir-sofosbuvir regimen proved to be well tolerated, safe, and free of any "clinically relevant" drug-drug interactions with the HIV antiretrovirals commonly prescribed in Thailand and Malaysia [34]. The most common adverse events to emerge during the treatments were pyrexia (12%), cough (9%), upper respiratory tract infection (8%), and headache (7%) [34]. There were no deaths or treatment discontinuations due to the study drugs. Similarly, some other investigational DAAs are in the pipeline, and clinical development. Their availability to treat difficult-to-cure HCV populations will help to achieve global HCV elimination. Those will also help in to search an effective antiviral treatment for acute HCV infection, establishing a strategy for pre-exposure prophylaxis, and ideally developing an effective HCV vaccine to prevent new HCV infections worldwide.

CONCLUSIONS

In 2014, the inclusion of the RNA-dependent polymerase inhibitor (*i.e.* sofosbuvir) to the treatment paradigm revolutionized the advent of DAAs for HCV therapeutics. After that, the manual of HCV-specific DAAs is consistently expanding and looming by achieving the cure of CHC for almost every person who is treated with those. Around 10 million people have been treated with DAAs achieving higher SVR rates and the lowest We have highly efficacious, well-tolerable, and pan-genotypic DAAs with cure rates of more than 95%. However; the availability, affordability, and accessibility of these costly regimens are still challenging in several LMICs where HCV is almost endemic. The promising real-world clinical data validate the pan-genotypic DAAs administration to all HCV GTs/subtypes infected individuals regardless of their infection status, absence, or presence of cirrhosis, HBV/HCV, HIV/HCV or HCV/CKD comorbid states, liver or kidney transplant patients, and as a retreatment option in previous treatment failures with IFN-free plus RBV or NS3-4A or NS5A failures. However, the treatment algorithms are yet to be defined for pregnant women, infants, and children. Similarly, DAAs efficacy in decompensated cirrhotic affected with HCV GT-3 and 4d are also not remarkably significant. RBV addition in some DAA regimens is also absolute which may lead to some SAEs in treated individuals and dosage adjustment is highly recommended in HCV/CKD coinfected patients. Despite the lack of an effective and protective vaccine model like HBV, the overall progress in HCV therapeutics based on DAAs administration is remarkably significant and still proving their worth to treat HCV; albeit the pace of DAAs availability and accessibility is slow to those who need them the most.

REFERENCES

[1] Shahid I, Ibrahim MM. All oral interferon-free direct-acting antivirals as combination therapies to cure hepatitis C. Curr Mol Med 2019; 18(7): 409-35.
[http://dx.doi.org/10.2174/1566524019666190104110439] [PMID: 30608042]

[2] Shahid I, ALMalki WH, Hafeez MH, Hassan S. Hepatitis C virus infection treatment: An era of game changer direct acting antivirals and novel treatment strategies. Crit Rev Microbiol 2016; 42(4): 535-47.
[http://dx.doi.org/10.3109/1040841X.2014.970123] [PMID: 25373616]

[3] Shahid I, AlMalki WH, Hassan S, Hafeez MH. Real-world challenges for hepatitis C virus medications: a critical overview. Crit Rev Microbiol 2018; 44(2): 143-60.
[http://dx.doi.org/10.1080/1040841X.2017.1329277] [PMID: 28539069]

[4] Shahid I, Alzahrani AR, Al-Ghamdi SS, Alanazi IM, Rehman S, Hassan S. Hepatitis C diagnosis: Simplified solutions, predictive brriers, and fuure promises. Diagnostics (Basel, Switzerland) 2021; 11(7).

[5] Forns X, Lee SS, Valdes J, *et al.* Glecaprevir plus pibrentasvir for chronic hepatitis C virus genotype 1, 2, 4, 5, or 6 infection in adults with compensated cirrhosis (EXPEDITION-1): a single-arm, open-label, multicentre phase 3 trial. Lancet Infect Dis 2017; 17(10): 1062-8.
[http://dx.doi.org/10.1016/S1473-3099(17)30496-6] [PMID: 28818546]

[6] Brown RS Jr, Buti M, Rodrigues L, *et al.* Glecaprevir/pibrentasvir for 8 weeks in treatment-naïve patients with chronic HCV genotypes 1 6 and compensated cirrhosis: The EXPEDITION-8 trial. J Hepatol 2020; 72(3): 441-9.
[http://dx.doi.org/10.1016/j.jhep.2019.10.020] [PMID: 31682879]

[7] Smith-Palmer J, Cerri K, Valentine W. Achieving sustained virologic response in hepatitis C: a systematic review of the clinical, economic and quality of life benefits. BMC Infect Dis 2015; 15(1):

19.
[http://dx.doi.org/10.1186/s12879-015-0748-8] [PMID: 25596623]

[8] Lawitz E, Gane E, Pearlman B, *et al.* Efficacy and safety of 12 weeks versus 18 weeks of treatment with grazoprevir (MK-5172) and elbasvir (MK-8742) with or without ribavirin for hepatitis C virus genotype 1 infection in previously untreated patients with cirrhosis and patients with previous null response with or without cirrhosis (C-WORTHY): a randomised, open-label phase 2 trial. Lancet 2015; 385(9973): 1075-86.
[http://dx.doi.org/10.1016/S0140-6736(14)61795-5] [PMID: 25467591]

[9] Highlights in Hepatitis C Virus From the 2017 AASLD Liver Meeting: A Review of Selected Presentations. The University of Texas Health, San AntonioSan Antonio, Texas. Gastroenterology and Hepatology. 2017; 13(12): 1-24.

[10] Simmons B, Saleem J, Heath K, Cooke GS, Hill A. Long-term treatment outcomes of patients infected with Hepatitis C virus: a systematic review and meta-analysis of the survival benefit of achieving a sustained virological response. Clin Infect Dis 2015; 61(5): 730-40.
[http://dx.doi.org/10.1093/cid/civ396] [PMID: 25987643]

[11] Feld JJ, Jacobson IM, Hézode C, *et al.* Sofosbuvir and Velpatasvir for HCV Genotype 1, 2, 4, 5, and 6 Infection. N Engl J Med 2015; 373(27): 2599-607.
[http://dx.doi.org/10.1056/NEJMoa1512610] [PMID: 26571066]

[12] Terrault NA, Zeuzem S, Di Bisceglie AM, *et al.* Effectiveness of Ledipasvir-Sofosbuvir Combination in Patients With Hepatitis C Virus Infection and Factors Associated With Sustained Virologic Response. Gastroenterology 2016; 151(6): 1131-1140.e5.
[http://dx.doi.org/10.1053/j.gastro.2016.08.004] [PMID: 27565882]

[13] Kowdley KV, Sundaram V, Jeon CY, *et al.* Eight weeks of ledipasvir/sofosbuvir is effective for selected patients with genotype 1 hepatitis C virus infection. Hepatology 2017; 65(4): 1094-103.
[http://dx.doi.org/10.1002/hep.29005] [PMID: 28027579]

[14] Bourlière M, Bronowicki JP, de Ledinghen V, *et al.* Ledipasvir-sofosbuvir with or without ribavirin to treat patients with HCV genotype 1 infection and cirrhosis non-responsive to previous protease-inhibitor therapy: a randomised, double-blind, phase 2 trial (SIRIUS). Lancet Infect Dis 2015; 15(4): 397-404.
[http://dx.doi.org/10.1016/S1473-3099(15)70050-2] [PMID: 25773757]

[15] Reddy KR, Bourlière M, Sulkowski M, *et al.* Ledipasvir and sofosbuvir in patients with genotype 1 hepatitis C virus infection and compensated cirrhosis: An integrated safety and efficacy analysis. Hepatology 2015; 62(1): 79-86.
[http://dx.doi.org/10.1002/hep.27826] [PMID: 25846144]

[16] Kwo PY, Poordad F, Asatryan A, *et al.* Glecaprevir and pibrentasvir yield high response rates in patients with HCV genotype 1 6 without cirrhosis. J Hepatol 2017; 67(2): 263-71.
[http://dx.doi.org/10.1016/j.jhep.2017.03.039] [PMID: 28412293]

[17] Afdhal N, Reddy KR, Nelson DR, *et al.* Ledipasvir and sofosbuvir for previously treated HCV genotype 1 infection. N Engl J Med 2014; 370(16): 1483-93.
[http://dx.doi.org/10.1056/NEJMoa1316366] [PMID: 24725238]

[18] Bourlière M, Gordon SC, Flamm SL, *et al.* Sofosbuvir, Velpatasvir, and Voxilaprevir for Previously Treated HCV Infection. N Engl J Med 2017; 376(22): 2134-46.
[http://dx.doi.org/10.1056/NEJMoa1613512] [PMID: 28564569]

[19] Poordad F, Felizarta F, Asatryan A, *et al.* Glecaprevir and pibrentasvir for 12 weeks for hepatitis C virus genotype 1 infection and prior direct-acting antiviral treatment. Hepatology 2017; 66(2): 389-97.
[http://dx.doi.org/10.1002/hep.29081] [PMID: 28128852]

[20] Lawitz E, Poordad FF, Pang PS, *et al.* Sofosbuvir and ledipasvir fixed-dose combination with and without ribavirin in treatment-naive and previously treated patients with genotype 1 hepatitis C virus infection (LONESTAR): an open-label, randomised, phase 2 trial. Lancet 2014; 383(9916): 515-23.

[http://dx.doi.org/10.1016/S0140-6736(13)62121-2] [PMID: 24209977]

[21] Poordad F, Felizarta F, Asatryan A, *et al.* Glecaprevir and pibrentasvir for 12 weeks for hepatitis C virus genotype 1 infection and prior direct-acting antiviral treatment. Hepatology 2017; 66(2): 389-97. [http://dx.doi.org/10.1002/hep.29081] [PMID: 28128852]

[22] Kohli A, Kapoor R, Sims Z, *et al.* Ledipasvir and sofosbuvir for hepatitis C genotype 4: a proof-of-concept, single-centre, open-label phase 2a cohort study. Lancet Infect Dis 2015; 15(9): 1049-54. [http://dx.doi.org/10.1016/S1473-3099(15)00157-7] [PMID: 26187031]

[23] HCV Guideline Committee of the New York State Department of Health AIDS Institute (NYSDOH AI). Treatment of Chronic HCV with Direct-Acting Antivirals. Baltimore (MD): Johns Hopkins University; 2020. Available from: https://www.ncbi.nlm.nih.gov/books/NBK559965/.

[24] Asselah T, Kowdley KV, Zadeikis N, Wang S, Hassanein T, Horsmans Y, *et al.* Efficacy of Glecaprevir/Pibrentasvir for 8 or 12 Weeks in Patients With Hepatitis C Virus Genotype 2, 4, 5, or 6 Infection Without Cirrhosis. Clinical gastroenterology and hepatology : the official clinical practice journal of the American Gastroenterological Association. 2018;16(3):417-26.

[25] Bourliere M, Sulkowski M, Omata M, *et al.* An integrated safety and efficacy analysis of >500 patients with compensated cirrhosis treated with ledipasvir/sofosbuvir with or without ribavirin. 65th Annual Meeting of the American Association for the Study of Liver Diseases. 2014 Nov 7-11; Boston, MA.

[26] AASLD-IDSA. HCV Guidance: Recommendations for testing, management, and treating hepatitis C. Retreatment of persons in whom prior therapy failed: Sofosbuvir-Based and Elbasvir/Grazoprevir Treatment Failures. [AASLD-IDSA Hepatitis C Guidance].

[27] AASLD-IDSA. HCV Guidance: Recommendations for testing, management, and treating hepatitis C. Retreatment of persons in whom prior therapy has failed: glecaprevir/pibrentasvir treatment failure (all genotypes). [AASLD-IDSA].

[28] Kowdley KV, Gordon SC, Reddy KR, *et al.* Ledipasvir and sofosbuvir for 8 or 12 weeks for chronic HCV without cirrhosis. N Engl J Med 2014; 370(20): 1879-88. [http://dx.doi.org/10.1056/NEJMoa1402355] [PMID: 24720702]

[29] Zeuzem S, Foster GR, Wang S, *et al.* Glecaprevir Pibrentasvir for 8 or 12 Weeks in HCV Genotype 1 or 3 Infection. N Engl J Med 2018; 378(4): 354-69. [http://dx.doi.org/10.1056/NEJMoa1702417] [PMID: 29365309]

[30] Reddy KR, Bourlière M, Sulkowski M, *et al.* Ledipasvir and sofosbuvir in patients with genotype 1 hepatitis C virus infection and compensated cirrhosis: An integrated safety and efficacy analysis. Hepatology 2015; 62(1): 79-86. [http://dx.doi.org/10.1002/hep.27826] [PMID: 25846144]

[31] Abergel A, Asselah T, Metivier S, *et al.* Ledipasvir-sofosbuvir in patients with hepatitis C virus genotype 5 infection: an open-label, multicentre, single-arm, phase 2 study. Lancet Infect Dis 2016; 16(4): 459-64. [http://dx.doi.org/10.1016/S1473-3099(15)00529-0] [PMID: 26803446]

[32] Heo J, Kim YJ, Lee JW, *et al.* Efficacy and Safety of Glecaprevir/Pibrentasvir in Korean Patients with Chronic Hepatitis C: A Pooled Analysis of Five Phase II/III Trials. Gut Liver 2021; 15(6): 895-903. [http://dx.doi.org/10.5009/gnl20321] [PMID: 34053916]

[33] Foster GR, Pianko S, Brown A, *et al.* Efficacy of sofosbuvir plus ribavirin with or without peginterferon-alfa in patients with hepatitis C virus genotype 3 infection and treatment-experienced patients with cirrhosis and hepatitis C virus genotype 2 infection. Gastroenterology 2015; 149(6): 1462-70. [http://dx.doi.org/10.1053/j.gastro.2015.07.043] [PMID: 26248087]

[34] AASLD-IDSA. HCV Guidance: Recommendations for testing, management, and treating hepatitis C. Retreatment of persons in whom prior therapy has failed: sofosbuvir/velpatasvir/voxilaprevir treatment failure (all genotypes).

CHAPTER 7

Consensus Treatment Guidelines and Recommendations to Treat Hepatitis-C Infected Populations

Abstract: Unlike other infectious diseases and viral infections, the long-term chronicity of hepatitis C infection could worsen or propagate to irreversible extra-hepatic manifestations like decompensated cirrhosis or the development of hepatocellular carcinoma. The recent real-world clinical data of hepatitis C patients treated with IFN-free DAAs are still fewer to conclude or decide the best treatment protocols and guidelines for those who are still awaiting the treatment. However; based on the clinical data retrieved from the diverse patient cohorts, multicenter and multinational clinical studies, and pre- and post-therapeutic monitoring of hepatitis C-treated patients enable the clinicians, physicians, and health care providers to sketch consensus treatment guidelines and recommendations for the safe administration of DAAs in general and vulnerable hepatitis C infected populations. Interestingly and luckily, the treatment guidelines and recommendations approved by the FDA and CDC are following and working well in real-world clinical, hospital, and primary health care centers to manage hepatitis C, infected individuals. Albeit; for certain special populations like pediatric and pregnant hepatitis C females, we do not have clear guidelines for DAAs usage and their therapeutic monitoring. Furthermore, certain DAAs are not recommended in decompensated cirrhotics, in HCV rebound patients, and in previous treatment failure with a DAAs regimen. In this book chapter, we enlist updated treatment guidelines and recommendations to treat general as well as special hepatitis C-infected populations with DAAs and will briefly portray an overview of the pros and cons of these recommendations in real-world clinical settings.

Keywords: HBV reactivation, Hepatic fibrosis, Hepatic cirrhosis, HCV coinfection, Liver enzymes management, Post-treatment care, Pre-treatment history, RBV dose adjustment, Treatment monitoring, Treatment efficacy, Treatment referral.

INTRODUCTION

Many lessons have been learned from the current ongoing Covid-19 pandemic for the healthcare system, policymakers, research institutes, pharmaceutical industry, and academia of every country about the diagnosis, treatment, and management of

Imran Shahid and Qaiser Jabeen

an unprecedented pandemic outbreak at any time in the future [1]. Unfortunately, the devastating impacts of the pandemic both on economies and health sector programs of every country are still wearing on and we do not know how long the pandemic will last [1]. It has also highlighted the urgent need to minimize the complex cascade of diagnosis and care for complicated and critical-care patients of other endemic, epidemics, or syndemic infections all around the world (Fig. **1**). Furthermore, up-to-date clinical practice guidelines to reduce pandemic transmission as well as to ensure optimized patient treatment outcomes need to continue to evolve and be upgraded [1]. Rational to Hepatitis C, 71.1 million people are infected with this silent epidemic worldwide which corresponds to 1.0% of global prevalence [2]. Generally, as well as in the current situation of the Covid-19 pandemic, simplification of HCV diagnosis and particular treatment or care cascade pathways are urgently required to minimize the effect of the Covid-19 pandemic on the outcomes of patients with hepatitis c [3]. Furthermore, HCV clinical practice guidelines have a key role in guiding how to simplify the treatment or cascade of care for hepatitis C infected patients based on available data from clinical trials as well as from real-world cohort studies (Fig. **1**) [4]. Furthermore, guidelines also drive the pathways to eliminate HCV by advocating for simple hepatitis C care cascades as a part of recent national and international policies. Despite the significant advancement and remarkable progress toward simplified diagnostic and treatment algorithms, there remain some gaps to fill both in diagnostic and treatment strategies of HCV and to remove complexity in the recommendations for harder-to-cure, vulnerable, and marginal HCV-affected populations. Therefore, up-to-date and consensus HCV treatment guidelines are in eager demand, will always remain a priority, and is a continuous process to evolve to ensure HCV elimination [5].

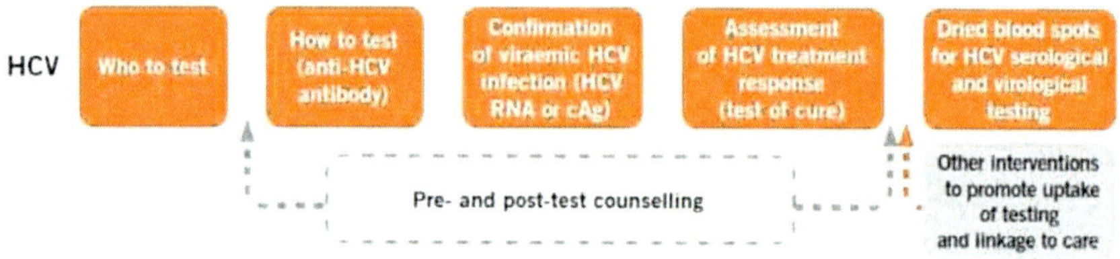

Fig. (1). A schematic diagram deciphering the importance of screening and treatment guidelines and pre-/post-test counseling for HCV patients [6]. HCV diagnostic and treatment guidelines play key roles in integrating HCV diagnosis and linkage to care. It may also be vital to promote the uptake of infection testing and enhance linkage to care. These guidelines may be very effective to bring more people to HCV testing and treatment while implementing pre-and post-test counseling.

Herein, we highlight consensus statements and current guidelines to consider for HCV treatment initiation decisions, monitoring during or after DAA treatment, post-treatment care, and post-treatment monitoring. Pre-treatment assessment of HCV-infected patients before recommendations for DAA administration is not a part of this book chapter, as already described in detail in chapter 4. Furthermore, we will not point out here recommendations of DAAs for general and vulnerable HCV-infected populations as already discussed in detail in chapters 5 and 6 respectively, however; we will only focus on special guidelines or considerations while administering DAAs in HCV-affected populations.

Strength of Recommendation	Quality of Supporting Evidence
A = Strong	1 = At least 1 randomized trial with clinical outcomes and/or validated laboratory endpoints.
B = Moderate	2 = One or more well-designed, nonrandomized trial or observational cohort studies with long-term clinical outcomes.
C = Optional	3 = Expert opinion

MEDICAL HISTORY AND PHYSICAL EXAMINATION

The patient's demographics, triage, sign, and symptoms are essential components of pretreatment assessment before setting a criterion to accept for hepatitis C treatment initiation (Table **1**). Enlists here key elements of the patient history and physical examination that may apply specifically to the pretreatment assessment of CHC-infected patients [7].

Table 1. Key elements of patient demographics before initiating HCV treatment [7].

Key Elements of a Pre-HCV Treatment Patient History and Physical Examination	
Elements of Patient History	**Rationale**
Previous treatment for HCV infection	• Previous regimen and treatment outcome will guide the choice and duration of therapy.
History of hepatic decompensation	• Warrants referral to a liver disease specialist.
History of renal disease	• Findings may influence the choice of regimen.
Medication history and current medications, including over-the-counter and herbal products	• Carefully consider drug-drug interactions with DAAs. See the Drug-Drug Interactions section of this guideline.
Pregnancy status and plans (see the Pregnancy and HCV section of this guideline)	• HCV treatment is deferred during pregnancy. • Birth control use is essential during HCV treatment and for 6 months after treatment if patients are receiving ribavirin (RBV).

(Table 1) cont.....

HIV infection	• If HIV infection is confirmed, offer the patient antiretroviral therapy (ART). • If the patient is being treated with antiretroviral medications, assess potential drug-drug interactions. See the Treatment of Patients with HIV/HCV > Drug-Drug Interactions between DAAs and ARVs section of this guideline. • Presence of HIV infection may influence fibrosis assessment modality, choice of treatment, duration, and monitoring.
History of infection/vaccination status	• Hepatitis A virus (HAV): Obtain HAV antibody (immunoglobulin [IgG] or total). • Hepatitis B virus (HBV): Obtain hepatitis B surface antigen (HBsAg), antibody to HB surface antigen (anti-HBs), and anti-hepatitis B core antibody (anti-HBc) (total). • Administer pneumococcal polysaccharide vaccination (PPSV23) as follows: 1- All patients with cirrhosis, which is associated with increased susceptibility to bacterial infections. 2- As indicated in the CDC/ACIP Recommended Immunization Schedule for Adults Aged 19 Years or Older. • Annual influenza: See U.S. Food and Drug Administration (FDA): Influenza Virus Vaccine Safety & Availability
Elements of a Pretreatment Physical Examination	**Clinical Details**
Presence or absence of ankle edema, abdominal veins, jaundice, palmar erythema, gynecomastia, spider telangiectasia, ascites, encephalopathy, and asterixis	Presence may suggest cirrhosis or decompensated cirrhosis and may require additional evaluation and management or treatment.
Presence or absence of physical signs related to extrahepatic manifestations of HCV, such as porphyria cutanea tarda, vasculitis, or lichen planus	Presence may increase the urgency of HCV treatment and may require additional evaluation and treatment needs. See, for instance, Medscape: Cutaneous Manifestations of HCV Clinical Presentation.
Liver size by palpation or auscultation for hepatomegaly or splenomegaly, as well as tenderness or hepatic bruits	Size and tenderness may suggest the severity of liver disease and may require additional evaluation.
Cardiac status	Findings may influence the choice of RBV-containing regimen, RBV dosing, or complete blood count (CBC) monitoring frequency.

CIRRHOSIS EVALUATION BEFORE INITIATING HCV TREATMENT

• To classify the severity of cirrhosis, the clinician should use the Model For End-Stage Liver Disease score (MELD) or the Child-Turcotte-Pugh (CTP) score [7].

• Clinicians should refer all patients with HCV-related cirrhosis for an upper endoscopy to screen for the presence of esophageal varices. (A3)

• Clinicians should screen for hepatocellular carcinoma (HCC) with ultrasound, computerized axial tomography (CT), or magnetic resonance imaging (MRI) every 6 months in patients with HCV-related bridging fibrosis or cirrhosis. (Table **2**) (A3). Alpha-fetoprotein (AFP) determination lacks adequate sensitivity and specificity for effective use in the surveillance and diagnosis of HCC because elevated AFP levels have been seen in HCV infection in the absence of HCC [7].

Table 2. Rationale for the evaluation of HCV cirrhosis before initiating DAA therapy [7].

Evaluation and Follow-Up Screening for Patients with Cirrhosis	
Type of Evaluation	**Rationale**
Assess for decompensation; refer to a liver disease specialist if history of decompensation or the Child's class B or C	• Decompensation is defined as the presence (or history) of 1 of the following: MELD score of >15. 1. Ascites. 2. Hepatic encephalopathy. 3. Portal hypertensive bleeding. 4. HCC. 5. Intractable pruritus. 6. Hepatopulmonary syndrome. 7. Portopulmonary hypertension.
Abdominal ultrasound to screen for HCC	• Ongoing HCC surveillance should be performed for patients with bridging fibrosis or cirrhosis according to standard guidelines every 6-12 months.

EVALUATION OF COMORBIDITIES STATUS IN HCV PATIENTS BEFORE INITIATING TREATMENT

Cardiac, renal, HAV/HCV or HBV/HCV co-infections, pregnancy, and metabolic status of HCV infected patients must be known and evaluated before initiating HCV treatment because;

• The administration of RBV-containing DAA regimens may worsen or exacerbate comorbid cardiac disease (*e.g.*, congestive heart failure, anemia) status in HCV-treated individuals [6, 7].

• DAAs dose adjustments in renal impairment HCV infected populations may affect comorbidities improvement while increasing or decreasing the elimination of therapeutic agents prescribed to be used for kidney diseases like glomerulonephritis, diabetes, and renal hypertension [7].

• Possible DDIs either between DAAs and cardiovascular drugs or DAAs and kidney disease drugs may also aggravate comorbid disease status or diminish the efficacies of DAAs in HCV-treated individuals [7, 8].

• Coinfection with HCV/HBV and either HCV or HAV may result in additional liver inflammation and pathology, and vaccination against HAV and HBV is important for patients with HCV infection to prevent acute decompensation and the sequelae of chronic superinfection by HBV. Approximately 40% to 50% of patients with HCV have no documented immunity against HAV or HBV [8, 9].

• HBV reactivation and HBV-related hepatic flares, sometimes fulminant, have been reported both during and after DAA therapy in patients who were not receiving concurrent HBV treatment. Studies have demonstrated that HCV has a suppressive effect on HBV replication, and previous interferon-based treatments were active against both viruses. However, unlike interferon, DAAs are not active against HBV, and when HCV is eradicated, HBV may be able to replicate [7, 10].

• The data on the use of DAA therapy in pregnancy is limited, and treatment of individuals who are pregnant is currently not recommended [11].

• Obesity does not affect the treatment of HCV with DAAs. Among individuals with HCV infection, both obesity and hepatic steatosis have been associated with the progression of fibrosis and increased risk of advanced liver disease [7, 12].

Table **3** illustrates the following guidelines/recommendations before initiating DAAs treatment in HCV-affected populations with cardiac, renal, or HAV/HCV or HBV/HCV comorbid infection status.

DAAS RECOMMENDATIONS IN HCV INFECTED PREGNANT WOMEN

The CDC recommends universal screening for hepatitis C infection in individuals who are pregnant or planning to get pregnant and that screening should be repeated during each pregnancy (Table **4**) [7]. Multiple studies on HCV care cascade models demonstrate the importance of this approach to ensure pregnant HCV women link with care, guide obstetric clinicians on the maternal and fetal risks in pregnant patients with hepatitis C and be cost-effective compared to current practice. However, no published data on DAA treatment for hepatitis C infection in pregnancy validate to recommend treatment of pregnant individuals. Furthermore, if a female becomes pregnant during DAA treatment, clinicians should discuss with the patient either the risks of DAAs on the fetus's health (although the information is scarce and clinical trials are underway) or the benefits (*e.g.*, probable HCV cure) of continuing treatment. However, during pregnancy in pregnant females, HCV infection is associated with higher incidences of intrahepatic cholestasis that cause significant maternal and fetal morbidity. Such high-risk pregnancies should be followed or managed by a liver specialist and/or experienced obstetricians. Other adverse maternal and fetal outcomes in pregnant females associated with hepatitis C include low birth weight, impaired intrauterine fetal growth, preterm delivery, miscarriage, and congenital anomalies [7].

Table 3. Rationale for the evaluation of comorbid infection status before initiating DAA treatment [7].

Cardiovascular Status
• For individuals with chronic HCV infection who are aged >50 years, clinicians should perform cardiovascular risk assessment before initiation of treatment with ribavirin (RBV). (A2)
Renal Status
• Clinicians should assess creatinine clearance in all patients with HCV infection. (A1)
• Clinicians new to HCV treatment should consult a liver disease specialist when treating patients with severe renal impairment (creatinine clearance <30 mL/min). (A3)
Hepatitis A (HAV) and/or Hepatitis B (HBV) Immunity Status
• Clinicians should obtain HAV antibodies (IgG or total) and administer the full HAV vaccine series in patients who are not immune to HAV. (A3)
• Clinicians should obtain HBV surface antigen (HBsAg), anti-hepatitis B surface (HBs), and anti-hepatitis B core antigen (HBc), total, and recommend administration of the anti-hepatitis B virus (HBV) vaccine series (0, 1, and 6 months) for HBV-susceptible patients (negative for all serologies). (A3)
1- In patients with positive HBsAg, clinicians should perform HBV DNA testing to assess for active HBV infection. (A1)
• For recommendations for patients with coinfection, see the Assessment of HBV Infection in Patients with HIV section of this guideline.
2- If HBV DNA is detectable, clinicians new to HCV treatment should consult a clinician experienced in the management of both HBV and HCV. (A1)
Pregnancy Status and Contraception (See the Pregnancy and HCV section of this guideline)
• Before initiating ribavirin (RBV), clinicians should (A2):
1- Confirm a negative pregnancy test.
2- Advise patients to use 2 methods of birth control to avoid pregnancy during therapy and for 6 months after completion of therapy.
3- Counsel female and male patients on effective contraceptive use.

GENERALLY ACCEPTED INDICATORS FOR HEPATITIS C TREATMENT

The recommendation to treat virtually all persons with acute or chronic HCV infection stems from multiple factors, including;

• To achieve very high sustained virologic response (SVR) rates with current DAA therapy,

Table 4. Guidelines for the initiation of DAA therapy in pregnant females [7].

Recommendations for DAAs treatment in pregnant women with HCV infection.
• Clinicians should perform HCV screening in all patients who are pregnant or planning to get pregnant. (B3) • Clinicians should advise pregnant patients with HCV to defer treatment with direct-acting antivirals (DAAs) until they are no longer pregnant or breastfeeding. (A2) • If an individual with HCV becomes pregnant during DAA treatment, clinicians should (A3): - Advise that the use of DAAs is not currently recommended during pregnancy because no data are currently available on the effects of medications on the fetus. - Discuss the risks and benefits of continuing treatment. • Clinicians should refer pregnant patients who are diagnosed with HCV (HCV antibody and HCV RNA positive), or who are known to have HCV and become pregnant before or during DAA treatment, to a specialist experienced in counseling about HCV in pregnancy. (A3) Specialists may include but are not limited to, hepatologists, gastroenterologists, infectious disease specialists, or high-risk obstetricians. • If a pregnant patient with HCV has a substance use disorder, the clinician should provide substance use treatment, including harm reduction services, or refer the patient for these services. (A3) • Clinicians should advise pregnant and postpartum individuals with HCV mono-infection that breastfeeding is considered safe, and HCV is not transmitted through breastmilk. (B3) • Clinicians should advise patients that if they have or develop cracked or bleeding nipples, breastfeeding should be discontinued, and milk should be expressed and discarded until the bleeding has resolved. (B3) • Clinicians should refer infants born to mothers with HCV to clinicians with experience in HCV care for further counseling and testing and notify the clinician of the mother's HCV status. (A3)

• To evaluate the safety and tolerability of DAA therapy, and the preponderance of data demonstrating benefits across a spectrum of clinical outcomes with the achievement of SVR in HCV patients [7, 13].

In addition to that, The AASLD-IDSA HCV guidance also addresses the following unique HCV populations that may require special considerations when weighing treatment decisions;

1) Individuals with HCV and HIV coinfection.

2) Individuals with HCV who have decompensated cirrhosis.

3) Individuals who develop HCV post-liver transplantation.

4) Individuals with HCV and renal impairment.

5) Individuals with HCV who are post-renal transplantation.

6) Individuals with acute HCV infection.

7) pregnant women with HCV.

8) Children with HCV.

CONTRAINDICATIONS FOR HEPATITIS C TREATMENT

Absolute Contraindications

With the advent and approvals of pan-genotypic DAAs to treat all HCV GTs/subtypes infected HCV patients irrespective of determining their hepatic fibrosis or cirrhosis status, few absolute contraindications for treatment initiation exist like;

• A short life expectancy that cannot be improved by HCV treatment (*i.e.*, according to AASLD-IDSA, only patients who are not candidates for treatment with DAAs are those with a life expectancy of less than 12 months or for whom treatment would not improve symptoms or prognosis) [13, 14].

• Liver transplantation.

• Another directed therapy.

Relative Contraindications

In contrast to absolute contraindications, several situations exist in relative contraindications where a clinician should exert careful considerations while initiating DAAs therapy [15, 16]. Those are described as follows;

• Active severe substance use disorder that would interfere with making follow-up appointments [17, 18].

• Psychiatric issues that are not well controlled [17]. Social issues that may negatively impact an individual's ability to adhere to therapy, make visits for monitoring treatment safety or show up for scheduled office visits [19].

• Initiation of HCV therapy before trying to conceive in WORA [20].

• For children with HCV, defer DAA therapy until at least 3 years of age [13, 16].

WHO TO ASSESS FOR TREATMENT

Acute HCV Infection

• Clinicians should suspect acute HCV infection if a patient who had a negative antibody test documented within the previous 6 months has a new positive antibody test or has detectable HCV RNA in the absence of a positive antibody test [13, 21]. (A3)

• Clinicians should not prescribe pre- or post-exposure prophylaxis to prevent HCV infection [22]. (A1)

• If chronic HCV infection is established, clinicians should evaluate patients for treatment (A1) [*i.e.*, pretreatment assessment; please see book chapter 4]) [23] and

• Clinicians should screen all patients with possible acute HCV infection for HIV, hepatitis A virus (HAV), and hepatitis B virus (HBV) infections, given the similar risk factors for acquisition [13, 24]. (A3)

Keypoints for Acute HCV Treatment

• Clinicians and their patients should determine the timing of HCV treatment concerning the likelihood of spontaneous clearance and patient or care provider concerns regarding the risk of transmission [7, 25, 26].

• Patient education should include the following information [27]:

1) If patients have acute HCV infection, they may be infectious and should take precautions to avoid transmitting HCV to others.

2) HCV infection may clear spontaneously (*i.e.*, without treatment).

• Treatment options are available if HCV infection is established [see chapter 6].

Chronic HCV Infection

Clinicians should assess all patients with a confirmed diagnosis of chronic HCV infection for treatment (Table **5**) [28]. (A1)

Referral to a Liver Specialist for Treatment Initiation

• Clinicians new to treating chronic HCV infection should consult with a liver disease specialist when treating chronic HCV infection in patients with any of the following conditions (Table **5**) (A3) [7, 29]:

1) Compensated and decompensated cirrhosis.

2) Concurrent hepatobiliary conditions.

• Extrahepatic manifestations of HCV, including renal, dermatologic, and rheumatologic manifestations [30].

3) Significant renal impairment (creatinine clearance <30 mL/min) or who are undergoing hemodialysis.

4) Active hepatitis B virus (HBV) infection, defined as HBV surface antigen-positive and detectable HBV DNA.

5) Ongoing HCV infection after failure of treatment with direct-acting antivirals (DAAs).

• Clinicians new to treating chronic HCV infection should consult with a liver disease specialist when evaluating patients for retreatment after any DAA treatment failure [31]. (B3)

• Clinicians should refer patients with chronic HCV infection and decompensated liver disease and patients who are pre- or post-transplant to a liver disease specialist [7, 32]. (A3)

Table 5. Key laboratory parameters to evaluate HCV patients for pre-treatment [7].

Baseline laboratory testing for pre-HCV treatment assessment	
Test	**Clinical Note**
HCV RNA quantification	• HCV RNA test confirms active HCV infection and determines HCV viral load.
Genotype/subtype	• Genotype and subtype guide choice of regimen.
Complete blood count (CBC)	• Low platelets (<140,000 platelets/μL) suggest cirrhosis and portal hypertension • Anemia may necessitate the choice of a regimen that does not contain ribavirin (RBV).
Serum electrolytes with creatinine	• Marked electrolyte abnormalities may suggest decompensated cirrhosis (*e.g.*, hyponatremia). • Renal function will influence the choice of regimen.
Hepatic function panel	• Elevated direct bilirubin suggests decompensated cirrhosis. • Markedly elevated transaminases may suggest comorbidities.
International normalized ratio (INR)	• Elevated INR suggests decompensated cirrhosis.
Pregnancy test for all individuals of childbearing potential (see Pregnancy and HCV section of this guideline)	• If pregnant, suggest treatment deferral.
Hepatitis A virus (HAV) antibodies	• Obtain HAV antibody (IgG or total) and administer the full HAV vaccine series in patients not immune to HAV.
Hepatitis B virus (HBV) antibodies	• Obtain HBsAg, anti-HBs, and anti-HBc (total) and recommend administration of the HBV vaccine series (0, 1, and 6 months) for HBV-susceptible patients (negative for all serologies): - In patients with positive HBsAg, perform HBV DNA testing to assess for active HBV infection. - If HBV DNA is detectable, care providers new to HCV treatment should consult a liver disease specialist regarding treatment for HBV and HCV.
HIV test if the status is unknown	• If HIV infection is confirmed, offer the patient antiretroviral therapy.

(Table 5) cont.....

Urinalysis	• Protein may suggest extrahepatic manifestation of HCV.
Fibrosis serum markers	• If not previously evaluated by biopsy or FibroScan.

KEY POINTS FOR PHYSICIANS, CLINICIANS, AND PATIENTS WHILE STARTING HCV TREATMENT

The main objective of HCV treatment initiation and its successful completion while achieving either higher SVR rates or HCV cure should include a pretreatment baseline evaluation, patient adherence to treatment, consideration of drug-drug interactions, evaluation of treatment response after therapy, and in some populations, monitoring for safety during treatment [7]. To achieve all this, we briefly highlight here the key considerations for the physicians, clinicians, and patients for DAAs treatment options, durations, and their successful completion [7].

Overall Considerations

• Clinicians can increase their patients' ability to understand treatment-related information and to participate in decision-making if they communicate with language that is clear, easily understood, jargon-free, and culturally sensitive [7].

• Sex, age, viral load levels, substance use disorders, mental health disorders, pill burden, and HIV coinfection are not considerations in selecting HCV treatment regimens [7].

• The most suitable DAAs regimen for any individual patient depends on the patient's preference and the clinician's assessment of comorbidities, such as chronic kidney disease, potential drug-drug interactions with the patient's current prescription and over-the-counter medications, medication tolerability, and adverse event profile, and duration of treatment [7].

• Patient preferences are central to all treatment decisions.

• The purpose of the DAAs adherence assessment is to optimize support, not to deny access to treatment.

• Though HCV treatment regimens are relatively short in duration, assessing a patient's readiness for treatment and ability to adhere to a medication regimen and medical care appointments before initiating DAA therapy is essential. After the pretreatment assessment and before treatment initiation, a plan can be developed with the patient to address potential barriers and/or to put support resources in place [7].

• Clinicians should obtain HCV GTs/subtype testing for all patients before starting treatment with DAAs. (A1)

• Clinicians should assess the degree of fibrosis in patients with chronic HCV infection to aid in determining the following (A1):

1. Need for pretreatment screening for varices and hepatocellular carcinoma (HCC).

2. Duration of antiviral treatment.

3. Need to include ribavirin (RBV) in the treatment regimen.

4. Need for post-treatment follow-up.

• Clinicians should assess patients with chronic HCV infection for decompensated liver disease. (A1)

• Clinicians should refer patients with decompensated cirrhosis to a liver disease specialist. (A3)

• Clinicians should refer all patients with HCV-related cirrhosis for an upper endoscopy to screen for the presence of esophageal varices. (A3)

• Clinicians should screen for hepatocellular carcinoma (HCC) with ultrasound, computerized axial tomography (CT), or magnetic resonance imaging (MRI) every 6 months in patients with HCV-related bridging fibrosis or cirrhosis. (A3) [7]

• Clinicians should assess creatinine clearance before initiating antiviral therapy. (A1)

• Clinicians new to HCV treatment should consult a liver disease or experienced viral hepatitis specialist when treating patients who:

1. Have severe renal impairment (creatinine clearance <30 mL/min) and/or are undergoing hemodialysis. (A3)

2. Require retreatment after treatment failure of any DAA regimen. (B3)

• Clinicians should prescribe ribavirin (RBV) with caution for patients with a creatinine clearance <50 mL/min. (A1)

1. If prescribed, a reduced dose of 200 mg per day is required.

2. Non-RBV-containing regimens can be prescribed without dose adjustments for patients with creatinine clearance ≥30 mL/min.

• Cardiac disease and other comorbidities may affect a patient's ability to tolerate RBV-induced anemia and should be considered before initiating an RBV-containing regimen.

• If a DAA regimen with weight-based ribavirin (RBV) is chosen, clinicians should dose as follows: (A1)

1. <75 kg: RBV 400 mg once daily plus 600 mg once daily (total daily dose: 1000 mg)

2. ≥75 kg: RBV 600 mg twice daily (total daily dose: 1200 mg)

• Based on the results of the pretreatment assessment, clinicians should choose from among the treatment regimens for patients with HCV GT-3.

• Clinicians should order NS5A testing in patients with HCV GT-3 who are being considered for 12 weeks of sofosbuvir/velpatasvir and are either treatment-naive and have cirrhosis, or are treatment-experienced and do not have cirrhosis. (A1)

1. If the Y93H resistance-associated substitution (RAS) is present, weight-based ribavirin should be added to the regimen or another regimen should be selected. (A1) [7]

• Clinicians new to HCV treatment should consult a liver disease or experienced viral hepatitis specialist when retreating patients in whom prior treatment with any DAA regimen has failed. (B3) [Failure is defined as detectable HCV RNA 12 weeks after the conclusion of HCV treatment] [7].

• For patients with active HBV infection, treatment of both HBV and HCV should be provided in consultation with a clinician experienced in the management of both HCV and HBV.

• All pregnant individuals should be tested for HCV during each pregnancy [7].

• If patients engage in ongoing high-risk behaviors during pregnancy, rescreening during pregnancy or the postpartum period is appropriate.

• Report perinatal exposure to ribavirin (RBV) to the *Ribavirin Pregnancy Registry*.

• It is important to recognize and acknowledge the influence of stigma when caring for patients in particular those who are pregnant or planning pregnancy and disclosure of positive results to an individual's OB-GYN and/or an HCV specialist but recognize the risk for stigma toward an individual who is pregnant and diagnosed with HCV. The effects of stigma cannot be underestimated. One cannot assume that HCV infection is associated with current or past injection drug use. Such assumptions can result in personal, family, and legal consequences for the patient, particularly among pregnant individuals [7].

Contraindications

• Clinicians should not prescribe RBV in the treatment of the following patients:

1. Female or male patients planning conception within 6 months of the last dose of RBV. (A2)

2. Male patients who have pregnant partners. (A2)

• RBV is contraindicated in female and male patients planning conception within 6 months of treatment.

• To use an RBV-containing DAA regimen in women of childbearing potential or in the male sex partners of these women, extreme care must be taken to avoid pregnancy during therapy and for 6 months after completion of therapy:

1. A negative pregnancy test is required immediately before initiation of therapy; and

2. Two forms of contraception or abstinence are advised during, and for 6 months after, therapy [7].

MONITORING DURING DAA TREATMENT

A typical schedule of a clinic visit for an HCV-treated individual with DAAs is based on treatment choice, patient mono-infection or comorbidities status, and duration of therapy [13, 33]. Generally, an 8- or 12-week DAA treatment course would consist of a baseline visit just before starting therapy, a follow-up visit at week 4 of therapy, an end-of-treatment visit, and a post-treatment visit 12 weeks after completing therapy [34, 35]. Depending on the patient's specific circumstances, follow-up visits may be done *via* phone calls or telehealth. However, for a longer treatment duration of 16 or 24 weeks, the clinicians may add one or more on-treatment visits [13, 35]. In unprecedented situations like developing a severe adverse event or complications during treatment, a patient must be evaluated as indicated [36]. Besides that, patients with compensated or decompensated cirrhosis or advanced hepatic manifestations may require more frequent follow-up. Herein we briefly address the recommendations monitoring for DAAs' safety and efficacy during treatment as well as considerations for monitoring patients after treatment [35, 36].

Monitoring for DAAs Treatment Efficacy

The gold standard approach to monitoring DAA treatment efficacy consists of repeated measurement of quantitative HCV RNA levels. Monitoring requires the use of a highly sensitive quantitative HCV RNA assay, typically with a lower limit of quantification (LLoQ) in the range of 12 to 25 IU/mL [37]. In addition, to minimize interassay and interlaboratory variation, monitoring should ideally utilize the same HCV RNA assay performed by the same laboratory. Three commercially available HCV RNA assays are widely used in the United States: Roche COBAS TaqMan Version 1.0, Roche COBAS TaqMan Version 2.0, and the Abbott RealTime HCV (ART) assay [13, 38].

The following definitions related to HCV RNA assay results are used in clinical practice and research studies;

Lower Limit of Quantification (LLOQ)

This is the lowest HCV RNA concentration that is within the validated range the assay can accurately quantify [33]. If HCV RNA is not quantifiable, the result is either HCV RNA detected but below the LLOQ or HCV RNA not detected. Note that the lower limit of quantification is not the same as the lower limit of detection.

Limit of Detection (LOD)

This value is the concentration of HCV RNA detectable at a rate of at least 95%. The ability of the assay to detect HCV RNA gradually decreases as the actual amount of HCV RNA in the sample approaches 0 IU/mL [34]. The result below the limit of detection is referred to as undetectable.

Target Detected (TD)

The HCV RNA is detected [35].

Target Not Detected (TND)

The HCV RNA is not detected [35].

RECOMMENDED SCHEDULE FOR HCV RNA MONITORING

For individuals receiving HCV therapy, the AASLD-IDSA HCV guidance recommends obtaining a quantitative HCV RNA level at baseline and 12 weeks after completing therapy, regardless of the treatment duration [13, 34].

Typical pangenotypic DAAs treatment durations are 8 weeks and 12 weeks [35].

On-Treatment HCV RNA Monitoring

For persons on DAA-based therapy, routine HCV RNA testing at week 4 is no longer recommended. Observational data from multiple studies suggest that detectable HCV RNA (15 IU/mL or greater) at week 4 may be associated with lower odds of sustained virologic response (SVR) at 12 weeks after completion of therapy [37, 39]. The AASLD-IDSA HCV guidance now advises against routine testing for HCV RNA level during treatment unless:

1. Alanine aminotransferase (ALT) fails to decline from baseline (in persons where hepatic function monitoring is indicated and ongoing) [13], or

2. There is concern regarding patient adherence to DAA therapy [40].

Furthermore, no valid data exist to support HCV treatment cessation or modification based on a detectable level at week 4 of treatment. It is also not clear that a detectable HCV RNA anytime during therapy reflects therapy nonadherence [35, 38].

On-Treatment Persistent Low-Level Viremia

The significance of on-treatment persistent low-level viremia (*i.e.*, that does not increase) is not known [13, 37]. There is no clear indication this represents a lack of adherence or likelihood of virologic relapse and routine treatment monitoring of HCV RNA levels is not indicated. Indeed, recent data involving patients receiving DAA sofosbuvir-containing therapy has shown that low-level quantifiable HCV RNA levels at week 4 were not clinically useful in predicting SVR12. Furthermore, the AASLD-IDSA guidelines do not provide a recommendation regarding stopping or extending therapy in the setting of stable low-level viremia [35, 37].

Determining Sustained Virologic Response

The recommended testing to determine whether the patient has achieved an SVR is a quantitative HCV RNA level 12 weeks after completing therapy [41]. An undetectable HCV RNA level 12 weeks after completing therapy is referred to as

SVR12 and this generally translates into a long-term cure of HCV infection [13, 42]. Some experts will obtain an HCV RNA level 24 weeks after completing treatment in selected patients, such as those with cirrhosis [43]. Research studies have utilized HCV RNA levels 4 weeks after completing therapy (SVR4), but the SVR4 is not considered as robust a marker for treatment response as an SVR12 [35, 44].

MONITORING FOR SAFETY DURING TREATMENT

Baseline Safety Laboratory Studies

The optimal and standard approach to monitoring for treatment safety depends on whether ribavirin is a component of the regimen [13]. The AASLD-IDSA HCV guidance, recommends obtaining the following baseline studies within 6 months before starting (the HCV RNA and HCV genotype can be obtained any time before treatment) DAAs treatment [35].

• Complete blood count (CBC).

• Hepatic function panel: albumin, total bilirubin, direct bilirubin, alanine aminotransferase (ALT).

• aspartate aminotransferase (AST), and alkaline phosphatase.

• Hepatitis B surface antigen (HBsAg), hepatitis B core antibody (anti-HBc), and hepatitis B surface antibody (anti-HBs).

• HCV RNA level.

• HCV genotype and subtype should be obtained if the planned treatment regimen is not a pangenotypic regimen.

• HIV-1/2 antigen-antibody immunoassay.

• International normalized ratio (INR).

• Serum creatinine level and calculated glomerular filtration rate.

• Serum pregnancy testing for women of childbearing age, especially if the HCV treatment regimen includes ribavirin.

Monitoring of Patients Taking RBV

• While patients are taking ribavirin (RBV), clinicians should perform hemoglobin testing at weeks 2 and 4 of treatment and every 4 weeks thereafter until therapy is complete [13].

Safety Laboratory Studies at Week 4 of Therapy

For patients receiving hepatitis C therapy, the AASLD-IDSA HCV guidance recommends obtaining the following laboratory studies 4 weeks after starting therapy [13]:

• Serum creatinine level and calculated glomerular filtration rate.

• Hepatic function panel: albumin, total bilirubin, direct bilirubin, ALT, AST, and alkaline phosphatase if the person has chronic hepatitis B.

• CBC if the person is taking ribavirin.

• Monitoring for hypoglycemia for individuals taking diabetes medications.

• Monitoring of INR in persons taking warfarin.

• Many experts continue to recommend monthly hepatic function test monitoring in cirrhotic patients and in those who are anti-HBc positive (regardless of anti-HBs status) while on therapy [35].

Management of Abnormal ALT During Therapy

Clinically significant hepatotoxicity has been reported with DAA therapy, specifically NS3-4A PIs, particularly for patients with advanced liver disease. The AASLD-IDSA HCV guidance advises against the use of NS3-4A PIs in patients with a Child-Turcotte-Pugh score of 7 or greater [13]. Elevations in ALT to greater than 5 times the upper limit of normal occur in up to 1% of all persons taking elbasvir-grazoprevir; therefore, hepatic panel monitoring for persons taking elbasvir-grazoprevir has been recommended by the manufacturer at week 8 and as clinically indicated during therapy (some experts recommend monitoring of ALT every 4 weeks while on elbasvir-grazoprevir) [35]. Due to the increased risk of hepatotoxicity, coadministration of Ethinyl estradiol with glecaprevir-pibrentasvir is not recommended. For individuals who have on-treatment increases in ALT levels at week 4, the AASLD-IDSA HCV guidance provides the following recommendations based on the severity of the ALT elevation and whether symptoms are present [13, 35].

A 10-fold or Greater Increase in ALT Levels

If a patient receiving treatment for HCV develops a 10-fold or greater increase in ALT levels, regardless of the presence of clinical symptoms, they should immediately stop HCV therapy and undergo close clinical and laboratory monitoring for liver toxicity [13, 35].

Clinical Symptoms and Increase in ALT Levels of Less than 10-Fold

If a patient receiving treatment for HCV has elevated ALT levels that are less than a 10-fold increase they should immediately stop therapy if they have either of the following [13, 35]:

1. Symptoms suggestive of acute hepatitis (weakness, nausea, vomiting, or jaundice), or

2. A significant increase in other hepatic function panel labs (bilirubin, alkaline phosphatase, or international normalized ratio). After stopping therapy, the individual should have close clinical and laboratory monitoring for liver toxicity. The AASLD-IDSA HCV guidance does not specify what degree of change in bilirubin, alkaline phosphatase, or international normalized ratio should be considered "significant". Most experts would use clinical judgment with this recommendation and not discontinue therapy with a low-level increase in ALT accompanied by a low-level increase in bilirubin or alkaline phosphatase [13, 35].

Asymptomatic Infection and Increases in ALT Levels Less than 10-Fold

Patients with an increase in ALT levels less than 10-fold, but without symptoms suggestive of acute hepatitis, should have close monitoring and repeat ALT levels checked at treatment weeks 6 and 8 [13]. If the ALT levels remain consistently elevated, discontinuation of therapy should be considered. Most experts in this situation would follow this general AASLD-IDSA recommendation but decide on a case-by-case basis, taking into account the degree of ALT elevation, the trend in ALT levels, and the presence or absence of underlying cirrhosis or symptoms of hepatic injury [35].

HEPATITIS B REACTIVATION ASSOCIATED WITH HCV DAA THERAPY

Chronic HCV has been known to suppress HBV replication in persons coinfected with HCV and reciprocal interaction between these viruses has long been postulated [45, 46]. The elimination of HCV can result in a potential loss of immunologic control of HBV infection and result in HBV reactivation. The U.S. Food and Drug Administration (FDA) issued a drug safety warning on October 4, 2016, for persons receiving DAA medications for the treatment of HCV [13, 47]. The FDA warning was based on several cases reported to the FDA and from published literature [48, 49]. The AASLD-IDSA HCV Guidance provides specific recommendations that address the risk of HBV reactivation following initiation of DAA treatment for HCV as summarized in the following list:

• In patients who are hepatitis B virus surface antigen (HBsAg) positive and have no detectable HBV DNA, clinicians should monitor for HBV reactivation by performing aspartate aminotransferase (AST), ALT, and HBV DNA tests every 4 weeks during HCV treatment [46, 49].

• Clinicians new to HCV treatment should consult a liver disease or experienced viral hepatitis specialist for further evaluation of patients who develop detectable HBV DNA [47].

POST-TREATMENT CARE

Approach to Monitoring After Receiving HCV Therapy

The approach to monitoring individuals following completion of a course of HCV therapy depends entirely on the person's response to therapy. Two main scenarios exist [9]:

1. The person achieved an SVR12, or

2. The person did not achieve an SVR, including persons who completed therapy, and persons who received an inadequate treatment course because of adherence problems, intolerance, or laboratory toxicity necessitating premature discontinuation of the treatment regimen [13, 49].

The AASLD-IDSA HCV guidance stratifies the follow-up for persons who achieve an SVR based on the degree of hepatic fibrosis and the risk of HCV reinfection (Table **6**) [35, 50].

Individuals with Minimal to Moderate Fibrosis (F0-F2)

These individuals do not need special monitoring or follow-up specifically for hepatitis C or liver care [13, 35]. This recommendation is based on data that show persons who achieve SVR following hepatitis C treatment generally do not have further progression of HCV-related liver fibrosis [50].

Individuals with Advanced Fibrosis (F3-F4)

Although fibrosis may improve in these individuals, they are considered to have a persistent risk for developing hepatocellular carcinoma (HCC) [51]. Accordingly,

1. These individuals should have continued surveillance for HCC with abdominal

ultrasound (with or without alpha-fetoprotein) every 6 months [13].

2. Persons with cirrhosis (F4 fibrosis) should have a baseline upper endoscopy to screen for varices unless this has previously been done [35].

3. Individuals identified with varices should receive appropriate management and follow-up [52].

Table 6. Key recommendations for post-treatment DAAs care for HCV patients [7].

Recommendations for post-treatment care.
Evaluating the Response to HCV Treatment • Clinicians should perform HCV RNA testing 12 weeks after treatment is complete to verify that a sustained virologic response (SVR) has been achieved. (A1) • If SVR is achieved, as established by undetectable HCV RNA at 12 weeks after treatment, clinicians should: - Inform their patients that the HCV infection has been cured. (A2) - Explain the risk of HCV reinfection and that HCV antibodies are not protective against reinfection. (A1) • To assess for reinfection in patients with ongoing risk factors, clinicians should perform follow-up screening with HCV RNA testing (not HCV antibody testing) at least annually, even with a history of an SVR. (A1) • If HCV RNA is detectable at 12 weeks after treatment, clinicians should: - Inform patients that treatment has failed. (A1) - If new to HCV treatment, consult with a liver disease specialist for retreatment evaluation. (B3) **Post-Treatment Monitoring** • For patients taking ribavirin (RBV)-containing HCV treatment regimens, clinicians should: - Advise female and male patients to take extreme care to avoid pregnancy for 6 months after completion of therapy. (A2) - Counsel female and male patients on effective contraceptive use. (A2) • If an individual becomes pregnant within 6 months of completing an RBV-containing HCV treatment, clinicians should discuss the risks of using DAAs and RBV during pregnancy. (A3) **Patients with Persistent Liver Disease** • Clinicians should evaluate patients with persistent abnormal transaminase levels after SVR for other causes of liver disease and consult with a liver disease specialist. (A3) • In patients with underlying bridging fibrosis or cirrhosis, clinicians should screen for hepatocellular carcinoma (HCC) every 6 months. (A1)

Individuals with Persistently Abnormal Liver Tests

Any person who has achieved an SVR12, but who has persistently elevated hepatic aminotransferase levels should undergo evaluation for possible other causes of liver disease, such as [13, 35];

1. Alcohol use,

2. Iron overload, or

3. Fatty liver disease

Persons with Ongoing Risk of HCV Reinfection

All persons with ongoing risk for acquiring HCV should have a periodic assessment for HCV reinfection and counseling on the prevention of reinfection.

1. At least annual HCV RNA screening (quantitative HCV RNA level) is recommended for persons who inject drugs and for men with HIV who have condomless sex with men, given the significant risk of HCV reinfection in these individuals.

2. Any elevation in hepatic aminotransferase levels should prompt evaluation for reinfection with a quantitative HCV RNA level [35].

Monitoring of Persons Who Do Not Achieve SVR

The AASLD-IDSA HCV guidance recommends the following for individuals who did not achieve an SVR with HCV therapy [13, 35]:

All Individuals

For all individuals who did not achieve an SVR and are awaiting or deferring retreatment:

1. Follow-up laboratory testing should occur every 6-12 months with a hepatic function panel, complete blood count, and international normalized ratio.

2. These patients must receive counseling for alcohol abstinence and avoidance of hepatotoxic medications.

Persons with Advanced Fibrosis (F3-F4)

These individuals should have [51, 52];

1. Surveillance for hepatocellular carcinoma with abdominal ultrasound, with or without serum alpha-fetoprotein, every 6 months.

2. Individuals with cirrhosis (F4 fibrosis) should have a baseline upper endoscopy to screen for varices unless this has previously been done.

3. Persons identified with varices should receive appropriate management and follow-up.

CONCLUSIONS

The selection of a simple care pathway for HCV-infected patients is a wise approach to drive HCV elimination, for which treatment guidelines and consensus-based statements may drive to establish a good physician-patient relationship from the initiation of treatment to post-therapy. However, healthcare providers are much more responsible for considering the medical history and physical examination of the patient before initiating the treatment. Hepatic cirrhosis evaluation and defined comorbid status before initiating treatment will pave the ways to prevent patient non-adherence to treatment and determine potential treatment outcomes and post-treatment SAEs. The physicians and clinicians while starting treatment for hepatitis C must bear in mind the general indicators for treatment including; the patient's eligibility, treatment indications/contraindications, assessment for treatment, and general considerations. Furthermore, the parameters of monitoring during treatment (*e.g.*, SVR, LOD and LLoQ of HCV RNA, persistent low-level viremia, *etc.*), patient safety, and approaches to monitoring after receiving HCV therapy (*e.g.*, fibrosis evaluation, ALT levels and HCV reinfection risk, *etc.*) must be clear and up-to-date. The treatment considerations are very specific and even not well defined for pregnant and liver transplant patients, so healthcare providers must be very careful while initiating treatment in such patient populations and make appropriate referrals for the liver transplant waiting patients.

REFERENCES

[1] Martinez MA, Franco S. Impact of COVID-19 in Liver Disease Progression. Hepatol Commun 2021; 5(7): 1138-50.
[PMID: 34533001]

[2] Shahid I, Alzahrani AR, Al-Ghamdi SS, Alanazi IM, Rehman S, Hassan S. Hepatitis C Diagnosis: Simplified Solutions, Predictive Barriers, and Future Promises. Diagnostics (Basel, Switzerland). 2021; 11, 7.

[3] Boettler T, Newsome PN, Mondelli MU, *et al.* Care of patients with liver disease during the COVID-19 pandemic: EASL-ESCMID position paper. JHEP Reports 2020; 2(3): 100113.
[PMID: 32289115]

[4] Yu ML, Chen PJ, Dai CY, Hu TH, Huang CF, Huang YH, *et al.* Taiwan consensus statement on the management of hepatitis C: Part (II) special populations. Journal of the Formosan Medical Association Taiwan 2020; 119(7): 1135-57.

[5] Yeon JE. Recent update of the 2017 Korean Association for the Study of the Liver (KASL) treatment guidelines of chronic hepatitis C: Comparison of guidelines from other continents, 2017 AASLD/IDSA and 2016 EASL. Clin Mol Hepatol 2018; 24(3): 278-93.
[PMID: 29716179]

[6] WHO guidelines on hepatitis B and C testing. Geneva: World Health Organization; 2017. Available from: https://www.who.int.

[7] HCV Guideline Committee of the New York State Department of Health AIDS Institute (NYSDOH AI). Treatment of Chronic HCV with Direct-Acting Antivirals. Baltimore (MD): Johns Hopkins University; 2020. Available from: https://www.ncbi.nlm.nih.gov/books/NBK559965/.

[8] Cacoub P, Desbois AC, Comarmond C, Saadoun D. Impact of sustained virological response on the extrahepatic manifestations of chronic hepatitis C: a meta-analysis. Gut 2018; 67(11): 2025-34. [PMID: 29703790]

[9] Morgan RL, Baack B, Smith BD, Yartel A, Pitasi M, Falck-Ytter Y. Eradication of hepatitis C virus infection and the development of hepatocellular carcinoma: a meta-analysis of observational studies. Ann Intern Med 2013; 158(5 Pt 1): 329-37. [PMID: 23460056]

[10] Tada T, Kumada T, Toyoda H, *et al.* Viral eradication reduces all-cause mortality, including non-live--related disease, in patients with progressive hepatitis C virus-related fibrosis. J Gastroenterol Hepatol 2017; 32(3): 687-94. [PMID: 27577675]

[11] U.S. Food and Drug Administration. FDA Drug Safety Communication: FDA warns about the risk of hepatitis B reactivating in some patients treated with direct-acting antivirals for hepatitis C. [U.S. Food and Drug Administration].

[12] Maylin S, Martinot-Peignoux M, Moucari R, *et al.* Eradication of hepatitis C virus in patients successfully treated for chronic hepatitis C. Gastroenterology 2008; 135(3): 821-9. [PMID: 18593587]

[13] Recommendations for Hepatitis C Screening. Washington University; 2022. Available from: https://www.hepatitisc.uw.edu/go/screening-diagnosis/recommendations-screening/core-concept/all.

[14] Feld JJ, Jacobson IM, Sulkowski MS, Poordad F, Tatsch F, Pawlotsky JM. Ribavirin revisited in the era of direct-acting antiviral therapy for hepatitis C virus infection. Liver international : official journal of the International Association for the Study of the Liver. 2017; 37(1): 5-18.

[15] Grebely J, Oser M, Taylor LE, Dore GJ. Breaking down the barriers to hepatitis C virus (HCV) treatment among individuals with HCV/HIV coinfection: action required at the system, provider, and patient levels. The Journal of infectious diseases. 2013; 207 Suppl 1(Suppl 1): S19-25.

[16] Meyer JP, Moghimi Y, Marcus R, Lim JK, Litwin AH, Altice FL. Evidence-based interventions to enhance assessment, treatment, and adherence in the chronic Hepatitis C care continuum. Int J Drug Policy 2015; 26(10): 922-35. [PMID: 26077144]

[17] Roberts SS, Miller RK, Jones JK, *et al.* The Ribavirin Pregnancy Registry: Findings after 5 years of enrollment, 2003-2009. Birth Defects Res A Clin Mol Teratol 2010; 88(7): 551-9. [PMID: 20564430]

[18] Ward RP, Kugelmas M. Using pegylated interferon and ribavirin to treat patients with chronic hepatitis C. Am Fam Physician 2005; 72(4): 655-62. [PMID: 16127955]

[19] Cacoub P, Desbois AC, Isnard-Bagnis C, Rocatello D, Ferri C. Hepatitis C virus infection and chronic kidney disease: Time for reappraisal. J Hepatol 2016; 65(1) (Suppl.): S82-94. [PMID: 27641990]

[20] Dore GJ, Altice F, Litwin AH, *et al.* Elbasvir-Grazoprevir to Treat Hepatitis C Virus Infection in Persons Receiving Opioid Agonist Therapy: A Randomized Trial. Ann Intern Med 2016; 165(9): 625-34. [PMID: 27537841]

[21] Hoofnagle JH. Course and outcome of hepatitis C. Hepatology 2002; 36(5) (Suppl. 1): S21-9. [PMID: 12407573]

[22] Maheshwari A, Ray S, Thuluvath PJ. Acute hepatitis C. Lancet 2008; 372(9635): 321-32. [PMID: 18657711]

[23] Micallef JM, Kaldor JM, Dore GJ. Spontaneous viral clearance following acute hepatitis C infection: a

systematic review of longitudinal studies. J Viral Hepat 2006; 13(1): 34-41.
[PMID: 16364080]

[24] Kamal SM. Acute hepatitis C: a systematic review. Am J Gastroenterol 2008; 103(5): 1283-97.
[PMID: 18477352]

[25] Grebely J, Page K, Sacks-Davis R, *et al.* The effects of female sex, viral genotype, and IL28B genotype on spontaneous clearance of acute hepatitis C virus infection. Hepatology 2014; 59(1): 109-20.
[PMID: 23908124]

[26] Blackard JT, Shata MT, Shire NJ, Sherman KE. Acute hepatitis C virus infection: a chronic problem. Hepatology 2008; 47(1): 321-31.
[PMID: 18161707]

[27] Newsum AM, Schinkel J, van de Laar TJW, van der Meer JTM, Prins M. Spontaneous Clearance of Hepatitis C Virus Infection Among Human Immunodeficiency Virus-Infected Men Who Have Sex With Men. Open Forum Infect Dis 2017; 4: 2.
[PMID: 28638847]

[28] Nguyen GC, Sam J, Thuluvath PJ. Hepatitis C is a predictor of acute liver injury among hospitalizations for acetaminophen overdose in the United States: a nationwide analysis. Hepatology 2008; 48(4): 1336-41.
[PMID: 18821593]

[29] Chou R, Wasson N. Blood tests to diagnose fibrosis or cirrhosis in patients with chronic hepatitis C virus infection: a systematic review. Ann Intern Med 2013; 158(11): 807-20.
[PMID: 23732714]

[30] Boursier J, de Ledinghen V, Zarski JP, *et al.* Comparison of eight diagnostic algorithms for liver fibrosis in hepatitis C: new algorithms are more precise and entirely noninvasive. Hepatology 2012; 55(1): 58-67.
[PMID: 21898504]

[31] Duarte-Rojo A, Altamirano JT, Feld JJ. Noninvasive markers of fibrosis: key concepts for improving accuracy in daily clinical practice. Ann Hepatol 2012; 11(4): 426-39.
[PMID: 22700624]

[32] Gara N, Zhao X, Kleiner DE, Liang TJ, Hoofnagle JH, Ghany MG. Discordance among transient elastography, aspartate aminotransferase to platelet ratio index, and histologic assessments of liver fibrosis in patients with chronic hepatitis C. Clinical gastroenterology and hepatology : the official clinical practice journal of the American Gastroenterological Association. 2013; 11(3): 303-8.

[33] Cloherty G, Cohen D, Sarrazin C, *et al.* HCV RNA assay sensitivity impacts the management of patients treated with direct-acting antivirals. Antivir Ther 2015; 20(2): 177-83.
[PMID: 24941124]

[34] Cobb B, Pockros PJ, Vilchez RA, Vierling JM. HCV RNA viral load assessments in the era of direct-acting antivirals. Am J Gastroenterol 2013; 108(4): 471-5.
[PMID: 23552304]

[35] AASLD-IDSA. HCV Guidance: Recommendations for testing, management, and treating hepatitis C. Monitoring patients who are starting HCV treatment, are on treatment, or have completed therapy. [AASLD-IDSA Hepatitis C Guidance].

[36] Strassl R, Rutter K, Stättermayer AF, *et al.* Real-Time PCR Assays for the Quantification of HCV RNA: Concordance, Discrepancies and Implications for Response Guided Therapy. PLoS One 2015; 10(8): e0135963.
[PMID: 26274922]

[37] Sidharthan S, Kohli A, Sims Z, *et al.* Utility of hepatitis C viral load monitoring on direct-acting antiviral therapy. Clin Infect Dis 2015; 60(12): 1743-51.

[PMID: 25733369]

[38] Childs-Kean LM, Hong J. Detectable Viremia at the End of Treatment With Direct-Acting Antivirals Can Be Associated With Subsequent Clinical Cure in Patients With Chronic Hepatitis C: A Case Series. Gastroenterology 2017; 153(4): 1165-6.
[PMID: 28881195]

[39] Steinebrunner N, Sprinzl MF, Zimmermann T, *et al.* Early virological response may predict treatment response in sofosbuvir-based combination therapy of chronic hepatitis c in a multi-center "real-life" cohort. BMC Gastroenterol 2015; 15: 97.
[PMID: 26239732]

[40] Backus LI, Belperio PS, Shahoumian TA, Loomis TP, Mole LA. Real-world effectiveness of ledipasvir/sofosbuvir in 4,365 treatment-naive, genotype 1 hepatitis C-infected patients. Hepatology 2016; 64(2): 405-14.
[PMID: 27115523]

[41] Morisco F, Granata R, Stroffolini T, *et al.* Sustained virological response: a milestone in the treatment of chronic hepatitis C. World J Gastroenterol 2013; 19(18): 2793-8.
[PMID: 23687416]

[42] Manns MP, Pockros PJ, Norkrans G, *et al.* Long-term clearance of hepatitis C virus following interferon α-2b or peginterferon α-2b, alone or in combination with ribavirin. J Viral Hepat 2013; 20(8): 524-9.
[PMID: 23808990]

[43] Simmons B, Saleem J, Hill A, Riley RD, Cooke GS. Risk of late relapse or reinfection with hepatitis C virus after achieving a sustained virological response: A systematic review and meta-analysis. Clin Infect Dis 2016; 62(6): 683-94.
[PMID: 26787172]

[44] Yoshida EM, Sulkowski MS, Gane EJ, *et al.* Concordance of sustained virological response 4, 12, and 24 weeks post-treatment with sofosbuvir-containing regimens for hepatitis C virus. Hepatology 2015; 61(1): 41-5.
[PMID: 25314116]

[45] Pisaturo M, Macera M, Alessio L, Calò F, Coppola N, Hepatitis B. Hepatitis B Virus (HBV) Reactivation Following Pharmacological Eradication of Hepatitis C Virus (HCV). Viruses 2019; 11(9): 850.
[PMID: 31540223]

[46] Ou P, Fang Z, Chen J. Hepatitis B reactivation in a chronic hepatitis C patient treated with ledipasvir and sofosbuvir: A case report. Clin Res Hepatol Gastroenterol 2017; 41(2): e17-8.
[PMID: 27601170]

[47] Takayama H, Sato T, Ikeda F, Fujiki S. Reactivation of hepatitis B virus during interferon-free therapy with daclatasvir and asunaprevir in patient with hepatitis B virus/hepatitis C virus co-infection. Hepatology research : the official journal of the Japan Society of Hepatology. 2016; 46(5): 489-91.

[48] Hayashi K, Ishigami M, Ishizu Y, *et al.* A case of acute hepatitis B in a chronic hepatitis C patient after daclatasvir and asunaprevir combination therapy: hepatitis B virus reactivation or acute self-limited hepatitis? Clin J Gastroenterol 2016; 9(4): 252-6.
[PMID: 27329484]

[49] Singal AG, Volk ML, Jensen D, Di Bisceglie AM, Schoenfeld PS. A sustained viral response is associated with reduced liver-related morbidity and mortality in patients with hepatitis C virus. Clinical Gastroenterology and Hepatology: Journal of the American Gastroenterological Association 2010; 8(3): 280-8.

[50] Welker MW, Zeuzem S. Occult hepatitis C: how convincing are the current data? Hepatology 2009; 49(2): 665-75.
[PMID: 19105211]

[51] Heimbach JK, Kulik LM, Finn RS, *et al.* AASLD guidelines for the treatment of hepatocellular carcinoma. Hepatology 2018; 67(1): 358-80.
[PMID: 28130846]

[52] Garcia-Tsao G, Abraldes JG, Berzigotti A, Bosch J. Portal hypertensive bleeding in cirrhosis: Risk stratification, diagnosis, and management: 2016 practice guidance by the American Association for the study of liver diseases. Hepatology 2017; 65(1): 310-35.
[PMID: 27786365]

CHAPTER 8

Treatment Recommendations for Harder-to-Cure and Vulnerable Populations

Abstract: Certain hepatitis C-infected populations are still challenging to treat in the era of all-oral interferon-free direct-acting antivirals (IFN-free DAAs), which are highly efficacious, well-tolerable, and relatively safe in treated individuals. Such difficult-to-treat patients were also challenging even to manage with pegylated interferon (PEG-IFN) plus a nucleoside analog ribavirin (RBV) once known as the "gold standard of hepatitis C care". People infected with hepatitis C genotype 3, decompensated cirrhosis, individuals with co-infection status (*e.g.*, HCV/HBV, HCV/HIV, HCV/CKD), hepatitis C patients with induction of hepatocellular carcinoma (HCC), previous treatment failure with PEG-IFN plus RBV or DAAs failures, and viral relapse patients with the use of one or more DAA combinations are even compromised to achieve higher SVR rates with IFN-free DAAs. Similarly, some DAAs have sub-optimal clinical efficacies in harder-to-cure populations and some are contraindicated and can worsen hepatitis C-associated hepatic pathological states if administered without drug monitoring. Interestingly, DAAs in clinical trials conducted for their administration approvals demonstrated to achieve satisfactory SVRs in hepatitis C-infected special populations. Recently, limited data from real-world cohorts depict the excellent efficacy and safety of IFN-free DAAs in real-life clinical situations, similar to clinical trials. It is still uncertain whether either viral or host factors are responsible for the trivial effectiveness of DAAs in such populations. In this chapter, we will discuss the management of harder-to-treat special populations with DAAs by exploring some real-world cohort data as well as the treatment algorithms, guidelines, and recommendations for those patients in real-world clinical settings.

Keywords: Acute HCV treatment, DAAs for pediatrics, Decompensated cirrhosis, Hepatocellular carcinoma, HCV viremic organ, HCV/HBV coinfection, HCV/HIV coinfection, HCV/CKD coinfection, HCV correctional populations, HCV occupational treatment, Post-liver transplantation, Renal impairment, Renal transplantation, Regimens for retreatment, Substance use disorders, Treatment failure.

Imran Shahid and Qaiser Jabeen

INTRODUCTION

HCV Treatment in Patients with Compensated or Decompensated Cirrhosis

Chronic hepatitis C-infected individuals with cirrhosis have an increased risk of developing severe hepatic clinical manifestations, including hepatic decompensation, HCC, and death. Therefore, CHC-infected patients with compensated cirrhosis are on high priority to initiate treatment immediately after diagnosis [1, 2]. It means that an important step of pretreatment assessment for HCV patients is to determine whether the cirrhosis is compensated or decompensated. However, the treatment goals for CHC patients with decompensated cirrhosis need modifications if the patients are on the waiting list for liver transplantation [2].

Compensated Cirrhosis

HCV patients with compensated cirrhosis have mild hepatic impairment (*i.e.*, CTP class A) and do not have clinical hepatic manifestations of decompensated cirrhosis like jaundice, ascites, variceal hemorrhage, or hepatic encephalopathy [3].

Decompensated Cirrhosis

HCV patients with decompensated cirrhosis have a moderate or severe hepatic disease (*i.e.*, CTP class B or C, or a score of 7 or higher) and experience one or more of the following hepatic manifestations; ascites, jaundice, variceal hemorrhage, or hepatic encephalopathy [4]. HCV patients who show significant clinical improvement after experiencing one clinical feature of decompensated cirrhosis should be evaluated for DAAs treatment on a case-by-case to determine whether to initiate treatment similar to patients with compensated cirrhosis [2]. It is because of shreds of evidence that even hepatic decompensation patients recover from the acute event, they are still considered to have decompensated cirrhosis [5, 6].

HCV TREATMENT IN PATIENTS WITH COMPENSATED CIRRHOSIS

Multiple studies reveal that the treatment of HCV patients with compensated cirrhosis with IFN-free DAAs would significantly decrease the incidences of subsequent cirrhosis-related complications, including hepatic failure, HCC, and hepatic-related mortalities (Table **1**) [6 - 9]. The studies also reveal that the treatment of CHC in hepatic decompensation with DAAs also remarkably improves the inflammatory grade of fibrosis following therapy and achieves higher SVR rates [10, 11]. Furthermore, it also substantially improves hepatic fibrosis following the achievement of an SVR with DAAs-based regimens [11].

Table 1. The available DAA options for HCV-infected patients with compensated cirrhosis [12].

HCV Genotype 1 population	Duration	Brands
Treatment naïve HCV GT-1/subtype 1a population:		
Glecaprevir 300 mg/pibrentasvir 120 mg once daily (A1)	8 weeks	GLE/PIB; (Mavyret®)
Ledipasvir 90 mg/sofosbuvir 400 mg once daily (A1)	12 weeks	LED/SOF; (multiple brands)
Sofosbuvir 400 mg/velpatasvir 100 mg once daily (A1)	12 weeks	SOF/VEL; (multiple brands)
Fixed-dose combination of elbasvir (50 mg)/grazoprevir (100 mg) one tablet once daily	12 weeks	(EBR/GZR); (Zepatier®)
Treatment naïve HCV GT-1/subtype 1b population:		
Glecaprevir 300 mg/pibrentasvir 120 mg once daily (A1)	8 weeks	GLE/PIB; (Mavyret®)
Ledipasvir 90 mg/sofosbuvir 400 mg once daily (A1)	12 weeks	LED/SOF; (multiple brands)
Sofosbuvir 400 mg/velpatasvir 100 mg once daily (A1)	12 weeks	SOF/VEL; (multiple brands)
HCV GT-2 population:		
Glecaprevir 300 mg/pibrentasvir 120 mg once daily (A1)	8 weeks	GLE/PIB; (Mavyret®)
Sofosbuvir 400 mg/velpatasvir 100 mg once daily (A1)	12 weeks	SOF/VEL; (multiple brands)
HCV GT-3 population:		
Glecaprevir 300 mg/pibrentasvir 120 mg once daily (A1)	8 weeks	GLE/PIB; (Mavyret®)
Sofosbuvir 400 mg/velpatasvir 100 mg once daily (A1)	12 weeks	SOF/VEL; (multiple brands)
• Sofosbuvir 400 mg/velpatasvir 100 mg one tablet once daily (A2); plus • Ribavirin 1000 mg if <75 kg or 1200 mg if ≥75 kg (the daily dose is given in two divided doses)	12 weeks	SOF/VEL; (multiple brands)
	12 weeks	RBV; (Copegus®)
Fixed-dose combination of sofosbuvir (400 mg)/velpatasvir (100 mg)/voxilaprevir (100 mg) one tablet once daily (A1);	12 weeks	SOF/VEL/VOX; (Vosevi®)

(Table 1) cont.....

HCV GT-4 population:		
Glecaprevir 300 mg/pibrentasvir 120 mg once daily (A1); This is taken as 3 tablets once daily with each fixed-dose tablet containing glecaprevir (100 mg)/pibrentasvir (40 mg).	8 weeks	GLE/PIB; (Mavyret®)
Fixed-dose combination of elbasvir (50 mg)/grazoprevir (100 mg) one tablet once daily (A1)	12 weeks	EBR/GZR; (Zepatier®)
Sofosbuvir 400 mg/velpatasvir 100 mg once daily (A1)	12 weeks	SOF/VEL; (multiple brands)
Ledipasvir 90 mg/sofosbuvir 400 mg once daily (A1)	12 weeks	(LED/SOF; (multiple brands)
HCV GT-5 or 6 population:		
Glecaprevir 300 mg/pibrentasvir 120 mg once daily (A1); This is taken as 3 tablets once daily with each fixed-dose tablet containing glecaprevir (100 mg)/pibrentasvir (40 mg).	8 weeks	GLE/PIB; (Mavyret®)
Fixed-dose combination of elbasvir (50 mg)/grazoprevir (100 mg) one tablet once daily (A1)	12 weeks	EBR/GZR; (Zepatier®)
Sofosbuvir 400 mg/velpatasvir 100 mg once daily (A1)	12 weeks	SOF/VEL; (multiple brands)
Ledipasvir 90 mg/sofosbuvir 400 mg once daily (A1)	12 weeks	(LED/SOF; (multiple brands)

HCV TREATMENT IN PATIENTS WITH DECOMPENSATED CIRRHOSIS

HCV treatment goal in patients with decompensated cirrhosis differs based on the candidacy for liver transplantation (Table **2**) [1 - 3]. The immediate or short-term goal for patients who are not potential candidates for liver transplantation should be to achieve an SVR, with the hope to reverse some degree of liver decompensation as a result of DAAs therapy, which may ultimately stabilize or improve their clinical condition [12]. However, the treatment model for HCV patients with decompensated cirrhosis and those on the waiting list for liver transplantation could be to achieve virologic clearance of hepatitis C before the liver transplantation [12]. Because it has been demonstrated that patients with detectable HCV RNA at the time of liver transplant will infect their new liver with HCV, which will ultimately reduce the life of the liver graft. In short, the primary goal to treat HCV before liver transplantation will be to minimize the risk of HCV reinfection of the new liver and thus improve post-transplantation outcomes [13]. Furthermore, pretransplantation HCV treatment seems a cost-effective approach in resource-rich nations as well as in resource-constraint nations, as some studies reveal that the treatment of pretransplantation hepatitis C patients with decompensated cirrhosis may prevent the further need for a liver transplant. One European study conducted in 103 HCV patients with decompensated cirrhosis and who were on an active liver transplant list showed that treatment with pangenotypic DAA regimens resulted in the delisting of 19% at 60 weeks posttreatment [14].

Table 2. The available DAA options for HCV-infected patients with decompensated cirrhosis [12 - 14].

<table>
<tr><th>HCV-affected populations:</th><th>Duration</th><th>Brands</th></tr>
<tr><th colspan="3">Treatment naïve and treatment-experienced HCV GT-1 & 4 populations</th></tr>
<tr><td rowspan="2">Ledipasvir 90 mg/sofosbuvir 400 mg once daily (A1); plus
Ribavirin 600 mg/day initially and after that titrated up as tolerated</td><td rowspan="2">12 weeks
or
24 weeks</td><td>LED/SOF;
(multiple brands)</td></tr>
<tr><td>RBV;
(Copegus®)</td></tr>
<tr><td rowspan="2">Sofosbuvir 400 mg once daily (A1) plus
Ribavirin 1,000 mg to 1200mg twice daily in divided doses</td><td rowspan="2">48 weeks</td><td>SOF;
(multiple brands)</td></tr>
<tr><td>RBV;
(Copegus®)</td></tr>
<tr><th colspan="3">Treatment naïve and treatment-experienced HCV GT-1, 2, 3, 4, or 6 populations</th></tr>
<tr><td rowspan="2">Sofosbuvir 400 mg/velpatasvir 100 mg once daily (A1); with or without
Ribavirin 1000 mg if <75 kg or 1200 mg if ≥75 kg (the daily dose is given in two divided doses)</td><td rowspan="2">12 weeks
or
24 weeks</td><td>SOF/VEL;
(multiple brands)</td></tr>
<tr><td>RBV;
(Copegus®)</td></tr>
</table>

HCV TREATMENT IN PATIENTS WITH HEPATOCELLULAR CARCINOMA (HCC)

The administration of PEG-IFN-free DAAs in HCV viremic patients with treated/inactive HCC demonstrates high SVR rates (*i.e.* 93-97%). However, since 2016, concerns have been raised about HCC recurrence risk following DAAs therapy in treated patients, with an estimated rate ranging from 0 to 59% due to the heterogeneity of the included studies [12, 15 - 17]. In contrast, all meta-analysis studies from different parts of the world focusing on HCC recurrence after DAA therapy, demonstrate no significant elevation of HCC recurrence risk in treated individuals compared to PEG-IFN treated or untreated HCV populations. Besides that, retrospective cohort studies also express no significant differences in HCC recurrence risk and patterns between DAAs-treated and untreated patient groups [17, 18]. Furthermore, retrospective cohort studies provide a piece of evidence about survival benefits associated with DAA therapy. Prospective cohort studies also exhibit an overall improved survival rate as well as a reduced rate of hepatic decompensation in DAA-treated individuals than to the propensity-score-matched untreated controls [14, 19]. The conclusions drawn from the recent studies support the clinical efficacy and safety of DAA regimens among hepatitis C patients with treated HCC and suggest no withholding of DAAs therapy in this population [15]. However, despite achieving an SVR rate in such patients, a persistent risk of HCC recurrence always remains in such individuals. For this reason, continued HCC surveillance is eagerly demanded especially for those patients who have already experienced multiple occurrences of HCC, high α-fetoprotein levels, and diabetes [15].

Equivocally, emerging studies conducted in HCV patients with active HCC demonstrate lower odds of achieving SVR rates in the era of pan-genotypic DAA regimens [17]. A recent meta-analysis conducted in 15 countries while including 49 studies, reported 73.1% SVR rates in HCV patients with active HCC, as compared to 92.6% in patients with treated HCC and 93.3% in HCV patients without HCC [17]. Hence, for HCV patients with active HCC, withholding DAA therapy is suggested until after a complete treatment response to HCC treatment is advised, provided that curative treatment is available [17]. How long to wait for optimal timing of DAA initiation therapy after HCC post-treatment response is still uncertain; however, a 3-6 months gap is considered sufficient and preferred to ensure sustained HCC response [14, 17].

The treatment initiation for HCV patients with treated HCC should be planned as recommended to the general population. However, if curative HCC treatment is available for active HCC, then it should be treated first and followed by HCV treatment 3-6 months later is advised [17]. If HCC is incurable then HCV treatment should be started immediately like the general population, regardless of considering HCC treatment [14, 17].

HCC TREATMENT FOR LIVER AND OTHER SOLID ORGAN TRANSPLANTATION

Detectable HCV RNA during liver transplantation of HCV-affected patients has universally encountered HCV recurrence post-liver transplantation which may ultimately lead to rapid progression of HCV-associated hepatic comorbidities [20]. However, the studies show the survival of a 3-year liver graft of a nonviremic HCV person by 4-fold for HCV viremic recipients in the DAA era as compared to the pre-DAA era [12, 19]. Hence, the use of DAA as a treatment for patients with HCV recurrence post-liver transplantation could be useful to improve overall liver health and prevent the deterioration of liver graft (Table **3**) [17]. However, the use of DAAs to prevent post-transplant HCV recurrence should be suggested with cautions, including potential drug-drug interactions (DDIs) between NS3/4A PIs and immunosuppressive agents like calcineurin inhibitors (*e.g.*, cyclosporine and tacrolimus) and mTOR inhibitors (*e.g.*, rapamycin) or NS5A inhibitors and everolimus. Similarly, the monitoring of plasma drug levels is also warranted because, with an improvement of liver function, the clearance of immunosuppressive agents is enhanced [13, 17].

Table 3. Treatment paradigms for HCV-infected patients awaiting for liver transplantation [12 - 14].

HCV treatment for post-liver transplantation recurrence		
	Duration	**Brands**
Recurrent HCV GT-1 to 6 infections post-liver transplantation, without cirrhosis or with compensated cirrhosis		
• Sofosbuvir 400 mg/velpatasvir 100 mg once daily (A1); • Addition of weight-based ribavirin (RBV)	12 weeks	SOF/VEL; (multiple brands)
		RBV; (Copegus®)
Recurrent HCV GT-1 to 6 infections post-liver transplantation, with decompensated cirrhosis		
Extension of sofosbuvir 400 mg/velpatasvir 100 mg once daily (B1) if RBV is not well tolerated	24 weeks	SOF/VEL; (multiple brands)
Recurrent HCV GT-1,2,4,5 or 6 infection post-liver transplantation, without cirrhosis or with compensated cirrhosis		
• Sofosbuvir 400 mg/velpatasvir 100 mg once daily (A1); • Addition of weight-based ribavirin (RBV)	12 weeks	SOF/VEL; (multiple brands)
		RBV; (Copegus®)
• Sofosbuvir 400 mg/velpatasvir 100 mg once daily (A1); without RBV	24weeks	SOF/VEL; (multiple brands)
Recurrent HCV GT-1 to 6 infections post-liver transplantation, without cirrhosis or with compensated cirrhosis		
Glecaprevir 300 mg/pibrentasvir 120 mg once daily (A1); This is taken as 3 tablets once daily with each fixed-dose tablet containing glecaprevir (100 mg)/pibrentasvir (40 mg).	12 weeks	GLE/PIB; (Mavyret®)
Recurrent HCV GT-1 to 4 infections post-liver transplantation, without cirrhosis or with compensated cirrhosis		
• Sofosbuvir 400 mg plus daclatasvir 60mg once daily; plus • weight-based ribavirin (RBV)	12 weeks	SOF plus DCV (multiple brands)
		RBV; (Copegus®)

To prevent HCV recurrence post-non-hepatic solid organ transplantation (*e.g.*, heart, kidney, lung, pancreas, or small bowel), the efficacy and tolerability of sofosbuvir (SOF)-based regimens have already been demonstrated before the approvals of pan-genotypic DAA regimens [17]. Although, pan-genotypic regimens are well tolerable, highly efficacious, and without any significant clinically relevant safety signals than SOF-based regimens (Table **4**); however, potential DDIs may happen between administered DAA and immunosuppressive agents. Close monitoring of drug levels and dosage adjustments is highly recommended in these clinical scenarios [14, 17].

Table 4. Treatment paradigms for HCV-infected patients awaiting for other non-hepatic solid organ transplantation [12 - 14].

HCV treatment for non-hepatic solid organ transplantation		
	Duration	**Brands**
Recurrent HCV GT-1,2,4,5 or 6 infections for non-hepatic solid organ transplantation		
Sofosbuvir 400 mg/velpatasvir 100 mg once daily (A1);	12 weeks	SOF/VEL; (multiple brands)
Recurrent HCV GT-1 to 6 infections for non-hepatic solid organ transplantation		
Ledipasvir 90 mg/sofosbuvir 400 mg once daily (A1); plus • weight-based ribavirin (RBV)	12 weeks	LED/SOF; (multiple brands) RBV; (Copegus®)
Glecaprevir 300 mg/pibrentasvir 120 mg once daily (A1); This is taken as 3 tablets once daily with each fixed-dose tablet containing glecaprevir (100 mg)/pibrentasvir (40 mg).	12 weeks	GLE/PIB; (Mavyret®)

TREATMENT FOR RECIPIENTS OF AN HCV VIREMIC ORGAN

A markedly increased rate of organ donation worldwide in recent years creates a huge discrepancy between the demand and supply of organs [12, 17]. To overcome these circumstances and expand the organ donor pool, the donation of transplanting an organ from an HCV viremic person to HCV-uninfected recipients has grabbed increased attention in various clinical settings [17]. However; this approach was strongly contraindicated in the past due to the 95% of HCV transmission risk from HCV viremic donors to HCV-uninfected recipients. Consequently, HCV viremic donor organs had to be discarded 2-6 times higher than nonviremic organs. Interestingly, in the post-DAAs era with the availability of treatment paradigms to prevent post-transplantation HCV recurrence, recent studies reveal that accepting HCV viremic organs may decrease waiting time for transplantation in patients who are on active transplantation lists with clinically meaningful survival benefits. Multiple small-scale studies express the feasibility of HCV viremic organ transplantation into HCV-uninfected recipients based on the favorable treatment outcomes of early DAA treatment in recipients of HCV viremic organs. This preemptive DAA treatment approach was found to achieve 100% SVR rates in post-transplantation organ recipients in two small clinical trials [13, 19]. However; despite promising preliminary findings, extensive research is required to elucidate this treatment approach on a larger scale to optimize treatment initiation timing and dosage algorithms for this population as well as to alluding the impact of DAA therapy on graft survival. Preemptive DAA therapy for a short duration of 4-8 weeks is recommended before transplantation. Furthermore, DAA regimens for HCV viremic organ recipients should be recommended like for patients with post-transplantation HCV recurrence [14, 19].

For other non-urgent non-hepatic solid organ transplantation, the risk of HCV transmission could be prevented from HCV viremic living donors by treating them with DAA before the transplantation [17]. However; for the urgent need for transplantation, HCV seronegative organ donors can be achieved by immediate suppression of HCV by DAA regimens to prevent HCV transmission risk [14, 17].

TREATMENT FOR HCV/HIV CO-INFECTED PATIENTS

The patients co-infected with HCV/HIV are always on high priority with DAA regimens because the studies evidence that coinfection with HIV accelerates the progression of hepatic fibrosis and ultimately results in a more aggressive course of hepatic disease [19]. Multiple studies reveal that hepatic cirrhosis in HCV/HIV coinfected patients was observed 12 to 16 years earlier than in those who had HCV mono-infection [12, 17, 21, 22]. It has also been noticed that hepatic-related mortalities in HIV/HCV coinfection is a prominent non-AIDS-related complication and up to 80 to 90% of deaths in those coinfected patients are attributable to hepatitis C infection [17, 22, 23]. Furthermore, HCV/HIV coinfected patients have decreased access to liver transplantation than those who have HCV mono-infection. Because of all these plausible justifications, it is recommended to initiate HCV/HIV coinfection treatment as early as possible [17, 24]. The following are the treatment recommendations for HCV/HIV coinfected patients infected with different hepatitis C GTs/subtypes (Table **5**).

Table 5. The available DAA options for HCV/HIV co-infected patients [12, 14].

HCV GT-1 population:	Duration	Brands
Treatment naïve HCV GTs-1a, 1b patients coinfected with HIV and without cirrhosis		
Ledipasvir 90 mg/sofosbuvir 400 mg once daily (A1)	12 weeks	LED/SOF; (multiple brands)
For patients who are black, HIV-infected, or have HCV RNA ≥6 million copies/mL		
Ledipasvir 90 mg/sofosbuvir 400 mg once daily (A1)	12 weeks	LED/SOF; (multiple brands)
For patients who are non-black, HIV-uninfected, and have HCV RNA <6 million copies/mL		

(Table 5) cont.....

Ledipasvir 90 mg/sofosbuvir 400 mg once daily (A1)	8 weeks	LED/SOF; (multiple brands)
Treatment naïve HCV GT-1a, 1b, 2, 3, and 4 populations coinfected with HCV/HIV and with compensated cirrhosis		
Glecaprevir 300 mg/pibrentasvir 120 mg once daily (A1)	12 weeks	GLE/PIB; (Mavyret®)
Treatment naïve HCV GT-5 and 6 populations coinfected with HCV/HIV and without or with compensated cirrhosis		
Glecaprevir 300 mg/pibrentasvir 120 mg once daily (A1)	12 weeks	GLE/PIB; (Mavyret®)

TREATMENT FOR HBV/HCV DUAL INFECTION

Several studies demonstrate comparably higher SVR rates in HCV/HBV coinfected patients despite the risk of HBV reactivation following DAA treatment in patients with HBV/HCV dual infection [25]. Therefore HCV patients with HBV coinfection should be assessed with HBsAg, anti-HBs, and anti-HBc testing before initiating DAA [26]. Worst histological and clinical outcomes have been reported in patients with HBV/HCV dual infection than in those with mono-infection [27]. Therefore treatment for HBV/HCV coinfected patients should be started with concurrent administration of anti-HBV therapy together with DAA regimens provided that such patients fulfill the criteria for HBV treatment [28]. Prophylactic nucleos(t)ide analog treatment for HBV is strongly recommended until 12-24 weeks post-DAA therapy to prevent HBV reactivation due to the risk of HBV flare with hepatic decompensation in HBV/HCV dual infected patients with HBsAg positivity and advanced fibrosis or cirrhosis [12, 13]. However, for patients without cirrhosis and positive HBsAg, prophylactic nucleos(t)ide anti-HBV therapy with close monitoring is suggested until week 12-24 post-DAA therapy (Table **6**). Furthermore, clinicians should be aware of HBV reactivation and pay close attention, especially to patients with advanced fibrosis and cirrhosis [13, 14].

Table 6. The treatment options for HBV/HCV co-infected patients [14].

HCV/HBV Dual Infection	Duration	Brands
Ledipasvir 90 mg/sofosbuvir 400 mg once daily (A1)	12 weeks	LED/SOF; (multiple brands)

TREATMENT OF HCV IN PATIENTS WITH RENAL IMPAIRMENT

Before defining DAAs treatment algorithms for HCV-infected individuals with renal disease, it is of prime importance to first assess the stage of the patient's kidney disease, which utilizes the following definitions of various kidney ailments [12, 29].

Chronic Kidney Disease (CKD)

Any kidney damage or decreased kidney function which persists for three or more months, irrespective of cause is classified as chronic kidney disease (CKD) [30].

Glomerular Filtration Rate (GFR)

The general gold reference standard to evaluate the best index of overall kidney function is the glomerular filtration rate (GFR); However, the test cutoff may vary in the normal individual by age and sex, dietary protein intake, and possibly by race-ethnicity [31 - 33]. The test index values are referred to as follows for the normal as well as for the diseased individuals;

1. Normal GFR value for men and women: 130 and 120 mL/min/1.73 m^2 respectively.
2. Threshold values for a decreased GFR function: 60 mL/min/1.73 m^2.
3. Kidney failure for a decreased GFR of less than 15 mL/min/1.73 m^2 or treatment by dialysis.

GFR values represent the total sum of the filtration rates in all of the functioning nephrons; however, GFR cannot be measured directly, and it is usually estimated from serum markers. The gold standard method for the assessment of GFR is the renal inulin clearance test, however, this method is too complicated and seems impractical for routine clinical purposes. Hence, several other methods including Chronic Kidney Disease Epidemiology Collaboration (CKD-EPI) and the Modification of Diet in renal disease (MDRD), have been utilized in clinical practice to estimate GFR [33].

Creatinine Clearance (CrCl)

The creatinine clearance is a good parameter to evaluate GFR; however, it overestimates the GFR since creatinine is both filtered by the glomeruli and secreted in the renal tubules [34]. The Cockcroft-Gault formula is commonly used in clinical practice to estimate creatinine clearance based on serum creatinine, patient age, body mass in kilograms, and sex. The normal cutoff values are 95 to 145 mL/min in males and 75 to 115 mL/min in females respectively. Albeit, this formula is less accurate in body weight extremes, another accurate but less practical determination of creatinine clearance can be made with a 24 hrs urine collection [34]. Hence CrCl is calculated by dividing the 24 hrs urine creatinine by the serum creatinine; which is equal to the urine creatinine concentration multiplied by urine volume. However, 24 hrs urine creatinine clearance has also some limitations which may cause inaccuracies like incomplete urine collection [34].

Staging of Kidney Disease

Staging of kidney disease before initiating DAAs treatment should be done according to the Kidney Disease Improving Global Outcomes (KDIGO) 2012 Clinical Practice Guideline for patients who are diagnosed with hepatitis C while using the criteria described above [35]. It includes the cause of disease, category of eGFR, and category of albuminuria with an overall prognosis of kidney function [35, 36].

DAAS DOSE ADJUSTMENTS IN HCV/CKD PATIENTS

DAAs Choice	Dose Adjustment
• Elbasvir-Grazoprevir (EBR/GZR; Zepatier®)	No dosage adjustment is needed for patients who have mild, moderate, or severe renal impairment, including individuals requiring dialysis.
• Glecaprevir-Pibrentasvir GLE/PIB; Mavyret®)	
• Ledipasvir-Sofosbuvir (LED/SOF; (multiple brands)	
• Sofosbuvir-Velpatasvir (SOF/VEL; (multiple brands)	
• Sofosbuvir-Velpatasvir-Voxilaprevir SOF/VEL/VOX; (Vosevi®)	

RIBAVIRIN DOSING IN PATIENTS WITH HCV/CKD CO-INFECTIONS

Being not a DAA, as well as with potential toxicities documented in many studies while administering RBV in HCV-affected populations, its use in patients with HCV/CKD requires special consideration independent of recommendations for IFN-free DAAs in CKD [13, 37]. In the current era of HCV treatment with PEG-IFN free DAAs, RBV is recommended for use in selected situations like;

- In combination with Ledipasvir-Sofosbuvir (LED/SOF) in patients with decompensated cirrhosis [38]; or
- In patients with HCV GT-1a infection receiving treatment with EBR/GZR and who have been detected with NS5A resistance-associated substitutions (RASs)

for elbasvir (EBR) [39].

However, in the case of HCV/CKD coinfections, the story is different where ribavirin administration is based on the use of generic or multiple companies' brand formulations [14]. As it is clinically evident that since ribavirin (RBV) levels will increase as renal function decreases, the use of RBV in patients with renal impairment becomes cautious. For example, brand names *Rebetol®* and *Ribasphere®*, do not recommend using RBV in patients with an eGFR rate of less than 50mL/min [14]. However; the prescriber's leaflet for *Copegus®* suggests the use of RBV in patients with an eGFR less than 50mL/min provided that the dose is reduced with careful treatment monitoring. Likely, the AASLD-IDSA HCV guidance recommends the use of RBV with reduced and alternating doses of 200 and 400 mg every other day (*e.g.*, 200 mg on Monday, 400 mg on Tuesday, 200 mg on Wednesday, *etc.*) in patients with creatinine clearance of 30 to 50 mL/min. The guidelines also recommend reducing the RBV dose to 200 mg in adult patients having severe renal diseases (CrCl < 30 mL/min), end-stage renal disease, or hemodialysis [14].

HCV TREATMENT IN PATIENTS WITH RENAL TRANSPLANTATION

Ideally, most clinicians recommend HCV treatment before renal transplant in patients who are renal transplantation candidates if possible [13, 40]. The rationale behind this approach reveals to give the potential for graft dysfunction in patients who received IFN-based therapy post-transplant and to improve clinical outcomes in those who underwent HCV clearance before transplantation [41]. Another point of view deciphers that pretransplant treatment has also been shown to prevent some hepatitis C-related renal complications like glomerulonephritis in the kidney transplant population [42]. The DAAs regimens recommended for patients waiting for renal transplants are the same as those prescribed for severe renal impairment (Table 7) [42]. However, it is not possible to treat HCV before renal transplantation in some circumstances [42]. Furthermore, DDIs studies are of extreme importance in the posttransplantation period, in particular with immunosuppressant calcineurin inhibitors, particularly cyclosporine and tacrolimus [13].

Table 7. DAAs option for HCV-infected patients with renal transplantation [13].

Treatment-naïve and non-DAA experienced HCV GTs 1 to 6 infected patients waiting for a renal transplant with or without compensated cirrhosis	Duration	Brands
Ledipasvir 90 mg/sofosbuvir 400 mg once daily (A1)	12 weeks	LED/SOF; (multiple brands)

(Table 7) cont.....

Glecaprevir 300 mg/pibrentasvir 120 mg once daily (A1)	12 weeks	GLE/PIB; (Mavyret®)
Sofosbuvir 400 mg/velpatasvir 100 mg once daily (A1)	12 weeks	SOF/VEL; (multiple brands)
Treatment-naïve and non-DAA experienced GTs 1 or 4 HCV patients waiting for a renal transplant with or without compensated cirrhosis		
*Fixed-dose combination of elbasvir (50 mg)/grazoprevir (100 mg) one tablet once daily (A1) *Provided that if they do not have any baseline NS5A resistance-associated substitutions for elbasvir.	12 weeks	EBR/GZR; (Zepatier)
Treatment-naïve and DAA experienced HCV GTs 1 to 6 infected patients waiting for a renal transplant with or without compensated cirrhosis		
• Fixed-dose combination of sofosbuvir (400 mg)/velpatasvir (100 mg)/voxilaprevir (100 mg) one tablet once daily (A1); • With or without RBV	12 weeks	SOF/VEL/VOX; (Vosevi)
	12 weeks	RBV; (Copegus)

TREATMENT OF HCV IN PATIENTS WITH SUBSTANCE USE DISORDERS

With the availability and effectiveness of pangenotypic DAAs, a widened space is available now to clinicians for treatment decisions in PWIDs, recent or past IDUs, or other substance abusers having hepatitis C infection (Table **8**). The AASLD-IDSA guidance suggests that recent or active IDU or alcohol use should not be considered an absolute contraindication to hepatitis C treatment and not necessary to discontinue illicit drug or alcohol use for pretreatment screening [13]. Nevertheless, the individuals having CHC infection with concomitant substance abuse (either past or present) including opioids, amphetamines, cannabis, alcohol, and other drugs would always remain relevant to the individual's overall health and medication access [13]. Similarly, the initiation of treatment of hepatitis C for individuals with a prior history of substance use including injecting drugs, or alcohol use should be the same as in patients with no history of drug use. Furthermore, studies explicit that abstinence of both injection-drug use and alcohol before initiating HCV treatment or duration of abstinence have found no significant impact on the likelihood of achieving SVR rates after completing IFN-free DAA-based therapy. It means that clinically no reason to ensure abstinence of any duration before initiating HCV treatment and it should not be a contraindication to HCV treatment [13].

Table 8. HCV treatment for patients who are substance abusers and for patients who inject drugs (PWIDs) [12, 14].

PWIDs who are on opiate agonist therapy and infected with HCV GT-1, 4, or 6	Duration	Brands
Fixed-dose combination of elbasvir (50 mg)/grazoprevir (100 mg) one tablet once daily (A1)	12 weeks	EBR/GZR; (Zepatier®)
PWIDs who are on opioid substitution therapy and infected with HCV GT-1		
Ledipasvir 90 mg/sofosbuvir 400 mg once daily (A1)	12 weeks	LED/SOF; (multiple brands)
Patients with recent injection drug use and infected with HCV GT-1 to 6		
Sofosbuvir 400 mg/velpatasvir 100 mg once daily (A1)	12 weeks	SOF/VEL; (multiple brands)
Patients on opioid substitution therapy during treatment and infected with HCV		
Sofosbuvir 400 mg/velpatasvir 100 mg once daily (A1)	12 weeks	SOF/VEL; (multiple brands)
Patients who are recent or current injection drug use and infected with HCV		
Glecaprevir 300 mg/pibrentasvir 120 mg once daily (A1)	8 or 12 weeks	GLE/PIB; (Mavyret®)

TREATMENT OF HCV IN CORRECTIONAL SETTINGS

Before initiating HCV treatment in inmates who are considered a high-risk reservoir for HCV transmission within their prison in jail or after release to communities, it is better to differentiate between jails and prisons. Most persons placed in jail are pre-adjudication or have received a conviction and are serving a brief sentence (*i.e.*, usually one year or less) [12, 43]. It means that jail houses innocent people as well as people who commit misdemeanors and felonies. Once sentenced, then the length of the sentence is the predominant factor to determine if a person is transferred to prison [44]. In contrast to a scenario with the situation in jails, a person is considered in prison when he or she is sentenced usually a couple of years, a time frame which seems sufficient to treat many incarcerated people for hepatitis C [45]. However, HCV treatment of inmates and incarcerated people depends on a lot of factors including HCV screening policies (*e.g.*, upon request, risk-based, opt-in, opt-out, and mandatory testing), cost of therapy, patient adherence to treatment, and release date [13, 46]. Hence, a variety of treatment models are utilized to provide hepatitis C treatment in correctional settings including; on-site correctional HCV specialists, on-site community HCV specialists, project [47] support, and community referral (Table **9**) [48]. Even though correctional settings could be an ideal environment to provide HCV treatment and with the availability of DAAs, many of the clinical barriers to treatment have been eliminated; interestingly, the real-world data from multiple studies predict that patient adherence to treatment as well as limited clinician capacity, and lack of perceived expertise among clinicians are still crosscutting barriers to treat and achieve high SVR rates in a large population of incarcerated people [14, 48].

Table 9. HCV treatment for patients who are inmates and in prison [12, 14].

Treatment-naïve and non-DAA Experienced HCV GTs-1 to 6 infected patients in jail with or without compensated cirrhosis	Duration	Brands
Ledipasvir 90 mg/sofosbuvir 400 mg once daily (A1)	12 weeks	LED/SOF; (multiple brands)
Sofosbuvir (400 mg) one tablet once daily	12 weeks	SOF; (multiple brands)
Prisoners with opioid use disorders and infected with HCV GT-1, 4, or 6	**Duration**	**Brands**
Fixed-dose combination of elbasvir (50 mg)/grazoprevir (100 mg) one tablet once daily (A1)	12 weeks	EBR/GZR; (Zepatier)
Ledipasvir 90 mg/sofosbuvir 400 mg once daily (A1)	12 weeks	LED/SOF; (multiple brands)
Sofosbuvir (400 mg) one tablet once daily	12 weeks	SOF; (multiple brands)

TREATMENT OF ACUTE HEPATITIS C INFECTION

Before starting treatment for acute hepatitis C infection, it must be accurately diagnosed because most acute HCV infections are subclinical and do not depend on the presence or absence of symptoms associated with infection (Table **10**) [49]. As most clinicians and infectious disease experts define acute infections as the 6 months following the acquisition of HCV, a preferred accepted laboratory diagnosis document either of the two following criteria [13, 50]:

1. A positive quantitative HCV RNA test in conjunction with a negative anti-hepatitis C Abs test; or
2. A positive anti-hepatitis C Abs test for a negative anti-hepatitis C Abs documented test of a person in the past 12 months [50].

Table 10. HCV treatment for patients who are acutely infected with the infection [12, 14].

Treatment for acute HCV infection	Duration	Brands
Pegylated interferon-alpha 2b injection/week	12 weeks	PEG-IFN-α-2b (multiple brands)

(Table 10) cont.....

Treatment for acute HCV infection infected with HCV GT-1 or 4 and having HIV infection		
Fixed-dose combination of elbasvir (50 mg)/grazoprevir (100 mg) one tablet once daily	8 weeks	(EBR/GZR); (Zepatier®)
Treatment for acute HCV infection infected with HCV GT-1 & MSM		
Glecaprevir 300 mg/pibrentasvir 120 mg once daily (A1)	6 weeks	GLE/PIB; (Mavyret®)
Treatment for acute HCV infection infected with HCV GT-1 with or without HIV infection		
Glecaprevir 300 mg/pibrentasvir 120 mg once daily (A1)	4 weeks	GLE/PIB; (Mavyret®)
Glecaprevir 300 mg/pibrentasvir 120 mg once daily (A1)	6 weeks	GLE/PIB; (Mavyret®)
Glecaprevir 300 mg/pibrentasvir 120 mg once daily (A1)	4 weeks	GLE/PIB; (Mavyret®)
Treatment for acute HCV GT-1 mono-infection		
Ledipasvir 90 mg/sofosbuvir 400 mg once daily	6weeks	(LED/SOF; (multiple brands)
Treatment for acute HCV infection infected with GT-1& 4 and with HIV infection		
Ledipasvir 90 mg/sofosbuvir 400 mg once daily (A1)	6 weeks	(LED/SOF; (multiple brands)
Treatment for acute HCV infection in PWIDs		
Sofosbuvir 400 mg/velpatasvir 100 mg once daily	6 or 12 weeks	SOF/VEL; (multiple brands)

HCV patients who achieve an SVR with DAAs will have always positive for anti-HCV Abs tests [49]. Hence, for such people who achieve SVR at 12 weeks or later after completing hepatitis C treatment, a diagnosis of reinfection must be based on the detection of HCV RNA [49]. It is also very important to mention here that reinfection after treating acute HCV infection is uncommon, but it can occur in people who continue high-risk activities at potential risk premises for acquiring HCV [14, 51]. Furthermore, distinguishing reinfection from viral relapse is also important following achieving an SVR at post-DAAs treatment [14, 51]. Hepatitis C viral relapse always occurs within the first 12 weeks after completing DAA therapy. Therefore, if a patient achieves SVR at 12 weeks or later after post-therapy and subsequently has detectable HCV RNA, it is an indication of a suspected HCV reinfection [51]. In this case, an HCV genotyping/subtyping test should be ordered and compared the results to HCV GTs in the initial infection [51]. The detection of distinct GTs/subtypes would confirm recent reinfection. It is also possible that the patient may reinfect with the same GTs/subtypes and thus finding of same GTs/subtypes does not rule out hepatitis C reinfection. For this purpose, viral genome sequencing could be a better option to differentiate HCV infections of the same GTs/subtypes, but it is not performed in routine clinical practice [52].

HCV TREATMENT FOR HEALTH CARE PROFESSIONALS WITH OCCUPATIONAL EXPOSURE

Hepatitis C exposure to health care professionals (HCPs) is well described with an estimated risk ranging from 0 to 10% following percutaneous exposure [53, 54]. However, this fraction varies according to the healthcare system, healthcare provider facilities, strict compliance to protective measures, and type of exposure. Interestingly, the risk of HCV infection through mucocutaneous exposure is estimated to be 0% [14, 55]. Although HCV RNA is detected in several body fluids including saliva, semen, and vaginal secretions; however, controversies exist about whether these secretions are capable to transmit HCV as a sufficient infectious HCV titer is needed for this purpose [53]. Consequently, the data are limited, murky, and inconclusive in this regard [53]. Ultimately, the approaches to managing occupational exposure to HCV in HCPs mostly rely on regular HCV screening and diagnosis monitoring [13, 54]. Similarly, the management of postexposure prophylaxis (PEP) in HCPs with DAA regimens is not recommended based on certain factors including [14, 53];

1. Hepatitis C infection risk is less following percutaneous or mucocutaneous exposure,
2. The high cost of DAA therapy, and
3. Lack of real-world clinical studies data to support the use and duration of DAAs for hepatitis C PEP [14, 53].

However, HCPs who seroconvert to HCV infection (i.e, confirmed by a positive HCV RNA qualitative or quantitative test) should be referred for treatment [56]. As DAAs are proving highly efficacious in curing both acute and chronic hepatitis C infections, the guidelines recommend early identification and treatment of hepatitis C (in most cases, "acute HCV infection") in a "test-to-treat" fashion for HCV RNA positive HCPs [56]. There are no significant differences in treatment recommendations (*e.g.*, DAAs used, treatment duration, *etc.*,) for both acute and chronic hepatitis C infection; however, shortened courses of DAAs regimens could be either cost or treatment effective in treating acute hepatitis C in HCPs [14, 56].

REGIMENS FOR RETREATMENT OF HCV IN TREATMENT-EXPERIENCED PATIENTS HAVING FAILURE WITH DAAS

Thanks to the approval and availability of pan-genotypic DAAs for the patients with HCV GTs 1 to 6 whose previous treatments with DAAs failed [57]. However; the dosage algorithms and duration of therapy in such a population are entirely based on previous exposure to either NS3/4A PIs or NS5A (Table **11**), or NS5B polymerase inhibitors along with PEG-IFN plus RBV failure (Table **12**) [13, 57]. Interestingly, DAAs regimens approved for retreatment after DAA treatment failure require no resistance testing to initiate HCV retreatment or the addition of RBV in dosage algorithms.

Table 11. DAA retreatment options for patients having the previous failure with NS5A inhibitors [13].

Retreatment for prior failure with an NS5A inhibitor-containing regimen*				
HCV Genotype	**Cirrhosis Status**	**DAA regimens**	**Duration**	**Brand**
1	No cirrhosis; or Compensated cirrhosis	**Retreatment options for HCV patients with no previous treatment with NS3/4A PIs§ [57]** Glecaprevir 300 mg/pibrentasvir 120 mg once daily	16 weeks	GLE/PIB; (Mavyret®)
3	Compensated cirrhosis	Sofosbuvir (400 mg)/velpatasvir (100 mg)/voxilaprevir (100 mg) one tablet once daily plus weight-based ribavirin twice daily [58]	12 weeks	SOF/VEL/VOX; (Vosevi®) RBV; (Copegus®)
1,2,3,4,5,6	No cirrhosis; Compensated cirrhosis	Sofosbuvir (400 mg)/velpatasvir (100 mg)/voxilaprevir (100 mg) one tablet once daily [58]	12 weeks	SOF/VEL/VOX; (Vosevi®)
*NS5A polymerase inhibitors: daclatasvir, elbasvir, ledipasvir, ombitasvir, pibrentasvir, and velpatasvir, §NS3/4A protease inhibitors: glecaprevir, grazoprevir, paritaprevir, and voxilaprevir				
Retreatment for prior failure with an NS3/4A PIs - regimens that did not contain an NS5A inhibitor*				
1	No cirrhosis; compensated cirrhosis	Glecaprevir 300 mg/pibrentasvir 120 mg once daily [57]	12 weeks	
	No cirrhosis; compensated cirrhosis	Sofosbuvir 400 mg/velpatasvir 100 mg once daily [58]	12 weeks	
	No cirrhosis	Ledipasvir 90 mg/sofosbuvir 400 mg once daily [59]	12 weeks	
	Compensated cirrhosis	Ledipasvir 90 mg/sofosbuvir 400 mg once daily plus weight-based ribavirin twice daily [60]	12 weeks	
	Compensated cirrhosis	Ledipasvir 90 mg/sofosbuvir 400 mg once daily [61]	24 weeks	

(Table 11) cont.....

1,2,3,4,5,6	No cirrhosis; compensated cirrhosis	Sofosbuvir (400 mg)/velpatasvir (100 mg)/voxilaprevir (100 mg) one tablet once daily [58]	12 weeks	
*NS3/4A protease inhibitors: glecaprevir, grazoprevir, paritaprevir, and voxilaprevir, §NS5A polymerase inhibitors: daclatasvir, elbasvir, ledipasvir, ombitasvir, pibrentasvir, and velpatasvir				

Table 12. DAA retreatment options for patients having the previous failure with NS5B inhibitors and having PEG-IFN/RBV failure [13].

Retreatment options for failure with SOF-containing regimens that did not contain an NS5A inhibitor*				
1	No cirrhosis	**Retreatment options for HCV patients with no previous treatment with NS3/4A PIs**§ Glecaprevir 300 mg/pibrentasvir 120 mg once daily [57]	12 weeks	GLE/PIB; (Mavyret®)
1	Compensated cirrhosis	**Retreatment options for HCV patients with no previous treatment with NS3/4A PIs**§ Glecaprevir 300 mg/pibrentasvir 120 mg once daily [57]	16 weeks	GLE/PIB; (Mavyret®)
1,2,3,4,5,6	No cirrhosis; Compensated cirrhosis	Sofosbuvir (400 mg)/velpatasvir (100 mg)/voxilaprevir (100 mg) one tablet once daily [58]	12 weeks	SOF/VEL/VOX; (Vosevi®)
*NS5A polymerase inhibitors: daclatasvir, elbasvir, ledipasvir, ombitasvir, pibrentasvir, and velpatasvir, §NS3/4A protease inhibitors: glecaprevir, grazoprevir, paritaprevir, and voxilaprevir				
Retreatment for prior failure with PEG-IFN plus RBV* and sofosbuvir				
1,2,4,5,6	No cirrhosis; compensated cirrhosis	Glecaprevir 300 mg/pibrentasvir 120 mg once daily [57]	12 weeks	GLE/PIB; (Mavyret®)
3		Glecaprevir 300 mg/pibrentasvir 120 mg once daily [57]	16 weeks	GLE/PIB; (Mavyret®)
1,2,3,4,5,6		Sofosbuvir (400 mg)/velpatasvir (100 mg)/voxilaprevir (100 mg) one tablet once daily [58]	12 weeks	SOF/VEL/VOX; (Vosevi®)
*Pegylated interferon plus ribavirin				

HCV TREATMENT FOR CHILDREN AND ADOLESCENTS

Worldwide, HCV infection occurs in nearly 3.5 million children and adolescents aged 1-19 years, among which 73-100% of cases are acquired through perinatal transmission [14, 62]. The perinatal risk of HCV acquisition was once estimated to be 6-11% corresponding to >1 infection in every 20 newborns delivered by hepatitis C viremic pregnant women [63]. Furthermore, other potential routes of HCV transmission among children and adolescents are mostly attributed to nosocomial and IDU transmission [63]. An advantage is a slow progression of hepatic fibrosis in children as compared to adults, unfortunately, the unknown infection status and untreated children (*i.e.*, approximately 30% cases) develop worsening hepatic fibrosis over 5 years [14, 63]. Obesity and HIV coinfection (*e.g.*, transmitted in children and adolescents majority by using drug syringe exchange) are predisposing factors to escalate the progression of hepatic comorbidities in children and adolescents. Therefore, HCV eradication in children and adolescents is of prime importance to reduce further transmission of HCV in other fractions of the population as well as to prevent the development of severe hepatic comorbidities (*e.g.*, cirrhosis, HCC, and end-stage liver disease) [14, 62].

At the time of writing this book chapter, only three IFN-free DAAs combinations are being used for hepatitis C treatment in children and/or adolescents (Table **13**). The clinical trials of these DAA combinations demonstrate their high efficacy, well tolerability, and fewer adverse events in children and adolescents. Sofosbuvir plus ribavirin safety profile was found considerably better than the other two DAAs combinations in children and adults [13, 17]. SVR rates were also achieved in all participants irrespective of the presence of baseline NS5A or NS5B resistance-associated substitutions (RAS).

Table 13. HCV treatment paradigms for children and adolescents [12 - 14].

DAA regimen	HCV GT	Age	Dose adjustment	Duration	Brand
Ledipasvir /sofosbuvir	1	≥3	Weight-based adjustment: ≥35 kg: 400mg/90mg 17-34kg: 200mg/45mg <17 kg: 150mg/33.75 mg	12 weeks; T.N without cirrhosis 12 weeks; T.N with compensated cirrhosis 12weeks; [a]T.E without cirrhosis 24 weeks; [a]T.E with compensated cirrhosis	(LED/SOF; (multiple brands)
	2,4,5,6			12 weeks	
Sofosbuvir + Ribavirin	2	≥3	Weight-based adjustment: ≥35 kg: 400mg SOF 17-34kg: 200mg SOF <17 kg: 150mg SOF	12 weeks	SOF; multiple brands + [b]RBV; (Copegus®)
	3			24 weeks	

(Table 13) cont.....

Glecaprevir /pibrentasvir	1,2,4,5,6	≥12	Glecaprevir 300 mg/pibrentasvir 120 mg once daily	8 weeks; T.N without cirrhosis 8 weeks; T.N with compensated cirrhosis 8 weeks; Prior treatment failure with PEG-IFN/RBV/SOF without cirrhosis 12 weeks: [c]Prior treatment failure with PEG-IFN/RBV/SOF with compensated cirrhosis	GLE/PIB; (Mavyret®)
	3			8 weeks; T.N without cirrhosis or with compensated cirrhosis 16 weeks: [c]Prior treatment failure with PEG-IFN/RBV/SOF without cirrhosis or with compensated cirrhosis	

DAA, direct-acting antiviral; GLE, glecaprevir; HCV, hepatitis C virus; LDV, ledipasvir; PegIFN, pegylated interferon; PI, protease inhibitor;
PIB, pibrentasvir; SOF, sofosbuvir; TE, treatment-experienced; TN, treatment-naı¨ve; RBV, ribavirin.
[a]TE refers to PegIFN _ RBV _ HCV PI.
[b]Weight-based adjustment for ribavirin daily dose: 1200 mg for >80 kg; 1000 mg for 66 to 80 kg; 800 mg for 50 to 65 kg; 600 mg for 47 to 49 kg; 15 mg/kg for <47 kg.
[c]PRS refers to prior treatment experience of PegIFN+RBV+SOF.

HCV TREATMENT IN PREGNANCY

Worldwide, the prevalence of HCV infection has dramatically increased in WORA as well as in pregnant women [12, 63]. It is estimated that 0.1-8% of pregnant women in the world are infected with hepatitis C infection. Multiple studies also predict that the newborn delivered by pregnant HCV-infected women is at a 6-11% risk of acquiring HCV through perinatal transmission [64]. For this reason, universal HCV screening/diagnosis in WORA or pregnant women before and during each pregnancy is highly recommended to improve linkage to care as well as to increase the HCV detection rate in neonates [64, 65]. Furthermore, currently, no DAAs have clear recommendations to be administered in pregnant women during pregnancy to treat HCV as well as to avoid adverse outcomes for the fetus. Much emphasis is given to hepatitis C diagnosis to prevent prenatal HCV transmission and the progression of advanced hepatic diseases in pregnant women. Ribavirin is a proven teratogenic. Hence RBV-containing regimens are strongly contraindicated in pregnant females [66]. Sofosbuvir-based regimens (*e.g.*, sofosbuvir/ledipasvir, sofosbuvir plus daclatasvir, and sofosbuvir/velpatasvir) are in different phases of their clinical trials to predict their clinical efficacies as well as safety in pregnant women and their birth defects on neonates and infants [65, 67]. Interestingly no significant association between HCV transmission risk and breastfeeding has been developed until now, therefore, breastfeeding is not contraindicated in HCV viremic females, unless the breast nipples are cracked, damaged, or bled out [12, 68]. However, DAAs may transfer to breast milk, as evidenced by some studies in the rat model. Hence the DAA's safety in breastfeeding women requires further elucidation.

CONCLUSIONS

The treatment paradigms for harder-to-cure and vulnerable HCV-affected populations will always remain a big challenge due to multiple reasons. Treatment non-adherence, and abstinence during or post-treatment monitoring are two big challenges with substance use disorders, PWIDs, and IDUs affected with HCV. Treatment options for correctional populations must be opted according to the facilities, upon request, risk-based, mandatory testing, and cost of therapy. Furthermore, treatment options are scarce for decompensated cirrhotics, HCV patients with HCC, and liver and solid organs awaiting transplantation. However; the pan-genotypic DAAs administration is effective to achieve reasonable SVRs in such patient populations to prevent liver transplantation while reducing the exacerbation of CHC to convert into end-stage liver disease, and increasing the QALY. The treatment recommendations for the recipient of viremic organs must also be followed in real-life clinical situations. The successful management of HCV patients suffering from other comorbidities with DAAs is also attainable provided that the treatment guidelines are properly followed in particular to prevent HBV reactivation, HCC occurrence, or recurrence in treated individuals. DAAs dose adjustment in particular with RBV administration should be performed carefully in treating HCV/CKD coinfection and renal transplant patients while monitoring GFR, CrCl, and other renal function tests. Acute HCV infection and occupational or accidental exposure to HCV also require immediate treatment attention in health care settings; however; it is based on regular HCV screening and diagnosis monitoring and postexposure prophylaxis (PEP) in HCPs with DAAs is usually not recommended. As mentioned elsewhere, treatment protocols are not well defined yet for pregnant women, infants, and children; hence, DAAs should not be administered in such patient populations except in extreme emergencies.

REFERENCES

[1] Garcia-Tsao G, Friedman S, Iredale J, Pinzani M. Now there are many (stages) where before there was one: In search of a pathophysiological classification of cirrhosis. Hepatology 2010; 51(4): 1445-9. [http://dx.doi.org/10.1002/hep.23478] [PMID: 20077563]

[2] Ge PS, Runyon BA. Treatment of Patients with Cirrhosis. N Engl J Med 2016; 375(8): 767-77. [http://dx.doi.org/10.1056/NEJMra1504367] [PMID: 27557303]

[3] D'Amico G, Garcia-Tsao G, Pagliaro L. Natural history and prognostic indicators of survival in cirrhosis: A systematic review of 118 studies. J Hepatol 2006; 44(1): 217-31. [http://dx.doi.org/10.1016/j.jhep.2005.10.013] [PMID: 16298014]

[4] D'amico G, Morabito A, Pagliaro L, Marubini E. Survival and prognostic indicators in compensated and decompensated cirrhosis. Dig Dis Sci 1986; 31(5): 468-75. [http://dx.doi.org/10.1007/BF01320309] [PMID: 3009109]

[5] Tada T, Kumada T, Toyoda H, *et al.* Viral eradication reduces all-cause mortality, including non-live--related disease, in patients with progressive hepatitis C virus-related fibrosis. J Gastroenterol Hepatol 2017; 32(3): 687-94. [http://dx.doi.org/10.1111/jgh.13589] [PMID: 27577675]

[6] Marcellin F, Roux P, Protopopescu C, Duracinsky M, Spire B, Carrieri MP. Patient-reported outcomes with direct-acting antivirals for the treatment of chronic hepatitis C: current knowledge and outstanding issues. Expert Rev Gastroenterol Hepatol 2017; 11(3): 1-10. [http://dx.doi.org/10.1080/17474124.2017.1285227] [PMID: 28116926]

[7] Akhtar E, Manne V, Saab S. Cirrhosis regression in hepatitis C patients with sustained virological response after antiviral therapy: a meta-analysis 2015. [http://dx.doi.org/10.1111/liv.12576]

[8] Chan J, Gogela N, Zheng H, *et al.* Direct-Acting Antiviral Therapy for Chronic HCV Infection Results in Liver Stiffness Regression Over 12 Months Post-treatment. Dig Dis Sci 2018; 63(2): 486-92. [http://dx.doi.org/10.1007/s10620-017-4749-x] [PMID: 28887750]

[9] Kobayashi N, Iijima H, Tada T, *et al.* Changes in liver stiffness and steatosis among patients with hepatitis C virus infection who received direct-acting antiviral therapy and achieved sustained virological response. Eur J Gastroenterol Hepatol 2018; 30(5): 546-51. [http://dx.doi.org/10.1097/MEG.0000000000001106] [PMID: 29494353]

[10] Singh S, Facciorusso A, Loomba R, Falck-Ytter YT. Magnitude and Kinetics of Decrease in Liver Stiffness After Antiviral Therapy in Patients With Chronic Hepatitis C: A Systematic Review and Meta-analysis. Clinical gastroenterology and hepatology : the official clinical practice journal of the American Gastroenterological Association. 2018; 16(1): 27-38.

[11] Tada T, Kumada T, Toyoda H, *et al.* Improvement of liver stiffness in patients with hepatitis C virus infection who received direct-acting antiviral therapy and achieved sustained virological response. J Gastroenterol Hepatol 2017; 32(12): 1982-8. [http://dx.doi.org/10.1111/jgh.13788] [PMID: 28299813]

[12] Recommendations for Hepatitis C Screening. Washington University; 2022. Available from: https://www.hepatitisc.uw.edu/go/screening-diagnosis/recommendations-screening/core-concept/all.

[13] HCV Guideline Committee of the New York State Department of Health AIDS Institute (NYSDOH AI). Treatment of Chronic HCV with Direct-Acting Antivirals. Baltimore (MD): Johns Hopkins University; 2020. Available from: https://www.ncbi.nlm.nih.gov/books/NBK559965/.

[14] AASLD-IDSA. HCV Guidance: Recommendations for testing, management, and treating hepatitis C. Unique populations: patients with decompensated cirrhosis. [AASLD-IDSA Hepatitis C Guidance]; accessed on 6th February 2022.

[15] ANRS collaborative study group on hepatocellular carcinoma (ANRS CO22 HEPATHER, CO12 CirVir and CO23 CUPILT cohorts). Lack of evidence of an effect of direct-acting antivirals on the recurrence of hepatocellular carcinoma: Data from three ANRS cohorts. J Hepatol 2016; 65(4): 734-40. [http://dx.doi.org/10.1016/j.jhep.2016.05.045] [PMID: 27288051]

[16] Shahid I, AlMalki WH, Hassan S, Hafeez MH. Real-world challenges for hepatitis C virus medications: a critical overview. Crit Rev Microbiol 2018; 44(2): 143-60. [http://dx.doi.org/10.1080/1040841X.2017.1329277] [PMID: 28539069]

[17] Yu ML, Chen PJ, Dai CY, Hu TH, Huang CF, Huang YH, *et al.* Taiwan consensus statement on the management of hepatitis C: Part (II) special populations. Journal of the Formosan Medical Association Taiwan 2020; 119(7): 1135-57.

[18] Yeon JE. Recent update of the 2017 Korean Association for the Study of the Liver (KASL) treatment guidelines of chronic hepatitis C: Comparison of guidelines from other continents, 2017 AASLD/IDSA and 2016 EASL. Clin Mol Hepatol 2018; 24(3): 278-93. [http://dx.doi.org/10.3350/cmh.2018.1002] [PMID: 29716179]

[19] Highlights in Hepatitis C Virus From the 2017 AASLD Liver Meeting: A Review of Selected Presentations. The University of Texas Health, San AntonioSan Antonio, Texas. Gastroenterology and Hepatology. 2017; 13(12): 1-24.

[20] WHO Guidelines Approved by the Guidelines Review Committee. Guidelines for the Screening Care and Treatment of Persons with Chronic Hepatitis C Infection: Updated Version. Geneva: World Health OrganizationCopyright © World Health Organization 2016.

[21] Crowell TA, Berry SA, Fleishman JA, LaRue RW, Korthuis PT, Nijhawan AE, *et al.* Impact of hepatitis coinfection on healthcare utilization among persons living with HIV. Journal of acquired immune deficiency syndromes (1999). 2015; 68(4): 425-31. [http://dx.doi.org/10.1097/QAI.0000000000000490]

[22] Kim AY, Onofrey S, Church DR. An epidemiologic update on hepatitis C infection in persons living with or at risk of HIV infection. The Journal of infectious diseases. 2013; 207 Suppl 1(Suppl 1): S1-6. [http://dx.doi.org/10.1093/infdis/jis927]

[23] Joshi D, O'Grady J, Dieterich D, Gazzard B, Agarwal K. Increasing burden of liver disease in patients with HIV infection. Lancet 2011; 377(9772): 1198-209. [http://dx.doi.org/10.1016/S0140-6736(10)62001-6] [PMID: 21459211]

[24] Rosenthal E, Roussillon C, Salmon-Céron D, *et al.* Liver-related deaths in HIV-infected patients between 1995 and 2010 in France: the Mortavic 2010 study in collaboration with the Agence Nationale de Recherche sur le SIDA (ANRS) EN 20 Mortalité 2010 survey. HIV Med 2015; 16(4): 230-9. [http://dx.doi.org/10.1111/hiv.12204] [PMID: 25522874]

[25] Pisaturo M, Macera M, Alessio L, Calò F, Coppola N, Hepatitis B. Hepatitis B Virus (HBV) Reactivation Following Pharmacological Eradication of Hepatitis C Virus (HCV). Viruses 2019; 11(9): 850. [http://dx.doi.org/10.3390/v11090850] [PMID: 31540223]

[26] Wang C, Ji D, Chen J, Shao Q, Li B, Liu J, *et al.* Hepatitis due to Reactivation of Hepatitis B Virus in Endemic Areas Among Patients With Hepatitis C Treated With Direct-acting Antiviral Agents. Clinical gastroenterology and hepatology : the official clinical practice journal of the American Gastroenterological Association. 2017; 15(1): 132-6.

[27] Belperio PS, Shahoumian TA, Mole LA, Backus LI. Evaluation of hepatitis B reactivation among 62,920 veterans treated with oral hepatitis C antivirals. Hepatology 2017; 66(1): 27-36. [http://dx.doi.org/10.1002/hep.29135] [PMID: 28240789]

[28] Serper M, Forde KA, Kaplan DE. Rare clinically significant hepatic events and hepatitis B reactivation occur more frequently following rather than during direct-acting antiviral therapy for chronic hepatitis C: Data from a national US cohort. J Viral Hepat 2018; 25(2): 187-97. [http://dx.doi.org/10.1111/jvh.12784] [PMID: 28845882]

[29] Nguyen DB, Gutowski J, Ghiselli M, *et al.* A Large Outbreak of Hepatitis C Virus Infections in a Hemodialysis Clinic. Infect Control Hosp Epidemiol 2016; 37(2): 125-33. [http://dx.doi.org/10.1017/ice.2015.247] [PMID: 26573412]

[30] Patel PR, Thompson ND, Kallen AJ, Arduino MJ. Epidemiology, surveillance, and prevention of hepatitis C virus infections in hemodialysis patients. Am J Kidney Dis 2010; 56(2): 371-8.

[http://dx.doi.org/10.1053/j.ajkd.2010.01.025] [PMID: 20570422]

[31] Botev R, Mallié JP, Couchoud C, *et al.* Estimating glomerular filtration rate: Cockcroft-Gault and Modification of Diet in Renal Disease formulas compared to renal inulin clearance. Clin J Am Soc Nephrol 2009; 4(5): 899-906.
[http://dx.doi.org/10.2215/CJN.05371008] [PMID: 19406960]

[32] Levey AS, Coresh J, Greene T, *et al.* Using standardized serum creatinine values in the modification of diet in renal disease study equation for estimating glomerular filtration rate. Ann Intern Med 2006; 145(4): 247-54.
[http://dx.doi.org/10.7326/0003-4819-145-4-200608150-00004] [PMID: 16908915]

[33] Levey AS, Stevens LA, Schmid CH, *et al.* A new equation to estimate glomerular filtration rate. Ann Intern Med 2009; 150(9): 604-12.
[http://dx.doi.org/10.7326/0003-4819-150-9-200905050-00006] [PMID: 19414839]

[34] Cockcroft DW, Gault H. Prediction of creatinine clearance from serum creatinine. Nephron 1976; 16(1): 31-41.
[http://dx.doi.org/10.1159/000180580] [PMID: 1244564]

[35] Covic A, Abramowicz D, Bruchfeld A, *et al.* Endorsement of the Kidney Disease Improving Global Outcomes (KDIGO) hepatitis C guidelines: a European Renal Best Practice (ERBP) position statement. Nephrol Dial Transplant 2008; 24(3): 719-27.
[http://dx.doi.org/10.1093/ndt/gfn608] [PMID: 19202192]

[36] Inker LA, Astor BC, Fox CH, *et al.* KDOQI US commentary on the 2012 KDIGO clinical practice guideline for the evaluation and management of CKD. Am J Kidney Dis 2014; 63(5): 713-35.
[http://dx.doi.org/10.1053/j.ajkd.2014.01.416] [PMID: 24647050]

[37] Maruyama A, Partovi N, Yoshida EM, Erb SR, Azalgara VM, Hussaini T. A review of direct-acting antivirals for the treatment of hepatitis C in patients with advanced chronic kidney disease. Nephrol Dial Transplant 2017; 32(1): 35-41.
[PMID: 26481484]

[38] Butt AA, Ren Y, Puenpatom A, Arduino JM, Kumar R, Abou-Samra A-B. Effectiveness, treatment completion and safety of sofosbuvir/ledipasvir and paritaprevir/ritonavir/ombitasvir + dasabuvir in patients with chronic kidney disease: an ERCHIVES study. Aliment Pharmacol Ther 2018; 48(1): 35-43.
[http://dx.doi.org/10.1111/apt.14799] [PMID: 29797514]

[39] Roth D, Nelson DR, Bruchfeld A, *et al.* Grazoprevir plus elbasvir in treatment-naive and treatment-experienced patients with hepatitis C virus genotype 1 infection and stage 4 5 chronic kidney disease (the C-SURFER study): a combination phase 3 study. Lancet 2015; 386(10003): 1537-45.
[http://dx.doi.org/10.1016/S0140-6736(15)00349-9] [PMID: 26456905]

[40] Fabrizi F, Penatti A, Messa P, Martin P. Treatment of hepatitis C after kidney transplant: A pooled analysis of observational studies. J Med Virol 2014; 86(6): 933-40.
[http://dx.doi.org/10.1002/jmv.23919] [PMID: 24610278]

[41] Terrault NA, Adey DB. The kidney transplant recipient with hepatitis C infection: pre- and posttransplantation treatment. Clin J Am Soc Nephrol 2007; 2(3): 563-75.
[http://dx.doi.org/10.2215/CJN.02930806] [PMID: 17699464]

[42] Wei F, Liu J, Liu F, Hu H, Ren H, Hu P. Interferon-based anti-viral therapy for hepatitis C virus infection after renal transplantation: an updated meta-analysis. PLoS One 2014; 9(4): e90611.
[http://dx.doi.org/10.1371/journal.pone.0090611] [PMID: 24699257]

[43] Varan AK, Mercer DW, Stein MS, Spaulding AC. Hepatitis C seroprevalence among prison inmates since 2001: still high but declining. Public health reports (Washington, DC : 1974). 2014; 129(2): 187-95.

[44] Weinbaum C, Lyerla R, Margolis HS. Prevention and control of infections with hepatitis viruses in

correctional settings. Centers for Disease Control and Prevention. MMWR Recommendations and reports : Morbidity and mortality weekly report Recommendations and reports. 2003; 52(Rr-1): 1-36; quiz CE1-4.

[45] Edlin BR, Eckhardt BJ, Shu MA, Holmberg SD, Swan T. Toward a more accurate estimate of the prevalence of hepatitis C in the United States. Hepatology 2015; 62(5): 1353-63. [http://dx.doi.org/10.1002/hep.27978] [PMID: 26171595]

[46] Spaulding AC, Anderson EJ, Khan MA, Taborda-Vidarte CA, Phillips JA. HIV and HCV in U.S. Prisons and Jails: The Correctional Facility as a Bellwether Over Time for the Community's Infections. AIDS Rev 2017; 19(3): 134-47. [http://dx.doi.org/10.24875/AIDSRev.M17000006] [PMID: 28926560]

[47] Tran L, Feldman R, Riley T III, Jung J. Association of the Extension for Community Healthcare Outcomes Project With Use of Direct-Acting Antiviral Treatment Among US Adults With Hepatitis C. JAMA Netw Open 2021; 4(7)e2115523 [http://dx.doi.org/10.1001/jamanetworkopen.2021.15523] [PMID: 34213557]

[48] Denniston MM, Jiles RB, Drobeniuc J, *et al.* Chronic Hepatitis C Virus Infection in the United States, National Health and Nutrition Examination Survey 2003 to 2010. Ann Intern Med 2014; 160(5): 293-300. [http://dx.doi.org/10.7326/M13-1133] [PMID: 24737271]

[49] Hajarizadeh B, Grebely J, Dore GJ. Case definitions for acute hepatitis C virus infection: A systematic review. J Hepatol 2012; 57(6): 1349-60. [http://dx.doi.org/10.1016/j.jhep.2012.07.007] [PMID: 22796896]

[50] Grebely J, Matthews GV, Dore GJ. Treatment of acute HCV infection. Nat Rev Gastroenterol Hepatol 2011; 8(5): 265-74. [http://dx.doi.org/10.1038/nrgastro.2011.32] [PMID: 21423258]

[51] Young J, Rossi C, Gill J, *et al.* Risk Factors for Hepatitis C Virus Reinfection After Sustained Virologic Response in Patients Coinfected With HIV. Clin Infect Dis 2017; 64(9): 1154-62. [http://dx.doi.org/10.1093/cid/cix126] [PMID: 28199495]

[52] Simmons B, Saleem J, Hill A, Riley RD, Cooke GS. Risk of Late Relapse or Reinfection With Hepatitis C Virus After Achieving a Sustained Virological Response: A Systematic Review and Meta-analysis. Clin Infect Dis 2016; 62(6): 683-94. [http://dx.doi.org/10.1093/cid/civ948] [PMID: 26787172]

[53] Moorman AC, de Perio MA, Goldschmidt R, Chu C, Kuhar D, Henderson DK, *et al.* Testing and Clinical Management of Health Care Personnel Potentially Exposed to Hepatitis C Virus - CDC Guidance, United States, 2020. MMWR Recommendations and reports: Morbidity and mortality weekly report Recommendations and reports. 2020; 69(6): 1-8.

[54] Naggie S, Holland DP, Sulkowski MS, Thomas DL, Hepatitis C. Hepatitis C Virus Postexposure Prophylaxis in the Healthcare Worker: Why Direct-Acting Antivirals Don't Change a Thing. Clin Infect Dis 2017; 64(1): 92-9. [http://dx.doi.org/10.1093/cid/ciw656] [PMID: 27682067]

[55] Egro FM, Nwaiwu CA, Smith S, Harper JD, Spiess AM. Seroconversion rates among health care workers exposed to hepatitis C virus contaminated body fluids: The University of Pittsburgh 13-year experience. Am J Infect Control 2017; 45(9): 1001-5. [http://dx.doi.org/10.1016/j.ajic.2017.03.011] [PMID: 28449917]

[56] Tomkins SE, Elford J, Nichols T, *et al.* Occupational transmission of hepatitis C in healthcare workers and factors associated with seroconversion: UK surveillance data. J Viral Hepat 2012; 19(3): 199-204. [http://dx.doi.org/10.1111/j.1365-2893.2011.01543.x] [PMID: 22329374]

[57] Poordad F, Felizarta F, Asatryan A, *et al.* Glecaprevir and pibrentasvir for 12 weeks for hepatitis C virus genotype 1 infection and prior direct-acting antiviral treatment. Hepatology 2017; 66(2): 389-97. [http://dx.doi.org/10.1002/hep.29081] [PMID: 28128852]

[58] Bourlière M, Gordon SC, Flamm SL, *et al.* Sofosbuvir, Velpatasvir, and Voxilaprevir for Previously Treated HCV Infection. N Engl J Med 2017; 376(22): 2134-46. [http://dx.doi.org/10.1056/NEJMoa1613512] [PMID: 28564569]

[59] Osinusi A, Kohli A, Marti MM, *et al.* Re-treatment of chronic hepatitis C virus genotype 1 infection after relapse: an open-label pilot study. Ann Intern Med 2014; 161(9): 634-8. [http://dx.doi.org/10.7326/M14-1211] [PMID: 25364884]

[60] Wyles D, Pockros P, Morelli G, *et al.* Ledipasvir-sofosbuvir plus ribavirin for patients with genotype 1 hepatitis C virus previously treated in clinical trials of sofosbuvir regimens. Hepatology 2015; 61(6): 1793-7. [http://dx.doi.org/10.1002/hep.27814] [PMID: 25846014]

[61] Bourlière M, Bronowicki JP, de Ledinghen V, *et al.* Ledipasvir-sofosbuvir with or without ribavirin to treat patients with HCV genotype 1 infection and cirrhosis non-responsive to previous protease-inhibitor therapy: a randomised, double-blind, phase 2 trial (SIRIUS). Lancet Infect Dis 2015; 15(4): 397-404. [http://dx.doi.org/10.1016/S1473-3099(15)70050-2] [PMID: 25773757]

[62] Patel AA, Bui A, Prohl E, *et al.* Innovations in Hepatitis C Screening and Treatment. Hepatol Commun 2021; 5(3): 371-86. [http://dx.doi.org/10.1002/hep4.1646] [PMID: 33681673]

[63] Pawlotsky JM, Ramers CB, Dillon JF, Feld JJ, Lazarus JV. Simplification of Care for Chronic Hepatitis C Virus Infection. Semin Liver Dis 2020; 40(4): 392-402. [http://dx.doi.org/10.1055/s-0040-1713657] [PMID: 32725611]

[64] Shahid I, Alzahrani AR, Al-Ghamdi SS, Alanazi IM, Rehman S, Hassan S. Hepatitis C Diagnosis: Simplified Solutions, Predictive Barriers, and Future Promises. Diagnostics (Basel, Switzerland). 2021; 11, 7.

[65] Terrault NA, Levy MT, Cheung KW, Jourdain G. Viral hepatitis and pregnancy. Nat Rev Gastroenterol Hepatol 2021; 18(2): 117-30. [http://dx.doi.org/10.1038/s41575-020-00361-w] [PMID: 33046891]

[66] Shahid I, ALMalki WH, Hafeez MH, Hassan S. Hepatitis C virus infection treatment: An era of game changer direct acting antivirals and novel treatment strategies. Crit Rev Microbiol 2016; 42(4): 535-47. [http://dx.doi.org/10.3109/1040841X.2014.970123] [PMID: 25373616]

[67] Chappell CA, Scarsi KK, Kirby BJ, *et al.* Ledipasvir plus sofosbuvir in pregnant women with hepatitis C virus infection: a phase 1 pharmacokinetic study. Lancet Microbe 2020; 1(5): e200-8. [http://dx.doi.org/10.1016/S2666-5247(20)30062-8] [PMID: 32939459]

[68] Freriksen JJM, van Seyen M, Judd A, *et al.* Review article: direct-acting antivirals for the treatment of HCV during pregnancy and lactation - implications for maternal dosing, foetal exposure, and safety for mother and child. Aliment Pharmacol Ther 2019; 50(7): 738-50. [http://dx.doi.org/10.1111/apt.15476] [PMID: 31448450]

CHAPTER 9

Real-World Therapeutic Outcomes of Direct-Acting Antiviral Regimens and Formidable Challenges

Abstract: Oral interferon-free DAAs (IFN-free DAAs) have proven their clinical and therapeutic worth in real-life situations by achieving higher sustained virologic response rates (SVRs >90%) in treated individuals. After their recommendations to be administered to hepatitis C-infected populations in 2017 more than 5 million hepatitis C-infected individuals have been treated across the world and the overall health care burden of active hepatitis C comorbidities and mortalities have been declined from 130 million hepatitis C patients to approximately 71 million. Despite these great achievements in hepatitis C therapeutics, certain patient-oriented, clinical, and societal challenges are still prevailing to accept IFN-free DAAs on the large scale clinical, hospital, and primary health care settings in low and middle-income countries as well as even in developed nations. High therapy costs, treatment access and monitoring, co-infection status of certain vulnerable hepatitis C infected populations, racial disparity, pre-, and post-therapeutic monitoring, and long-term follow-ups are potential barriers to consensually implementing uniform treatment algorithms and accessibility to DAAs regimens worldwide. Furthermore, recurrence of hepatitis C infection, reactivation risks of co-infections (*e.g.*, HCV/HIV, HCV/HBV or HCV/CKD), minefield risks of hepatocellular carcinoma (HCC) rebound, and surveillance of hepatitis C liver transplant recipients which are on treatment with IFN-free DAAs also limit the administration of these regimens to every hepatitis C infected individual. In this book chapter, we will explore all these real-world challenges and will discuss/suggest the strategies to coup them in clinical, hospital, and community settings to improve the cascades of care and scale-up HCV cure.

Keywords: Clinical efficacy, Cascades of care, Dose algorithms, Direct-acting antivirals, Drug-drug interactions, Formidable challenges, HBV reactivation, Hepatocellular carcinoma, Resistance-associated substitutions, Resistance-associated variants, Real-world challenge, Retreatment, Sustained virologic response, Severe adverse events, Therapy cost, Treatment access, Treatment monitoring, Transplant recipients, Treatment failure, Viral fitness.

Imran Shahid and Qaiser Jabeen

INTRODUCTION

With the rapid advancement in HCV treatment by the advent and approvals of oral IFN-free DAAs in the last decade, clinicians have seen therapeutic outcomes they never thought possible in real-world clinical settings [1]. Furthermore, liver specialists and infectious disease experts are also cautiously optimistic that more harder-to-cure and challenging populations are also responding to DAA regimens [2]. Multiple studies from real-world clinical settings are deciphering the strong potential of pan-genotypic DAAs (Table **1**) to cure the general HCV-infected population as well as achieve higher SVR rates in difficult-to-treat fractions of HCV-infected individuals and among HCV patients with advanced hepatitis C associated comorbidities (*e.g.*, decompensated cirrhosis, hepatocellular carcinoma, *etc.*) [3 - 5]. The big picture on a clinic canvas in real-life situations reveals that 95 to 100% of patients treated for hepatitis C can be cured [5, 6]. Although, treatment choices can be tricky in certain classifications of HCV-infected populations; however, the end therapeutic outcome would be an SVR12 at the end of treatment either after 12 or 16 weeks, albeit, some clinicians monitor out to 24 weeks [7]. Interestingly, more than 99% of patients who achieved SVR rates will remain negative. Despite these higher SVR rates and significant cures of HCV in real-world clinical settings, the availability, accessibility, and affordability of DAAs regimens are still challenging in LMICs and even in resource-replete nations that prohibit treating everyone who is in need [4]. Furthermore, treatment-associated barriers in the form of pretreatment assessment, treatment monitoring during therapy, and post-treatment assessment/follow-ups are also influencing challenges to patient treatment adherence as well as to achieving successful SVR rates at post-treatment completion [4]. In addition to that, potential drug-drug interactions (DDIs) and DAAs incompatibility with certain other medications taken by HCV comorbid patients (*e.g.*, HCV/HBV or HCV/HIV or HCV/CKD) while treated by DAAs, as well as DAAs induced severe adverse events (*e.g.*, Abnormal ALTs, worsening of hepatic fibrosis or cirrhosis, HBV reactivation, and HCC recurrence), also pose hurdles to achieve hepatitis C cure in a large number of patients who receive active treatment for HCV [8]. Subsequently, HCV reinfections, virologic breakthrough, viral relapse, and treatment failure have also been demonstrated in general as well as harder-to-treat HCV individuals (*e.g.*, HCV GT 1a and 3 cirrhotic patients, MSM, IDUs, homeless HCV/HIV co-infection, and HCV infected liver transplant patients) with DAAs in real-world clinical settings [8]. Furthermore, DAA dosage algorithms and recommendations for administration to women of reproductive age (WORA), pregnant females, neonates, infants, children, and adolescents are not defined yet; although, various clinical trials are underway in this direction [9].

It is not possible in this book chapter to discuss real-world cohort studies in detail while covering every aspect of baseline HCV-infected patient demographics, DAAs treatment strategies, and outcomes of the treatment; however, we present some selected studies from real-world clinical experiences in tabulated form projecting DAAs therapeutic outcomes, efficacies, and safety in HCV infected populations as well as other comorbid conditions (Table **1**). We will also confine while discussing formidable challenges in HCV therapeutics that present potential barriers to overcoming the HCV healthcare burden in clinics, hospitals, and healthcare services providing centers as well as those hamper the efforts to eliminate this silent epidemic worldwide.

Table 1. The real-world therapeutic outcomes of DAAs against the hepatitis C virus in various parts of the world. T.N; treatment naïve, T.E; treatment-experienced, SVR; sustained virologic response, HIV; human immunodeficiency virus, GT; genotype, SOF; sofosbuvir, DCV; daclatasvir, LDV; ledipasvir, VEL; velpatasvir, RBV; ribavirin, EBR; elbasvir, GZR; grazoprevir; PrOD; paritaprevir, r; ritonavir, O; ombitasvir, D; dasabuvir, GLE; glecaprevir, PIB; pibrentasvir, VOX; voxilaprevir, RAS; resistance-associated substitution, PWID; patient who inject drugs, PEG-IFN; pegylated interferon, SMV; simeprevir.

Study (Year)	Study Country	Reference	Patient Demographics					Regimen	Treatment Duration (Week)	SVR12 (n/N)
			HIV (%)	Cirrhosis Status	PWID (%)	T.N/ T.E	GT			
1. Real-world effectiveness and safety of sofosbuvir and nonstructural protein 5A inhibitors for chronic hepatitis C genotype 1, 2, 3, 4, or 6: a multicentre cohort study [10]										
2020	Thailand	Phunchai Charatcharoenwitthaya *et al.*	2.1%	Compensated	-	T.N + T.E	1/2/3/4/6	SOF +DCV ± RBV	12/24	98.0%
								LDV/SOF±RBV		97.9%
								VEL/SOF ±RBV		96.5%
2. Efficacy and safety of ledipasvir/sofosbuvir in 5028 Mongolian patients infected with genotype 1 hepatitis C virus: A multicenter study [11]										
2020	Mongolia	Oidov Baatarkhuu *et al.*	-	Compensated	-	T.N + T.E	1	LDV/SOF	12	99.6% (5008/5028)
3. Treatment outcomes in hepatitis C virus genotype 1a infected patients with and without baseline NS5A resistance□associated substitutions [12]										
2020	Germany	Julia Dietz *et al.*	-	Compensated	-	T.N	1a	In the absence of RAS Overall SVR12:		
								EBR/GZR	12	97%
								LDV/SOF±RBV	12	99%
								GLE/PIB	12	99%
								PrOD + RBV	12	99%
								VEL/SOF	12	99%
								In the presence of RAS Overall SVR12:		
								LDV/SOF	12	100%
								GLE/PIB	12	83%
								PrOD + RBV	12	100%
								VEL/SOF	12	100%
								SMV/SOF	12	100%
								EBR/GZR+RBV	16	100%
4. Efficacy of direct-acting antivirals: UK real-world data from a well-characterized predominantly cirrhotic HCV cohort [13]										
2019	UK	Lucia macken *et al.*	-	Compensated	-	T.N + T.E	1	LDV/SOF ± RBV	12	Overall 91% (819/900)
								OBV/PTV/DSV/± RBV		
							3	SOF+ DCV + RBV	12	Overall 87% (396/455)
								SOF/PEG-IFN/RBV		

(Table 1) cont.....

5. Direct-Acting Antivirals: Efficacy in a Real-World, Urban, Undeserved, HIV-HCV Co-Infected Population [14]										
2018	USA	Sarah Michienzi *et al.*	97%	Compensated	-	T.N	1a	LDV/SOF	12	93% (37/40)
								LDV/SOF + RBV	12	75% (3/4)
								SMV+ SOF	12	100% (6/6)
								SOF/VEL	12	100% (6/6)
								EBR/GZR	12	100% (4/4)
6. A Collaborative Drug Therapy Management Model for the Treatment of Hepatitis C Virus (HCV) in an Urban Clinic [15]										
2018	USA	Sonia Vibhakar *et al.*	94.6%	Compensated	-	T.N	1	LDV/SOF	12	Overall: 93.5% (402/430)
										HCV/HIV: 94.6% (192/203)
										Monoinfection: 92.5% (210/227)
7. Real-world use, effectiveness, and safety of antiviral treatment in chronic hepatitis C genotype 3 infection [[16]]										
2017	Germany	M. Cornberg *et al.*	-	Compensated	-	T.N + T.E	3	PegIFN+RBV	12	80.9%
								PegIFN+RBV+SOF		96.1%
								SOF+RBV		68%
								DCV+SOF±RBV	24	90-95%
								LDV/SOF±RBV	24	>95%
8. Effectiveness and safety of sofosbuvir-based regimens plus an NS5A inhibitor for patients with HCV genotype 3 infection and cirrhosis. Results of a multicenter real-life cohort [[17]]										
2016	Spain	Sebastian Alonso *et al.*	-	compnsated + decompensated	-	T.N + T.E	3	DCV+SOF	12	Overall: 93.8%
										94%
								LDV/SOF		93.5%
9. Direct-Acting Antivirals in Hepatitis C Virus (HCV)-Infected and HCV/HIV-Coinfected Patients [18]										
2017	Italy	L Milazzo *et al.*	53%	Compensated	-	T.N + T.E	1a/1b/2/3	SOF+SMV	12	Overall SVR in HCV mono- or HCV/HIV co-infection: 91% to 95%
								SOF+DCV		
								LDV/SOF		
								PrOD		
								SOF+ RBV		
10. Efficacy and safety of direct-acting antivirals in elderly with chronic hepatitis C: results from a retrospective cohort study [19]										
2018	Italy	R. Villani *et al.*	-	Compensated	-	T.N + T.E	1/2/3/4	SOF+SMV ± RBV	12/24	Overall SVR in SOF-based regimens: 97.2% to 100%
								SOF+DCV ± RBV		
								LDV/SOF ± RBV		
								SOF+ RBV		
								PrOD ± RBV	12/24	Overall SVR in non-SOF-based regimens: 100%
								PrO ± RBV		
11. Successful prolonged treatment of glecaprevir/pibrentasvir for chronic hepatitis C patient with treatment failure after 8-week therapy: a case report [20]										
2019	Japan	Atsushi Naganuma *et al.*	-	Non-cirrhotic	-	T.E with GLE/PIB for 8 week	2a	GLE/PIB	12	100%
12. Glecaprevir and Pibrentasvir for Japanese Patients with Human Immunodeficiency Virus and Genotype 3 Hepatitis C Virus Coinfection: A Report of Three Cases [21]										
2018	Japan	Takuya Sho *et al.*	+	compensated	-	T.N + T.E	3a	GLE/PIB	12	100%

(Table 1) cont.....

13. Effect of the baseline Y93H resistance-associated substitution in HCV genotype 3 for direct-acting antiviral treatment: real-life experience from a multicenter study in Sweden and Norway [22]										
2019	Sweden & Norway	Midori Kjellin *et al.*	-	compensated	-	T.N	3a	SOF+ PEG-IFN/RBV	12	95.4% (124/130)
								DCV + SOF	16	100% (5/5)
								VEL/SOF ± RBV	24	98% (98/100)
14. Real-world effectiveness of sofosbuvir/velpatasvir/voxilaprevir in 573 direct-acting antiviral experienced hepatitis C patients [23]										
2019	USA	Pamela S. Belperio *et al.*	-	compensated	-	T.E	1/2/3/4	SOF/VEL/VOX	12	GT1: 90.7%
										GT2: 90.0%
										GT3: 91.3%
										GT4: 100.0%
15. Real-world safety and effectiveness of ombitasvir/paritaprevir/ritonavir ± dasabuvir ± ribavirin in hepatitis C virus genotype 1- and 4-infected patients with diverse comorbidities and comedications [24]										
2019	Multiple countries	Peter Ferenci *et al.*	-	compnsated + decompensated	-	T.N + T.E	1a/1b/4	PrOD ± RBV	12	1a: 93% 1b: 97% 4: 94%
16. Low Recurrence Rate of Hepatocellular Carcinoma Following Ledipasvir and Sofosbuvir Treatment in a Real-world Chronic Hepatitis C Patients Cohort [25]										
2019	Tukey	Ramazan Idilman *et al.*	-	compensated	-	T.N	1a/1b/4	LDV/SOF ± RBV	24	Overall SVR with per protocol (PP) analysis: 98.3%
17. SVR12 Higher than 97% in GT3 Cirrhotic Patients with Evidence of Portal Hypertension Treated with SOF/VEL without Ribavirin: A Nation-Wide Cohort Study [26]										
2019	Italy	Alessandra Mangia *et al.*	-	compensated	-	T.N	3	SOF/VEL	12	Overall SVR: 97.6%
18. Sofosbuvir-Based Therapies for Patients with Hepatitis C Virus Infection: Real-World Experience in China [27]										
2018	China	Chengguang Hu *et al.*	-	Without cirrhosis	-	T.N + T.E	1b/2a/3/6a	DCV+SOF	12	100%
								LDV/SOF	12	96%
								SOF/VEL	12	100%
19. Sofosbuvir, Velpatasvir, and Voxilaprevir for Treatment of Recurrent Hepatitis C Virus Infection After Liver Transplantation [28]										
2018	USA	Maria G. Cardona-Gonzalez *et al.*	-	compensated	-	T.E	3	SOF/VEL/VOX ± RBV	16	100%
20. Eight-Week Hepatitis C Treatment with New Direct Acting Antivirals Has a Better Safety Profile While Being Effective in the Treatment-Naive Geriatric Population Without Liver Cirrhosis and Hepatitis C Virus-RNA < 6 Million IU/mL [29]										
2018	USA	Beshoy Yanny *et al.*	-	Without cirrhosis	-	T.N	1	LDV/SOF	8	93%
									12	95%
21. HCV kinetic and modeling analyses project shorter durations to cure under combined therapy with daclatasvir and asunaprevir in chronic HCV-infected patients [30]										
2017	Japan	Laetitia Canini *et al.*	-	compensated	-	T.N+ T.E	1b	DCV + ASV	12	94%
22. Effectiveness and safety of elbasvir/grazoprevir therapy in patients with chronic HCV infection: Results from the Spanish HEPA-C real-world cohort [31]										
2018	Spain	Marta Hernández-Conde *et al.*	-	compensated	-	T.N+ T.E	1a/1b/4	EBR/GZR ± RBV	12	96.9%
23. Effectiveness of chronic hepatitis C treatment with direct-acting antivirals in the Public Health System in Brazil [32]										
2018	Brazil	Iandra Holzmann *et al.*	-	compensated	-	T.N+ T.E	1/2/3	PEG-IFN/RBV/SOF	12	Overall SVR rates: GT 1: 94.7% GT 2: 91.7% GT 3: 91.4%
								SOF+DCV± RBV		
								SOF+SMV± RBV		
24. Real-life data confirm the efficacy of elbasvir/grazoprevir in HCV patients with severe kidney disease [33]										
2018	Italy	M. G. Rumi *et al.*	-	-	-	T.N	1/4	EBR/GZR ± RBV	12	Overall SVR rates: 99%
25. Direct-Acting Antivirals in Chronic Hepatitis C Genotype 4 Infection in Community Care Setting [34]										
2018	USA	Vijay Gayam *et al.*	-	compensated	-	T.N+T.E	4·	LDV/SOF± RBV	12	Overall SVR rates: 94%
								PrOD ± RBV		
								SOF/VEL		

(Table 1) cont.....

26. Direct-acting Antiviral Agents in Hepatitis C Virus-infected Renal Allograft Recipients: Treatment and Outcome Experience from Single Center [35]										
2018	India	N. Prasad *et al.*	-	Compensated + decompensated	-	T.N+ T.E	1/2/3/4/6	SOF+RBV SOF+DCV+RBV LDV/SOF+ RBV	12 or 24 weeks	Overall SVR rates: 100%
27. Real-World Clinical Efficacy and Tolerability of Direct-Acting Antivirals in Hepatitis C mono-infection Compared to Hepatitis C/Human Immunodeficiency Virus Coinfection in a Community Care Setting [7]										
2018	USA	Vijay Gayam *et al.*	23%	Compensated	-	T.N+ T.E	1/2/3/4	SOF+RBV LDV/SOF LDV/SOF+RBV EBR/GZR SOF/VEL PrOD PrOD+RBV DCV+RBV SMV/SOF	12 or 24 weeks	Overall HCV-mon- -infection SVR rates:94%, Overall HCV/HIV coinfection SVR rates:84%
28. Real-world virological efficacy and safety of elbasvir and grazoprevir in patients with chronic hepatitis C virus genotype 1 infection in Japan [36]										
2018	Japan	Hidenori Toyoda *et al.*	-	compensated	-	T.N+ T.E	1	EBR/GZR	12	Overall SVR rates: 97.4%
29. Ledipasvir–Sofosbuvir for 8 Weeks in Non-Cirrhotic Patients with Previously Untreated Genotype 1 HCV Infection–HIV-1 Co-Infection [37]										
2017		Vasily Isakov *et al.*	46.82%	No cirrhosis	-	T.N	1	LDV/SOF	8	Overall HCV-mon- -infection SVR rates:100%, Overall HCV/HIV coinfection SVR rates:97%
30. Real-world Effectiveness of Elbasvir/Grazoprevir in HCV-infected Patients in the US Veterans Affairs Healthcare System [38]										
2018	USA	J. R. Kramer *et al.*	3.0%	compensated	50%	T.N+ T.E	1a/1b	EBR/GZR EBR/GZR+RBV EBR/GZR+SOF EBR/GZR+SOF±RBV	12 or 16 weeks	Overall SVR rates: 95.6%
31. Generic Sofosbuvir-based Direct-acting Antivirals in Hepatitis C Virus-infected Patients With Chronic Kidney Disease [39]										
2018	India	Manoj Kumar *et al.*	-	compensated	-	T.N+T.E	1a/1b/3	SOF+RBV SOF+DCV SOF+LDV	24 12 12	Overall SVR rates in GT 1 & 3: 100%
32. Eight Weeks of Paritaprevir/r/Ombitasvir + Dasabuvir in HCV Genotype 1b With Mild-moderate Fibrosis [40]										
2018	Spain	Marc Puigvehí *et al.*	-	mild liver fibrosis (F0-F1) + moderate fibrosis (F2)	-	T.N	1b	PrOD	8	Overall SVR rates: 100%
33. All-Oral Direct-Acting Antiviral Therapy Against Hepatitis C Virus (HCV) in Human Immunodeficiency Virus/HCV–Coinfected Subjects in Real-World Practice: Madrid Coinfection Registry Findings [41]										
2018	Spain	Juan Berenguer *et al.*	98%	Compensated+ decompensated	52.8%	T.N+T.E	1a/1b/2/3/4	SOF+LDV±RBV SOF+DCV±RBV PrOD ± RBV PrO ± RBV SOF+SMV ±RBV SOF+RBV	8 /12/16/24 12/16/24 8/12/24 12/24 12/24 12/16/24	Overall SVR rates: 92%, no cirrhosis:93.8%, compensate cirrhosis:91.0%, decompensated cirrhosis: 80.8%
34. Safety and Efficacy of Combined Sofosbuvir/Daclatasvir Treatment of Children and Adolescents With Chronic Hepatitis C Genotype 4 [42]										
2019	Egypt	Tawhida Y. Abdel Ghaffar *et al.*	-	No cirrhosis	-	T.N	4	SOF+DCV	12/24	SVR rates at week12: 97.5%, SVR rates at week 24: 95%.
35. All-oral direct antiviral treatment for hepatitis C chronic infection in a real-life cohort: The role of cirrhosis and comorbidities in treatment response [43]										

(Table 1) cont.....

2018	Brazil	Noelle Miotto *et al.*	-	Compensated	-	T.N+T.E	1/2/3	SOF+DCV± RBV	12 or 24	Overall SVR rates: 90.5% (ITT) and 96.0% (mITT)
								SOF + SMV ± RBV		
36. Real-world outcomes of unrestricted direct-acting antiviral treatment for hepatitis C in Australia: The South Australian statewide experience [44]										
2018	Australia	J. Haridy *et al.*	1.4%	Compensated	77.6%	T.N+T.E	1/2/3/4/6	SOF/LDV±RBV	8/12/24	Overall SVR rates: 95.7%
								SOF+DCV± RBV	12/24	
								SOF+ RBV	12	
								EBR/GZR	12	
								PrOD	12	
37. Integrated analysis of 8-week glecaprevir/pibrentasvir in Japanese and overseas patients without cirrhosis and with hepatitis C virus genotype 1 or 2 infection [45]										
2019	Japan	Atsushi Naganuma *et al.*	-	no cirrhosis	-	T.N+T.E	1/2	GLE/PIB	8	Overall SVR rates: 98.9%
38. Treatment of HCV genotype 2 with sofosbuvir and ribavirin results in lower sustained virological response rates in real life than expected from clinical trials [46]										
2017	Germany	Frank Tacke *et al.*	-	Compensated	-	T.N+T.E	2	SOF + RBV	12	Overall SVR rates: 83%
39. Real-world cure rates for hepatitis C virus treatments that include simeprevir and/or sofosbuvir are comparable to clinical trial results [47]										
2017	USA	Kian Bichoupan *et al.*	-	Compensated	-	T.N+T.E	1/2/3/4	SMV+SOF ± RBV	12	86%
								SOF+RBV		62%
								SOF+PEG-IFN+RBV		78%
40. Real-World Single-Center Experience with Sofosbuvir-Based Regimens for the Treatment of Chronic Hepatitis C Genotype 1 Patient [48]										
2017	USA	Hyun Phil Shin *et al.*	1%	Compensated + decompensated	-	T.N+T.E	1	SOF/LDV	12	92.2%
								SMV+SOF		87.0%
								SOF+PEG-IFN+RBV		82.4%

FORMIDABLE CHALLENGES TO DAAS THERAPY IN REAL-LIFE CLINICAL SETTINGS

Oral-IFN-free DAAs are promising to achieve higher SVR rates and infection cure while administered to HCV-infected individuals as large data both from clinical trials and real-world clinical cohort studies reveal their excellent efficacy and safety [4]. However, it should be noted here that progress toward reducing hepatitis C transmission, eliminating CHC infection, and reducing both morbidity and mortality attributed to CHC infection could be impeded by certain systemic barriers. The notable problems and pitfalls in eradicating infection from society and eliminating the HCV epidemic worldwide could be included; a lack of disease surveillance data, failure to enroll confirmed HCV-infected patients to linkage to care, complicated infection screening & cascade of care, DAAs cost, treatment access, treatment adherence, treatment-associated SAEs and significant DDIs with comedications, social stigma, racial disparity toward infection diagnosis and treatment access, lack of motivation in society to prevent infection progression, and deficit of national and international health care policy [4, 49]. It is not a subject of the matter here to discuss in detail every aspect of potential hurdles that impede achieving the global goal of HCV elimination; however, we will adhere to highlight here the potential pitfalls attributed to DAAs while treating HCV-infected individuals in real-world clinical settings with shreds of evidence from real-life clinical data.

DAAs Cost

Simplified solutions to diagnose HCV infections and bringing confirmed infected patients to care could be significantly helpful to reduce HCV disease burden in healthcare settings (*e.g.*, hospitals, clinics, community health centers, *etc.*), healthcare services provider centers, and in communities with high-risk of HCV prevalence in a country [4]. however; to eliminate HCV, the most promising tool would be the treatment access and affordability in terms of DAAs administration that elicit SVR rates in more than 95% of patients [4]. With the advent and approvals of pan-genotypic DAA regimens, cure rates are similar across all HCV GTs/subtypes with some exceptions of GT-3 infected patients either treatment naïve or who failed prior treatment with PEG-IFN/RBV or first and second-generation DAAs [4]. It seems that effective HCV treatment is now a reality; however, treatment costs and access are still poor in particular to LMICs and even in resource-replete nations [4]. A study finding in the USA reveals that more than a third of patients with hepatitis C submitting prescriptions for DAAs are denied coverage by private and public insurers in the country [50]. It is a big barrier to curative treatment that persists in the US where private and public insurers reimburse DAAs cost to those patients only who are on the prioritized list of receiving treatment (*e.g.*, patients infected with CHC and fibrosis score F3-F4) [50]. The prospective cohort study included data from 9025 patients with chronic HCV who submitted a DAA prescription to diplomat Pharmacy Inc, a national provider of HCV medications, between January 2016 and April 2017 [50]. The investigators were surprised to find that 3200 patients overall (35.5%; 95% CI, 34.5% - 36.5%) were denied treatment approval, including 52.4% of those with private insurance, 34.5% of those with Medicaid, and 14.7% of those insured by Medicare [50]. Furthermore, the absolute denial rate rose in each quarter of the 16-month study period, increasing from 27.7% in the first quarter to 43.8% in the last (test for trend $P < .001$), and it also rose for each of the three insurance types (test for trend $P < .001$ for each type) [50]. The study results run counter to the investigators' working hypothesis that access would likely have increased in the previous 2 years, thanks to advocacy efforts, threatened lawsuits, more options, greater price competition, and some relaxation of reimbursement requirements. Although DAA therapy has a cure rate of at least 95% and reduces healthcare and economic costs overall, its high price had led to tough criteria for coverage, including advanced hepatic fibrosis, specialist consultation, and/or abstinence from alcohol and illicit drugs [50]. Whatever the reasons, the adverse consequences could be many from a clinical standpoint, patients who are denied access to hepatitis C treatment are going to remain at risk for the development of liver complications like cirrhosis, hepatic decompensation, and liver cancer [50]. Furthermore, the denial of this treatment can also lead to ongoing hepatitis C-associated hepatic and systemic inflammation, which could increase the risk of other extra-hepatic complications (*e.g.*, cardiovascular disease, bone, and joint disease, and kidney disease) [50].

DAAs Were Quite Expensive a Few Years Ago

In 2018, while discussing real-world clinical challenges to dispense DAAs to HCV-treating individuals, we mentioned costs per treatment course for 12, 16, and 24 weeks respectively of various brand DAA regimens including; SMV (US$ 66,360/-/85,000), SOF (US$84,000/-/168,000), SOF plus SMV (US$150,000/-/300,000), DCV (US$63000/-/-), DCV plus SOF (US$147,000/-/294,000), LDV/SOF (US$94500/-/189,000), SOF/VEL (US$74,760/-/149,520), EBR/GZR (US$54,600/72,800/-), PrO (US$76,653/-/153,306), and PrOD (US$83,319/-/166,638) based on the wholesale acquisition cost (WAC) [4]. We also demonstrated that in the UK, the government cannot afford to treat everyone immediately based on these DAA regimen prices [4]. A similar was the situation in Europe, where DAAs to treat HCV are only available after price negotiations. It works to be successful for some countries but not all 26 European countries where prices for DAAs are kept confidential [51]. Subsequently, a few European countries are on the WHO track to eliminate HCV by 2030 and others are still far away from the goal [51]. However, the planning and launching of cheap generic versions of costly DAA brands have slashed the cost of cure in many European countries as well as escalated the treatment outcomes in LMICs and resource-limited settings where logistical and financial barriers are much higher than the developed nations [51]. Furthermore, the findings of a series of REDEMPTION-clinical trials encouraged the use of DAAs generics by clinicians to cut the cost of cure in patients at the cost of brand-name regimens [52, 53]. Indeed, the data from interim REDEMPTION-1 clinical trials showed higher SVR rates (*i.e.* 94.4%) at 4 weeks of generic treatments of CHC infection [54]. Similarly, the REDEMPTION-2 and -3 clinical trials assessed generic DAAs' tolerability and safety while evaluating adverse event profiles and on-treatment viral load of various DAAs' generic combinations [4]. However, the major limitation of the REDEMPTION-1 clinical trial is to evaluate SVR rates at week 4 instead of at week 12 after completion of therapy for almost every brand DAA regimen [52]. It also does not make sense to treat CHC patients for 4, 6, or even 8 weeks as DAAs only inhibit an HCV protein and do not destroy the whole virus [52]. Consequently, virus immune response recovery is of prime importance along with DAAs actions to clear HCV from resting infected hepatocytes. Generally, recovery and activation of innate immune responses following DAAs treatment take a mean of 8 weeks to clear the virus. In addition to that, 4 weeks of treatment is not feasible by some triple (*e.g.*, SOF/VEL/VOX) or Quadruple (*e.g.*, PrOD) DAAs to achieve significantly higher SVR rates as recently published data suggest [4]. It may also result in treatment failure for many patients who could not reach that SVR point which determines infection cure; albeit, some acute or other HCV infected patients need only 4 to 6 weeks for recovery. Perhaps, 4 or 8-week treatment of HCV by generic DAAs seems only for cost-effectiveness or based on patient treatment economy, not scientific. Moreover, very limited studies with a small number of patient cohorts support the shortening of HCV treatment with generic DAAs less than 12 weeks [52].

DAAs are Now Cheap but Accessibility is Still an Issue in Many LMICs and Even in Resource Replete Nations

Recent research comparatively analyzes the cost of production and current prices for DAAs in 50 countries [51]. According to the study, median originator prices per standard course were US$ 40,502 for SOF, US$ 26,928 for DCV, US$ 46,812 for SOF/LDV, US$ 34,381 for SOF/VEL, and US$ 30,710 for GLE/PIB. The estimated cost-based generic prices for a 12-week course were US$ 28 for SOF, US$ 31 for LDV, US$ 58 for VEL, and US$ 4 for DCV. For fixed-dose combinations, estimated cost-based prices were US$ 58 for SOF/LDV, US$ 85 for SOF/VEL, and US$ 31 for SOF/DCV [51]. The study findings also reveal that prices of DAAs significantly vary between resource-rich nations and LMICs due to a lack of correlation between DAA prices, country GDP, and viremic populations [51]. A sudden fall in prices among resource-rich nations was noticed as income levels rise and most probably due to a wealthier commitment to negotiate prices. However, prices are still sky-high for DAAs brands in many countries including LMICs and resource-constraint nations that represent a key barrier to access for many patients to the continuum of care and scale-up HCV cure in many national health programs. The estimation of a 2018 study found that at least 22 European have restrictions on DAA reimbursement based on disease stage [55]. Subsequently, there is no alternative to administering generic versions of DAAs brand in many low-income countries to treat hepatitis C. However, it is only feasible in the premises where local production or importation of generics is warranted under voluntary or compulsory licensing agreements and where DAAs are not under patent protection [55]. One good example in this regard is Pakistan, where local manufacturing of generic DAAs is allowed, and prices have fallen to US$ 34 for a 12-week course of SOF plus DCV and US$ 92 for SOF/VEL. Similarly, the combination of SOF plus DCV is also cheap in Russia to date (*i.e.*, the estimated cost of 378000 rubles) for 12 weeks [51, 56]. However, the same combination in 2019 was available in India for 135 US dollars in the commercial market (estimated cost of 10500 rubles). Kazakhstan purchases generics of SOF plus DCV combination for 12 weeks course for less than 100 US dollars for the state hepatitis C treatment program. It is clear that the potential for price reduction and production of generics is enormous, but its implementation demands national production of quality generics in countries where the HCV disease burden and new infection rates are significantly higher [51]. Furthermore, issuing the compulsory licensing agreement (although, it seems an uphill task to negotiate with patent holders on licensing) and negotiations on price reduction while procuring bulk volume are also vital in this direction (it is already experienced in Australia and Portugal). It would be very interesting to mention here that 60% of people containing HCV live in countries that can procure generic DAAs. However, unfortunately, several middle-income countries with significant HCV burdens have not been included in voluntary licensing agreements notably Brazil, China, Colombia, Kazakhstan, and Mexico [51].

DAAs are State-of-the-Art Regimens but Drug Innovation is Slow

Equivocally, not everyone believes that the prices of DAAs are too high or unsustainable. Three counter-arguments are presented to support this statement [4, 51, 55]. First, despite the sticker-shock prices of DAAs, they are cost-effective for treating HCV GT-1 patients, the most prevalent GT worldwide (*i.e.*, even at that high price, the benefits from treatment outweigh the costs) [4]. To treat treatment-naïve HCV GT-1 patients with SOF-based therapies, the incremental cost-effectiveness ratio ranged from US$31,452 to US$9,703 per quality-adjusted life-year (QALY) as compared to older IFN-based therapies. It has been estimated based on paying for one QALY (*i.e.*, US$ 100,000 is common if conservative) that treating 1.6 million HCV GT-1 infected individuals with DAAs would cost about US$49 billion, as compared to paying the benefits of treatment that are US$88 billion, exceeding the costs by US$39 billion [51]. The second argument supports the current high-pricing DAAs model to encourage innovation. Most economists postulate that lowering DAAs prices will escalate trade-offs which will ultimately improve access to existing treatments but reduce the pace of innovation or access to future HCV treatments [51]. It is due to this fact that most countries have patent regimens that encourage innovation and allow the patent holders to charge higher prices and increase revenues from new products for the length of the patent. How the patent length may affect innovation, the data are scarce; however, multiple studies demonstrate that pharmaceutical research and development are responsive to revenues or market size. Some estimates predict that a 10% change in market size leads to about a 30% change in innovation measured as new drug approvals [51]. The third argument states that the initial high prices of the DAAs were temporary, as new regimens are approved and launched in the market, the prices dropped down; however, such price models are thought to encourage competition among pharmaceutical industries to design and develop new treatment paradigms. One good example is that when pan-genotypic DAAs regimens were introduced in the market, discounted prices or revenue per patient initiating therapy with SOF or SOF/LDV has fallen from US$75,000 in 2014 to US$52,000 in 2015 [4]. Despite all these plausible qualms and justifications, universal treatment access to everyone who is in need would be very crucial to achieve the WHO's ambitious goal of HCV elimination by 2030 or beyond that. Similarly, reducing DAA costs will link more patients to care, adhere to therapy as well as complete the treatment [4]. Furthermore, DAAs affordability could be improved in areas with a high disease burden of HCV infection [4].

Availability, Accessibility, and Affordability of DAAs in LMICs and Resource-Rich Nations

The clinicians are cautiously optimistic that with the availability of pan-genotypic DAA regimens, HCV elimination is feasible by 2030; albeit, the new hepatitis C infection ratio is continued to outpace the number of people treated annually [54]. An estimation of WHO predicts that 71 million people were infected with HCV worldwide in 2015 and 2016, among that 1.10-1.76 million initiated DAAs treatment, and there were approximately 1.75 million new HCV infections were reported annually [52]. The world health organization (WHO) with the cooperation of its member states put forward a global health sector strategy in 2016 to eliminate HCV by 2030 by setting some ambitious goals. The strategy aims to reduce the number of new hepatitis C infections by 80% and to reduce the mortality rate from hepatitis C by 65% while increasing HCV diagnoses from <5% to 90% and treatment from <1% to 80% to eligible patients in the period between 2015 and 2030 [49]. However, in several parts of the world, the estimation and implementation of WHO strategy was carried out taking into account the costs of patient informing, screening, and treating HCV infections while considering not the viral relapse, viral breakthrough, treatment failure, or reinfections cases [51]. Based on the median estimate of originator prices per standard course of DAA revealed that even national hepatitis C programs for developed and resource-rich nations would require extremely high amounts to billions of dollars and Euros [51]. It means that national hepatitis C programs of various countries belonging to LMICs and resource-poor nations who are off track to GHSS of HCV elimination by 2030 must be able to access affordable, safe, and efficacious generic versions of original DAAs brands [51]. It can be learned from the experiences of some countries (*e.g.*, Egypt, Georgia, Taiwan, Belarus, Kazakhstan, and Kyrgyzstan) that initiated national micro-and macro-HCV elimination programs by massive HCV screening by POC-RDTs as well as treatment with generic DAAs brands [56]. It significantly paved the way to ensure the availability of low-cost DAAs to treatment access for everyone who was diagnosed with active infection status [56, 57]. These models can be adopted and implemented in the national hepatitis plan of countries that are scarce in resources and where health infrastructure is poorly installed and lacks HCV diagnostic and treatment algorithms.

DAAs Associated Adverse Events and Potential Drug-Drug Interactions (DDIs)

DAAs Associated Adverse Events

Initially, severe adverse events (SAEs) were reported in high frequency and ratio while treating HCV individuals with first and second-generation DAAs [4]. Multiple studies of telaprevir, boceprevir, and simeprevir (first-generation DAAs as well as NS3-4A PIs) administration both in clinical trials and real-world clinical settings demonstrate a high frequency of SAEs that were sometimes unmanageable as compared to unaffected HCV patients [58]. That's why, the incidences of treatment non-adherence, treatment discontinuation, viral relapse, virologic breakthrough, and virologic failure were also noticed very high in hepatitis C-treated patients [4]. However, with the advent of NS5B RdRp inhibitors (*e.g.*, sofosbuvir), next-generation NS3-4A PIs, NS5A inhibitors, and pangenotypic regimens, the ratio of treatment-associated adverse events gradually decreased and manageable during or after the therapy [59]. The frequency of adverse events associated with pan-genotypic DAAs administration is very low and manageable. However, co-administration of RBV with DAAs may cause insomnia in treating patients, and adjustment of the timing of the dose earlier in the afternoon can avoid any sleep disruption [59]. Table **2** enlists the most commonly observed adverse events associated with DAA in an observed proportion.

HBV reactivation and HBV-related hepatic flare may occur both during or after treatment in HCV/HBV co-infection patients if not receiving HBV treatment [59]. The US FDA emphasizes red box warnings on the packing and information leaflet of currently used DAAs regarding these risks. DAAs-induced activation of HCC, or recurrence of HCC in HCV patients treated with current DAAs also causes treatment non-adherence, treatment withdrawal, and treatment failure in real-life clinical situations [5]. Both these issues are discussed in the later section of this book chapter.

Table 2. Commonly associated adverse events (AEs) with current DAAs observed as proportion in different populations [60]. Most of the AEs associated with DAAs administration are quite manageable during treatment or disappear after treatment completion.

Adverse events associated with DAAs	
Drug or Combination (Brand Name)	**Most Common Adverse Reactions (Proportion Observed)**
Elbasvir/grazoprevir (ELB/GRZ; Zepatier)	• Fatigue, headache, nausea, insomnia, and diarrhea (≥5%). • With ribavirin: anemia and headache (≥5%).

(Table 2) cont.....

Glecaprevir/pibrentasvir (GLE/PIB; Mavyret)	• Headache and fatigue (>10%).
Ledipasvir/sofosbuvir (LED/SOF; multiple brands)	• Asthenia, headache, and fatigue (≥10%).
Ribavirin (Copegus	• Fatigue/asthenia, pyrexia, myalgia, and headache in adults receiving combination therapy (>40%).
Sofosbuvir/velpatasvir (SOF/VEL; multiple brands)	• With velpatasvir/sofosbuvir: headache and fatigue (≥10%, all grades). • With velpatasvir/sofosbuvir and ribavirin in patients with decompensated cirrhosis: fatigue, anemia, nausea, headache, insomnia, and diarrhea (≥10%, all grades).
Sofosbuvir/velpatasvir/voxilaprevir (SOF/VEL/VOX; Vosevi)	• Headache, fatigue, diarrhea, and nausea (≥10%).
Sources: [FDA 2011a, 2015b, 2016b, 2016c; Hayashi, *et al.* 2016; FDA 2017, 2019]	

DAAs Interactions with Other Primary Care Medications

The clinical efficacy and safety studies of DAAs both in clinical trials and real-world clinical settings while treating various HCV-infected populations provide valuable and significant pieces of evidence on the interaction between DAAs and common primary care medications [60]. Although these recommendations and guidance can be helpful to treatment choice, treatment initiation, treatment duration, and patient management; however, they cannot be a substitute for sound clinical judgment and practice in HCV therapeutics. Furthermore, the DAA interactions with some medications reported in clinical trials could be of no use as in some cases, those medications are labeled as contraindicated in the US FDA labeling for the medication, or that label may state in some other clinical scenarios that co-administration is not recommended [60]. For some drugs, either the recommendation may be to "avoid co-administration", or in some clinical situations "to be administered concurrently". In such circumstances, the clinicians are recommended to consult additional references attributed to drug administration in comorbid conditions or a liver or infectious disease expert for more guidance. Furthermore, significant drug-drug interactions between DAAs and drugs used commonly in the management of substance use disorders are unlikely; even then, the clinicians should always monitor for excess sedation and drowsiness when altering the patient's DAA therapy while he/she is receiving methadone, buprenorphine, naltrexone, and naloxone [60]. Herein we mention co-administration or avoid co-administration of DAAs with common primary care medication including potential clinical outcomes in a tabulated form (Tables **3**, **4**, **5**, **6** and **7**). As boceprevir, telaprevir, and simeprevir administration is discontinued and obsolete, we will emphasize only the current regimens while discussing DAAs drug interactions and their compatibility with other primary care medications.

Table 3. Non-compliance of various primary care medications with GLE/PIB in HCV-treated patients with possible side effects [60].

Glecaprevir/Pibrentasvir (Mavyret) drug-drug interactions	
Avoid co-administration; see clinical comments	
Class (medications)	Clinical Comments
Anticonvulsants (carbamazepine, phenobarbital, phenytoin)	• Carbamazepine: Significant decrease in glecaprevir/pibrentasvir levels expected. • Phenobarbital, phenytoin: Significant decrease in glecaprevir/pibrentasvir levels possible.
Antimycobacterial (rifampin)	• Significant decrease in glecaprevir/pibrentasvir levels expected.
Ethinyl estradiol	• Increased risk of ALT elevations.
Herbal therapy (St John's Wort)	• Decreased glecaprevir/pibrentasvir levels expected.
HIV medications (efavirenz, atazanavir, darunavir, lopinavir, saquinavir, tipranavir)	• Efavirenz: Significant decrease in glecaprevir/pibrentasvir levels expected. • Atazanavir: Significant increase in glecaprevir/pibrentasvir levels expected; increased ALT elevations. • Darunavir, lopinavir/ritonavir, and other HIV protease inhibitors: Significant increase in glecaprevir/pibrentasvir levels expected.
HMG-CoA reductase inhibitors (atorvastatin, lovastatin, simvastatin)	• Increased levels of atorvastatin, lovastatin, and simvastatin are expected; do not co-administer. • See the note below regarding the use of alternative statins.

Table 4. Possible co-administration of certain primary care medications with GLE/PIB in HCV-treated patients [60].

Co-administration possible; see clinical comments	
Class (medications)	**Clinical Comments**
Antiarrhythmic (digoxin)	• Increased digoxin levels likely; reduce digoxin dosage 50%. • Measure serum digoxin level before initiating therapy with glecaprevir/pibrentasvir.
Anticoagulant (dabigatran etexilate)	• Refer to dabigatran prescribing information; follow dosage recommendations for concurrent use with P-glycoprotein inhibitors.
HMG-CoA reductase inhibitors (fluvastatin, pitavastatin, pravastatin, rosuvastatin)	• Fluvastatin, pitavastatin: Increased statin levels likely; use the lowest statin dosage and monitor for adverse events (e.g., myopathy). • Pravastatin: Increased statin level likely; reduce pravastatin dosage by 50% before initiating therapy with glecaprevir/pibrentasvir. • Rosuvastatin: Increased statin level likely; do not exceed rosuvastatin 10 mg daily when combined with glecaprevir/pibrentasvir.

(Table 4) cont.....

Immunosuppressant (cyclosporine)	• Increased levels of glecaprevir/pibrentasvir are expected; do not co-administer in patients requiring cyclosporine doses >100 mg daily.
Source: FDA. Mavyret (glecaprevir and pibrentasvir) tablets, for oral use. http://www.natap.org/2017/HCV/mavyret_pi.pdf	

Table 5. Possible co-administration and non-compliance of various primary medications with LDV/SOF in HCV-treated patients along with their undesirable effects [60].

Ledipasvir/sofosbuvir (multiple brands) drug-drug interactions	
Avoid co-administration; see clinical comments	
Class (medications)	**Clinical Comments**
Antiarrhythmic (amiodarone)	• Significant bradycardia, especially in patients who are taking beta-blockers, have underlying cardiac abnormalities or have advanced liver disease. • If concurrent use is required, cardiac monitoring is recommended. • See package insert for additional information.
Herbal product (St John's wort)	• Significant decrease in ledipasvir/sofosbuvir levels.
Anticonvulsants (carbamazepine, oxcarbazepine, phenobarbital, phenytoin)	• Significant decrease in ledipasvir/sofosbuvir levels.
Antimycobacterials (rifampin, rifabutin, rifapentine)	• Significant decrease in ledipasvir/sofosbuvir levels.
HMG-CoA reductase inhibitor (rosuvastatin)	• Significant increases in rosuvastatin level.
NS3/4A HCV protease inhibitor (simeprevir)	• Significant increases in ledipasvir levels.
Co-administration possible; see clinical comments	
Class (medications)	**Clinical Comments**
Antacids	• Ledipasvir solubility decreases as pH increases. • Separate administration of aluminum- and magnesium-containing antacids and ledipasvir/sofosbuvir by 4 hours.
Antiarrhythmic (digoxin)	• Increase in digoxin level expected. • Monitor digoxin level.
H2-receptor antagonists	• Administer simultaneously with, or 12 hours apart from, ledipasvir/sofosbuvir. • Do not exceed doses comparable to famotidine 40 mg twice daily.
Proton-pump inhibitors	• If co-administration is required, doses comparable to omeprazole 20 mg or lower can be administered simultaneously with ledipasvir/sofosbuvir under fasting conditions.
Source: FDA. Harvoni (ledipasvir and sofosbuvir) tablets, for oral use. https://www.accessdata.fda.gov/drugsatfda_docs/label/2017/205834s024lbl.pdf	

Table 6. Possible co-administration and non-compliance of various primary medications with SOF/VEL in HCV-treated patients along with their potential side effects [60].

Sofosbuvir/velpatasvir (multiple brands) drug-drug interactions	
Avoid co-administration; see clinical comments	
Class (medications)	**Clinical Comments**
Antiarrhythmic (amiodarone)	• Significant bradycardia, especially in patients who are taking beta-blockers, have underlying cardiac abnormalities or have advanced liver disease. • If concurrent use is required, cardiac monitoring is recommended. • See package insert for additional information.
Anticonvulsants (carbamazepine, oxcarbazepine, phenobarbital, phenytoin)	• Significant decrease in sofosbuvir level expected, leading to reduced sofosbuvir and/or velpatasvir drug levels.
Antimycobacterials (rifampin, rifabutin, rifapentine)	• Potential significant decrease in sofosbuvir and/or velpatasvir drug levels.
Herbal product (St John's wort)	• May significantly decrease sofosbuvir and/or velpatasvir drug levels.
Co-administration possible; see clinical comments	
Class (medications)	**Clinical Comments**
Antacids (aluminum and magnesium hydroxide)	• May decrease the concentration of velpatasvir. • Separate administration of antacid and velpatasvir/sofosbuvir by 4 hours.
Antiarrhythmic (digoxin)	• Increase in digoxin level expected. • Monitor digoxin level.
Anticancer (topotecan)	• Significant increase in topotecan expected.
H2-receptor antagonist (famotidine)	• Velpatasvir solubility decreases as pH increases. • May decrease the concentration of velpatasvir. • H2-receptor antagonists may be administered simultaneously with, or 12 hours apart from velpatasvir/sofosbuvir, at a dose that does not exceed doses comparable to famotidine 40 mg twice daily.
HMG-CoA reductase inhibitor (rosuvastatin)	• May significantly increase the concentration of rosuvastatin, which is associated with an increased risk of myopathy, including rhabdomyolysis. • Rosuvastatin may be administered at a dose not greater than 10 mg daily.
Proton-pump inhibitor (omeprazole)	• May decrease the concentration of velpatasvir. • Proton-pump inhibitor doses comparable to omeprazole 20 mg or lower can be administered simultaneously with velpatasvir/sofosbuvir under fasting conditions.
Source: FDA. Epclusa (sofosbuvir and velpatasvir) tablets, for oral use. https://www.accessdata.fda.gov/drugsatfda_docs/label/2016/208341s000lbl.pdf	

Table 7. Possible non-compliance and co-administration of various primary medications with SOF/VEL/VOX in HCV-treated patients along with their potential side effects [60].

Sofosbuvir/velpatasvir/voxilaprevir (Vosevi) drug-drug interactions	
Avoid co-administration; see clinical comments	
Class (medications)	**Clinical Comments**
Antiarrhythmic (amiodarone)	• Potential for significant bradycardia, especially in patients who are taking beta-blockers, have underlying cardiac abnormalities or have advanced liver disease. If concurrent use is required, cardiac monitoring is recommended
Herbal product (St John's wort)	• Significant decrease in sofosbuvir/velpatasvir/voxilaprevir levels.
Anticonvulsants (carbamazepine, oxcarbazepine, phenobarbital, phenytoin)	• Significant decrease in sofosbuvir/velpatasvir/voxilaprevir levels.
Antimycobacterials (rifampin, rifabutin, rifapentine)	• Significant decrease in sofosbuvir/velpatasvir/voxilaprevir levels.
HIV medications (efavirenz, atazanavir, tipranavir)	• Efavirenz: Significant decrease in velpatasvir and voxilaprevir levels expected. • Atazanavir: Significant increase in voxilaprevir level expected. • Tipranavir: Significant decrease in sofosbuvir and voxilaprevir levels expected
HMG-CoA reductase inhibitor (pitavastatin, rosuvastatin)	• Significant increase in pitavastatin and rosuvastatin levels expected when combined with sofosbuvir/velpatasvir/voxilaprevir.
Immunosuppressant (cyclosporine)	• Significant increases in cyclosporine level expected.
Co-administration possible; see clinical comments	
Class (medications)	**Clinical Comments**
Acid-reducing medications: • Aluminum- and magnesium hydroxide-containing antacids • H2-receptor antagonists • Proton pump inhibitor	• Separate administration of antacids and sofosbuvir/velpatasvir/voxilaprevir by 4 hours. • H2-receptor antagonists may be administered simultaneously with or staggered from sofosbuvir/velpatasvir/voxilaprevir at a dose that does not exceed a comparable dose of famotidine 40 mg twice daily. • Omeprazole 20 mg can be administered with sofosbuvir/velpatasvir/ voxilaprevir: - Use with other proton pump inhibitors has not been studied. - Use with the lowest doses of other proton pump inhibitors is unlikely to interact.
Antiarrhythmic (digoxin)	• Sofosbuvir/velpatasvir/voxilaprevir may increase digoxin levels; monitor digoxin levels closely before and during therapy.
HIV medication (tenofovir disoproxil fumarate [TDF])	• Significant increase in TDF levels expected; monitor for tenofovir-related adverse events.

(Table 7) cont.....

HMG-CoA reductase inhibitor (atorvastatin, fluvastatin, lovastatin, pravastatin, simvastatin)	• Atorvastatin, fluvastatin, lovastatin, simvastatin: Potential increase levels of statins when combined with sofosbuvir/velpatasvir/voxilaprevir; use lowest statin dosage. • Pravastatin: Potential increased levels of pravastatin when combined with sofosbuvir/velpatasvir/voxilaprevir; do not exceed pravastatin 40mg daily when combined.
Source: FDA. Vosevi (sofosbuvir and velpatasvir and voxilaprevir) tablets, for oral use. https://www.accessdata.fda.gov/drugsatfda_docs/label/2017/209195s000lbl.pdf	

DDIs Between DAAs and Antiretroviral Therapy (ART)

As previously mentioned in chapter 6, HCV/HIV co-infected patients represent a harder-to-treat fraction of HCV infected population even treated with pan-genotypic DAAs [60]. Concurrent administration of DAAs with ART may lead to clinically relevant drug interactions in HCV/HIV co-infection patients that may potentially contribute to less cure rates after post-completion therapy, patient non-adherence to therapy during treatment, or discontinuation of treatment at any moment (Tables **8** and **9**) [61]. The DDIs and non-compatibilities between DAAs and ART may lead to potential hepatic and renal drug toxicities which can cause above mentioned three treatment relapse possibilities [61].

Table 8. Possible non-compliance and co-administration of various primary medications with ELB/GRZ in HCV-treated patients along with their potential side effects [60].

Elbasvir/Grazoprevir (Zepatier) drug-drug interactions	
Avoid co-administration; see clinical comments	
Class (medications)	**Clinical Comments**
Anticonvulsants (carbamazepine, phenytoin)	• Significant decrease in elbasvir/grazoprevir levels.
Antimycobacterial (rifampin)	• Significant decrease in elbasvir/grazoprevir levels.
Herbal product (St John's wort)	• Significant decrease in elbasvir/grazoprevir levels.
HIV medications (efavirenz, atazanavir, darunavir, lopinavir, saquinavir, tipranavir)	• Efavirenz: Significant decrease in elbasvir/grazoprevir levels. • Atazanavir, darunavir, lopinavir, saquinavir, tipranavir: Significant increase in grazoprevir level. - May lead to ALT elevation.
Immunosuppressant (cyclosporine)	• Significant increase in grazoprevir level. - May lead to ALT elevation.
Co-administration possible; see clinical comments	
Class (medications)	**Clinical Comments**
Antibiotic (nafcillin)	• Decreased concentrations of elbasvir/grazoprevir levels.

(Table 8) cont.....

Antifungal (ketoconazole)	• Significant increase in elbasvir/grazoprevir levels. • Increased risk of hepatotoxicity.
Endothelin antagonist (bosentan	• Significant decrease in elbasvir/grazoprevir levels.
HMG-CoA reductase inhibitors (atorvastatin, fluvastatin, lovastatin, rosuvastatin, simvastatin)	• Increase in statin drug levels expected. • Atorvastatin: Maximum daily dose 20 mg. • Fluvastatin, lovastatin, or simvastatin: Use the lowest doses possible; titrate with close monitoring. • Rosuvastatin: Maximum daily dose 10 mg.
Immunosuppressant (tacrolimus)	• Significant increase in tacrolimus level expected. • Frequent monitoring is required for tacrolimus level, changes in renal function, and tacrolimus-associated adverse events.
Wakefulness-promoting agent (modafinil)	• Significant decrease in elbasvir/grazoprevir levels.
Source: U.S. Food and Drug Administration. Zepatier (elbasvir and grazoprevir) tablets, for oral use. https://www.accessdata.fda.gov/drugsatfda_docs/label/2016/208261Orig1s000lbl.pdf	

Table 9. Compatibility of Select ART and DAA Regimens for Non-Pregnant Adults (June 2019).

ART Regimen	Concurrent DAA Regimen and Clinical Comment
ABC/3TC/DTG (Triumeq) [a] • Preferred initial ART regimen [b] • Initiate only in patients with CrCl ≥50 mL/min • Initiate only in patients negative for HLA-B*5701	• All DAA regimens are compatible.
TAF 25 mg/FTC/BIC (Biktarvy) • Initiate only in patients with CrCl ≥30 mL/min	• All DAA regimens are compatible.
TAF 10 mg/FTC/COBI/EVG (Genvoya) [c,d] • Preferred initial ART regimen [b] • Initiate only in patients with CrCl ≥30 mL/min	• Do not co-administer with GRZ/ELB.
TAF 25 mg/FTC and DTG (Descovy and Tivicay) [d] • Preferred initial ART regimen [b] • Initiate only in patients with CrCl ≥30 mL/min	• All DAA regimens are compatible.
TAF 25 mg/FTC and RAL HD (Descovy and Isentress) [d,e] • Preferred initial ART regimen [b] • Initiate only in patients with CrCl ≥30 mL/min	• All DAA regimens are compatible

(Table 9) cont.....

TAF 25 mg/FTC/RPV (Odefsey) [d, f] • Alternative initial ART regimen [b] • Initiate only in patients confirmed to have: CrCl of ≥30 mL/min CD4 count ≥200 cells/mm3 Viral load	• Do not co-administer with GRZ/ELB.
TDF/FTC/COBI/EVG (Stribild) [c] • Alternative initial ART regimen [b] • Initiate only in patients with CrCl >70 mL/min	• Do not co-administer with GRZ/ELB. • When combining TDF/FTC/COBI/EVG with either LED/SOF, SOF/VEL/VOX, or SOF/VEL, plasma levels of tenofovir are increased and may lead to tenofovir-related renal side effects. Consider switching TDF to TAF, substituting ABC if the patient is HLAB*5701 negative and has no evidence of ABC resistance, or using a different DAA regimen.
TDF/FTC and DRV/COBI (Truvada and Prezcobix) [c] • Alternative initial ART regimen [b] • Initiate only in patients with CrCl ≥70 mL/min	• Do not co-administer with GRZ/ELB or GLE/PIB. • When combining TDF/FTC and DRV/COBI with either LED/SOF, SOF/VEL/VOX, or SOF/VEL, plasma levels of tenofovir are increased and may lead to tenofovir-related renal side effects. Consider switching TDF to TAF, substituting ABC if the patient is HLAB*5701 negative and has no evidence of ABC resistance, or using a different DAA regimen.
TDF/FTC and DRV and RTV (Truvada and Prezista and Norvir) [c]	• Do not co-administer with GRZ/ELB or GLE/PIB.
• Alternative initial ART regimen [b] • Initiate only in patients with CrCl ≥50 mL/min	• When combining TDF/FTC, DRV, and RTV with either LED/SOF, SOF/VEL/VOX, or SOF/VEL plasma levels of tenofovir are increased and may lead to tenofovir-related renal side effects. Consider switching TDF to TAF, substituting ABC if the patient is HLAB*5701 negative and has no evidence of ABC resistance, or using a different DAA regimen.
TDF/FTC and DTG (Truvada and Tivicay) • Alternative initial ART regimen [b] • Initiate only in patients with CrCl ≥50 mL/min	• When combining TDF with SOF/VEL/VOX, levels of tenofovir are increased and may lead to tenofovir-related renal side effects. Consider switching TDF to TAF, substituting ABC if the patient is HLAB*5701 negative and has no evidence of ABC resistance, or using a different DAA regimen.
TDF/FTC and RAL HD (Truvada and Isentress HD) • Alternative initial ART regimen [b] • Initiate only in patients with CrCl ≥50 mL/min	• When combining TDF with SOF/VEL/VOX, levels of tenofovir are increased and may lead to tenofovir-related renal side effects. Consider switching TDF to TAF, substituting ABC if the patient is HLAB*5701 negative and has no evidence of ABC resistance, or using a different DAA regimen.
TAF 25 mg/FTC and RAL (Truvada and Isentress HD) • Alternative initial ART regimen • Initiate only in patients with CrCl ≥30 mL/min	• All DAA regimens are compatible.

(Table 9) cont.....

a. In all cases, FTC and 3TC are interchangeable when not being used in fixed-dose combinations. b. See the NYSDOH AI guideline Selecting an Initial ART Regimen. c. Because of their drug-interaction profiles, COBI and RTV should not be considered interchangeable. d. TAF 10 mg and TAF 25 mg are not interchangeable. e. When dosing RAL once daily use the HD formulation of 600 mg tablets dosed at 1200 mg. f. When a "rapid start" or "test and treat" initiation of ART occurs before a patient's viral load and CD4 count is available, avoid the use of RPV. **ARV abbreviation key:** Abacavir (ABC); bictegravir (BIC); cobicistat (COBI); darunavir (DRV); dolutegravir (DTG); elvitegravir (EVG); emtricitabine (FTC); lamivudine (3TC); raltegravir (RAL); rilpivirine (RPV); ritonavir (RTV); tenofovir alafenamide (TAF); tenofovir disoproxil fumarate (TDF) **DAA abbreviation key:** Elbasvir (ELB); glecaprevir (GLE); grazoprevir (GRZ); ledipasvir (LED); paritaprevir/ritonavir/ombitasvir/dasabuvir (PrOD); sofosbuvir (SOF); pibrentasvir (PIB); velpatasvir (VEL); voxilaprevir (VOX)

Multiple studies showed that the use of tenofovir (*i.e.*, a nucleoside reverse transcriptase inhibitor used extensively in the treatment of HIV/HBV) as in the disoproxil fumarate form (TDF)), with VEL or LDV increases drug levels of TDF [62]. When LDV/SOF is administered with TDF concurrently with efavirenz or ritonavir-boosted atazanavir or darunavir to HCV/HIV co-infected patients, TDF levels increase even further and may cause TDF-related nephrotoxicity [63]. A report from the US FDA also confirms these interactions likely to occur with SOF/VEL combination [63]. Furthermore, some studies also reveal that TDF levels are also increased while using TDF with SOF/VEL/VOX fixed-dose combination [64]. Monitoring for adverse renal effects and close monitoring of creatinine clearance (CrCl) is recommended in these patient settings while co-administering LDV/SOF, SOF/VEL, or SOF/VEL/VOX with TDF and efavirenz or ritonavir-boosted PIs [65]. The clinicians should consider altering the patient's ART regimen by switching from TDF to tenofovir alafenamide (TAF) or TDF to Abacavir (ABC) which show a beneficial effect on bone and kidney toxicity)) if HIV is susceptible to these drugs [66]. Furthermore, TAF is also associated with much less serum tenofovir concentrations and current FDA-label drugs recommend TAF formulations to be used in patients whose CrCl is as low as 30mL/min [63]. In addition to that, as the new drug development and approval for both HIV and HCV continue, clinicians stay current on potential DDIs. Table **10** enlists the compatibility of preferred initial ART regimens with concurrent DAA regimens for nonpregnant HCV adults [60].

The Emergence of Resistance-Associated Substitutions (RAS) and Resistance-Associated Variants (RAV) with DAAs Treatment

The high replication rate of the HCV genome, poor fidelity, and lack of a proof-reading mechanism of HCV RNA-dependent RNA polymerase (RdRp) enzyme during replication generates various nucleotide mismatches or mutations in the HCV genome [67]. These nucleotide mutations are subsequently configured as various genotypes and subtypes (8 HCV GTs and 67 subtypes have been confirmed to date) in the virus genome which differ by > 30% at the GT level, > 15% at the subtypes level, and < 15% within a specific genotype (*i.e.*, quasispecies) in an HCV infected individual [68]. This HCV genome variation at GTs and subtypes level that is very much attributed to nucleotide substitutions during virus replication is considered one of the key factors to evolve/emerge or originate pre-existing/baseline or treatment-emergent resistance-associated substitutions (RASs) in HCV-infected patients on treatment with DAAs (Table **11**) [69]. The existence of baseline HCV genome polymorphism, pre-existing HCV RASs, and treatment-emergent RASs with DAAs are the main clinical diagnostic considerations for the care provider while deciding, choosing, and initiating IFN-free DAAs therapy either in treatment naïve or treatment-experienced/or failure HCV patients [70]. Meanwhile, RAS and resistance-associated variants (RAV) are two major terms which frequently but misconceptually used in hepatitis C therapeutics while treating infected patients with DAAs [71].

Table 10. Compatibility of alternative anti-HIV antivirals with concurrent DAA regimens for nonpregnant HCV adults [60].

Compatibility of Select ART and DAA Regimens for Non-Pregnant Adults (October 2021)	
ART Regimen	**Concurrent DAA Regimen and Clinical Comment**
Preferred Initial regimens	
Abacavir/lamivudine/dolutegravir (ABC/3TC/DTG; Triumeq)	All DAA regimens are compatible.
Lamivudine/dolutegravir (3TC/DTG; Dovato) [d,e,f]	All DAA regimens are compatible.
Tenofovir alafenamide/emtricitabine/ bictegravir (TAF 25 mg/FTC/BIC; Biktarvy)	All DAA regimens are compatible but see note [g] regarding the concomitant use of LED or VEL and tenofovir.
Tenofovir alafenamide/emtricitabine or tenofovir disoproxil fumarate/ emtricitabine and dolutegravir (TAF 25 mg/FTC or TDF 300 mg/FTC and DTG; Descovy or Truvada and Tivicay)	All DAA regimens are compatible but see note [g] regarding the concomitant use of LED or VEL and tenofovir.
Tenofovir alafenamide/emtricitabine or tenofovir disoproxil fumarate/ emtricitabine and raltegravir HD (TAF 25 mg/FTC or TDF 300 mg/FTC and RAL HD; Descovy or Truvada and Isentress HD)	• All DAA regimens are compatible. • GLE/PIB may increase the serum concentration of RAL but no action is needed. • See note [g] regarding the concomitant use of LED or VEL and tenofovir.

(Table 10) cont.....

Alternative Initial ART Regimens	
Tenofovir alafenamide/emtricitabine/ darunavir/cobicistat (TAF 10 mg/FTC/ DRV/ COBI/; Symtuza) [e]	• Do not co-administer with GLE/PIB. • When combining SOF/VEL/VOX with COBI-boosted DRV, levels of VOX may be increased. Until more safety data become available, patients who are taking the combination should be monitored for hepatotoxicity during therapy. • See note [g] regarding the concomitant use of LED or VEL and tenofovir
Tenofovir alafenamide/emtricitabine/ elvitegravir/cobicistat (TAF 10 mg/FTC/ EVG/COBI/; Genvoya) [e]	• When combining GLE/PIB with COBI-boosted EVG, levels of GLE/PIB may be increased. Until more safety data become available, patients who are taking the combination should be monitored for hepatotoxicity during therapy. • See note [g] regarding the concomitant use of LED or VEL and tenofovir.
Tenofovir alafenamide/emtricitabine/ rilpivirine (TAF 25 mg/FTC/RPV; Odefsey)	All DAA regimens are compatible but see note [g] regarding the concomitant use of LED or VEL and tenofovir.
Tenofovir disoproxil fumarate/lamivudine/ doravirine (TDF/3TC/DOR; Delstrigo)	• All DAA regimens are considered to be compatible, but limited data are evaluating the use of DOR with SOF/VEL or GLE/PIB. • See note [g] regarding the concomitant use of LED or VEL and tenofovir.
Abacavir/lamivudine and doravirine (ABC/3TC and DOR; Epzicom and Pifeltro)	All DAA regimens are considered to be compatible, but limited data are evaluating the use of DOR with SOF/VEL or GLE/PIB.
Tenofovir alafenamide/emtricitabine and doravirine (TAF 25 mg/FTC and DOR; Descovy and Pifeltro)	• All DAA regimens are considered to be compatible, but limited data are evaluating the use of DOR with SOF/VEL or GLE/PIB. • See note [g] regarding the concomitant use of LED or VEL and tenofovir.
Tenofovir disoproxil fumarate/ emtricitabine and raltegravir (TDF/FTC and RAL; Truvada and Isentress)	All DAA regimens are compatible but see note [g] regarding the concomitant use of LED or VEL and tenofovir.

(Table 10) cont.....

Abbreviations: 3TC, lamivudine; ABC, abacavir; BIC, bictegravir; COBI, cobicistat; DRV, darunavir; DTG, dolutegravir; EVG, elvitegravir; FTC, emtricitabine; RAL, raltegravir; RPV, rilpivirine; TAF, tenofovir alafenamide; TDF, tenofovir disoproxil fumarate.
Notes: a. Refer to DHHS for ART regimens for individuals of childbearing potential: Recommendations for the Use of Antiretroviral Drugs in Pregnant Women with HIV Infection and Interventions to Reduce Perinatal HIV Transmission in the United States.
b. See the NYSDOH AI guideline Selecting an Initial ART Regimen.
c. **Available DAA regimens as of October 2021:** Glecaprevir/pibrentasvir (GLE/PIB; Mavyret); ledipasvir/sofosbuvir (LED/SOF; multiple brands); sofosbuvir/velpatasvir (SOF/VEL; multiple brands); sofosbuvir/velpatasvir/voxilaprevir (SOF/VEL/VOX; Vosevi).
d. See Use of Dolutegravir in Individuals of Childbearing Capacity.
e. Substitutions: In all cases, FTC and 3TC are interchangeable; TAF 10 mg and TAF 25 mg are not interchangeable.
f. For dose adjustments, refer to the NYSDOH AI guideline Selecting an Initial ART Regimen > Table 9: Recommended Dose Adjustments for Use of Selected Fixed-Dose Combination Antiretroviral Medications in Patients With Hepatic or Renal Impairment.
g. **Concomitant use of LED or VEL and tenofovir:** When using TAF or TDF concurrently with a DAA regimen containing LED or VEL, renal function should be evaluated with CrCl testing at baseline and 4 weeks after the start of DAA treatment. When LED or VEL is taken with TDF or TAF, the serum concentration of tenofovir may be increased, which may lead to tenofovir-related renal side effects. Concurrent use of a LED- or VEL-containing DAA and TDF should be avoided in patients with a CrCl < 50 mL/min. Options include switching TDF to TAF [c], substituting ABC if the patient is HLAB*5701 negative and has no evidence of ABC resistance, or using a different DAA regimen.

Table 11. RAS associated with different DAA classes targeting different regions of the HCV genome.

Common RASs with reduced sensibility to DAAs according to HCV GTs/subtypes			
a. RASs associated with NS3/4A PIs acting on NS3 protein of the hepatitis C virus			
RASs	**Reduced sensibility to**	**HCV Genotype/subtypes**	**References**
V36M/A/G/L	Paritaprevir, Asunaprevir, Simeprevir, Grazoprevir, Vaniprevir, Glecaprevir Voxilaprevir	HCV GT-1 (1a/1b) HCV GT-6	[77]
Q41R/K	Simeprevir, Vaniprevir Voxilaprevir	HCV GT-1 (1a/1b) HCV GT-3 HCV GT-4 HCV GT-6	[78]
V55A	Paritaprevir Asunaprevir	HCV GT-1 (1a/1b)	[79]
Y56H/F/L	Asunaprevir, Paritaprevir, Grazoprevir, Glecaprevir, Voxilaprevir, Sovaprevir	HCV GT-1 (1a/1b) HCV GT-3 HCV GT-4 HCV GT-6	[80]

(Table 11) cont.....

Q80K/L/R/G, H	Simeprevir, Asunaprevir, Paritaprevir, Grazoprevir, Vaniprevir,Voxilaprevir,	HCV GT-1 (1a/1b) HCV GT-3	[81]
S122G/R/A/I/T/D/N	Simeprevir, Asunaprevir	HCV GT-1 (1a/1b)	[82]
I132V	Simeprevir	HCV GT-1 (1a)	[83]
R155K/T/Q/G/W/C/ I/S/L	Simeprevir, Asunaprevir Paritaprevir, Vaniprevir Grazoprevir, Voxilaprevir	HCV GT-1 (1a/1b) HCV GT-4	[84]
A156S/G/T/A/E/F/H/ N/V/Y/K/Y	Asunaprevir, Simeprevir Paritaprevir, Grazoprevir Vaniprevir, Voxilaprevir	HCV GT-1 (1a/1b) HCV GT-3 HCV GT-4 HCV GT-5 HCV GT-6	[85]
D168A/C/E/G/H/Q/T/ V/Y/N/F/I/K/S/R/L	Asunaprevir, Simeprevir Paritaprevir, Grazoprevir Vaniprevir,Voxilaprevir	HCV GT-1 (1a/1b) HCV GT-2 (2a/2b) HCV GT-3 HCV GT-4 HCV GT-5 HCV GT-6	[86]
I/V170A/T/M	Asunaprevir, Simeprevir Danoprevir, Voxilaprevir	HCV GT-1 (1b)	[87]
V36A/M+R155K/T	Asunaprevir, Simeprevir Paritaprevir, Vaniprevir Grazoprevir	HCV GT-1 (1a/1b)	[88]
F43S + D168E F43S+A156G F43S+Q80R	Simeprevir	HCV GT-1 (1b)	[84]
Q80H/K/L+D168E/ V/Y	Asunaprevir, Simeprevir	HCV GT-1 (1b)	[89]
Q80K/R+R155K	Simeprevir, Paritaprevir	HCV GT-1 (1a/1b)	[90]
Q80K/R/L+D168V/ Y/E	Asunaprevir Simeprevir	HCV GT-1 (1a/1b)	[89]
Q80K+V170T Q80L/R/K+R155K/W Q80R+A156V S122G/R+R155K	Simeprevir Simeprevir Simeprevir Simeprevir	HCV GT-1 (1a/1b) HCV GT-1 (1a/1b) HCV GT-1 (1b) HCV GT-1 (1a/1b)	[88]
R155K/Q/W+D168/A/ N/V/H/E	Simeprevir Grazoprevir Vaniprevir	HCV GT-1 (1a/1b)	[91]
R155K+I/V170T/A	Simeprevir Asunaprevir	HCV GT-1 (1a/1b)	[91]

(Table 11) cont.....

A156V+D168V	Simeprevir Glecaprevir	HCV GT-1 (1b)	[89]
Q80K/ R+R155K+D168E	Simeprevir	HCV GT-1 (1b)	[84]
Y56H+D/Q168A/V/ Y/N/R	Paritaprevir Grazoprevir Glecaprevir	HCV GT-1 (1a/1b) HCV GT-3a HCV GT-4a/4d	[92]
P89L/R+A156V/T	Glecaprevir	HCV GT-1 (1a/1b)	[93]
b. RASs associated with NS5A inhibitors acting on the NS5A protein of the hepatitis C virus			
K/Q/S24R/H/G/N/Q/K	Daclatasvir, Ledipasvir Ombitasvir, Velpatasvir Pibrentasvir	HCV GT-1 (1a/1b) HCV GT-3 HCV GT-4	[84]
M/L/F/28/A/T/V/G/M/C/I/V/F/S	Daclatasvir, Ledipasvir Ombitasvir, Elbasvir Velpatasvir, Pibrentasvir	HCV GT-1 (1a/1b) HCV GT-2 HCV GT-4	[94]
P29S/DELETION	Daclatasvir	HCV GT-1 (1b)	[92]
Q/R/K/A/L30D/E/G/H/K/L/N/R/T/Y/A/S	Ledipasvir, Ombitasvir Elbasvir, Velpatasvir Pibrentasvir	HCV GT-1 (1a/1b) HCV GT-3 HCV GT-4	[94]
L31M/I/V/F	Daclatasvir, Ledipasvir Elbasvir	HCV GT-1 (1a/1b) HCV GT-3a	[95]
P32L/S/A	Daclatasvir, Ledipasvir Ombitasvir, Velpatasvir	HCV GT-1 (1a/1b) HCV GT-6	[96]
P/H/T58D/A/L/S/N/R/T/G/H/D/P	Daclatasvir, Ledipasvir Ombitasvir, Elbasvir Velpatasvir	HCV GT-1 (1a/1b) HCV GT-3a HCV GT-4a HCV GT-6	[97]
A/C/E92K/R/T/S	Daclatasvir, Ledipasvir Ombitasvir,Velpatasvir	HCV GT-1 (1a/1b) HCV GT-2 (2a/b/c) HCV GT-6	[98]
T/Y93C/F/H/N/S/I/R/W/T/L/A	Daclatasvir, Ledipasvir Ombitasvir, Elbasvir Velpatasvir, Pibrentasvir	HCV GT-1 (1a/1b) HCV GT-2 (2a/b/c) HCV GT-3a HCV GT-4a/d HCV GT-6	[77]
M/L28A/M/T/V+Q/L30R/A/H/T/V/K/S	Daclatasvir, Ledipasvir, Elbasvir	HCV GT-1 (1a) HCV GT-4a/d	[99]
L/F28M/V+L/T31M/F/S	Daclatasvir, Ombitasvir	HCV GT-2 (2a/b/c) HCV GT-4a/d	[100]
F/M28+Y93H	Daclatasvir	HCV GT-1 (1a) HCV GT-2 (2a/b/c) HCV GT-3a	[101]
R/L/Q/A30R/Q/H+M/L31F/V/M	Daclatasvir, Ledipasvir Velpatasvir, Elbasvir	HCV GT-1 (1a/1b) HCV GT-4 (4a/d)	[100]

(Table 11) cont.....

Q30R+H58D	Daclatasvir, Elbasvir	HCV GT-1 (1a)	[102]
Q30R+H58D	Daclatasvir	HCV GT-1 (1a)	[99]
/A/L/Q30Q/L/H/I/A/V/R/S/D/K+Y93H/R/T/S/C/N	Daclatasvir, Ledipasvir Ombitasvir, Elbasvir Velpatasvir, Pibrentasvir	HCV GT-1 (1a/1b) HCV GT-3 HCV GT-4 (4a/d)	[103]
L31F/V/P/H58L/P/S	Daclatasvir Ombitasvir	HCV GT-1 (1a/1b) HCV GT-3 HCV GT-4 (4a/d)	[99]
L31F/M/V/I+Y93H/N	Ombitasvir, Daclatasvir Elbasvir, Pibrentasvir	HCV GT-1 (1a/1b)	[99]
P/H58S/P/A/L+Y93H/D	Daclatasvir, Ombitasvir Pibrentasvir	HCV GT-1 (1a/1b) HCV GT-3a	[31, 102]
A/S62T+Y93H F28L+L31M+C92S	Daclatasvir Daclatasvir	HCV GT-3a HCV GT-2 (2a/b/c)	[100, 102]
L28M+L/R30H/Q/S+Y93W/S/H	Daclatasvir, Ombitasvir	HCV GT-1 (1b) HCV GT-4 (4a/d)	[104]
L/M28M/T/V+Q/L30S/H+M/R31V	Daclatasvir, Elbasvir	HCV GT-1 (1a) HCV GT-4 (4a/d)	[103]
A/R30K/Q+L31M+Y93H	Daclatasvir, Pibrentasvir	HCV GT-1 (1b) HCV GT-3a	[105]
L31V+Q54H+Y93H L31M+P58L+Y93H	Daclatasvir	HCV GT-1 (1b)	[105]
L28I/V+P/T58L/S	Ombitasvir	HCV GT-4 (4a/d)	[106]
K24Q+T58P+Y93H	Ombitasvir	HCV GT-4 (4d)	[107]
K/S24F/T+M28T/K+Q/A30R/K	Elbasvir, Pibrentasvir	HCV GT-1 (1a) HCV GT-3a	[103]
M28T+Q30R+L31V+Y93H	Elbasvir	HCV GT-1 (1a)	[103]
S24F+M28K	Pibrentasvir	HCV GT-3a	[93]
c. RASs associated with NS5B inhibitors acting on the NS5B protein of the hepatitis C virus			
L159F	Sofosbuvir	HCV GT-1 (1a/1b) HCV GT-2 (2a/b/c) HCV GT-3 (3a)	[84]
E237G	Sofosbuvir	1a-3a-4a/d HCV GT-1 (1a) HCV GT-3 (3a) HCV GT-4 (4a/d)	[77]
S282 R/T/G	Sofosbuvir	HCV GT-1 (1a/1b) HCV GT-2 (2a/b/c) HCV GT-3 (3a) HCV GT-4 (4a/d) HCV GT-5 HCV GT-6	[108]

(Table 11) cont.....

C316F/H/N/Y	Sofosbuvir Dasabuvir	HCV GT-1 (1a)	[24]
L320F V321A/I	Sofosbuvir	HCV GT-1 (1a) HCV GT-1 (1a) HCV GT-3 (3a)	[109]
S368T A395G M414I/T/V C445F E446K/Q Y448C/H/R C451S A553T/V G554S/D S556G/N/R G558R D559G Y561H S565F	Dasabuvir	HCV GT-1 (1b) HCV GT-1 (1a) HCV GT-1 (1a/b) HCV GT-1 (1b) HCV GT-1 (1b) HCV GT-1 (1a/b) HCV GT-1 (1b) HCV GT-1 (1a/b) HCV GT-1 (1a) HCV GT-1 (1a/b) HCV GT-1 (1a) HCV GT-1 (1b) HCV GT-1 (1a) HCV GT-1 (1a)	[110, 111]
L159F+C316N L159F+L320F L159F+S282T L320F+S282T L159F+S282T+L320F	Sofosbuvir	HCV GT-1 (1a/1b) HCV GT-2 (2a/b/c) HCV GT-3 (3a) HCV GT-1 (1a/1b) HCV GT-3 (3a) HCV GT-1 (1a/1b) HCV GT-1 (1a) HCV GT-1 (1b)	[112]

Potential Implications of RAS on DAAs Efficacy

Molecular virology of HCV, genetic heterogeneity, and molecular phylogeny studies reveal that nucleotide mismatches or mutations within the virus genome make it less susceptible to DAAs inhibitory effects [70, 71]. It was concluded after many studies that HCV monotherapy could result in the selection of mutations within the HCV genome that enhance virus replication even in the presence of the drug [70 - 72]. HCV resistance against administered drugs occurs when nucleotide substitutions or mutations appear throughout the virus genome with each replication cycle [73]. Some of these mutations by chance intrude on that part of the genome where specific anti-HCV agents (*i.e.* DAAs) bind to their specific protein target and ultimately generate HCV-resistant variants [74]. HCV-*resistant variants* are virus clones that grow better than prototype viruses in the presence of a DAA agent [70]. These variant virus clones are themselves resistant but not involved in resistance emergence. Specific nucleotide substitutions from HCV genome sequencing of a patient may be identified which are the main culprit to evolving anti-HCV drug resistance; however, when a specific HCV clone with those resistance generating nucleotide substitutions would grow before DAA treatment, during DAA treatment, or post-completion DAA treatment is not exactly known [75]. For simplicity, the identification of RAV is not possible in HCV-affected individuals [70]. However, the identification of nucleotide mismatches or mutations that are potentially involved to emerge as anti-HCV drug resistance is possible through traditional genome sequencing methods or by next-generation sequencing (NGS; also known as deep sequencing); hence the term RAS was coined [76]. In clinical practice, RAV is a feasible term for *in-vitro* HCV-related studies, while RAS is preferred to genome sequencing findings and its interpretations from an infected HCV patient [76]. In addition to that, the RASs may be specific to a whole drug class or individual-specific drugs and maybe HCV GT or subtype-specific [70, 76]. It is very important to mention here that the administered DAAs do not produce or evolve RASs, they just select resistance-associated nucleotide substitutions within the virus genome [68, 70].

Virus fitness against DAAs

Nucleotide substitutions or mutations occur very randomly during HCV genome replication and most of them impair the virus genome fitness (i.e, the capability of a virus genome that how well it replicates) [70]. Virus variant clones with RAS possess a fitness advantage in the presence of a DAA regimen; however, most of them are outcompeted by wild or prototype HCV clones in the absence of a DAA agent [113]. This virus fitness with specific RAS probably determines that either RAS will persist after unsuccessful DAA therapy or they will exist at baseline in treatment-naïve HCV patients [113]. Interestingly, RAS within the HCV genome are specific to different DAAs classes and express markedly different virus fitness against each class [70]. One classical example is attributed to SOF-associated RAS (*i.e.* S282T) which replicates very poorly and is quickly out-grown by prototype virus clones [70]. It is due to this reason that such substitution is never detected or seen even after unsuccessful SOF-based treatment [113]. RASs related to NS3-4A PIs also express a low level of virus fitness; however; may be detected for some time after a specific PI treatment, but rarely occur at baseline and eventually revert to low or even undetectable levels of treatment [114]. Equivocally, RASs attributed to NNIs (non-nucleos(t)ide inhibitors)) express intermediate virus fitness that may persist after DAAs therapy but is found uncommon and irrelevant in treatment-naïve HCV patients [113]. Interestingly, RASs attributed to NS5A inhibitors show strong virus fitness (*i.e.* very minimum replication impairment; in other words, these RASs replicate very well in the variant virus clones) while competing for prototype virus clone replication and are very commonly found at baseline in treatment-naïve patients against NS5B inhibitors [115]. It has been estimated that approximately 10-15% of NS5A-associated RAS are found in HCV GT-1 patients [116]. These RASs usually persist for a long term after treatment failure with an NS5A-based DAA regimen [116]. The clinical relevance of NS5A-associated RASs is quite significant both at baseline and post-treatment levels because NS5A inhibitors are the active component of currently approved pan-genotypic DAA regimens to treat both general, as well as harder-to-treat HCV, infected populations [116].

RAS Interpretation also Contain Flaws and Cumbersome

The story does not end here just to handle the issue of RAS *vs.* RAV but the resistance testing, reporting, and interpretation are also confusing and cumbersome in literature and somehow in treatment guidelines [117]. The knowledge of RASs and information about their dealing while treating either treatment-naïve or treatment-experienced HCV patients in terms of selecting a DAA for treatment initiation according to the severity of disease (*i.e.* presence or absence of cirrhosis), altering a DAA regimen to compete for RAS, the inclusion of RBV is specific difficult-to-treat subpopulations, and most importantly to choose DAA regimens for retreatment [118]. On the flip side of the coin, the RAS impact on DAAs' treatment outcomes is also murky, where some RASs potentially affect the treatment outcomes of all DAAs including in one class, whereas some RASs have variable resistance impact on different DAAs' therapeutic outcomes within the same class [119]. In addition to that, RASs prevalence and influence on achieving SVR rates also vary in different HCV infected populations, infection kinetics, and current infection status (*i.e.*, RAS impact differently in emergence and treatment outcomes (variable SVR rates) within different HCV GTs/subtypes and quasispecies dynamics of infection), and remain more relevant for treatment-experienced and cirrhotic patients) [120].

RAS Identification is Not an Authentic Tool to Know DAAs Sensitivity or Resistance Against HCV

HCV genome sequencing identifies possible RASs but does not give any information about their effects on DAAs' sensitivity or resistance [121]. *In vitro,* DAAs susceptibility testing is difficult to do because that may introduce particular mutations into the tested HCV replicon system and reproduce the effect of different drug concentrations on virus replication [122]. At the same time, the correlation between *in vitro* data and *in vivo* significance is not perfect [123]. The traditional PCR-based Sanger sequencing (Dideoxy method; also known as population sequencing) is technically easier, robust, and straightforward, and many labs practically do it, but will only detect RASs accounting for 15% to 20% of the prevalence of the virus population [124]. Next-generation sequencing (NGS; also known as deep sequencing) is technically very sound and pragmatic to detect minority RAS species down to 1% and more likely to identify RASs unless account for at least 15% to 20% of the virus population [125]. However, it requires efficient bioinformatics expertise to interpret the sequencing data. Interestingly, it is also still ambiguous when DAA resistance testing should be recommended for HCV patients [123]. The available data collected from multiple studies about RASs are DAAs class-specific rather than individual DAAs specific and often at low threshold (1% *vs.* 15%) in difficult-to-treat or poorly defined HCV affected populations (*i.e.* HCV GT 1/subtype 1a/1b patients, T.N vs T.E, and cirrhotic *vs.* non-cirrhotic patients) [126]. With the advent and approvals of pan-genotypic DAAs regimens, baseline RAS testing is becoming almost irrelevant as these regimens are highly efficacious against almost all HCV GTs 1 through 6 infected patients [127]. Furthermore, the current treatment guidelines issued by the US FDA and AASLD-IDSA skip the resistance testing during or after the post-treatment completion of DAAs therapy except in the cases of viral breakthrough, viral relapse, or treatment failure with a pangenotypic regimen [128]. For example, NS5A RASs testing in HCV GT-1 patients with a previous treatment failure (*i.e.*, an NS5A inhibitor) and with or without hepatic cirrhosis is recommended to initiate retreatment therapy with a pan-genotypic DAA regimen (*e.g.*, either to start LDV/SOF or EBR/GZR combination as the retreatment option) [129]. Similarly, HCV GT-3 infected patients who had compensated cirrhosis and who are previously treatment-experienced (either with an NS3-4A PIs or an NS5B inhibitor with lower SVR rates) are recommended for RAS testing before initiating retreatment with a pan-genotypic regimen [129, 130]. RAS testing is also recommended in HCV GT-3 patients for the inclusion of RBV in active DAA regimens while treating decompensated cirrhotic patients [129]. Meanwhile, EASL recommendations about RAS testing raise concerns including the limited accessibility and affordability to reliable HCV RAS testing, limited consensus on the techniques used, sequencing analysis, data interpretations, and reported results [129]. On the other hand, EASL does not endorse baseline RAS testing before treatment initiation except recommending only for treatment-experienced and treatment-failure patients with PEG-IFN plus RBV, PEG-IFN plus RBV plus SOF, and SOF plus RBV-based regimens [129].

Baseline HCV Resistance Testing

Although, baseline RASs testing is not considered valuable while treating general HCV-infected populations with pan-genotypic DAAs unless the treatment outcomes reveal a potential change in clinical management [118]. For HCV GT-1b, 2, 4, and 6 affected patients, baseline RASs testing is not warranted because it does not affect the overall treatment responses [119]. However, for some harder-to-treat HCV GTs, (*e.g.*, 1a and 3) baseline RASs ultimately affect SVR rates of certain DAAs regimens in the treated population [120]. It has been reported that baseline RASs against EBR/GZR combination impair treatment response in HCV

GT-1a patients [120]. In such situations, the inclusion of weight-based RBV and extended treatment duration of up to 16 weeks will nullify the baseline RASs effects on therapy response and the patient may achieve higher SVR rates [120]. Similarly, it has been noticed that certain RASs against LDV/SOF combination affect HCV GT-1a patients' retreatment outcomes who had no treatment response to prior PEG-IFN/RBV therapy as well as in treatment-naive patients with cirrhosis [131]. Likewise, the selection of EBR/GZR as a retreatment regimen, the inclusion of RBV in the active regimen, and the extension of treatment duration in such treatment-experienced populations also neutralize the effects of baseline RAS [121]. however; the current data are limited and eagerly demand extensive clinical studies in this direction. For recently approved pan-genotypic DAA regimens (*e.g.* GLE/PIB) having a high genetic barrier to resistance and no inclusion of RBV in active regimens, the baseline RASs have minimal impact on treatment outcomes in HCV GT-1a patients [132].

In ASTRAL-3 clinical trials, baseline Y93 RAS in HCV cirrhotic patients infected with GT-3 declined SVR12 rates from 97% to 88% when administered to SOF/VEL combination [133]. Surprisingly, the same findings were not noticed in POLARIS-3 trials despite the same treatment plan of SOF/VEL administration with similar patient demographics as in ASTRAL-3 studies (*i.e.* SVR12 rates were achieved 97% without any significant decline in the presence of Y93 RAS) [134]. The reason behind this difference is not clear. The AASLD guidelines recommend the baseline Y93 RAS testing in cirrhotic patients and the addition of RBV for clinical management. The ASTRAL-4 clinical trials showed that the addition of RBV along with active regimens in GT-3 decompensated cirrhotics achieved the best response rates [135].

Equivocally, the counterarguments subside the importance of baseline RASs testing even in harder-to-treat HCV subpopulations because the treatment non-responders with baseline RASs are too small to affect the overall treatment response population percentage and it could be a potential barrier to treatment access and infection cure [136]. Similarly, testing costs, limited access in developing and poor third-world countries, and hard-to-interpret intermingled data/reports are also against the RASs testing procedures [137]. Baseline RASs might be useful at the individual patient level to impact and improve the SVR rates, although the approval of pan-genotypic regimens with a strong barrier to resistance makes it of no value in the future [138]. The reporting standard should also be needed to improve and must align clinical practice guidelines with recommended clinical management and treatment modifications (i.e, either to add RBV or extend treatment duration) [138].

HCV Retreatment is a Rare Emergency for Prior Treatment Failures with the Presence of Pre-existing, Baseline, or Treatment Acquired RASs

The phase III clinical trials and real-world clinical data of HCV-infected patients with prior treatment failure with DAA-containing regimens are promising but not so extensive that to broadly conclude or to build standard recommendations for retreatment of all HCV GTs/subtypes treatment failure patients [70]. Furthermore, the available retreatment options were evaluated in small patient cohorts, and RAS specific against one HCV protein target, and some are still under investigation for their efficacies and safety [70]. In this scenario, two big questions arise; first, does it (retreatment) work for all treatment-failure HCV subpopulations within a specific GT/subtypes, and secondly does RAS testing (either pre-existing RAS, or baseline RAS) helpful to retreat [139]. As mentioned earlier the AASLD guidelines somehow recommend RAS testing in all DAAs treatment failures before retreatment; however, the treatment strategies with current pan-genotypic DAAs regimens to overcome RAS are not accessed in large patient populations for retreatment settings [129]. For this reason, retreatment could be an emergency to manage the vulnerable HCV-infected populations with prior DAA-treatment failure as this fraction of the population would be a continuous reservoir of HCV transmission to generally unaffected individuals if remain untreated. Currently, the efficacy data of multiple salvage therapies administered to DAA-based treatment failure patients with RASs achieved excellent SVR rates that suggest their potential use in real-life situations rather than to be treated such patient populations with existing therapies or addition of RBV in active regimens [140]. However, weight-based RBV may be added for 24 weeks to retreat from SOF-based treatment failure unless contraindicated. SOF-based dual or triple DAA combination including an NS5A inhibitor (*e.g.*, velpatasvir; VEL) or the inclusion of an NS3-4A PIs (*e.g.*, voxilaprevir; VOX) along with RBV for 12 or 24 weeks are also good choices for the retreatment of previous treatment failures with first or second-generation NS3-4A PIs or NS5A inhibitors containing pre-existing or treatment-emergent RASs [140 - 142]. Likewise, for SOF and SMV failure, LDV/SOF or SOF/DCV administration for 24 weeks may achieve higher SVR rates in cirrhotic patients and including RBV, the treatment duration may shorten up to 12 weeks [143]. For SOF-RBV treatment failure, the retreatment strategies can be the inclusion of PEG-IFN (*i.e.*, SOF/ plus PEG-IFN plus RBV) for 12 weeks or with SOF/RBV for 24 weeks [143]. PEG-IFN plus RBV along with SOF is also suggested for LDV/SOF treatment failure with NS5B associated RAS for 12 weeks [143].

NS5A Associated RAS are More Prone to DAAs Resistance

As previously mentioned, RASs associated with NS5A inhibitors show maximum virus fitness and persist for a long time after treatment failure, some recently published data suggest retreatment strategies against the treatment failure of first-generation NS5A inhibitor regimens (*e.g.*, daclatasvir: DCV) [129]. In POLARIS-1 clinical trials, treatment-failure patients with an NS5A inhibitor have retreated with a combination of SOF/VEL/VOX for 12 weeks [144]. Overall SVR rates were achieved 96%, from which 83% of patients had NS3/NS5A RASs (SVR rates were achieved 97%) and 17% had no RAS (SVR rates 98%). SVR rates were achieved at 99% in non-cirrhotics, 93% in cirrhotics, and 95% in GT3 patients [144]. In contrast to POLARIS-1, POLARIS-4 studies were conducted in T.E patients who previously failed to an NS3 and/or NS5B inhibitors and were retreated with a combination of SOF/VEL/VOX or SOF/VEL for 12 weeks [145]. Overall SVR rates were achieved at 98% with SOF/VEL/VOX combination versus 90% with SOF/VEL [145]. However, the achieved SVR rates were not impacted by HCV GTs/subtypes, patient cirrhotic status, and NS3/ or NS5A-associated RASs [145]. In MAGELLAN-1 clinical trials, 16 weeks of administration of GLE/PIB combination achieved high SVR rates (*i.e.*, 100%) in HCV GT-1 patients who had a previous treatment failure with an NS5A and/or NS3-4A PIs [146]. However, the EASL guidelines recommend that this DAAs combination does not possess a high genetic barrier-to-resistance against previous treatment failures with an NS5A inhibitor and fails to achieve optimal SVR rates in treatment-experienced patients with NS5A-associated RASs [129]. In parallel to that, HCV patients without cirrhosis or having compensated cirrhosis and treatment failure with a PI and/or/NS5A inhibitor should retreat with SOF/VEL/VOX combination for 12 weeks [129]. SOF plus the fixed-dose combination of GLE/PIB should be administered for 12 weeks in patients who are predictors of lower treatment responses (*e.g.*, advanced hepatic disease, treatment-failure with multiple courses of DAA-based regimens, and having complex NS5A-associated RAS profile) [129]. For very difficult-to-cure populations based on complex RAS profiles (*e.g.*, patients with NS5A RASs who failed twice to achieve SVR rates with a PI and/or an NS5A inhibitor), the combination of SOF/VEL/VOX or SOF plus GLE/PIB can be given for 12 weeks with weight-based RBV and/or treatment duration can be prolonged from 12 to 16 or 24 weeks while excluding RBV [144].

Hepatitis B virus (HBV) Reactivation Risk with DAAs

HBV reactivation associated with severe hepatitis C flare has been increasingly recognized as a potential AEs associated with HCV DAA therapies [147]. Previous studies have demonstrated HBV reactivation with PEG-IFN-based therapy; however, in those prior cases, clinically significant HBV flare was rare [148]. The link between DAAs and the reactivation of hepatitis B virus (HBV) is very controversial; however, the clinical data and real-world findings support the phenomenal reactivation of HBV with concurrent DAAs administration in patients with a past or current HBV infection either on active treatment with anti-HBV drugs or not [149]. An ample understanding of this potential flare is still not very much clear although it is assumed that when DAAs drive an immediate drop in HCV virus, it can cause hepatitis B to flare [150]. Similarly, it is postulated that CHC infection suppresses HBV replication in patients coinfected with HCV and reciprocal interaction between these two viruses is also well characterized [151]. The cure of HCV by DAAs may result in a potential loss of immunologic control of HBV infection and result in HBV reactivation [151]. This trend has increased in the past year or so and clinicians are highly recommended that if you are treating a patient for HCV, make sure you check them for HBV infection [151]. The US FDA in 2016 reported 24 cases of confirmed reactivation of HBV infection in patients receiving DAA regimens for treatment of HCV [152]. In October 2016, the FDA issued a boxed warning on all DAAs because two patients required liver transplants or died because of HBV reactivation [152]. This safety warning by FDA was issued based on several cases reported with severe hepatitis B viremia and from published literature [152]. In addition to that, a prospective study from China also revealed 30% of HBsAg-positive patients (3 of 10) experienced a hepatitis flare with HBV reactivation versus none of the 317 who were HBsAg-negative, including 124 with occult HBV infection [153]. Overall 327 patients in an HBV-endemic area were scheduled to receive DAAs therapy for CHC infection cure. For the 3 patients who developed a hepatitis flare, the median time for onset of the flare was calculated to be 8 weeks [153]. In contrast, two retrospective studies from the US Veterans Affairs concluded that HBV reactivation is a rare event in HBV/HCV co-infection patients who are administered with HCV DAAs to cure CHC infection and most likely to occur in HBsAg-positive patients [154, 155].

HBV Screening For All HCV Affected or HBV/HCV Co-infected Patients

The US FDA advises clinicians to screen all patients for evidence of current or prior infection with the hepatitis B virus (HBV) before initiating treatment with DAAs [152]. Individuals with a positive HBsAg should receive therapy for HBV to prevent reactivation during HCV DAA therapy as this patient population has a significant risk for HBV flare with concomitant administration of HCV DAA therapy [129]. Furthermore, individuals who are anti-HBV core positive, but HBsAg and anti-HBs negative may have the risk of HBV reactivation during HCV DAA therapy, but the risk is likely significantly lower than in persons who are HBsAg positive [129]. For such patients, a quantitative HBV DNA level test is recommended before initiating anti-HBV therapy. If the HBV DNA is detectable, start the anti-HBV therapy. However, for the anti-HBs positive individuals, HBsAg negative, and anti-HB core positive, no HBV DNA testing or treatment to prevent HBV reactivation is recommended [129]. HBV reactivation monitoring is also not recommended in individuals who have a positive anti-HBs and negative anti-HB core (*i.e.* individuals who received the hepatitis B vaccine but have never been exposed to HBV infection naturally) [129].

HCV DAAs and Cancer Risk

Despite their overall efficacies and safety both in clinical trials and real-world administration to treat HCV patients, controversies still exist that whether the use of DAAs cut the risk of liver cancer, or increases the cancer risk in treated HCV patients [156]. Multiple studies point to heightened cancer risk, whereas various counter studies find no elevated cancer risk or cut the risk of liver cancer [157 - 159]. General speculation states that 'DAAs do not appear to increase the risk of liver cancer in a patient with HCV infection and cirrhosis; however, the drugs could make existing but previously undetected cancers worse and harder to treat [4]. Furthermore, advanced fibrosis and cirrhosis could be the driving factor to propagate cancer risk [159]. Clinical evidence in the literature and the buzz also generates regarding the fact that treatment with DAAs is associated with an increased recurrence rate of HCC in patients with hepatitis C cirrhosis [4, 159].

Liver Cancer Risk and HCC Recurrence with DAAs

Hepatocellular carcinoma (HCC), which has an annual incidence rate of 1%-4%, is a potential complication of HCV cirrhosis owing to a multistep carcinogenesis pathway [4]. Previous HCV treatment with IFN-based therapies was associated with poor cure rates and was limited to individuals with early fibrosis or well-compensated cirrhosis. Such therapy, however, also led to a decrease in HCC after an SVR rate [159]. Although remarkable progress has occurred in curing HCV in the current DAAs era, there is controversy regarding the associated risk of patients developing either incident (new, de novo) or recurrent HCC after DAA treatment [160]. Additional data also suggest a lower SVR rate in patients with HCC [4, 161].

Studies Evidence of No Difference in HCC Risk with DAAs

Given the IFN-era data, the assumption was that HCV cure *via* DAA treatment would also translate to a reduced incidence of HCC [162]. However, this was challenged by a 2016 publication that retrospectively compared HCV people with cirrhosis treated with DAAs. The investigators looked at 285 patients without HCC and 59 with HCC (*i.e.* previously treated and under complete response before HCV therapy) [163]. An ultrasound was performed at the end of therapy as well as 12 and 24 weeks later. At the final follow-up, HCC was detected in nine patients without previous HCC (3.16%; 95% confidence interval [CI], 1.45-5.90) and 17 with previous HCC (28.81%; 95% CI, 17.76-42.07). Given that these rates of de novo and recurrent cancers are similar to the historical data in patients with HCV cirrhosis, the study investigators concluded that SVR with DAAs does not reduce the occurrence of HCC [163]. This finding was further supported by a prospective multicentre cohort study in 2019, from Latin America regarding the risk of developing HCC after treatment with DAAs [164]. The data propose cumulative incidence and associated risk factors for de novo HCC [164]. Data from 1400 F1-F4-treated patients with DAAs (F3-F3; n= 1017) were analyzed to evaluate independent associated variables with HCC [164]. The study used Cox proportional regression models (hazard ratios (HR), and 95% CI)) to evaluate independent associated variables with HCC. The study findings describe that during a median follow-up of 16 months since DAA initiation, the overall cumulative incidence of HCC was 0.02 (CI 0.01; 0.03) at 12 months and 0.04 (CI 0.03; 0.06) at 24 months. Cumulative incidence of HCC in HCV cirrhotic patients (n = 784) was 0.03 (CI; 0.02-0.05) at 12 months and 0.06 (CI; 0.04-0.08) at 24 months of follow-up. Failure to achieve SVR was independently associated with de novo HCC with an HR of 4.9 (CI 1.44; 17.32), after adjusting for diabetes mellitus (DM), previous IFN-non-responder, CTP, and clinically significant portal hypertension [164]. SVR rates presented an overall relative risk reduction for de novo HCC of 73% (CI; 15%-91%), and 17 patients were needed to be treated to prevent one case of de novo HCC in this cohort. In addition to that, the study cautiously concluded that achieving SVR rates with DAA regimens could be significant to decrease the risk of HCC recurrence but does not eliminate the overall risks [164]. Furthermore, HCC risk remains high in HCV patients with advanced fibrosis, thus suggesting continuous surveillance strategies in this population even achieving high SVR rates after post-treatment [164].

Studies Evidence of Higher HCC Risk with DAAs

However, the research conducted in the same year (*i.e.* 2016 and 2017) by some investigators, concluded that there is a high rate of HCC recurrence following previous complete response to resection, ablation, or transarterial chemoembolization after treatment with DAAs. In a multicenter, retrospective evaluation of 77 patients with HCC under complete response before starting DAAs, the investigators noted a recurrence rate of 27.3% (21/77) with a median follow-up from the initiation of DAA therapy of 8.2 months [165]. The study was limited by the brief follow-up, small sample size, and short duration of recurrence, suggesting that recurrent tumors were developing at the initiation of HCV DAA treatment but were not causally related [165]. The major criticism of this position is that patients may have small tumors before therapy that are only detected after they complete three months of treatment. Therefore, the investigators and clinicians must complete a rigorous assessment to ensure that no residual tumor remains before DAA therapy [165].

There are other studies published as letters and small retrospective datasets that support an increased incidence of recurrent HCC after complete response, but no robust data showing an increased risk for incident tumors [166, 167]. The mechanism by which patients with cirrhosis potentially experience a higher HCC rate may be related to DAA therapy's ability to reduce the tumor-specific immune response, specifically of HCC-specific CD8+ T cells [167]. This reduced immune theory is also implicated in the risk for HBV reactivation in patients with HCV treated with DAAs [167]. In addition, an abstract described HCV's epigenetic effects, noting that the marked changes in histone modifications by chronic HCV are only partially reversed by viral cure by DAAs [168]. This abnormal transcription may drive HCC tumorigenesis.

Studies Evidence of Lower HCC Risk with DAAs

The initial data supporting a decreased HCC risk in HCV patients treated with DAA were presented at the 2016 annual meeting of the American Association for the Study of Liver Diseases [169]. The investigators found incidence rates that ranged from 0.23 per 100 person-years (PY) in patients without cirrhosis to 1.93 per 100 PY for those with cirrhosis, as compared with 2.8 per 100 PY among untreated HCV patients [169]. However, they also found that those who developed incident cancers demonstrated aggressive infiltrative and multinodular phenotypes [169].

The most robust data to support a lower rate of HCC risk with DAAs come from the French ANRS (France Recherche Nord & sud Sida-HIV Hépatites) agency. This group assessed the risk for HCC recurrence in three large prospective studies (*i.e.* HEPATHER, CirVir, and CULPIT) of HCV-infected patients treated with DAAs [170 - 173]. In the study cohorts, patients with HCC and treated by using curative procedures (hepatic resection, percutaneous ablation, or liver transplantation) were included for analysis; while those treated with chemoembolization were excluded. There was a lower rate of HCC recurrence in patients with DAAs treatment as compared with those not treated with DAAs among those in the HEPATHER (N = 267) cohort (24/189 [12.7%] vs 16/78 [20.5%]) and in the CirVir (N = 79) cohort (1/13 [7.7%] vs 31/66 [47%]). In the CUPILT (N = 314) cohort, the recurrence rate was 7/314 (2.2%). However, the study found the limitation of the registry nature of the cohort, which reduces its ability to identify relevant confounders [170, 171, 173]. The analysis of the CirVir cohort concluded that factors other than DAA treatment predict HCC recurrences, such as age older than 50 years, heavy alcohol use, and decompensated liver disease [173]. This study and other reports as mentioned above clearly demonstrate that the strongest risk for HCC development is an advanced hepatic disease (*e.g.*, advanced hepatic fibrosis (F3-F4) and cirrhosis)) [173]. Interestingly, the study findings also suggested that HCV-infected patients who were not candidates for IFN-based therapy previously because of advanced liver disease can now be treated with DAA therapy [173]. However, the patients in this cohort of study probably have a higher risk for HCC in real-life clinical settings. An additional study demonstrates a low risk of HCC dropout due to neoplastic progression in HCV-HCC patients treated with DAAs who is awaiting a liver transplant [174].

Several other abstract studies supported a lower incidence of HCC in DAAs treated patients as compared with interferon treatment [175, 176]. However, these data are limited by their retrospective single-center design, small sample sizes, and short follow-up. In a regression meta-analysis of 26 studies of liver cancer occurrence and 15 studies of hepatic cancer recurrence (3875 participants overall), the adjusted relative risk of DAA versus IFN-based treatment was 0.75 for initial hepatic cancer occurrence and 0.62 for hepatic cancer recurrence [176].

Large retrospective data of hospital populations from the Veterans Health Administration, USA also support a reduced rate of hepatic cancer in HCV patients treated with DAAs [177]. In one report, among 22,500 patients (39% with hepatic cirrhosis) from 129 institutions, patients with higher SVR rates had a significantly reduced risk for HCC (0.90 HCC/100 PY) compared with patients without SVR (3.45 HCC/100 PY; hazard ratio, 0.28; 95% CI, 0.22-0.36). In another report of 15,059 patients with advanced liver disease, HCC rates were 1.9 HCC/100 PY for patients with SVR and 11.5 HCC/100 PY for patients without SVR, an 83.5% reduction ($P < .001$) of HCC occurrence in the overall patient population.

Impact of HCC Occurrence or Recurrence on DAAs Achieved SVR rates

In addition to the potential effect of DAA treatment on HCC risk, HCC appears to affect the rate of SVR with DAA treatment [178 - 180]. In a retrospective report of 421 HCV-infected patients with cirrhosis (33% with a previous or active HCC status), 21% treatment relapse (*i.e.* failure to achieve SVR rates) was found in patients with active HCC as compared with 12% of HCV-infected patients without HCC ($P = .009$) [181]. Furthermore, in 27 out of 29 patients (93%) treatment relapse occurred only due to the presence of an active tumor. However, DAA regimens achieved excellent SVR rates in patients with an inactive tumor or after the removal of the tumor (*i.e.* resection/transplant) similar to those without HCC ($P < .0001$) [181].

In conclusion, these emerging data and comprehensive discussion about DAAs' risk of HCC occurrence or recurrence and impact on SVR rates in HCV-infected patients leave some fantabulous lessons to learn and recommendations to healthcare providers (HCPs), while treating HCV patients with current DAA regimens. Herein we briefly mention the followings;

1. The potential risk for HCC development or recurrence in HCV-infected patients (either having a previous history of HCC with treatment or active HCC) is the advanced hepatic disease (*e.g.*, advanced hepatic fibrosis (F3-F4) or decompensated cirrhosis).

2. The multicenter cohort studies and robust clinical data support a decreased incident (new, de novo) of the HCC rate in HCV-cirrhotic patients with HCV after achieving excellent SVR rates with DAA regimens.

3. Clinical data from multiple prospective and retrospective studies suggest that when individuals develop HCC after DAA therapy, tumors demonstrate a more aggressive phenotype, which appears to be an immunologic phenomenon.

4. HCV-infected patients with active HCC are more labile to achieve lower SVR rates with current DAA regimens.

Consensus Guidelines For HCV Treatment in HCV-Induced HCC Patients

The US FDA, AASLD/IDSA, EASL, and EMA recommend no treatment withhold for HCV-infected cirrhotic patients with DAA due to the risk of HCC [152]. Thorough surveillance of hepatic cancer or HCC recurrence is highly recommended immediately before initiating DAA therapy and 3 months after therapy [129]. This clinical evaluation may include; ultrasonography and alpha-fetoprotein (AFP) levels for those without HCC, and axial computer tomography (CT scan) or MRI and AFP levels for those with a history of HCC [129].

If an HCV-infected patient is diagnosed with HCC, the HCP should treat HCC first and wait 3-6 months after a complete response before initiating DAA regimens. Patients with HCV cirrhosis and HCC awaiting liver transplant should be considered for delay of HCV treatment until after transplant due to the decreased rate of SVR with HCC, the potential risk for aggressive HCC recurrence, and access to HCV-positive organ donors. HCV-infected patients with advanced fibrosis and without HCC should have ongoing monitoring for HCC after achieving SVR with DAA therapy [129].

Last but not the least, future randomized prospective trials and large database studies are eagerly needed, not only to better quantify the risk for HCC occurrence and recurrence in HCV-infected cirrhotic treatment naïve or treatment-experienced patients but also to identify HCV-infected patients who may be predisposed to the development of an aggressive HCC phenotype.

Other Clinical Challenges

HCV-infected patients with decompensated cirrhosis will remain a potential challenge even with excellent SVR outcomes in small patient cohorts with pan-genotypic DAAs in real-world clinical settings [129]. However, treatment recommendations are still precautiously recommended in HCV subtype 1a and GT-3 decompensated cirrhotic patients [182]. A couple of years ago, in the pre-DAAs era, clinicians were not able to treat these patients, and treatment with PEG-IFN plus RBV-based regimens made decompensated cirrhosis worse [182]. HCV-infected patients with renal disease are also an issue in particular HCV-infected patients who are on hemodialysis as well as patients co-infected with chronic kidney disease. It has been estimated that about 8% of dialysis patients in the United States have hepatitis C; and in some pockets of the world, that rate is closer to 40% to 50% [183]. Unfortunately, SOF-based regimens are not renal-friendly in such patient populations [184]. Recent clinical trial data about the use of EBR/GZR for 12 weeks in HCV/CKD co-infection patients showed excellent efficacy, even in patients on dialysis, who are quite sick and can better tolerate this regimen [185 - 187]. Portal hypertension could be an integral factor of mortalities in HCV cirrhotic patients [188]. However, pan-genotypic DAAs could be effective to treat HCV along with reducing the rate of portal hypertension in cirrhotic patients [189]. A recent study showed no increase in 104 patients with portal hypertension induced by HCV, and 63% experienced a reduction in hypertension while treated with current DAAs regimens [189]. Some studies suggest that catching earlier HCV-cirrhotic patients to initiate DAAs treatment, will prevent the clinical development of portal hypertension, as well as being able to reduce hypertension and all other associated complications [189]. Similarly, HCV patients with orthotopic liver transplantation should be started HCV treatment as soon as possible and not wait long for graft stability as these individuals if not started immediate treatment may progress to cirrhosis and ultimately the SVR outcomes would be lowered (*i.e.*, SVR outcomes would be similar to patients with cirrhosis and without cirrhosis, provided that the patient has developed no decompensated cirrhosis) [189].

Whether HCV patients with compensated cirrhosis who are treated with DAAs can become decompensated, is still not certain; however, the natural history of compensated cirrhosis conversion to decompensation is recorded from 4% to 7%

per year [173]. Do DAAs themselves contribute to this conversion is still uncertain and needs to figure out. We should be patient as we do not know everything about DAAs medications. Another challenge that could be faced after achieving successful SVR rates and HCV cure, is how long to follow patients after DAAs treatment. There is no clear answer and variable responses have been reported from different clinicians and care providers. Some clinicians evaluate quantitative HCV RNA levels at 1, 3, and 6 months post-DAAs therapy and hepatic fibrosis score [173]. If RNA LLOD is undetectable and the patient has fibrosis stage 0 to 2 by a FibroScan (*i.e.* transient elastography exam), the patient may discharge from further follow-ups; however, if the patient has stage 3 or 4 fibrosis, then they are kept for long-term follow-ups. For some patients with more advanced HCV-associated comorbidities (*e.g.*, decompensated cirrhosis or HCC), longer-treatment monitoring is warranted [173]. The US FDA and other treatment guidelines for DAAs administration accept SVR rates at 12 weeks post-treatment completion; however, 1% of HCV treatment relapse occurs between weeks 12 and 24, so those patients have to come back at 24 weeks for follow-ups [152].

CONCLUSIONS

A paradigm shift in the cascade of HCV care after the inclusion of pan-genotypic DAAs to treat all hepatitis C GTs and subtypes affected individuals a couple of years ago has raised the hopes to achieve the WHO ambitious goal of HCV elimination by 2030. The available real-world clinical data across the world also project their capability to treat all vulnerable, at-risk, high-risk, or vulnerable HCV-affected individuals, provided that the treatment is initiated in time, and treatment monitoring is accurate. Furthermore, disease assessment and monitoring, treatment indications, and post-treatment follow-ups also matter for successful HCV treatment. Certain challenges are still existing in real-life to overcome while linking every HCV-diagnosed one to the cascade of care and ultimately cure. Million undiagnosed HCV cases worldwide represent an important obstacle to the WHO objectives of HCV elimination by 2030. Although technical advances in HCV RDT in HCV infections are likely to improve and simplify access to testing and promote linkage to care, many vulnerable undiagnosed fractions of HCV-affected population in remote and harder-to-reach premises are still reluctant and difficult to approach for HCV diagnosis and linkage to care. Furthermore, certain pitfalls and potential gaps remain to fill between HCV diagnostic algorithms and cascade of care to find missing millions living with undiagnosed infections and to treat them respectively. DAAs cost would always be a bone of contention among manufacturers, health policymakers, government price negotiators, and procurement agencies of a country to manage their availability and accessibility. Although the current and steep innovation in DAAs development has slowed down the prices of certain DAAs in various

LMICs, nevertheless the prices are not at a level that can be easily managed by the government and health policymakers to dispense HCV-infected individuals. Hence, government, insurance companies, and the healthcare system are always under huge pressure to reimburse DAAs costs not even in many LMICs but also in resource-replete nations.

HBV reactivation is also a potential challenge and is the land on which hepatocellular carcinoma may occur in HCV/HBV coinfection patients even without reaching an end-stage liver disease and treating with pan-genotypic DAAs regimens. Its management is also cumbersome in a lot of HCV/HBV coinfection patients as many patients are reported with treatment non-adherence, loss in follow-ups, and treatment relapse even post-completion DAAs therapy. Indeed, the hypothesis of functional and virologic cure and mechanistic studies of oncogenesis propagation are desperately needed in such patient populations. Similarly, managing HCV infection in pregnancy requires assessing the risk of transmission to the baby, determining the gestational age at the time of infection, balancing mother-to-child transmission risk and sequelae, and understanding the pros and cons of treatments.

Virus fitness is still successful to evolve resistance-associated substitutions (RASs) in treated individuals even despite the advent and administration of pan-genotypic DAAs. These RASs are a potential cause of treatment failure in many individuals treated with first and second-generation NS3-4A Pis or NS5A inhibitors. Consequently, retreatment options are still fewer for previous treatment failure patients or treatment-experienced with undesirable SVRs. Furthermore, if retreatment options are not successful, those subpopulations could be a hidden reservoir of HCV transmission to other fractions of the population. After the approval of pan-genotypic DAAs to be given to HCV-infected individuals, baseline RAS testing before treatment initiation is meaningless and not recommended. Similarly, HCV genotyping/subtyping is not recommended in international guidelines for patients administering pan-genotypic DAAs. However; it is still suggested for patients with previous treatment failure with NS5A inhibitors and when the retreatment option contains an NS5A inhibitor.

The most controversial debate in HCV therapeutics with DAAs is attributed to liver cancer risk or recurrence of hepatocarcinogenesis even after HCV eradication. Intermingled, murky, and inconclusive data exist on the risk for liver cancer diminishing for patients with HCV for whom the virus is eliminated with DAA drugs, and these patients are not out of the woods, and those who do not have an SVR are at substantially higher risk of developing HCC. In contrast, multiple studies favor the lower risk of HCC occurrence or recurrence and an optimum set of studies augment no risk of hepatocarcinogenesis with DAAs.

These patients must be monitored for signs of cancer, and are usually recommended for long-term follow-ups even achieving HCV eradication with DAAs. In this decade, we must foresee novel and rapid diagnostic methods, improved management protocols, minimum effective vaccine models, and disease burden simulation studies to eliminate HCV by 2030 despite the ways paved by the pan-genotypic DAA drugs to achieve HCV cure.

REFERENCES

[1] Li DK, Chung RT. Overview of Direct-Acting Antiviral Drugs and Drug Resistance of Hepatitis C Virus. Methods Mol Biol 2019; 1911: 3-32.
[http://dx.doi.org/10.1007/978-1-4939-8976-8_1] [PMID: 30593615]

[2] de Gennaro N, Diella L, Monno L, Angarano G, Milella M, Saracino A. Efficacy and tolerability of DAAs in HCV-monoinfected and HCV/HIV-coinfected patients with psychiatric disorders. BMC Infect Dis 2020; 20(1): 196.
[http://dx.doi.org/10.1186/s12879-020-4922-2] [PMID: 32138757]

[3] Shahid I, Ibrahim MM. All oral interferon-free direct-acting antivirals as combination therapies to cure Hepatitis C. Curr Mol Med 2019; 18(7): 409-35.
[http://dx.doi.org/10.2174/1566524019666190104110439] [PMID: 30608042]

[4] Shahid I, AlMalki WH, Hassan S, Hafeez MH. Real-world challenges for hepatitis C virus medications: a critical overview. Crit Rev Microbiol 2018; 44(2): 143-60.
[http://dx.doi.org/10.1080/1040841X.2017.1329277] [PMID: 28539069]

[5] Scotto R, Buonomo AR, Moriello NS, *et al.* Real-World Efficacy and Safety of Pangenotypic Direct-Acting Antivirals Against Hepatitis C Virus Infection. Rev Recent Clin Trials 2019; 14(3): 173-82.
[http://dx.doi.org/10.2174/1574887114666190306154650] [PMID: 30848211]

[6] Chang KC, Tung SY, Wei KL, *et al.* Real-world efficacy and safety of pangenotypic direct-acting antivirals against hepatitis C virus infection in Taiwan. Sci Rep 2021; 11(1): 13543.
[http://dx.doi.org/10.1038/s41598-021-93095-x] [PMID: 34188161]

[7] Gayam V, Hossain MR, Khalid M, *et al.* Real-World Clinical Efficacy and Tolerability of Direct-Acting Antivirals in Hepatitis C Monoinfection Compared to Hepatitis C/Human Immunodeficiency Virus Coinfection in a Community Care Setting. Gut Liver 2018; 12(6): 694-703.
[http://dx.doi.org/10.5009/gnl18004] [PMID: 29938459]

[8] Hézode C. Treatment of hepatitis C: Results in real life. Liver international : official journal of the International Association for the Study of the Liver. 2018;38 Suppl 1:21-7.

[9] Martin MT, Deming P. Closing the Gap: The Challenges of Treating Hepatitis C Virus Genotype 3 Infection. Pharmacotherapy 2017; 37(6): 735-47.
[http://dx.doi.org/10.1002/phar.1933] [PMID: 28374965]

[10] Charatcharoenwitthaya P, Wongpaitoon V, Komolmit P, *et al.* Real-world effectiveness and safety of sofosbuvir and nonstructural protein 5A inhibitors for chronic hepatitis C genotype 1, 2, 3, 4, or 6: a multicentre cohort study. BMC Gastroenterol 2020; 20(1): 47.
[http://dx.doi.org/10.1186/s12876-020-01196-0] [PMID: 32138687]

[11] Baatarkhuu O, Lee JS, Amarsanaa J, *et al.* Efficacy and safety of ledipasvir/sofosbuvir in 5,028 Mongolian patients infected with genotype 1 hepatitis C virus: A multicenter study. Clin Mol Hepatol 2021; 27(1): 125-35.
[http://dx.doi.org/10.3350/cmh.2020.0023] [PMID: 33242929]

[12] Dietz J, Vermehren J, Matschenz K, Buggisch P, Klinker H, Schulze Zur Wiesch J, *et al.* Treatment outcomes in hepatitis C virus genotype 1a infected patients with and without baseline NS5A resistance-associated substitutions. Liver international : official journal of the International

Association for the Study of the Liver. 2020.

[13] Macken L, Gelson W, Priest M, *et al.* Efficacy of direct-acting antivirals: UK real-world data from a well-characterised predominantly cirrhotic HCV cohort. J Med Virol 2019; 91(11): 1979-88. [http://dx.doi.org/10.1002/jmv.25552] [PMID: 31329295]

[14] Michienzi S, Burgos R, Smith R, Martin M. 2236. Direct-Acting Antivirals: Efficacy in a Real-World, Urban, Undeserved, HIV-HCV Co-Infected Population. Open Forum Infect Dis 2018; 5 (Suppl. 1): S661-2.
[http://dx.doi.org/10.1093/ofid/ofy210.1889]

[15] Vibhakar S, Nowicki D, Huhn G, Goldberg R, Adeyemi O. A Collaborative Drug Therapy Management Model for the Treatment of Hepatitis C Virus (HCV) in an Urban Clinic. Open forum infectious diseases. 2018; 5(suppl_1): S661-S.

[16] Cornberg M, Petersen J, Schober A, *et al.* Real-world use, effectiveness and safety of anti-viral treatment in chronic hepatitis C genotype 3 infection. Aliment Pharmacol Ther 2017; 45(5): 688-700. [http://dx.doi.org/10.1111/apt.13925] [PMID: 28078723]

[17] Alonso S, Riveiro-Barciela M, Fernandez I, *et al.* Effectiveness and safety of sofosbuvir-based regimens plus an NS5A inhibitor for patients with HCV genotype 3 infection and cirrhosis. Results of a multicenter real-life cohort. J Viral Hepat 2017; 24(4): 304-11.
[http://dx.doi.org/10.1111/jvh.12648] [PMID: 27935168]

[18] Milazzo L, Lai A, Calvi E, *et al.* Direct-acting antivirals in hepatitis C virus (HCV)-infected and HCV/HIV-coinfected patients: real-life safety and efficacy. HIV Med 2017; 18(4): 284-91.
[http://dx.doi.org/10.1111/hiv.12429] [PMID: 27477612]

[19] Villani R, Donatiello I, Barone F, Cavallone F, Fioravanti G, Cosimo F, *et al.* Efficacy and safety of direct-acting antivirals in elderly with chronic hepatitis C: Results from a retrospective cohort study. Journal of Gerontology and Geriatrics 2018; 66: 46-55.

[20] Naganuma A, Sato K, Fukuchi T, *et al.* Successful prolonged treatment of glecaprevir/pibrentasvir for chronic hepatitis C patient with treatment failure after 8-week therapy: a case report. Clin J Gastroenterol 2019; 12(6): 592-7.
[http://dx.doi.org/10.1007/s12328-019-01029-y] [PMID: 31376076]

[21] Sho T, Suda G, Kimura M, *et al.* Glecaprevir and pibrentasvir for japanese patients with human immunodeficiency virus and genotype 3 hepatitis c virus coinfection: a report of three cases. Intern Med 2019; 58(6): 797-802.
[http://dx.doi.org/10.2169/internalmedicine.1856-18] [PMID: 30449808]

[22] Kjellin M, Kileng H, Akaberi D, *et al.* Effect of the baseline Y93H resistance-associated substitution in HCV genotype 3 for direct-acting antiviral treatment: real-life experience from a multicenter study in Sweden and Norway. Scand J Gastroenterol 2019; 54(8): 1042-50.
[http://dx.doi.org/10.1080/00365521.2019.1652846] [PMID: 31424972]

[23] Belperio PS, Shahoumian TA, Loomis TP, Backus LI. Real-world effectiveness of sofosbuvir/velpatasvir/voxilaprevir in 573 direct-acting antiviral experienced hepatitis C patients. J Viral Hepat 2019; 26(8): jvh.13115.
[http://dx.doi.org/10.1111/jvh.13115] [PMID: 31012179]

[24] Ferenci P, Bourgeois S, Buggisch P, *et al.* Real-world safety and effectiveness of ombitasvir/paritaprevir/ritonavir ± dasabuvir ± ribavirin in hepatitis C virus genotype 1- and 4-infected patients with diverse comorbidities and comedications: A pooled analysis of post-marketing observational studies from 13 countries. J Viral Hepat 2019; 26(6): 685-96.
[http://dx.doi.org/10.1111/jvh.13080] [PMID: 30739368]

[25] Idilman R, Demir M, Aladag M, *et al.* Low recurrence rate of hepatocellular carcinoma following ledipasvir and sofosbuvir treatment in a real-world chronic hepatitis C patients cohort. J Viral Hepat 2019; 26(6): 666-74.
[http://dx.doi.org/10.1111/jvh.13075] [PMID: 30740820]

[26] Mangia A, Cenderello G, Copetti M, *et al.* SVR12 Higher than 97% in GT3 Cirrhotic Patients with Evidence of Portal Hypertension Treated with SOF/VEL without Ribavirin: A Nation-Wide Cohort Study. Cells 2019; 8(4): 313.
[http://dx.doi.org/10.3390/cells8040313] [PMID: 30987413]

[27] Hu C, Yuan G, Liu J, *et al.* Sofosbuvir-based therapies for patients with hepatitis c virus infection: real-world experience in China. Can J Gastroenterol Hepatol 2018; 2018: 1-8.
[http://dx.doi.org/10.1155/2018/3908767] [PMID: 30538973]

[28] Cardona-Gonzalez MG, Goldman JD, Narayan L, Brainard DM, Kowdley KV. Sofosbuvir, velpatasvir, and voxilaprevir for treatment of recurrent hepatitis c virus infection after liver transplantation. Hepatol Commun 2018; 2(12): 1446-50.
[http://dx.doi.org/10.1002/hep4.1280] [PMID: 30556034]

[29] Yanny B, Saab S, Durazo F, *et al.* Eight-Week Hepatitis C Treatment with New Direct Acting Antivirals Has a Better Safety Profile While Being Effective in the Treatment-Naïve Geriatric Population Without Liver Cirrhosis and Hepatitis C Virus-RNA < 6 Million IU/mL. Dig Dis Sci 2018; 63(12): 3480-6.
[http://dx.doi.org/10.1007/s10620-018-5283-1] [PMID: 30259281]

[30] Canini L, Imamura M, Kawakami Y, *et al.* HCV kinetic and modeling analyses project shorter durations to cure under combined therapy with daclatasvir and asunaprevir in chronic HCV-infected patients. PLoS One 2017; 12(12): e0187409.
[http://dx.doi.org/10.1371/journal.pone.0187409] [PMID: 29216198]

[31] Hernández-Conde M, Fernández I, Perelló C, *et al.* Effectiveness and safety of elbasvir/grazoprevir therapy in patients with chronic HCV infection: Results from the Spanish HEPA-C real-world cohort. J Viral Hepat 2019; 26(1): 55-64.
[http://dx.doi.org/10.1111/jvh.13008] [PMID: 30265418]

[32] Barcaui HS, Tavares GC, May SB, Brandão-Mello CE, Amendola Pires MM, Barroso PF. Low rates of sustained virologic response with peginterferon plus ribavirin for chronic hepatitis C virus infection in HIV infected patients in Rio de Janeiro, Brazil. PLoS One 2013; 8(7): e67734.
[http://dx.doi.org/10.1371/journal.pone.0067734] [PMID: 23874441]

[33] Rumi MG, Occhipinti V. Editorial: real-life data confirm efficacy of elbasvir/grazoprevir in HCV patients with severe kidney disease. Aliment Pharmacol Ther 2018; 48(2): 226-7.
[http://dx.doi.org/10.1111/apt.14792] [PMID: 29939410]

[34] Gayam V, Khalid M, Mandal AK, *et al.* Direct-Acting Antivirals in Chronic Hepatitis C Genotype 4 Infection in Community Care Setting. Gastroenterol Res 2018; 11(2): 130-7.
[http://dx.doi.org/10.14740/gr999w] [PMID: 29707080]

[35] Prasad N, Patel MR, Pandey A, *et al.* Direct-acting antiviral agents in Hepatitis C Virus-infected renal allograft recipients: Treatment and outcome experience from single center. Indian J Nephrol 2018; 28(3): 220-5.
[http://dx.doi.org/10.4103/ijn.IJN_190_17] [PMID: 29962673]

[36] Toyoda H, Atsukawa M, Takaguchi K, *et al.* Real-world virological efficacy and safety of elbasvir and grazoprevir in patients with chronic hepatitis C virus genotype 1 infection in Japan. J Gastroenterol 2018; 53(12): 1276-84.
[http://dx.doi.org/10.1007/s00535-018-1473-z] [PMID: 29740665]

[37] Isakov V, Gankina N, Morozov V, *et al.* Ledipasvir Sofosbuvir for 8 Weeks in Non-Cirrhotic Patients with Previously Untreated Genotype 1 HCV Infection ± HIV-1 Co-Infection. Clin Drug Investig 2018; 38(3): 239-47.
[http://dx.doi.org/10.1007/s40261-017-0606-0] [PMID: 29177645]

[38] Kramer JR, Puenpatom A, Erickson KF, *et al.* Real-world effectiveness of elbasvir/grazoprevir In HCV-infected patients in the US veterans affairs healthcare system. J Viral Hepat 2018; 25(11): 1270-9.

[http://dx.doi.org/10.1111/jvh.12937] [PMID: 29851265]

[39] Manoj K, Nayak SL, Gupta E, Kataria A, Sarin SK. Generic sofosbuvir-based direct-acting antivirals in hepatitis C virus-infected patients with chronic kidney disease. Liver international : official journal of the International Association for the Study of the Liver. 2018; 38(12): 2137-48. [http://dx.doi.org/10.1111/liv.13863]

[40] Puigvehí M, De Cuenca B, Viu A, Diago M, Turnes J, Gea F, *et al.* Eight weeks of Paritaprevir/r/Ombitasvir + Dasabuvir in HCV genotype 1b with mild-moderate fibrosis: Results from a real-world cohort. Liver international : official journal of the International Association for the Study of the Liver. 2019; 39(1): 90-7.

[41] Berenguer J, Gil-Martin Á, Jarrin I, *et al.* All-oral direct-acting antiviral therapy against hepatitis C virus (HCV) in human immunodeficiency virus/HCV-coinfected subjects in real-world practice: Madrid coinfection registry findings. Hepatology 2018; 68(1): 32-47. [http://dx.doi.org/10.1002/hep.29814] [PMID: 29377274]

[42] Abdel Ghaffar TY, El Naghi S, Abdel Gawad M, *et al.* Safety and efficacy of combined sofosbuvir/daclatasvir treatment of children and adolescents with chronic hepatitis C Genotype 4. J Viral Hepat 2019; 26(2): 263-70. [http://dx.doi.org/10.1111/jvh.13032] [PMID: 30380158]

[43] Miotto N, Mendes LC, Zanaga LP, *et al.* All-oral direct antiviral treatment for hepatitis C chronic infection in a real-life cohort: The role of cirrhosis and comorbidities in treatment response. PLoS One 2018; 13(7): e0199941. [http://dx.doi.org/10.1371/journal.pone.0199941] [PMID: 29990371]

[44] Haridy J, Wigg A, Muller K, *et al.* Real-world outcomes of unrestricted direct-acting antiviral treatment for hepatitis C in Australia: The South Australian statewide experience. J Viral Hepat 2018; 25(11): 1287-97. [http://dx.doi.org/10.1111/jvh.12943] [PMID: 29888827]

[45] Naganuma A, Chayama K, Notsumata K, *et al.* Integrated analysis of 8-week glecaprevir/pibrentasvir in Japanese and overseas patients without cirrhosis and with hepatitis C virus genotype 1 or 2 infection. J Gastroenterol 2019; 54(8): 752-61. [http://dx.doi.org/10.1007/s00535-019-01569-7] [PMID: 30868245]

[46] Tacke F, Günther R, Buggisch P, Klinker H, Schober A, John C, *et al.* Treatment of HCV genotype 2 with sofosbuvir and ribavirin results in lower sustained virological response rates in real life than expected from clinical trials. Liver international : official journal of the International Association for the Study of the Liver. 2017; 37(2): 205-11. [http://dx.doi.org/10.1111/liv.13206]

[47] Bichoupan K, Tandon N, Crismale JF, *et al.* Real-world cure rates for hepatitis C virus treatments that include simeprevir and/or sofosbuvir are comparable to clinical trial results. World J Virol 2017; 6(4): 59-72. [http://dx.doi.org/10.5501/wjv.v6.i4.59] [PMID: 29147645]

[48] Shin HP, Burman B, Kozarek RA, *et al.* Real-World Single-Center Experience with Sofosbuvir-Based Regimens for the Treatment of Chronic Hepatitis C Genotype 1 Patients. Gut Liver 2017; 11(5): 711-20. [http://dx.doi.org/10.5009/gnl16447] [PMID: 28651301]

[49] Shahid I, Alzahrani AR, Al-Ghamdi SS, Alanazi IM, Rehman S, Hassan S. Hepatitis C Diagnosis: Simplified Solutions, Predictive Barriers, and Future Promises. Diagnostics (Basel, Switzerland). 2021; 11, 7.

[50] Gowda C, Lott S, Grigorian M, *et al.* Absolute Insurer Denial of Direct-Acting Antiviral Therapy for Hepatitis C: A National Specialty Pharmacy Cohort Study. Open Forum Infect Dis 2018; 5(6): ofy076. [http://dx.doi.org/10.1093/ofid/ofy076] [PMID: 29977955]

[51] Barber MJ, Gotham D, Khwairakpam G, Hill A. Price of a hepatitis C cure: Cost of production and

current prices for direct-acting antivirals in 50 countries. J Virus Erad 2020; 6(3): 100001. [http://dx.doi.org/10.1016/j.jve.2020.06.001] [PMID: 33251019]

[52] Hill A, Khwairakpam G, Wang J, *et al.* High sustained virological response rates using imported generic direct acting antiviral treatment for hepatitis C. J Virus Erad 2017; 3(4): 200-3. [http://dx.doi.org/10.1016/S2055-6640(20)30324-1] [PMID: 29057082]

[53] Hill A, Khoo S, Fortunak J, Simmons B, Ford N. Minimum costs for producing hepatitis C direct-acting antivirals for use in large-scale treatment access programs in developing countries. Clin Infect Dis 2014; 58(7): 928-36. [http://dx.doi.org/10.1093/cid/ciu012] [PMID: 24399087]

[54] Hill AM, Nath S, Simmons B. The road to elimination of hepatitis C: analysis of cures versus new infections in 91 countries. J Virus Erad 2017; 3(3): 117-23. [http://dx.doi.org/10.1016/S2055-6640(20)30329-0] [PMID: 28758018]

[55] Marshall AD, Cunningham EB, Nielsen S, *et al.* Restrictions for reimbursement of interferon-free direct-acting antiviral drugs for HCV infection in Europe. Lancet Gastroenterol Hepatol 2018; 3(2): 125-33. [http://dx.doi.org/10.1016/S2468-1253(17)30284-4] [PMID: 28986139]

[56] Kochneva G, Kartashov M, Krivosheina E, Kuznetsov AI, Chub E, Sivolobova GF, *et al.* On the possibility of eradicating hepatitis C in Russia. Mol Gen Microbiol Virol 2021; 39: 31.

[57] He T, Lopez-Olivo MA, Hur C, Chhatwal J. Systematic review: cost-effectiveness of direct-acting antivirals for treatment of hepatitis C genotypes 2-6. Aliment Pharmacol Ther 2017; 46(8): 711-21. [http://dx.doi.org/10.1111/apt.14271] [PMID: 28836278]

[58] Shahid I, ALMalki WH, Hafeez MH, Hassan S. Hepatitis C virus infection treatment: An era of game changer direct acting antivirals and novel treatment strategies. Crit Rev Microbiol 2016; 42(4): 535-47. [http://dx.doi.org/10.3109/1040841X.2014.970123] [PMID: 25373616]

[59] Schillie S, Wester C, Osborne M, Wesolowski L, Ryerson AB. CDC Recommendations for Hepatitis C Screening Among Adults - United States, 2020. MMWR Recommendations and reports : Morbidity and mortality weekly report Recommendations and reports. 2020; 69(2): 1-17.

[60] HCV Guideline Committee of the New York State Department of Health AIDS Institute (NYSDOH AI). Treatment of Chronic HCV with Direct-Acting Antivirals. Baltimore (MD): Johns Hopkins University; 2020. Available from: https://www.ncbi.nlm.nih.gov/books/NBK559965/.

[61] Kosloski MP, Oberoi R, Wang S, *et al.* Drug-Drug Interactions of Glecaprevir and Pibrentasvir Coadministered With Human Immunodeficiency Virus Antiretrovirals. J Infect Dis 2020; 221(2): 223-31. [http://dx.doi.org/10.1093/infdis/jiz439] [PMID: 31504702]

[62] Vega AD, Hynicka LM, Claeys K, Chua JV, Heil EL. Effectiveness of 8 weeks of ledipasvir/sofosbuvir for hepatitis C in HCV-HIV-coinfected patients. Antivir Ther 2019; 24(1): 11-7. [http://dx.doi.org/10.3851/IMP3263] [PMID: 30192231]

[63] Soeiro CASP, Gonçalves CAM, Marques MSC, *et al.* Glomerular filtration rate change during chronic hepatitis C treatment with Sofosbuvir/Ledipasvir in HCV/HIV Coinfected patients treated with Tenofovir and a boosted protease inhibitor: an observational prospective study. BMC Infect Dis 2018; 18(1): 364. [http://dx.doi.org/10.1186/s12879-018-3278-3] [PMID: 30075765]

[64] Gao LH, Nie QH, Zhao XT. Drug drug interactions of newly approved direct-acting antiviral agents in patients with Hepatitis C. Int J Gen Med 2021; 14: 289-301. [http://dx.doi.org/10.2147/IJGM.S283910] [PMID: 33536776]

[65] Bunnell KL, Vibhakar S, Glowacki RC, Gallagher MA, Osei AM, Huhn G. Nephrotoxicity associated with concomitant use of ledipasvir-sofosbuvir and tenofovir in a patient with hepatitis c virus and

human immunodeficiency virus coinfection. Pharmacotherapy 2016; 36(9): e148-53. [http://dx.doi.org/10.1002/phar.1803] [PMID: 27459733]

[66] Abutaleb A, Sherman KE. A changing paradigm: management and treatment of the HCV/HIV-co-infected patient. Hepatol Int 2018; 12(6): 500-9. [http://dx.doi.org/10.1007/s12072-018-9896-4] [PMID: 30238230]

[67] Shahid I, Almalki WH, Ibrahim MM, *et al.* Characterization of *in vitro* inhibitory effects of consensus short interference RNAs against non-structural 5B gene of hepatitis C virus 1a genotype. Indian J Med Microbiol 2018; 36(4): 494-503. [http://dx.doi.org/10.4103/ijmm.IJMM_17_146] [PMID: 30880695]

[68] AlMalki WH, Shahid I, Abdalla AN, Johargy AK, Ahmed M, Hassan S. Virological surveillance, molecular phylogeny, and evolutionary dynamics of hepatitis C virus subtypes 1a and 4a isolates in patients from Saudi Arabia. Saudi J Biol Sci 2021; 28(3): 1664-77. [http://dx.doi.org/10.1016/j.sjbs.2020.11.089] [PMID: 33732052]

[69] AlMalki WH, Shahid I, Abdalla AN, Johargy AK, Ahmed M, Hassan S. Consensus small interfering RNA targeted to stem-loops II and III of IRES structure of 5′ UTR effectively inhibits virus replication and translation of HCV sub-genotype 4a isolates from Saudi Arabia. Saudi J Biol Sci 2021; 28(1): 1109-22. [http://dx.doi.org/10.1016/j.sjbs.2020.11.041] [PMID: 33424405]

[70] Sagnelli E, Starace M, Minichini C, *et al.* Resistance detection and re-treatment options in hepatitis C virus-related chronic liver diseases after DAA-treatment failure. Infection 2018; 46(6): 761-83. [http://dx.doi.org/10.1007/s15010-018-1188-3] [PMID: 30084057]

[71] Di Stefano M, Faleo G, Farhan Mohamed AM, *et al.* Resistance Associated Mutations in HCV Patients Failing DAA Treatment. New Microbiol 2021; 44(1): 12-8. [PMID: 33453702]

[72] Paolucci S, Premoli M, Novati S, *et al.* Baseline and Breakthrough Resistance Mutations in HCV Patients Failing DAAs. Sci Rep 2017; 7(1): 16017. [http://dx.doi.org/10.1038/s41598-017-15987-1] [PMID: 29167469]

[73] Sorbo MC, Cento V, Di Maio VC, Howe AYM, Garcia F, Perno CF, *et al.* Hepatitis C virus drug resistance associated substitutions and their clinical relevance: Update 2018. Drug resistance updates : reviews and commentaries in antimicrobial and anticancer chemotherapy. 2018; 37: 17-39.

[74] Paolucci S, Fiorina L, Piralla A, *et al.* Naturally occurring mutations to HCV protease inhibitors in treatment-naïve patients. Virol J 2012; 9(1): 245. [http://dx.doi.org/10.1186/1743-422X-9-245] [PMID: 23095680]

[75] Costantino A, Spada E, Equestre M, *et al.* Naturally occurring mutations associated with resistance to HCV NS5B polymerase and NS3 protease inhibitors in treatment-naïve patients with chronic hepatitis C. Virol J 2015; 12(1): 186. [http://dx.doi.org/10.1186/s12985-015-0414-1] [PMID: 26577836]

[76] Wei B, Kang J, Kibukawa M, *et al.* Development and Validation of a Template-Independent Next-Generation Sequencing Assay for Detecting Low-Level Resistance-Associated Variants of Hepatitis C Virus. J Mol Diagn 2016; 18(5): 643-56. [http://dx.doi.org/10.1016/j.jmoldx.2016.04.001] [PMID: 27393904]

[77] Di Maio VC, Cento V, Lenci I, Aragri M, Rossi P, Barbaliscia S, *et al.* Multiclass HCV resistance to direct-acting antiviral failure in real-life patients advocates for tailored second-line therapies 2017. [http://dx.doi.org/10.1111/liv.13327]

[78] Verbinnen T, Van Marck H, Vandenbroucke I, *et al.* Tracking the evolution of multiple *in vitro* hepatitis C virus replicon variants under protease inhibitor selection pressure by 454 deep sequencing. J Virol 2010; 84(21): 11124-33. [http://dx.doi.org/10.1128/JVI.01217-10] [PMID: 20739521]

[79] Boglione L, De Nicolò A, Cardellino CS, Ruggiero T, Ghisetti V, Cariti G, *et al.* Relationship between the early boceprevir-S isomer plasma concentrations and the onset of breakthrough during HCV genotype 1 triple therapy 2015.
[http://dx.doi.org/10.1016/j.cmi.2014.07.009]

[80] Kumada H, Chayama K, Rodrigues L Jr, *et al.* Randomized phase 3 trial of ombitasvir/paritaprevir/ritonavir for hepatitis C virus genotype 1b infected Japanese patients with or without cirrhosis. Hepatology 2015; 62(4): 1037-46.
[http://dx.doi.org/10.1002/hep.27972] [PMID: 26147154]

[81] McPhee F, Hernandez D, Yu F, *et al.* Resistance analysis of hepatitis C virus genotype 1 prior treatment null responders receiving daclatasvir and asunaprevir. Hepatology 2013; 58(3): 902-11.
[http://dx.doi.org/10.1002/hep.26388] [PMID: 23504694]

[82] Lenz O, Verbinnen T, Fevery B, *et al.* Virology analyses of HCV isolates from genotype 1-infected patients treated with simeprevir plus peginterferon/ribavirin in Phase IIb/III studies. J Hepatol 2015; 62(5): 1008-14.
[http://dx.doi.org/10.1016/j.jhep.2014.11.032] [PMID: 25445400]

[83] Ruggiero T, Proietti A, Boglione L, *et al.* Predominance of hepatitis C virus Q80K among NS3 baseline-resistance-associated amino acid variants in direct-antiviral-agent-naïve patients with chronic hepatitis: single-centre experience. Arch Virol 2015; 160(11): 2881-5.
[http://dx.doi.org/10.1007/s00705-015-2563-3] [PMID: 26249823]

[84] Dietz J, Susser S, Vermehren J, *et al.* Patterns of resistance-associated substitutions in patients with chronic hcv infection following treatment with direct-acting antivirals. Gastroenterology 2018; 154(4): 976-988.e4.
[http://dx.doi.org/10.1053/j.gastro.2017.11.007] [PMID: 29146520]

[85] Jensen SB, Serre SBN, Humes DG, *et al.* Substitutions at NS3 residue 155, 156, or 168 of hepatitis c virus genotypes 2 to 6 induce complex patterns of protease inhibitor resistance. Antimicrob Agents Chemother 2015; 59(12): 7426-36.
[http://dx.doi.org/10.1128/AAC.01953-15] [PMID: 26392503]

[86] Soumana DI, Ali A, Schiffer CA. Structural analysis of asunaprevir resistance in HCV NS3/4A protease. ACS Chem Biol 2014; 9(11): 2485-90.
[http://dx.doi.org/10.1021/cb5006118] [PMID: 25243902]

[87] Suzuki Y, Ikeda K, Suzuki F, *et al.* Dual oral therapy with daclatasvir and asunaprevir for patients with HCV genotype 1b infection and limited treatment options. J Hepatol 2013; 58(4): 655-62.
[http://dx.doi.org/10.1016/j.jhep.2012.09.037] [PMID: 23183526]

[88] Ali A, Aydin C, Gildemeister R, *et al.* Evaluating the role of macrocycles in the susceptibility of hepatitis C virus NS3/4A protease inhibitors to drug resistance. ACS Chem Biol 2013; 8(7): 1469-78.
[http://dx.doi.org/10.1021/cb400100g] [PMID: 23594083]

[89] Verbinnen T, Fevery B, Vijgen L, Jacobs T, De Meyer S, Lenz O. *In Vitro* Activity of Simeprevir against Hepatitis C Virus Genotype 1 Clinical Isolates and Its Correlation with NS3 Sequence and Site-Directed Mutants. Antimicrob Agents Chemother 2015; 59(12): 7548-57.
[http://dx.doi.org/10.1128/AAC.01444-15] [PMID: 26392483]

[90] Pilot-Matias T, Tripathi R, Cohen D, *et al. In vitro* and *in vivo* antiviral activity and resistance profile of the hepatitis C virus NS3/4A protease inhibitor ABT-450. Antimicrob Agents Chemother 2015; 59(2): 988-97.
[http://dx.doi.org/10.1128/AAC.04227-14] [PMID: 25451053]

[91] Fridell RA, Qiu D, Valera L, Wang C, Rose RE, Gao M. Distinct functions of NS5A in hepatitis C virus RNA replication uncovered by studies with the NS5A inhibitor BMS-790052. J Virol 2011; 85(14): 7312-20.
[http://dx.doi.org/10.1128/JVI.00253-11] [PMID: 21593143]

[92] Lontok E, Harrington P, Howe A, *et al.* Hepatitis C virus drug resistance-associated substitutions: State of the art summary. Hepatology 2015; 62(5): 1623-32.
[http://dx.doi.org/10.1002/hep.27934] [PMID: 26095927]

[93] Zeuzem S, Foster GR, Wang S, *et al.* Glecaprevir Pibrentasvir for 8 or 12 Weeks in HCV Genotype 1 or 3 Infection. N Engl J Med 2018; 378(4): 354-69.
[http://dx.doi.org/10.1056/NEJMoa1702417] [PMID: 29365309]

[94] Karino Y, Toyota J, Ikeda K, *et al.* Characterization of virologic escape in hepatitis C virus genotype 1b patients treated with the direct-acting antivirals daclatasvir and asunaprevir. J Hepatol 2013; 58(4): 646-54.
[http://dx.doi.org/10.1016/j.jhep.2012.11.012] [PMID: 23178977]

[95] Asselah T, Reesink H, Gerstoft J, de Ledinghen V, Pockros PJ, Robertson M, *et al.* Efficacy of elbasvir and grazoprevir in participants with hepatitis C virus genotype 4 infection: A pooled analysis 2018.
[http://dx.doi.org/10.1111/liv.13727]

[96] Walker J, Crosby R, Wang A, *et al.* Preclinical characterization of GSK2336805, a novel inhibitor of hepatitis C virus replication that selects for resistance in NS5A. Antimicrob Agents Chemother 2014; 58(1): 38-47.
[http://dx.doi.org/10.1128/AAC.01363-13] [PMID: 24126581]

[97] Wong KA, Worth A, Martin R, *et al.* Characterization of Hepatitis C virus resistance from a multiple-dose clinical trial of the novel NS5A inhibitor GS-5885. Antimicrob Agents Chemother 2013; 57(12): 6333-40.
[http://dx.doi.org/10.1128/AAC.02193-12] [PMID: 23877691]

[98] Zhou N, Hernandez D, Ueland J, *et al.* NS5A Sequence Heterogeneity and Mechanisms of Daclatasvir Resistance in Hepatitis C Virus Genotype 4 Infection. J Infect Dis 2016; 213(2): 206-15.
[http://dx.doi.org/10.1093/infdis/jiv379] [PMID: 26170396]

[99] Wang C, Valera L, Jia L, Kirk MJ, Gao M, Fridell RA. In vitro activity of daclatasvir on hepatitis C virus genotype 3 NS5A. Antimicrob Agents Chemother 2013; 57(1): 611-3.
[http://dx.doi.org/10.1128/AAC.01874-12] [PMID: 23089758]

[100] Zhou N, Han Z, Hartman-Neumann S, *et al.* Characterization of NS5A polymorphisms and their impact on response rates in patients with HCV genotype 2 treated with daclatasvir-based regimens. J Antimicrob Chemother 2016; 71(12): 3495-505.
[http://dx.doi.org/10.1093/jac/dkw336] [PMID: 27605597]

[101] Wang C, Jia L, Huang H, *et al.* In vitro activity of BMS-790052 on hepatitis C virus genotype 4 NS5A. Antimicrob Agents Chemother 2012; 56(3): 1588-90.
[http://dx.doi.org/10.1128/AAC.06169-11] [PMID: 22203595]

[102] Hernandez D, Zhou N, Ueland J, Monikowski A, McPhee F. Natural prevalence of NS5A polymorphisms in subjects infected with hepatitis C virus genotype 3 and their effects on the antiviral activity of NS5A inhibitors 2013.
[http://dx.doi.org/10.1016/j.jcv.2012.12.020]

[103] Lahser FC, Bystol K, Curry S, *et al.* The Combination of Grazoprevir, a Hepatitis C Virus (HCV) NS3/4A Protease Inhibitor, and Elbasvir, an HCV NS5A Inhibitor, Demonstrates a High Genetic Barrier to Resistance in HCV Genotype 1a Replicons. Antimicrob Agents Chemother 2016; 60(5): 2954-64.
[http://dx.doi.org/10.1128/AAC.00051-16] [PMID: 26926625]

[104] Rockstroh JK, Nelson M, Katlama C, *et al.* Efficacy and safety of grazoprevir (MK-5172) and elbasvir (MK-8742) in patients with hepatitis C virus and HIV co-infection (C-EDGE CO-INFECTION): a non-randomised, open-label trial. Lancet HIV 2015; 2(8): e319-27.
[http://dx.doi.org/10.1016/S2352-3018(15)00114-9] [PMID: 26423374]

[105] Fridell RA, Wang C, Sun JH, *et al.* Genotypic and phenotypic analysis of variants resistant to hepatitis C virus nonstructural protein 5A replication complex inhibitor BMS-790052 in Humans: *In Vitro* and *In Vivo* Correlations. Hepatology 2011; 54(6): 1924-35.
[http://dx.doi.org/10.1002/hep.24594] [PMID: 21809362]

[106] Yoshimi S, Imamura M, Murakami E, *et al.* Long term persistence of NS5A inhibitor-resistant hepatitis C virus in patients who failed daclatasvir and asunaprevir therapy. J Med Virol 2015; 87(11): 1913-20.
[http://dx.doi.org/10.1002/jmv.24255] [PMID: 25954851]

[107] Hézode C, Asselah T, Reddy KR, *et al.* Ombitasvir plus paritaprevir plus ritonavir with or without ribavirin in treatment-naive and treatment-experienced patients with genotype 4 chronic hepatitis C virus infection (PEARL-I): a randomised, open-label trial. Lancet 2015; 385(9986): 2502-9.
[http://dx.doi.org/10.1016/S0140-6736(15)60159-3] [PMID: 25837829]

[108] Xu S, Doehle B, Rajyaguru S, *et al.* In vitro selection of resistance to sofosbuvir in HCV replicons of genotype-1 to -6. Antivir Ther 2017; 22(7): 587-97.
[http://dx.doi.org/10.3851/IMP3149] [PMID: 28248189]

[109] Tong X, Le Pogam S, Li L, *et al.* In vivo emergence of a novel mutant L159F/L320F in the NS5B polymerase confers low-level resistance to the HCV polymerase inhibitors mericitabine and sofosbuvir. J Infect Dis 2014; 209(5): 668-75.
[http://dx.doi.org/10.1093/infdis/jit562] [PMID: 24154738]

[110] Sulkowski MS, Eron JJ, Wyles D, *et al.* Ombitasvir, paritaprevir co-dosed with ritonavir, dasabuvir, and ribavirin for hepatitis C in patients co-infected with HIV-1: a randomized trial. JAMA 2015; 313(12): 1223-31.
[http://dx.doi.org/10.1001/jama.2015.1328] [PMID: 25706092]

[111] Lemm JA, Liu M, Gentles RG, *et al.* Preclinical characterization of BMS-791325, an allosteric inhibitor of hepatitis C Virus NS5B polymerase. Antimicrob Agents Chemother 2014; 58(6): 3485-95.
[http://dx.doi.org/10.1128/AAC.02495-13] [PMID: 24733465]

[112] Svarovskaia ES, Dvory-Sobol H, Parkin N, *et al.* Infrequent development of resistance in genotype 1-6 hepatitis C virus-infected subjects treated with sofosbuvir in phase 2 and 3 clinical trials. Clin Infect Dis 2014; 59(12): 1666-74.
[http://dx.doi.org/10.1093/cid/ciu697] [PMID: 25266287]

[113] Sarrazin C. Treatment failure with DAA therapy: Importance of resistance. J Hepatol 2021; 74(6): 1472-82.
[http://dx.doi.org/10.1016/j.jhep.2021.03.004] [PMID: 33716089]

[114] Szymanek A, Krzysztof S. HCV drug resistance and DAA agents. Przegl Epidemiol 2013; 67(3): 403-406, 513-515.
[PMID: 24340550]

[115] Gottwein JM, Pham LV, Mikkelsen LS, *et al.* Efficacy of NS5A Inhibitors Against Hepatitis C Virus Genotypes 1 7 and Escape Variants. Gastroenterology 2018; 154(5): 1435-48.
[http://dx.doi.org/10.1053/j.gastro.2017.12.015] [PMID: 29274866]

[116] Sharafi H, Alavian SM. Hepatitis C resistance to NS5A inhibitors: Is it going to be a problem? World J Hepatol 2018; 10(9): 543-8.
[http://dx.doi.org/10.4254/wjh.v10.i9.543] [PMID: 30310532]

[117] Rossetti B, Paglicci L, Di Maio VC, *et al.* Prevalence of resistance-associated substitutions to NS3, NS5A and NS5B inhibitors at DAA-failure in hepatitis C virus in Italy from 2015 to 2019. Infez Med 2021; 29(2): 242-51.
[PMID: 34061790]

[118] Papaluca T, O'Keefe J, Bowden S, Doyle JS, Stoove M, Hellard M, *et al.* Prevalence of baseline HCV NS5A resistance associated substitutions in genotype 1a, 1b and 3 infection in Australia. Journal of

clinical virology : the official publication of the Pan American Society for Clinical Virology. 2019; 120: 84-7.

[119] Safarnezhad Tameshkel F, Karbalaie Niya MH, Khoonsari M, *et al.* Effect of Baseline Resistance-Associated Substitutions on Thalassemia Patients with Chronic HCV Infection: A Two-Year Follow-Up. Middle East J Dig Dis 2021; 13(1): 27-34.
[http://dx.doi.org/10.34172/mejdd.2021.200] [PMID: 34712435]

[120] Safarnezhad Tameshkel F, Karbalaie Niya MH, Zamani F, *et al.* Resistance-associated substitutions (RASs) to HCV direct-acting antivirals (DAAs) at baseline of treatment in thalassemia patients: a referral center study. Arch Virol 2020; 165(10): 2193-203.
[http://dx.doi.org/10.1007/s00705-020-04728-x] [PMID: 32638116]

[121] Hinrichsen H, Stoehr A, Cornberg M, *et al.* Utilization and effectiveness of elbasvir/grazoprevir and adoption of resistance-associated substitutions testing in real-world treatment of hepatitis C virus genotype 1A infection: results from the German Hepatitis C-Registry. Eur J Gastroenterol Hepatol 2021; 33(3): 415-23.
[http://dx.doi.org/10.1097/MEG.0000000000001759] [PMID: 32345848]

[122] Morsica G, Vercesi R, Hasson H, Messina E, Uberti-Foppa C, Bagaglio S. Compartmentalization of Resistance-Associated Substitutions in HIV/HCV-Infected Patients: Possible Correlation with Infecting HCV Genotype. Viruses 2021; 13(8): 1486.
[http://dx.doi.org/10.3390/v13081486] [PMID: 34452351]

[123] Fadl N, Salem TZ. Hepatitis C genotype 4: A report on resistance-associated substitutions in *NS3*, *NS5A*, and *NS5B* genes. Rev Med Virol 2020; 30(4): e2120.
[http://dx.doi.org/10.1002/rmv.2120] [PMID: 32478480]

[124] Cabral BCA, Ramos JA, Silveira ALM, Nascimento É. Frequency distribution of HCV resistance-associated variants in infected patients treated with direct-acting antivirals. International journal of infectious diseases : IJID : official publication of the International Society for Infectious Diseases. 2022; 115: 171-7.

[125] Bagaglio S, Messina E, Hasson H, Galli A, Uberti-Foppa C, Morsica G. Geographic Distribution of HCV-GT3 Subtypes and Naturally Occurring Resistance Associated Substitutions. Viruses 2019; 11(2): 148.
[http://dx.doi.org/10.3390/v11020148] [PMID: 30754682]

[126] Isakov V, Hedskog C, Wertheim JO, Hostager RE, Parhy B, Schneider AB, *et al.* Prevalence of resistance-associated substitutions and phylogenetic analysis of hepatitis C virus infection in Russia 2021.
[http://dx.doi.org/10.1016/j.ijid.2021.09.041]

[127] Garcia-Cehic D, Rando A, Rodriguez-Frias F, *et al.* Resistance-associated substitutions after sofosbuvir/velpatasvir/voxilaprevir triple therapy failure. J Viral Hepat 2021; 28(9): 1319-24.
[http://dx.doi.org/10.1111/jvh.13497] [PMID: 33720484]

[128] Loggi E, Vukotic R, Andreone P. Managing HCV treatment failure and the potential of resistance testing in informing second-line therapy options. Expert Rev Anti Infect Ther 2018; 16(11): 833-8.
[http://dx.doi.org/10.1080/14787210.2018.1538783] [PMID: 30336699]

[129] Yeon JE. Recent update of the 2017 Korean Association for the Study of the Liver (KASL) treatment guidelines of chronic hepatitis C: Comparison of guidelines from other continents, 2017 AASLD/IDSA and 2016 EASL. Clin Mol Hepatol 2018; 24(3): 278-93.
[http://dx.doi.org/10.3350/cmh.2018.1002] [PMID: 29716179]

[130] Hézode C. Pan-genotypic treatment regimens for hepatitis C virus: Advantages and disadvantages in high- and low-income regions. J Viral Hepat 2017; 24(2): 92-101.
[http://dx.doi.org/10.1111/jvh.12635] [PMID: 27862695]

[131] Hsu SJ, Enkhzaya S, Lin YY, Tseng TC, Khosbayar T, Tsai CH, *et al.* Resistance-associated substitution and ledipasvir/sofosbuvir therapy in Mongolian chronic hepatitis C patients. Journal of the

Formosan Medical Association = Taiwan yi zhi. 2020; 119(3): 712-9.

[132] Singh AD, Maitra S, Singh N, *et al.* Systematic review with meta-analysis: impact of baseline resistance-associated substitutions on the efficacy of glecaprevir/pibrentasvir among chronic hepatitis C patients. Aliment Pharmacol Ther 2020; 51(5): 490-504. [http://dx.doi.org/10.1111/apt.15633] [PMID: 31943236]

[133] Younossi ZM, Stepanova M, Sulkowski M, *et al.* Ribavirin-Free Regimen With Sofosbuvir and Velpatasvir Is Associated With High Efficacy and Improvement of Patient-Reported Outcomes in Patients With Genotypes 2 and 3 Chronic Hepatitis C: Results From Astral-2 and -3 Clinical Trials. Clin Infect Dis 2016; 63(8): 1042-8. [http://dx.doi.org/10.1093/cid/ciw496] [PMID: 27444413]

[134] Chahine EB, Kelley D, Childs-Kean LM. Sofosbuvir/Velpatasvir/Voxilaprevir: A Pan-Genotypic Direct-Acting Antiviral Combination for Hepatitis C. Ann Pharmacother 2018; 52(4): 352-63. [http://dx.doi.org/10.1177/1060028017741508] [PMID: 29115151]

[135] Chahine EB, Sucher AJ, Hemstreet BA. Sofosbuvir/Velpatasvir. Ann Pharmacother 2017; 51(1): 44-53. [http://dx.doi.org/10.1177/1060028016668897] [PMID: 27609942]

[136] Ren S, Wei F, Jin Y, *et al.* Baseline resistance-associated substitutions may impact DAA response among treatment failure chronic hepatitis C patients with pegylated interferon and ribavirin in real life. Antivir Ther 2020; 25(5): 245-55. [http://dx.doi.org/10.3851/IMP3369] [PMID: 32936785]

[137] Carrasco I, Arias A, Benítez-Gutiérrez L, *et al.* Baseline NS5A resistance associated substitutions may impair DAA response in real-world hepatitis C patients. J Med Virol 2018; 90(3): 532-6. [http://dx.doi.org/10.1002/jmv.24971] [PMID: 28990680]

[138] Pérez AB, Chueca N, Macías J, *et al.* Prevalence of resistance associated substitutions and efficacy of baseline resistance-guided chronic hepatitis C treatment in Spain from the GEHEP-004 cohort. PLoS One 2019; 14(8): e0221231. [http://dx.doi.org/10.1371/journal.pone.0221231] [PMID: 31469856]

[139] Liu Z, Mao X, Yu K, *et al.* Prevalence of HCV resistance-associated substitutions among treatment-failure patients receiving direct-acting antiviral agents. J Viral Hepat 2020; 27(6): 585-92. [http://dx.doi.org/10.1111/jvh.13270] [PMID: 32049405]

[140] Akuta N, Sezaki H, Suzuki F, *et al.* Ledipasvir plus sofosbuvir as salvage therapy for HCV genotype 1 failures to prior NS5A inhibitors regimens. J Med Virol 2017; 89(7): 1248-54. [http://dx.doi.org/10.1002/jmv.24767] [PMID: 28079269]

[141] Tergast TL, Kordecki N, Ohlendorf V, Beier C, Sandmann L, Wedemeyer H, *et al.* Z Gastroenterol 2021. [Glecaprevir/Pibrentasvir + Sofosbuvir + Ribavirin as a salvage regimen after Sofosbuvir + Velpatasvir + Voxilaprevir re-treatment failure].

[142] Voaklander R, Jacobson IM. Sofosbuvir, velpatasvir and voxilaprevir combination for the treatment of hepatitis C. Expert Rev Gastroenterol Hepatol 2017; 11(9): 789-95. [http://dx.doi.org/10.1080/17474124.2017.1351295] [PMID: 28673106]

[143] Abdurakhmanov DT, Rozina TP, Nikulkina EN, Nabatchikova EA, Chulanov VP, Moiseev SV. Sofosbuvir-based salvage therapy for HCV infection in cirrhotic patients with DAA failure and multidrug resistance. Antivir Ther 2018; 23(8): 705-8. [http://dx.doi.org/10.3851/IMP3266] [PMID: 30265242]

[144] Bourlière M, Gordon SC, Flamm SL, *et al.* Sofosbuvir, Velpatasvir, and Voxilaprevir for Previously Treated HCV Infection. N Engl J Med 2017; 376(22): 2134-46. [http://dx.doi.org/10.1056/NEJMoa1613512] [PMID: 28564569]

[145] Zuckerman A, Chastain CA, Naggie S. Retreatment Options Following HCV Direct-Acting Antiviral Failure. Curr Treat Options Infect Dis 2017; 9(4): 389-402.

[http://dx.doi.org/10.1007/s40506-017-0136-6] [PMID: 29242710]

[146] Poordad F, Felizarta F, Asatryan A, *et al.* Glecaprevir and pibrentasvir for 12 weeks for hepatitis C virus genotype 1 infection and prior direct-acting antiviral treatment. Hepatology 2017; 66(2): 389-97. [http://dx.doi.org/10.1002/hep.29081] [PMID: 28128852]

[147] Abdelaal R, Yanny B, El Kabany M. HBV/HCV Coinfection in the Era of HCV-DAAs. Clin Liver Dis 2019; 23(3): 463-72. [http://dx.doi.org/10.1016/j.cld.2019.04.003] [PMID: 31266620]

[148] Smalls DJ, Kiger RE, Norris LB, Bennett CL, Love BL, Hepatitis B. Hepatitis B Virus Reactivation: Risk Factors and Current Management Strategies. Pharmacotherapy 2019; 39(12): 1190-203. [http://dx.doi.org/10.1002/phar.2340] [PMID: 31596963]

[149] Calvaruso V, Ferraro D, Licata A, *et al.* HBV reactivation in patients with HCV/HBV cirrhosis on treatment with direct-acting antivirals. J Viral Hepat 2018; 25(1): 72-9. [http://dx.doi.org/10.1111/jvh.12754] [PMID: 28703895]

[150] Blackard JT, Sherman KE. Hepatitis B virus (HBV) reactivation-The potential role of direct-acting agents for hepatitis C virus (HCV). Rev Med Virol 2018; 28(4): e1984. [http://dx.doi.org/10.1002/rmv.1984] [PMID: 29761585]

[151] Mohamed SY, Gaballah BA, Mohamed Elsadek H, Hassan Emara M, Hamed EF. Resolved HBV behavior during the treatment of chronic HCV infection with direct-acting antivirals. Gastroenterol Hepatol Bed Bench 2019; 12(4): 301-8. [PMID: 31749918]

[152] WHO Guidelines Approved by the Guidelines Review Committee. Guidelines for the Screening Care and Treatment of Persons with Chronic Hepatitis C Infection: Updated Version. Geneva: World Health OrganizationCopyright © World Health Organization 2016.

[153] Jiang XW, Ye JZ, Li YT, Li LJ. Hepatitis B reactivation in patients receiving direct-acting antiviral therapy or interferon-based therapy for hepatitis C: A systematic review and meta-analysis. World J Gastroenterol 2018; 24(28): 3181-91. [http://dx.doi.org/10.3748/wjg.v24.i28.3181] [PMID: 30065564]

[154] Belperio PS, Shahoumian TA, Mole LA, Backus LI. Evaluation of hepatitis B reactivation among 62,920 veterans treated with oral hepatitis C antivirals. Hepatology 2017; 66(1): 27-36. [http://dx.doi.org/10.1002/hep.29135] [PMID: 28240789]

[155] Mücke MM, Mücke VT, Peiffer KH, *et al.* Absence of HBV Reactivation in Patients With Resolved HBV Infection Following DAA Therapy for Hepatitis C: A 1-Year Follow-up Study. Open Forum Infect Dis 2019; 6(1): ofy340. [http://dx.doi.org/10.1093/ofid/ofy340] [PMID: 30648130]

[156] Sanduzzi-Zamparelli M, Mariño Z, Lens S, Sapena V, Iserte G, Pla A, *et al.* Liver cancer risk after HCV cure in patients with advanced liver disease without non-characterized nodules. J Hepatol 2021. [PMID: 34856322]

[157] Piscaglia F, Granito A, Bolondi L. DAAs for HCV and risk of hepatocellular carcinoma: current standpoint. Lancet Gastroenterol Hepatol 2018; 3(11): 736-8. [http://dx.doi.org/10.1016/S2468-1253(18)30238-3] [PMID: 30353852]

[158] Morisco F, Federico A, Marignani M, *et al.* Risk Factors for Liver Decompensation and HCC in HCV-Cirrhotic Patients after DAAs: A Multicenter Prospective Study. Cancers (Basel) 2021; 13(15): 3810. [http://dx.doi.org/10.3390/cancers13153810] [PMID: 34359711]

[159] Hamdane N, Jühling F, Crouchet E, *et al.* HCV-Induced Epigenetic Changes Associated With Liver Cancer Risk Persist After Sustained Virologic Response. Gastroenterology 2019; 156(8): 2313-2329.e7. [http://dx.doi.org/10.1053/j.gastro.2019.02.038] [PMID: 30836093]

[160] Rinaldi L, Nevola R, Franci G, *et al.* Risk of Hepatocellular Carcinoma after HCV Clearance by Direct-Acting Antivirals Treatment Predictive Factors and Role of Epigenetics. Cancers (Basel) 2020; 12(6): 1351.
[http://dx.doi.org/10.3390/cancers12061351] [PMID: 32466400]

[161] Singal AG, Rich NE, Mehta N, *et al.* Direct-Acting Antiviral Therapy Not Associated With Recurrence of Hepatocellular Carcinoma in a Multicenter North American Cohort Study. Gastroenterology 2019; 156(6): 1683-1692.e1.
[http://dx.doi.org/10.1053/j.gastro.2019.01.027] [PMID: 30660729]

[162] Tampaki M, Savvanis S, Koskinas J. Impact of direct-acting antiviral agents on the development of hepatocellular carcinoma: evidence and pathophysiological issues. Ann Gastroenterol 2018; 31(6): 670-9.
[http://dx.doi.org/10.20524/aog.2018.0306] [PMID: 30386116]

[163] Buonfiglioli F, Conti F, Andreone P, *et al.* Development of Hepatocellular Carcinoma in HCV Cirrhotic Patients Treated with Direct Acting Antivirals. J Hepatol 2016; 64(2): S215.
[http://dx.doi.org/10.1016/S0168-8278(16)00183-5]

[164] You MW, Kim KW, Shim JJ, Pyo J. Impact of liver-stiffness measurement on hepatocellular carcinoma development in chronic hepatitis C patients treated with direct-acting antivirals: A systematic review and time-to-event meta-analysis. J Gastroenterol Hepatol 2021; 36(3): 601-8.
[http://dx.doi.org/10.1111/jgh.15243] [PMID: 32875681]

[165] Reig M, Mariño Z, Perelló C, *et al.* Unexpected high rate of early tumor recurrence in patients with HCV-related HCC undergoing interferon-free therapy. J Hepatol 2016; 65(4): 719-26.
[http://dx.doi.org/10.1016/j.jhep.2016.04.008] [PMID: 27084592]

[166] Piñero F, Mendizabal M, Ridruejo E, Herz Wolff F, Ameigeiras B, Anders M, *et al.* Treatment with direct-acting antivirals for HCV decreases but does not eliminate the risk of hepatocellular carcinoma 2019.

[167] Tamaki N, Higuchi M, Kurosaki M, *et al.* Risk assessment of hepatocellular carcinoma development by magnetic resonance elastography in chronic hepatitis C patients who achieved sustained virological responses by direct-acting antivirals. J Viral Hepat 2019; 26(7): 893-9.
[http://dx.doi.org/10.1111/jvh.13103] [PMID: 30974045]

[168] Tsai PC, Huang CF, Yu ML. Unexpected early tumor recurrence in patients with hepatitis C virus-related hepatocellular carcinoma undergoing interferon-free therapy: Issue of the interval between HCC treatment and antiviral therapy. J Hepatol 2017; 66(2): 464.
[http://dx.doi.org/10.1016/j.jhep.2016.10.035] [PMID: 27840227]

[169] Spârchez Z, Mocan T. Hepatocellular carcinoma occurrence and recurrence after antiviral treatment in HCV-related cirrhosis. Are outcomes different after direct antiviral agents? a review. J Gastrointestin Liver Dis 2017; 26(4): 403-10.
[http://dx.doi.org/10.15403/jgld.2014.1121.264.hcv] [PMID: 29253056]

[170] Carrat F, Fontaine H, Dorival C, *et al.* Clinical outcomes in patients with chronic hepatitis C after direct-acting antiviral treatment: a prospective cohort study. Lancet 2019; 393(10179): 1453-64.
[http://dx.doi.org/10.1016/S0140-6736(18)32111-1] [PMID: 30765123]

[171] Poynard T, Lacombe JM, Deckmyn O, Peta V, Akhavan S, de Ledinghen V, *et al.* External validation of LCR1-LCR2, a multivariable HCC risk calculator, in patients with chronic HCV 2021.
[http://dx.doi.org/10.1016/j.jhepr.2021.100298]

[172] Brichler S, Nahon P, Zoulim F, *et al.* Non-virological factors are drivers of hepatocellular carcinoma in virosuppressed hepatitis B cirrhosis: Results of ANRS CO12 CirVir cohort. J Viral Hepat 2019; 26(3): 384-96.
[http://dx.doi.org/10.1111/jvh.13029] [PMID: 30380181]

[173] Lack of evidence of an effect of direct-acting antivirals on the recurrence of hepatocellular carcinoma:

Data from three ANRS cohorts. J Hepatol 2016; 65(4): 734-40.
[http://dx.doi.org/10.1016/j.jhep.2016.05.045] [PMID: 27288051]

[174] Lim N, Singh D, Jackson S, Lake JR. Recurrence of Hepatocellular Carcinoma in Hepatitis C Virus (HCV) Liver Transplant Recipients Treated with Pretransplant Direct-Acting Antiviral (DAA) Therapy. Gastrointest Tumors 2020; 7(4): 134-43.
[http://dx.doi.org/10.1159/000510341] [PMID: 33173777]

[175] Søholm J, Hansen JF, Mössner B, *et al.* Low incidence of HCC in chronic hepatitis C patients with pretreatment liver stiffness measurements below 17.5 kilopascal who achieve SVR following DAAs. PLoS One 2020; 15(12): e0243725.
[http://dx.doi.org/10.1371/journal.pone.0243725] [PMID: 33301499]

[176] Singh S, Nautiyal A, Loke YK. Oral direct-acting antivirals and the incidence or recurrence of hepatocellular carcinoma: a systematic review and meta-analysis. Frontline Gastroenterol 2018; 9(4): 262-70.
[http://dx.doi.org/10.1136/flgastro-2018-101017] [PMID: 30245788]

[177] Kanwal F, Kramer JR, Asch SM, Cao Y, Li L, El-Serag HB. Long-Term Risk of Hepatocellular Carcinoma in HCV Patients Treated With Direct Acting Antiviral Agents. Hepatology 2020; 71(1): 44-55.
[http://dx.doi.org/10.1002/hep.30823] [PMID: 31222774]

[178] Roche B, Coilly A, Duclos-Vallee JC, Samuel D. The impact of treatment of hepatitis C with DAAs on the occurrence of HCC 2018.
[http://dx.doi.org/10.1111/liv.13659]

[179] Butt AS, Sharif F, Abid S. Impact of direct acting antivirals on occurrence and recurrence of hepatocellular carcinoma: Biologically plausible or an epiphenomenon? World J Hepatol 2018; 10(2): 267-76.
[http://dx.doi.org/10.4254/wjh.v10.i2.267] [PMID: 29527262]

[180] Dash S, Aydin Y, Widmer KE, Nayak L. Hepatocellular Carcinoma Mechanisms Associated with Chronic HCV Infection and the Impact of Direct-Acting Antiviral Treatment. J Hepatocell Carcinoma 2020; 7: 45-76.
[http://dx.doi.org/10.2147/JHC.S221187] [PMID: 32346535]

[181] Frazzoni L, Sikandar U, Metelli F, *et al.* Hepatocellular Carcinoma Recurrence after Hepatitis C Virus Therapy with Direct-Acting Antivirals. A Systematic Review and Meta-Analysis. J Clin Med 2021; 10(8): 1694.
[http://dx.doi.org/10.3390/jcm10081694] [PMID: 33920785]

[182] Highlights in Hepatitis C Virus From the 2017 AASLD Liver Meeting: A Review of Selected Presentations. The University of Texas Health, San AntonioSan Antonio, Texas. Gastroenterology and Hepatology. 2017; 13(12): 1-24.

[183] Zubkin ML, Shchepetkova GS, Balkarova OV, Chervinko VI, Kryukov EV. Successful Hepatitis C Virus Eradication in a Hemodialysis Patient With 2k/1b Chimera Genotype: A Case Report and Literature Review. Gastroenterol Res 2019; 12(3): 176-80.
[http://dx.doi.org/10.14740/gr1171] [PMID: 31236161]

[184] Li C, Liang J, Xiang H, Chen H, Tian J. Effectiveness of direct-acting antivirals in maintenance hemodialysis patients complicated with chronic hepatitis C. Medicine (Baltimore) 2020; 99(48): e23384.
[http://dx.doi.org/10.1097/MD.0000000000023384] [PMID: 33235113]

[185] Pol S, Parlati L. Treatment of hepatitis C: the use of the new pangenotypic direct-acting antivirals in "special populations". Liver international : official journal of the International Association for the Study of the Liver. 2018;38 Suppl 1:28-33.

[186] Choi DT, Puenpatom A, Yu X, *et al.* Effectiveness of Elbasvir/Grazoprevir in patients with hepatitis C virus genotype 1 infection and chronic kidney disease in the United States veterans population.

Antiviral research. 2020;174:104698.

[187] Reddy KR, Roth D, Bruchfeld A, *et al*. Elbasvir/grazoprevir does not worsen renal function in patients with hepatitis C virus infection and pre-existing renal disease. Hepatology research : the official journal of the Japan Society of Hepatology. 2017;47(12):1340-5.

[188] Yu ML, Chen PJ, Dai CY, *et al*. Taiwan consensus statement on the management of hepatitis C: part (I) general population. Journal of the Formosan Medical Association = Taiwan yi zhi. 2020;119(6):1019-40.

[189] Yu ML, Chen PJ, Dai CY, *et al*. Taiwan consensus statement on the management of hepatitis C: Part (II) special populations. Journal of the Formosan Medical Association = Taiwan yi zhi. 2020;119(7):1135-57.

CHAPTER 10

Appling Drug Discovery in HCV-therapeutics: A snapshot from the past and glimpse into the future

Abstract: The ongoing COVID-19 pandemic with its devastating impacts in terms of huge disease burden and patient management on the world's leading healthcare systems and jolting the world's biggest economies, has leveraged the lesson that to prevent the transmission and elimination of a viral pandemic, endemic, or epidemic in future, a prophylactic or protective vaccine would be indispensable. In this scenario, DAAs regimens alone would not be sufficient to eliminate the HCV epidemic by 2030 or beyond and there would always be the demand for a prophylactic or protective vaccine to prevent the transmission of this epidemic again from vulnerable populations. The anti-mRNA-based treatment strategies (*e.g.*, anti-HCV protein-specific oligonucleotides, RNA interference (RNAi), and micro RNA (miRNA)), and some potential anti-hepatitis C vaccine models have been widely and extensively studied as an alternative or adjuvant therapeutic approaches for hepatitis C in the recent past and some of those models are still in the pipeline. The approval of the first RNAi therapy against a hereditary protein deposition disorder has urged investigators to refocus this approach against hepatitis C because it represents the most thoroughly studied treatment strategy against hepatitis C in the last two decades. Furthermore, some emerging approaches like host targeting agents (HTA), nanoparticles-containing immunogens, and nanomedicine-based therapeutic agents are also in their full investigative form. In this book chapter, we will discuss and highlight emerging hepatitis C treatment approaches that could be the game-changer to vanquishing HCV by 2030 while used as an adjuvant or compensatory regimen with DAAs.

Keywords: Antisense Oligonucleotides, Anti-HCV Vaccines, Controlled Infection Models, Distinct Conceptualization, Dnazymes, Emerging Therapeutics, Host Targeting Agents, Inorganic Nanoparticles, Micro-RNA, MiRNA Inhibitors, Monoclonal Antibodies, Nanozymes, Nanoparticle Immunogens, Nanomedicine, RNA Interference, Traditional Immunization Models.

INTRODUCTION

Since its initial discovery in 1989 through non-traditional virological techniques, remarkable progress has been made in hepatitis C biology, virology, immunology, diagnostics, and therapeutics. From that time until now, it would not be an exaggeration if we say that every notable discovery and invention in virology was

Imran Shahid and Qaiser Jabeen

tried to link hepatitis C research to comprehensively elucidating HCV infection cycle in host cells, generation of efficient *in vitro* cell culture systems, development of rapid molecular tests and simplified HCV screening and diagnostic algorithms to identify HCV infected persons, and the most important effective HCV therapeutics that can achieve SVR rates >95% of treated infections [1]. For example, in the last two decades, the world has never seen so much rapid advancement and revolution in diagnostics and therapeutics of any other infectious or contagious virus infection except the ongoing COVID-19 pandemic, where we have reached a point to eradicate this 'silent epidemic' with the help of the state-of-the-art IFN-free DAAs and some other emerging therapeutic paradigms in the late-stage of development [1]. This journey does not seem so easy and incredible success in HCV diagnostics and therapeutics involved the dedicated and untired contributions of so many famous and renowned investigators and scientists around the world. Subsequently, the participation and contributions of these efforts in HCV discovery and characterization were evident and admitted last year while awarding the Noble Prize in Medicine or Physiology to Micheal Houghton, Charles Rice, and Harvey Alter.

HCV DIAGNOSIS AND DRUG DISCOVERY-A CONTINUED JOURNEY

Despite these many successes while starting from interferon as an initial therapy to treat HCV-infected patients to promising pan-genotypic DAAs, which are highly efficacious with a cure rate of more than 95%, and transferring from initial HCV screening by a traditional ELISA test to digital self-test HCV diagnostic technologies, HCV research unfortunately yet could not succeed to deliver on one of its principles promises critical to achieving global elimination [2]. A key lack in HCV therapeutics is the deficiency of a prophylactic or protective vaccine. This failure is not due to a lack of trying, as multiple studies were carried out in the last 30 years to understand the kinetics of adaptive immune responses in the spontaneous clearance of acute HCV infection during 6 months in the majority of individuals and trying to translate this knowledge into the designing of a preventive vaccine [2]. Although; this knowledge was quite useful to understand the fundamental insights of protective HCV immunity (*i.e.* role of T cells) to achieve virus clearance, however, still not converted or transformed to develop an effective anti-HCV vaccine [2]. Consequently, significant barriers hinder global elimination efforts in the absence of a preventive anti-HCV vaccine to eradicate HCV by the year 2030 [1]. As HCV disease progression from acute infection to chronic and ultimately to end-stage liver disease (*e.g.*, HCC; hepatic failure) takes years to decades to develop, therapeutic termination of infection with promising anti-HCV agents (*e.g.*, current DAAs) represent a conceptually feasible strategy to prevent and probably eliminate hepatitis C and associated comorbidities [3]. However, it also seems an uphill task despite the remarkable efficacy of DAA treatment because of their existing limitations such as difficult access to these expensive regimens in LMICs and resource-poor nations, the emergence of RASs, and DAAs associated with high risks of developing or recurrence of HCC in treated individuals [1]. Furthermore, inadequate infection surveillance programs, poor treatment adherence within harder-to-treat subpopulations, and the fear of remaining immunologically susceptible to reinfection even cured with pan-genotypic DAAs also complicate the elimination of HCV from the vulnerable fraction of populations (*e.g.*, IDUs, sex workers, MSM, opiate use disorders, and illegal immigrants with HCV/HIV co-infection) [1].

ANTI-MRNA BASED TREATMENT STRATEGIES

In the postgenomic era, the knowledge of the physiological functions of the genome has become the rate-limiting step in the quest to develop "gene-based therapies" [4]. The discovery of RNA interference (RNAi) technology known as once," one of the most exciting discoveries in biology in the last couple of decades", and 'breakthrough of the year' became rapidly one of the key methods in functional genomics and played a pivotal role in the validation of novel 'gene-based drugs' [5]. RNA interference (RNAi) is a fundamental cellular mechanism for silencing gene expression through a sequence-specific double-strand RNA degradation process to inhibit genome replication and treat various diseases. Since its discovery, the technology has been widely used to develop RNAi-based drugs (*e.g.*, small interference RNA (siRNA) and short hairpin RNA (shRNA)) to treat and prevent various human diseases like tumors, metabolic disorders, genetic diseases, and certain viral infections [5]. Furthermore, the mechanistic approach of this technology to be more effective while knocking-out gene functions in the cell cytoplasm, makes it the most gene-based therapy studied against HCV replication and translation inhibition in both *in vitro* and *in vivo* cell culture and animal models [5]. However, certain crosscutting barriers related to effective siRNA delivery to their target hepatic cells, siRNA toxicities, and their potential impact on immune systems prevented this technology from being effectively tested in humans. Recently, the approval of the first siRNA-based treatment (Patisiran: ONPATTRO™) by the US FDA against a hereditary protein deposition disorder (*i.e.* hereditary transthyretin-mediated amyloidosis) has sparked the researchers to refocus this approach against hepatitis C [6].

Like RNAi, a similar discovery of another small RNA, *i.e.* microRNA (miRNA) has also revolutionized our understanding of gene regulation while studying their pivotal roles as an important regulator in human development, cellular differentiation, adaptation to the environment, oncogenesis, and host cell interactions with pathogens [7]. Furthermore, the development of methods to measure and regulate microRNA activities also offer a new set of tools to be used in improving our understanding and classification of many diseases and their treatment [7]. Several pieces of evidence collected from both healthy and diseased human tissues unveiled that there may be well over 500 distinct miRNAs in the human genome [8]. Some of the roles of these miRNAs, either in normal human biology or in various diseases, immediately came into focus after their discovery. Multiple studies provide evidence that either up-regulation or down-regulation of miRNAs expression and manipulation of their activities may prove a valuable aspect in hepatitis C treatment and other HCV-associated comorbidities [8].

Although extensively studied and broadly trialed both in *in vitro* and *in vivo* studies since HCV discovery to yet, these two broad classes of anti-hepatitis C regimens including gene-based therapies (*i.e.* siRNA and miRNA inhibitors) and directly targeted HCV-protein agents (*i.e.* IFN-based regimens and DAAs) have encountered several challenges to be safely delivered to their targeted sites (*e.g.*, gene-based therapies) and to easily accessible, without developing the risk of adverse events and the emergence of RASs (*i.e.* DAAs) in treated individuals. To overcome these hurdles, new therapeutic options were also tailored and are still in the pipeline in the form of host-targeting agents (HTAs), monoclonal antibodies, nano-based medicine, and phytochemicals with some unique characteristics [9, 10]. In this book chapter, we will comprehensively overview these novel therapeutic options which can be used as adjuvant therapy with DAAs or may act synergistically with DAAs to offer opportunities to overcome DAAs-based limitations and improve therapeutic outcomes and patient survival in real-world clinical settings.

RNA Interference (RNAi) is Still Infancy for HCV Treatment

RNA interference (RNAi) privilege is still in its infancy as the field has grown into a substantial enterprise that impacts both biomedical and therapeutic research. The technology uses small interfering RNAs (siRNAs; also known as short-interference RNA) either chemically synthesized siRNA or vector-based short hairpin RNAs (shRNAs) to target the mRNA genome of potentially infectious or contagious viruses as well as other genetic disorders and cancers [11]. The diverse clinical trial applications of RNAi also impart their optimistic approach to treating other diseases than virus infection [6]. It was evident from multiple studies that almost all viruses are susceptible to RNAi, which further made the technology a powerful therapeutic tool against viral infections in humans, invertebrates, plants, and even bacteria [4]. Human infectious, contagious, or disease-associated viruses are intracellular obligate parasites that direct infected host cellular machinery under the command of their DNA or RNA genome to synthesize virus proteins, new virus genome, and virus structural parts to assemble as new virion particles and infect other healthy cells after their egress from an infected cell [12]. The virus genome and viral proteins involved in HCV replication or polyprotein processing are unique in the characteristics of preventing themselves by off-target effects with host proteins or host cell receptors as well as even from direct targeting drug molecules to generate virus resistance against treatment and emergence of novel virus mutants [12]. Consequently, most virus infections propagate from acute to chronic stage and then ultimately to severe comorbidities [12].

RNAi-A powerful Therapeutic Tool Against Single-Strand RNA Viruses

Since RNAi is genome-specific thus does not interfere with other normal cell metabolism and cell signaling pathways [6]. The RNAi function is mediated by the insertion of a long double-strand RNA (dsRNA; either siRNA or shRNA) in host cells to target mRNA. This dsRNA undergoes processing in the cytoplasm by an RNaseIII-like ribonuclease enzyme called Dicer comprising one helicase and two RNaseIII domains. After this processing, a dsRNA of 21-23 nucleotides in length is formed which is known as a functional siRNA. This siRNA forms a multi-subunit RISC (RNA-induced silencing complex) with intracellular host proteins which also possess nuclease and helicase activities and altogether drive this siRNA-RISC complex to target recognition of intracellular mRNA. The antisense strand of siRNA guides RISC leading to target complementary RNA and the nuclease protein of the siRNA-RISC complex cleaves the target RNA in a sequence-specific manner. In addition to that RNAi works in mammalian cell cytoplasm to degrade targeted mRNA mediated by either chemically synthesized siRNA or vector-based shRNAs; however, in the latter case, shRNAs are first exported from the cell nucleus to the cytoplasm *via* exportin-5, and GTP-bound form of its cofactor Ran. The resting cascade of targeted mRNA degradation by shRNA utilizes the same step as siRNA does [6]. The cytoplasmic mRNA degradation by RNAi implies that the RNA will become "diluted" as cells undergo division and ultimately reduce the chances of cytotoxicity [4]. siRNA silencing effects both on genome replication and translation phenomena are transient and generally effective for approximately 3-7 days and then naturally degraded or disappear so few chances of deposition in cells and drug-deposition toxicities as seen with other therapeutic regimens [4].

HCV mRNA-A potential Candidate for siRNA Therapeutics

HCV RNA genome is an attractive target for RNAi by both chemically synthesized siRNA and shRNA [13]. HCV genome replicates in the cytoplasm of the hepatic cells which makes it a suitable candidate for RNAi phenomena as Dicer and the siRNA-RISC work efficiently in the cell cytoplasm. This functional activity also makes RNAi technically easier than other gene silencing methods that attempt gene knock-out function at the cell nuclear levels [13]. Many studies reported in the last two decades have shown potential antiviral effects of siRNAs against all major HCV GTs/sub-genotypes in an *in vitro* human hepatoma cell culture system, and *in vivo* mouse, and chimpanzee animal models [4, 5, 12, 13]. HCV full-genome replicon, subgenomic replicon, stable cell lines expressing different HCV genome regions, HCV pseudo particles, and HCV infectious clones all represent efficient culture systems to carry out siRNA-mediated viral replication and translation inhibition studies [14, 15]. Prabhu *et al.* demonstrated effective translation inhibition of major six HCV GTs while targeting 5' untranslated region (5' UTR with siRNAs [16]. They also showed effective siRNA-induced silencing of HCV 1a infectious clones by targeting E2, NS3, and NS5B regions of the virus genome. However; such an approach is not fruitful against other viral strains where sequence variations within target sites hinder siRNA silencing function [17]. Some other studies explore this antiviral approach to be very effective by yielding 100-fold inhibition of virus replication [18]. Ansar *et al.* elucidated full-length HCV subtype 1a particle inhibition targeted by siRNAs [12]. We have also shown siRNA-mediated gene silencing of HCV subtype 1a nonstructural genome regions in a stable Huh-7 cell culture system [3]. Khaliq *et al.* explicated effective virus replication and translation inhibition of HCV subtype 3a strains from the Pakistani population by targeting variable genome regions through chemically synthesized and vector-based siRNAs [19]. Some studies explore viral replication and translation inhibition of HCV GT-4 Egyptian strains by siRNA and antisense oligonucleotide [20]. All these glimpses of widely studied siRNA gene silencing impacts on HCV replication and translation made it of paramount interest to many investigators and researchers to sort out it as a potent alternate or adjuvant treatment against HCV. It would also be valuable to test siRNAs against harder-to-treat HCV GTs (*e.g.*, GT-1 and 3) which show low SVR rates against certain IFN-free DAAs in treated individuals, and to circumvent the problem of IFN resistance with GT-4 derived subtypes. Despite multiple studies of *in vitro*, *in vivo* animal trials, and a few clinical trials (*i.e.*, two clinical trials (NCT01899092, NCT02315638) were conducted to evaluate the efficacy of TT-034 as effective siRNA to treat CHC; however, the trials were discontinued as a result of commercial issues), no antiviral siRNA-based therapy has been approved for clinical use against HCV due to certain challenges [6].

Approval of First siRNA Therapy: A Ray of Hope to Refocus the Tool Against HCV

The recent approval of Patisiran® (ONPATTRO™) by the US FDA against a hereditary protein deposition disorder has raised the hopes of the investigators to refocus siRNA against HCV replication and translation inhibition in humans [6].

The rationale behind this approach is evident by the fact that patisiran® targets hepatocytes and silences a sequence within the transthyretin (TTR) messenger RNA that is conserved across wild-type and all TTR variants to decrease hepatic production of mutant and wild-type TTR. Second, as discussed in chapter 2, HCV infection mainly targets hepatocytes, hence effective anti-HCV therapy should target Fas in hepatocytes or FAS L in immune cells [6]. Several lines of evidence indicate that immune cells expressing Fas L activate and trigger hepatitis with cells infiltrating the liver resulting in the upregulation of death receptor Fas in hepatocytes which are prime targets for immune-mediated apoptosis [6].

Crosscutting Barriers to Reinvigorate siRNA Therapy

However, certain challenges also limit the evaluation of siRNAs effectiveness both *in vitro* and in clinical trials to be an effective anti-mRNA-based treatment approach against hepatitis C [6]. First, to be an effective anti-HCV siRNA, it must reach the cell cytoplasm to mediate RNAi pathways. For this purpose, siRNAs have to travel *via* the bloodstream by avoiding serum nucleases in blood, evading immune recognition by circulating immune cells, crossing the cell membrane, and subverting cell endosomal entrapment. Parenteral (*i.e.* either intravenous (IV) or intramuscular (IM)) administration of siRNA does not seem feasible as it directly contacts blood containing serum nucleases as well as immune cells that degrade siRNA itself or siRNA carrier as well. IV administration of siRNAs also seems less practical as the patients would require to travel to hospitals/clinics, which may be time-consuming and not cost-effective. Aerosolized delivery of siRNA is difficult for infants and children. Similarly, siRNAs cannot be administered orally because of their first-pass effect in the liver. Naked, unmodified siRNAs molecules remain unstable in the bloodstream and serum nucleases recognize them immediately and mediate rapid renal clearance of siRNA molecules after degradation. Similarly, long duplex siRNA (*i.e.* >30 bp) triggers the innate immune responses as toll-like receptors (TLR) 3, 7, and 8 embedded in immune cells recognize siRNA-specific sequences. Ultimately, siRNAs are degraded by immune-activated cells before reaching their target. In addition to that, repeat administration can be required to achieve a therapeutic dose level as siRNAs are diluted during each cell division. The chemical stability of siRNA is also generally compromised as being negatively charged, their passage through the negatively charged phospholipid bilayer of the cell membrane of the host cells is also difficult. The processing of RNAi can also sometimes degrade essential host mRNAs as siRNA can bind to non-target mRNAs with partial complementarity. Subsequently, the resultant siRNA-RISC complex may target essential host mRNAs [6].

Even though overcoming the above-mentioned challenges, there are several other barriers to break while considering siRNAs for anti-HCV therapeutics. As genome mutations evolve many HCV GTs and further subtypes, the virus develops resistance against specific siRNAs, which may further limit both activity and efficacy of siRNAs. In addition to that, RNAi activity by siRNA is more pronounced in those viruses that actively replicate than the latent viruses which express decreased siRNA effects against their target genome [4].

Strategies to Overcome Challenges to Revive siRNA Therapeutic Potential

How to overcome these challenges or at least to minimize the level at which siRNA could be refocused as adjuvant therapy or used in combinations with other treatment regimens against HCV both *in vitro* and *in vivo* studies seem tricky [6]. However, the siRNAs efficacy can be increased by improving their stability, facilitating their delivery to target sites, and using multiplex siRNAs targeting various regions of the HCV genome.

Structural Configuration

The structural configuration and designing of siRNA can be modified and improved to protect it against nuclease degradation and evasion of an immune response after their administration [6]. These modifications include the replacement of hydrogen at 2'-OH ribose with 2'-OMe, 2'-F substitutions, or 2'-O-methoxymethyl. These residues are vital for the conformational analysis of siRNA. The seed region of siRNA hangs on the 5' end of the antisense strand from nucleotide 2-8 that interacts with target mRNA and can be altered with a 2'-O-methyl modification. This modification may be helpful to reduce the off-target effects of siRNA. Furthermore, siRNA designing between 21-23 nucleotide base pairs also prevents or limits siRNA immune recognition by TLR of immune cells. Other chemical modifications include the use of nucleic acid analog at the 2'-OH position of siRNA which results in derivatives of the ribose structure. These include cyclohexenic (CeNa), locked nucleic acids (LNA), unlocked nucleic acids (UNA), and glycolic nucleic acid (GNA). Cyclohexenic modification increases the resistance against serum nuclease degradation of siRNA while locked nucleic acids on the 5' end of the passenger strand of siRNA prevent its incorporation into RISC thereby preventing off-target effects. Other nucleic acid analogs like UNA or GLA also increase the siRNA specificity toward their target mRNA and prevents its off-target effects. One of the most important chemical modification of the phosphodiester linkage of siRNA nucleic acid is phosphorothioate (PS) which effectively facilitate the delivery of siRNAs to the cell cytoplasm. Other chemical modifications like the inclusion of an amide bond between base pairs 10-12 may also be helpful to increase the inhibitory effects of siRNA against their target mRNA [6].

Bioconjugation

Bioconjugation is also considered an effective approach by which a siRNA is conjugated with some biomolecules which bind specifically to cell membrane receptors [6]. These include antibodies, aptamers, peptides, and cell ligands (*e.g.*, cholesterol and lipid molecules). Bioconjugation of siRNA probably facilitates the mechanisms to bind cell surfaces and entrapment of siRNA inside the cell by endocytosis by using some cell surface peptides and proteins. Specific Abs and aptamers can also be used to enhance and improve the delivery of siRNAs to the target cell. However, despite the potential benefit of chemical modifications to enhance siRNA specificity, delivery to target cells, and avoiding off-target effects, these alterations may impact RNAi development for clinical use. First, the number and locations of chemical modifications should be carefully considered on the siRNA duplex as those will impact the overall efficacy of siRNA. Second, many chemical modifications may result in cytotoxicities and decrease the inhibitory effects of siRNA. Third and most importantly, the high cost of these chemical modifications on large-scale production may contribute toward the slow progress of RNAi therapeutics [6].

Robust and Durable siRNA Delivery Vehicles

As previously described, siRNA delivery to the target cells is a major hurdle to developing an effective siRNA therapy, because being negatively charged, siRNA alone cannot cross the negatively charged phospholipid bilayer of the cell membrane of the mammalian cells without using a carrier or a delivery vector [6]. Furthermore, most of the siRNA transfection methods used in *in-vitro* studies are not applicable to use in *in-vivo* or animal studies. This problem can be solved by the use of different siRNA delivery vehicles like lipidosome, cationic and biodegradable polymers having positive charge for efficient delivery of siRNA *in vivo* for long-lasting RNAi activity. Some delivery vectors also protect siRNA from cellular degradation, reduce cytotoxicity, and may prevent kidney filtration. Herein, we briefly highlight some promising siRNA delivery vectors experienced for other viral infections that could be the rationale for anti-HCV siRNA delivery in hepatocytes [6].

Dendriplexes

Dendrimers were evaluated as siRNA delivery vectors in HIV-infected peripheral blood mononuclear cells (PBMCs) for targeting NEF protein (negative factor protein indispensable for HIV-1 replication) [6]. The dendrimers with a higher positive charge (50%) carrying siRNAs against NEF were noticed to be more effective as compared to dendrimers with a lower positive charge (25%). The choice of dendrimer as a siRNA delivery vehicle also impacted the study outcomes where reduced p24 antigen production was noticed in PBMCs targeted with high positive charge dendrimer delivery vector carrying siRNAs against NEF protein. Another HIV study validates the potential of dendrimers as an effective and robust siRNA delivery vector where high fluorescence levels indicated that dendriplexes were successfully delivered to the brain spots. This approach may be useful for other viruses where the blood-brain barrier (BBB) could be a problem delivering siRNA at the target site. Pegylated PEI-siRNA polymers were also evaluated as an effective siRNA delivery vector against the HIV genome in cell culture and demonstrated inhibitory effects to the same extent as AZT (zidovudine) [6].

Cationic Lipophilic Modifications

siRNA delivery vectors for the viruses that affect hepatocytes (*e.g.*, HBV and HCV) were based on a pH-sensitive cationic lipophilic modification [6]. Cationic lipid-siRNA complexes which delivered siRNA specific to the HBV genome in cell culture or mice were developed to improve gene silencing with a single dose treatment. In one study such carriers were effective to reduce both HBV DNA and antigen when compared to entecavir. Similarly, cholesterol-conjugated siRNA complexes were used for anti-HCV genome siRNA delivery in hepatocytes which highly express low-density or high-density lipoprotein (LDL or HDL) receptors. siRNA conjugated to bile-salt derivatives of long-chain fatty acids were also found to trigger RNAi in hepatocytes *in vivo*. One study also showed that α-tocopherol-conjugated siRNAs (Toc-siRNA) specific to apolipoprotein B (apoB) were effectively delivered and processed by DICER in livers of mice without stimulating IFN production [6].

Dynamic Polyconjugates

A novel technology called dynamic polyconjugates (DPCs) addresses the issues of cell-specific targeting and endosomal escape of anti-HCV siRNA [6]. DPCs consist of the hepatocyte targeting ligand N-acetylgalactosamine conjugated to polyethylene glycol (PEG; used as a shielding agent to prevent non-specific interactions of the nanoparticle) and to an endosomolytic polymer that is activated only in the acidic environment of the endosome. By using this technique an IV injection administration of anti-apoB siRNA reported specific inhibition of apoB mRNA in the hepatocytes only not in kupffer cells. Another strategy that encapsulates siRNA into SiO_2 capsules and targets the virus nucleoprotein region in cell culture also proved more effective and superior than siRNA/PEI complexes. Furthermore, encapsulated siRNA remained stable and survived degradation for all-time study findings [6].

Use of Multiplexed siRNAs to Prevent the Emergence of Virus Escape Mutants

The high replication rate of HCV under the regulation of an RNA-dependent RNA-polymerase (RdRp) produces 10^{10}-10^{12} virions per day in a CHC patient with an estimated $1.5–2.0 \times 10^{3}$ base substitutions per genome site per year [6]. This poor fidelity of HCV polymerase enzyme results in a high degree but a mix of distinct but closely related virion populations in infected individuals that are subsequently known as HCV GTs, subtypes, or mixed infections (*i.e.* quasispecies). Furthermore, the lack of an efficient proofreading mechanism of the RdRp enzyme incorporates mismatch nucleotides in the new virus genome during RNA replication. These nucleotide substitutions or mutations are picked by administered HCV treatment either in the form of DAAs or anti-mRNA-based treatment strategies under selection pressure. Consequently, these resistance-associated substitutions (RASs) of the viral genome pose a big hurdle to achieving higher SVR rates or cures in HCV-treated individuals either with DAAs or anti-mRNA-based therapies. Sometimes these RASs may also contribute to viral relapse, viral breakthrough, or treatment failure. We have discussed in detail the RASs' potential impact on treatment outcomes with DAAs in chapter 7 and herein will briefly discuss their limitations on RNAi [6].

It has been demonstrated that prolonged administration of highly sequence-specific siRNAs may evolve the emergence of siRNA-resistant virus variants, especially for viruses that encode a polymerase enzyme that lack proofreading capabilities [4]. There is a shred of strong experimental evidence in the literature that continuous administration of one siRNA against the NS5B region of the HCV genome in a replicon accumulated multiple point mutations [5]. Hence, there must be some strategies to prevent virus-escape mutants with siRNA treatment as well as to increase the effectivity of siRNAs against viral variants [6]. The best strategy to way out virus-escape mutants can be the use of combinatorial siRNAs that target multiple regions of the HCV genome and the selection of that region of the genome comprising minimum mutation rate for siRNA designing [6]. siRNA combinations have been alluded to significantly reduce HCV RNA levels in the replicon system not only by silencing 5' and 3' UTRs but also by inhibiting other coding regions of the HCV genome [6]. An Australian-based company (BLT-HCV, Benitec Ltd.) first time reported the importance of a multi-targeted approach of three siRNAs in a combination by targeting different HCV genome regions to prevent the virus-escape mutants [13]. After that multiple studies evidenced the underlying importance of this approach where hairpin ribozymes targeted against 5' and 3' UTRs efficiently inhibited replication of the HCV genome in a replicon [19]. Multiplexed siRNA (tandem siRNA or tsiRNA) were designed to target HCV structural (*e.g.*, E2) and nonstructural proteins (*e.g.*, NS3) in full-length HCV replicon while efficiently reducing the probability of the virus-escape mutants [21]. A siRNA cocktail targeting against multiple sites of untranslated regions (UTRs) of HCV genome in cell culture was designed which effectively silenced RNA replication and a reduction in resistant variants was also noted [22].

Another suitable way to reduce the emergence of virus-escape mutants is to choose the highly conserved region of the HCV genome to synthesize siRNA or shRNA while comparing the sequence conservation analysis of different HCV GTs and subtypes [4]. In this prospect, nucleotide BLAST (Basic Local Alignment Search Tool) studies indicate that IRES sites within the 5' UTR and HCV antigen protein core (C) region are highly conserved among all HCV GTs/subtypes while NS3, NS5A, and NS5B coding regions and 3'UTR are of the relatively low degree of conservation [13]. Furthermore, multiplexed siRNA in combination with other anti-HCV agents acting by some other mechanism may enhance their individual antiviral effects. It was documented in one study where multiplexed siRNA along with IFN-α enhanced the individual antiviral effects of IFN in HCV replicon [23].

Gaps Need to Fill and Some Tricky Questions Must be Answered Prior to Consider siRNA as an Anti-HCV Therapy

However, despite all these plausible qualms, justifications, and even surmounting the barriers, the acceptance of RNAi in real-world clinical practice as a powerful therapeutic tool or as an adjuvant or combination therapy with other drugs does not seem so easy and demands a lot of investigations [4]. Indeed certain molecular, genetic, and immunological aspects of RNAi phenomena are still unclear and RNAi-triggered genetic regulation is ambiguous, murky, and inconclusive [11]. Similarly, we do not have a clear picture of the full extent of this RNAi-based genetic regulation, why these RNAi-based modalities exist, and how they interact with intracellular host genetic machinery [6]. Furthermore, some more questions are still answerable before their inclusion into current gene-based therapeutics to treat rare genetic anomalies, metabolic disorders, cancers, and virus infections [13]. We may find some surprises in RNAi technology while doing extensive and thoughtful research work on these fundamental queries discussed somewhere else like; How do some organisms encapsulate RNA triggers to produce a systemic response? How are long-term RNAi effects perpetuated? What is the link between RNAi and immunity? What biological effects will come from the selective or global inactivation or augmentation of the RNAi pathway? How can we best use RNAi to discover the most sensitive and critical targets for biological investigation and drug development? Can we cure diseases by specifically triggering the RNAi pathway to attack errant genes? Can we treat other diseases by up-or down-regulating components of the RNAi machinery itself in specific cell types? How will cells and organisms respond in the long term to continuous modulation or use of the RNAi machinery? All these questions must be addressed as the field of RNAi is rapidly growing both in search of fundamental mechanisms of immune responses against diseases in plants, invertebrates, and worms, as well as the development of anti-mRNA-based treatment strategies against certain uncurable disorders and virus infection in humans [5].

Micro RNAs (miRNAs) and miRNA inhibitors

As described earlier miRNAs act as key mediators of HCV infection and associated hepatic comorbidities (*e.g.*, HCC); therefore miRNAs can act as a liable therapeutic target for their inhibitors in the field of gene therapy [24]. The active involvement of miRNAs to propagate HCV infection and associated hepatic diseases was evident by many pathways analysis of targeted genes performed by using infection-associated miRNAs. It was unveiled that proteasome, lipid metabolism activation, immune responses, and antigen presentation were predominantly regulated by their miRNAs in HCV-infected liver. miRNA levels responsible for all those modalities were measured in Huh7.5 cells in which HCV infectious clones can be replicated. How miRNA regulates these cellular pathways remains controversial as the miRNA mechanism of action is still not fully understood. Until now, very small numbers of *in vivo* functions of miRNAs have been documented in many organisms. Unlike siRNAs, it is postulated that miRNAs work as either translation inhibition or mRNA degradation. In animals, miRNA inhibits mRNA translation of target genes through imperfect base-pairing with 3' UTR of target mRNA; however, alternate mechanisms suggest direct mRNA cleavage, as well as mRNA stability. How many target genes can be regulated by one miRNA *in vivo* is largely unknown, although it is preassumed that one to a hundred target genes can be modulated for a given miRNA based on miRNA target prediction by using a variety of bioinformatics software [24].

miRNAs Modulation in Hepatitis C Infection

How HCV-infected liver is susceptible to miRNA functionality was evident by accumulated studies of miRNA in liver disease which indicates that the unique vasculature of hepatocytes makes it an ideal candidate for the efficient and rapid accumulation of exogenous small RNAs [25]. Various miRNAs modulating the kinetics of HCV infection have been deeply studied, that manipulate CHC infection in the risk of developing hepatic cirrhosis and HCC [25]. It has been estimated that almost 70% of miRNAs manipulates in the liver and the most abundant one, specifically expressed in the human liver is miR-122 [26]. It plays an important role in lipid and cholesterol metabolism, and adipocyte differentiation which is considered a predisposing factor for fatty liver disease (steatosis) [27]. Hence, illustrates a good effective target to ameliorate hepatic steatosis. Besides that, it has an essential role in the progression of several hepatic diseases like NAFLD (non-alcoholic fatty liver disease), HCV, and HCV-associated HCC [27]. Therefore, its inhibition could be a good therapeutic approach in HCV-targeted therapy as many studies show its role in the production of neutralizing antagomirs (*i.e.* neutralizing inhibitors of miRNA). Considering miRNAs as a key target for HCV gene-based therapeutics indirectly way outs other liable possibilities either to target other HCV-induced comorbidities (*e.g.* HCC) or to reduce the risk of comorbidities progression and mortality upon CHC infection [27].

miRNA Kinetics in Hepatitis C Infection Progression

The most important role of liver-specific miRNA, miR-122 in HCV replication was noticed in the human hepatoma (Huh-7) cell line [28]. It interacts directly with the 5' UTR of the HCV genome to enhance its replication although the precise mechanism is not fully understood. It also explains the first link between endogenous miRNA expression and infectious disease. Furthermore, the identification of miR-122 as a critical host factor for HCV genome replication is also implicated in the discovery and development of a novel therapeutic strategy against HCV infection [28]. Based on the miR-122 knock-out therapeutic strategy by using an antisense oligonucleotide, a significant reduction in the expression of HCV mRNA was demonstrated in one study [29]. Another study also reported that IFN-β treatment was significantly associated with a decreased expression of miR-122. This finding supported the assumption that mammalian cells, through the IFN system, use cellular miRNAs to mount an anti-viral response; however, it was not conclusive and refuted by further studies [30]. Similarly, some studies postulate that miR-122 has been involved to elevate both replication and translation of HCV mRNA, independently from virus replication. Up-regulation of HCV translation steps through miR-122 dependent pathways was demonstrated both in reporter and full-length HCV genome constructs [31].

miR-122- A Key Regulator of HCV Replication in Host Cells

miR-122 is the finest studied HCV-related miRNA that is potentially involved in virus genome replication; however, other miRNAs modulate HCV infection progression and associated comorbidities (Table **1**) [32]. For example, miR-199a directly recognizes 5' UTR and regulates HCV replication [7]. Hence its down-regulation could be an effective therapeutic approach to decrease virus replication and suppress viral titers. miR-196 downregulates Bach1 protein (*i.e.* a transcription regulator protein) and HCV gene expression in Huh-7 cells which suggests that overexpression of miR-196 holds promise as a potential novel strategy to prevent or ameliorate HCV infection and protect against liver injury in CHC infection [33]. Furthermore, some immune regulatory miRNAs (*e.g.*, miR-155) are induced by antiviral TLR 3 or 4 cell signaling pathways [34]. Up-regulated miR-155 levels are inversely proportional to serum HCV loads, which signifies its relevant antiviral effect by suppression of Tim-3 (T-cell immunoglobulin and mucin-domain containing-3), also known as HAVCR2; Hepatitis A virus cellular receptor 2) that acts as an immune signaling modulator which is elevated in NK (natural killer) cells of hepatitis C infected patients [34]. Elevated miR-155 levels in CHC-infected patients lead to inhibition of Tim-3 that causes enhanced production of IFN-γ. miR-155 also exhibits antiviral effects against other viruses like HIV infection by modulating TLR3/TLR4 cell signaling pathways that prevent macrophage infiltration by HIV [34]. Another miRNA *i.e.*, miR-21 is self-induced by HCV infection that facilitates HCV replication by escaping the immune response through directly suppressing interleukin-1 receptor-associated kinase 1 (IRAK1) and myeloid differentiation factor 88 (MyD88) [35]. This factor is very much important to induce IFN type 1 response upon HCV infection in immune cells. Last but not the least, a recent study predicts that miR-99a restricts HCV replication by targeting the mammalian target of rapamycin (mTOR) and de novo lipogenesis by regulating mTOR/SREBP-1c and causes inefficient replication and packaging of intracellular HCV [7]. mTOR is considered one of the major cell signaling pathways involved in the regulation of HCV infection. Furthermore, a previous study provides evidence about a potential role of mTORC1 protein of mTOR complex in lipogenesis and found that rapamycin blocked the expression of genes involved in lipogenesis by impairing nuclear accumulation of the sterol regulatory element-binding proteins (SREBPs; membrane-bound transcription factors that activate genes involved in lipid synthesis [7].

Surprisingly, it was found that more than half of the human miRNA genes are located at sites known to be involved in cancers (*e.g.*, fragile sites, minimal regions of loss of heterozygosity, minimal regions of amplification, or common breakpoint regions) [36]. The existence of some miRNAs in these locations provides a hint about their involvement in tumorigenesis. Multiple studies focused on hepatic miRNA (*e.g.*, miR-122) suggested the significant impact of this specific miRNA in several hepatic diseases including NAFLD, HCV, and liver cancers (*i.e.* HCC). Some studies suggest the let-7a, miR-21, miR-23, miR-130, miR-190, and miR-92a family of genes were upregulated, while miR-122 was downregulated in animals with HCC (Table **1**) [37]. Differential expression of miR-122 in HCV-induced HCC in humans has been revealed in many studies

[37]. Overexpression of miR-122 in hepatic tumors along with two other miRNAs (*i.e.* miR-100 and 10a) were also found to be overexpressed in hepatitis C-associated HCC [38]. Table **1** enlists various miRNAs involved in CHC infection and their association with HCC.

Table 1. A list of potential miRNAs involved in HCV infections' progression to hepatic fibrosis, cirrhosis, and subsequently HCC.

<table>
<tr><th colspan="4">miRNAs Involved in CHC-induced Hepatic Cirrhosis and Further Progression to HCC</th></tr>
<tr><th>miRNAs
(Up-regulation)</th><th>Target
Genes</th><th>miRNAs
(Down-regulation)</th><th>Target
Genes</th></tr>
<tr><td>miR-602</td><td>RASSF1A</td><td>miR-23
miR-26</td><td>STAT3, MYC, RAS, HMGA2</td></tr>
<tr><td>Let-7c
miR-10a</td><td>STAT3, MYC, Casp3, RAS, HMGA2</td><td>miR-27a</td><td>PTEN</td></tr>
<tr><td>miR-21
miR-23
miR-25</td><td>PTEN</td><td>miR-122
miR-145</td><td>CAT-1, Cyclin G1, HCV RNA, HO-1</td></tr>
<tr><td>miR-34a
miR-92a
miR-96
miR-99a</td><td>c-Met</td><td>miR-152
miR-199b</td><td>DNMT-1</td></tr>
<tr><td>miR-122a
miR-125b
miR-143
miR-150</td><td>CAT-1, CyclinG1, HCV RNA, HO-1</td><td>-</td><td>-</td></tr>
<tr><td>miR-223
miR-342
miR-375
miR-423</td><td>STMN1</td><td>-</td><td>-</td></tr>
<tr><td>miR-602</td><td>RASSF1A</td><td>-</td><td>-</td></tr>
<tr><th colspan="4">miRNAs involved in HCV-induced steatohepatitis</th></tr>
<tr><th>miRNAs (up-regulation)</th><th colspan="2">miRNAs (down-regulation)</th><th>miRNAs
(dysregulation)</th></tr>
<tr><td>miR-17, miR-24, miR-27, miR-34a, miR-103, miR-107, miR-122</td><td colspan="2">miR-21, miR-29a, miR-130a, miR-185, miR-205, miR-206, miR-378, miR-451</td><td>miR-21, miR-33a/b, miR-122, miR-155</td></tr>
<tr><th colspan="4">miRNAs involved in HCV infection</th></tr>
<tr><td>miR-21, miR-122, miR-141, miR-146a, miR-192, miR-215, miR-491</td><td colspan="2">Let-7, miR-17, miR-27a, miR-29a,b,c, miR-130a, miR-155, miR-181a, miR-194, miR-196, miR-199a, miR-221</td><td>miR-126, miR-192, miR-198, miR-345</td></tr>
<tr><th colspan="4">miRNAs involved in HCC progression</th></tr>
</table>

(Table 1) cont.....

miR-18a, miR-21, miR-92a, miR-130b, miR-141, miR-155, miR-181, miR-195, miR-221, miR-222, miR-224, miR-494, miR-1269	Let-7, miR-1, miR-15a, miR-16, miR-26a, miR-29, miR-34a, miR-101, miR-122, miR-124, miR-125b, miR-126, miR-138, miR-141, miR-145, miR-146a, miR-148, miR-195, miR-199, miR-200, miR-223, miR-375	miR-233

miRNA Knockdown Models

Consequently, miRNA regulation studies in HCV-infected populations were also carried out and are still carrying on to be considered as an alternative therapeutic approach in translational medicine to inhibit hepatitis C replication as well as to prevent the progression of acute/chronic HCV infection to severe hepatic comorbidities (*e.g.*, cirrhosis and HCC) [38]. For this purpose, potential inhibitors of some miRNAs that encode some integral proteins essential for virus replication and translation could be considered prospective therapeutic agents [39]. Several approaches have been deeply studied including direct delivery of miRNA-ASO or expressing it *via* mini-circle or viral vectors, which have been recognized as effective miRNA knockdown models *in vitro* and *in vivo* [39, 40]. Later on, miR-ASO-based therapy was suggested to be applied in humans for liver sickness and promising clinical trials are ongoing [39].

Host-Targeting Agents (HTA) for HCV Treatment

As described earlier host-targeting antivirals could be another promising anti-HCV therapeutic option to overcome limitations associated with both IFN-free DAAs and anti-mRNA-based treatment strategies against hepatitis C infection [41]. Furthermore, HTA could be tested in harder-to-treat populations by acting through complementary mechanisms [9]. Herein we will discuss the latest and most relevant studies about host cellular factors involved in HCV infection progression as well as explore targets for HTA. Briefly, we will highlight the most important HTA evaluated in preclinical and clinical development and also their pivotal role to be considered as an alternative adjuvant or complementary therapeutics against HCV infection and associated comorbidities (Table **2**) [9].

HCV shows narrow host-tropism and only exploits hepatocytes extensively to complete its replication and translation cycle to establish persistent infection [42]. Despite the lack of an *in vivo* disease model, the ample understanding of the HCV life cycle both at structural and functional levels in cell culture systems and experimental animal models through functional genomics screening (*e.g.*, genome-wide siRNA and genome-scale CRISPR-Cas screens) unveils obligatory HCV-host interactions involving various virus and host-encoded factors in each step of HCV life cycle [43]. The information regarding the kinetics and dynamics of these host-virus factors (also known as host-virus dependencies) not only provides critical insights into the underlying mechanisms of HCV molecular pathogenesis but also evolves novel candidates for antiviral therapy research [44].

An effective regimen to cure HCV infection relies on two important factors including a potent antiviral activity and a high genetic barrier to viral resistance [45]. Indeed certain key advantages of HTA over DAAs demonstrate that, unlike DAAs which target HCV proteins of high variability, most HTAs are supposed to maintain a high genetic barrier to resistance as targeted host factors are less prone to mutations [46]. Furthermore, HTAs are generally HCV GTs /subtypes independent, and thus may exhibit an oval pan-genotypic anti-HCV activity. However, HTA may intervene physiological functions of targeted host factors, which may induce cellular toxicity and side effects [46]. Table **2** enlists the most promising HTAs evaluated against HCV host-cell factors and their current development phase.

HTAs Against Hepatitis C Entry into Host Cells

As discussed earlier in chapter 1, HCV entry into host cells involves a highly orchestrated process involving mainly virus envelope glycoproteins (E1 and E2) and four transmembrane host-cellular receptors (Please see Fig. **4** in chapter 1). A genome-scale CRISPR/Cas9 knockout screening of HCV in human cell culture system demonstrates that these 4 host cell receptors (*i.e.*, SR-BI, CD81, CLDN1, and OCLN) are integral for HCV infection *in vivo* as well as to determining the virus tropism for human cells [47].

Table 2. A list of potential HTAs against HCV host cell factors and their current development phase.

Host Targeting Agents (HTAs) Directed Against HCV with Targeted Host-cell Factors and Current State of Clinical Development			
Host Cell Factors	**Host Cell Factors Targeting Agent**	**HTAs Development Phase**	**References**
HTAs against host cell factors involved in HCV entry into the cells			
Scavenger receptor BI (SR-BI)	ITX-5061	Phase II clinical trials	[48, 49]
Human cluster of differentiation 81 (CD81)	Anti-CD81 mAbs	Preclinical	[50]
Claudin-1 (CLDN1)	Anti-CLDN1 mAbs (OM-7D--B3, H3L3)	Preclinical	[51 - 54]
Occludin (OCLN)	Anti-OCLN mAbs (Xi 1-3, Xi 37-5)	Preclinical	[55]
Epidermal growth factor receptor (EGFR)	Erlotinib	Preclinical	[56]

(Table 2) cont.....

Nieman-Pick C1-Like 1 (NPC1L1)	Ezetimibe	Phase I clinical trials	[57, 58]
HTAs against host cell factors involved in HCV replication			
Cyclophilin A	Alisporivir	Phase III clinical trials (halted)	[59 - 63]
	NIM811	Phase II clinical trials	[64]
	SCY-635	Phase IIa clinical trials	[65, 66]
microRNA-122	Miravirsen/ SPC3649	Phase IIa clinical trials	[67 - 70]
	RG-101	Phase Ib clinical trials	[71 - 73]
HTAs against host cell factors involved in virus assembly			
Diglyceride acyltransferase I (DGAT-I)	siRNA	Preclinical	[74]
	Quercetin	Phase I clinical trials	[75, 76]
	LCQ908/Pradigastat	Phase II clinical trials	[77]
HTAs against host cell factors involved in virus assembly/Egress			
Acyl coenzyme A: cholesterol acyltransferase (ACAT)	Avasimibe	Preclinical	[78, 79]
Adaptor-associated kinase 1 (AAK1)	Sunitinib	Preclinical	[80]
Cyclin-associated kinase (GAK)	Erlotinib	Preclinical	[81]
	Isothiazolo [5,4-b] pyridine	Preclinical	[118]

HTA evaluated against HCV entry into host cells blocks the beginning of the HCV life cycle intracellularly before initiation of virus replication and translation which may prevent cell-to-cell signaling transmission, new virion spread, and ultimately persistent infection [48, 49]. Most importantly, viral entry blockade by HCV-entry inhibitors could be useful to prevent graft reinfection in hepatitis C-infected end-stage liver disease patients who are waiting for liver transplantation because viral entry plays an integral role in liver graft re-infection during transplantation [48, 49]. However, additional studies are eagerly required in this direction to establish a place for HCV entry inhibitors in the management of HCV graft infection.

ITX-5061

Many compounds have been investigated for their potential to act as HCV entry inhibitors (Table **2**). The most studied one is ITX-5061 which acts as an antagonist of SR-BI and reduces SR-BI-mediated lipid transfer inside the host cell membrane [48, 49]. During HCV attachment to hepatocytes, SR-BI binds HDL and delivers lipids inside the hepatic cells which are very important for HCV entry into hepatocytes. Hence reducing the lipid transfer capability of SR-BI by ITX-5061 could be one possible mechanism to reduce HCV entry. *In vitro* studies have demonstrated an efficient reduction of HCV entry by ITX-5061 for all HCV GTs. Furthermore, the phase I clinical trials reveal good tolerability in noncirrhotic CHC-infected patients over 4 weeks of administration except for high serum levels of high-density lipoproteins (HDLs). Similarly, Phase I clinical studies showed limited efficacy of ITX-5061 against enrolling CHC patients. Furthermore, long-term administration of ITX-5061 in cell culture (*i.e.in vitro* studies) resulted in the emergence of escape mutants against E2 envelope glycoproteins. However, escape mutations were only limited to *in vitro* studies because these mutations also showed increased sensitivities to neutralizing antibodies and might not arise *in vivo*. Another in vitro study demonstrates that ITX-5061 functions synergistically with PIs (*e.g.*, telaprevir), and no cross-resistance is expected between ITX-5061, and PIs or RdRP inhibitors. ITX-5061 is in the pipeline for phase II clinical studies for safety and efficacy in large HCV-infected populations [48, 49].

Neutralizing Monoclonal Antibodies (mAbs)

Specific monoclonal antibodies (mAbs) targeting HCV-entry receptors have been shown potent antiviral effects in preclinical mouse studies [50]. These specific neutralizing mAbs bind to CD81, CLDN1, and SR-BI host cell receptors and block their attachment with HCV. mAbs targeting CD81 has been shown their potent antiviral effects in preclinical mouse studies. Anti-CLDN1 mAbs were able to cure CHC infection in the albumin enhancer-promoter-driven urokinase-type plasminogen activator/severe combined immunodeficiency (uPA/SCID) liver chimeric mouse model [51]. After that, preclinical development of a rodent anti-CLDN1 mAb (OM-7D3-B3) also demonstrated a potent antiviral response against HCV in primary human hepatocytes (PHHs) and human liver-chimeric mice [51, 52]. For clinical translation in humans, Colpitts and colleagues successfully humanized this mAb into a human IgG4 isotype, designed as H3L3 [53]. H3L3 exhibited pan-genotypic antiviral activity against HCV entry without evolving escape mutants both *in vitro* and in the mouse model [53, 54]. Moreover, a synergistic potential of this mAb was also unveiled with DAAs inhibitors (*e.g.*, SOF and DCV). Such synergism between an HTA and DAAs can allow shortening of treatment duration against HCV and thus could be cost-effective as well as without any severe adverse events (SAEs) [54]. HCV entry into host cells through OCLN attachment may also be considered a potential antiviral target [55]. Until now, two successful human-rat chimeric mAbs have been developed against OCLN, which showed complete inhibition of HCV infection *in vitro* and human liver-chimeric mice without SAEs [55].

Ezetimibe and Erlotinib

Other promising HCV entry inhibitors of kinases and host-cell pathways have also been evaluated *in vitro* and mouse models with their potent antiviral potential and are now in phase I/II clinical trials to prove their clinical worth (Table **2**) [57]. These include Nieman-Pick C1-Like 1 (NPC1L1) inhibitor (ezetimibe) and epidermal growth factor receptor (EGFR) inhibitor (erlotinib). The clinically approved EGFR inhibitor (erlotinib), prevents the formation of the CLDN1-CD81 receptor complex, and NPC1L1 inhibitor (ezetimibe), decreases systemic cholesterol deposition in hepatocytes of HCV-infected patients [57, 58]. The uPA-SCID mouse model studies of these two inhibitors demonstrated markedly impaired establishment of HCV infection in mouse hepatocytes. Erlotinib has been entered into phase I/II clinical trials (NCT01835938) to evaluate its antiviral potential against HCV-infected patients. However; Ezetimibe elicited only a minor reduction in HCV viral loads of two HCV patients before undergoing liver transplantation in phase I clinical trials [56].

HTAs to Inhibit HCV Replication

Cyclophilin A (CypA) Inhibitors

Not only for HTAs but also for the discovery and development of DAAs and anti-mRNA-based treatment strategies, HCV replication inhibition always remained a hot-spot drug discovery target (Table **2**). The most well-studied HTAs against HCV RNA replication belong to cyclophilin A (CypA) inhibitors and antagomirs of miR-122 [59, 60]. CypA is an essential proviral factor that interacts with HCV NS5A protein to establish a replicase membrane web complex that facilitates/promotes HCV RNA replication. Inhibition of CypA/NS5A replication complex by an immunosuppressive CypA inhibitor (*e.g.*, cyclosporin A (CsA)) demonstrated suppression of viral replication *in vitro* and in liver transplantation awaiting recipients in earlier studies [60]. However, because of both the immunosuppressive and antiviral kinetics of cyclosporine A, non-immunosuppressive antiviral derivatives of Cyclosporine A were designed and developed including Alisporiver (ALV)/Debio-025, N-Methyl-4-isoleucne-cyclosporin (NIM811), and SCY-635 [61]. So far, these three molecules have exhibited clinical efficacy against both HCV treatment naïve or treatment-experienced patients either with PEG-IFN plus RBV or IFN-free DAA regimens. However, major safety concerns have delayed their clinical development and further studies are extensively needed in this regard to be well tolerable in HCV-treating individuals. The CypA inhibitors inhibit virus replication by two distinct approaches [64]. One like cyclosporine A prevents the interaction between CypA and NS5A protein to form a replicase membrane web complex thus disrupting

HCV replication, and the second by restoration of the innate immune responses against HCV. However, treatment-emergent RASs with CsA also evolved to Alisporiver and NIM811. However, a comparative analysis of both CypA inhibitors against adaptive mutations showed that Alisporiver has a high genetic barrier to resistance than NIM811 [65]. The anti-HCV potential of ALV on HCV GT-1a/1b was confirmed in chimeric mice with human hepatocytes. After that, the drug entered into clinical development, and was evaluated in phase II clinical trials, where a combination of ALV plus PEG-IFN-α plus RBV to treatment naïve HCV GT-1 patients achieved SVR rates of 69-76% as compared to 55% in the patient group receiving only PEG-IFN-α plus RBV [61]. ALV was also evaluated in HCV GT- 2 and 3 infected patients in combination with other IFN-free DAAs and achieved overall SVR rates of 80-85% at post-completion therapy. However, the development of ALV/Debio-025 was halted because of severe adverse events in seven patients reported to suffer from acute pancreatitis [61]. Furthermore, the phase III clinical trials for ALV efficacy and safety were also postponed or discontinued. Surprisingly, it was noticed that ALV exhibited inhibition of HIV replication both *in vitro* and *in vivo* by inhibiting CyPA-HIV capsid protein interaction. The rationale for this approach, a novel CypA inhibitor named CPI-431-32 demonstrated more efficient and rapid inhibition of HCV and HIV replication than ALV. This finding supports the notion that CyPA inhibitors may be of interest to treat HCV/HIV coinfected patients [62].

MicroRNA-122 (miR-122) Inhibitors

We have deeply discussed above the role of miRNAs as key regulators of both HCV replication and to somehow mRNA translation in CHC-infected individuals as well as their support to progress CHC infection into cirrhosis and HCC. Herein we will briefly overview that sequestering of miR-122 using some specific anti-sense oligonucleotides or inhibitors could repress HCV replication (Table **2**).

Miravirsen/SPC3649

Miravirsen/SPC3649 represents a locked nucleic acid-modified DNA antisense oligonucleotide that contains the capability to sequester mature miR-122 in a highly stable heteroduplex, thereby inhibiting its function to augment HCV RNA replication [67]. Since miR-122 binding sites are highly conserved among all HCV GTs, miravirsen demonstrated pan-genotypic antiviral effects against all HCV GTs *in vitro* [68]. Furthermore, it was found safe, well tolerable, and elicited a dose-dependent reduction in HCV viral titers in infected patients without any SAEs [69]. In Phase 2a clinical studies conducted in 36 HCV GT-1 patients, miravirsen showed a significant decrease in HCV RNA levels without any evidence of resistant mutations and SAEs. Although both *in vitro* and clinical studies data predict a high genetic barrier to viral resistance for this miR-122 inhibitor, some individuals experienced viral rebound within 14 weeks after treatment cessation [70]. It indicated that might be miravirsen as monotherapy could not be so much effective, but rather in combination with other HTAs or DAAs. In this regard, promising findings of an additive effect exerted by miravirsen and DAAs combination alluded that miravirsen is fully effective against DAA-resistant HCV variants. Some studies correlate prolonged reduction in lipid levels with miravirsen treatment in line with the regulatory role of miR-122 on cholesterol metabolism [70].

RG-101

Another miR-122 inhibitor (*i.e.* RG-101) is a hepatocyte-targeted N-acetylgalactosamine conjugated oligonucleotide that antagonizes miR-122 [71]. The safety, tolerability, and antiviral potential of RG-101 were evaluated in 32 HCV GTs-1,3, or 4 infected patients in the phase 1B study [71]. The treatment was considered safe and well tolerable with a substantial reduction in HCV viral load of all treated patients within 4 weeks and achieved SVR rates in 3 individuals at week 76 of follow-up [72]. However, viral rebound was detected in six patients infected with HCV GT-1 within weeks 5 and 12 which might be due to nucleotide substitutions in miR-122 binding sites in the HCV genome. Another phase 1B clinical trial assessed the impact of RG-101 on antiviral immunity in CHC-infected patients and revealed that a single dose of RG-101 led to a decrease in HCV viral titers and achieved SVR rates in three patients after prolonged treatment of more than 76 weeks [72]. However, the combination regimens including either miravirsen or RIG-101 and highly potent DAAs could potentially shorten HCV treatment duration. Recently two clinical studies were conducted to evaluate the potential of RG-101 and an NS5A inhibitor (GSK2878175) in combination as a single-visit curative regimen for CHC [73].

NS5A inhibitor (GSK2878175) demonstrates pan-genotypic antiviral activity, especially against harder-to-treat HCV GT-3 patients with acceptable safety and tolerability [73]. The findings of the clinical studies described that daily oral administration of GSK2878175 plus a single dose of RG-101 resulted in high cure rates in treatment-naïve, non-cirrhotic HCV GT-1 and 3 infections with a treatment duration of more than 9 weeks [73]. These findings illuminate miR-122 inhibitors to be considered as a complementary therapeutic approach that could be valuable in combination with DAAs to cure difficult-to-treat HCV patients [73]. However, multiple studies are still required to evaluate their safety and tolerability as so far no SAEs have been observed after administration of miR-122 inhibitors. Furthermore, the long-term administration of these therapies should be investigated because persistent lower hepatic miR-122 levels have been documented with other hepatic disease progression and development of HCC [73].

HTAs Against HCV Assembly

A close correlation exists between new HCV virion formation and host-cell lipid metabolism [74]. HCV virion circulates as lipo-viral particles (LVPs) in the systemic circulation of an infected individual. Hence, targeting host-cell lipid biogenesis and metabolism pathways may provide a potential therapeutic option (Table **2**) [74].

DGAT-I Inhibitors

A key enzyme diglyceride acyltransferase I (DGAT-I) directly interacts with the hepatitis C core protein and facilitates its trafficking to lipid droplets (LD). Either the inhibition of DGAT-I enzymatic activity or RNAi-mediated knockdown severely disrupts infectious viral particle production *in vitro* without affecting lipid droplet (LD) production [74, 75]. Hence DGAT-I inhibition represent another HTAs for HCV antiviral therapy. Quercetin, a natural flavonoid possessing DGAT-I inhibitory potential showed anti-HCV properties in clinical trials [75]. In a phase I dose-escalation study, quercetin showed high safety and potential antiviral efficacy up to 5g/day dose in CHC-infected patients. It is cheap and widely available and thus could be considered an inexpensive adjuvant for HCV therapy [75]. The antiviral efficacy of another DGAT-I inhibitor (LCQ908/pradigastat) was evaluated against HCV patients in phase II clinical studies [77]. However, no significant clinical efficacy was demonstrated with treatment by any change in serum HCV RNA levels in treated individuals than placebo although the regimen was safe and well tolerable. Further studies are needed to infer whether DGAT-I inhibitors could be evaluated in combination with DAAs against HCV [77].

AAKI and GAK Inhibitors

HCV virion assembly relies on several host factors, including clathrin assembly protein complex 2 medium-chain μ1 (AP2M1), that directly interacts with core protein and recruits it from LD to the HCV assembly site [78]. Furthermore, some other cellular factors like adaptor-associated kinase 1 (AAK1) and cyclin-associated kinase (GAK) regulate this core-AP2M1 interaction and are essential for HCV assembly. Hence, inhibition of both AAK1 and GAK enzymes could block HCV assembly [79]. Two already approved anticancer drugs sunitinib and erlotinib were assessed for their anti-HCV assembly effects. However, these compounds induced adverse effects in treated patients because of a lack of specificity or drug off-target effects [80]. To overcome this limitation, a specific

GAK inhibitor (isothiazolo [5,4-b]pyridine]) was developed that efficiently disrupts HCV entry and assembly *in vitro* with limited drug off-target effects [81, 82].

HTAs Against HCV Assembly and Release

Citrus Flavonoids

Before release or egress from infected host cells, HCV virions adopt VLDL pathways during the later stage of their assembly which requires microsomal triglyceride transfer protein (MTP) to traffic more LDL and VLDL to LVPs [83]. These apolipoproteins (*e.g.*, ApoE, ApoB, and ApoA1) are considered essential for the formation of infectious HCV particles as numerous studies have evidenced that highly infectious LVPs are usually associated with more lipoproteins [84]. Furthermore, MTP incorporates more triglycerides into nascent LD and mediates apolipoprotein B (ApoB) loading in the endoplasmic reticulum. Thus, inhibitors of VLDL assembly pathways like MTP or ApoB inhibitors could prevent the assembly of more infectious VLPs and their release [85]. In this respect, a natural grapefruit flavonoid (naringenin) possessing MTP inhibitor characteristics, has been shown to prevent VLDL secretion both *in vitro* and *in vivo* and even HCV secretion in cell culture [85]. A study published in 2011, further expanded the mechanistic approach of this flavonoid to disrupt HCV assembly by activating the peroxisome proliferator-activated receptor α (PPARα) in hepatitis C-infected cells. PPARα belongs to a family of nuclear transcription factors that regulates several aspects of lipid metabolism in hepatic cells [86]. Activation of PPARα notably increases lipid oxidation and impairment of virion assembly and release [85]. HCV core protein inhibits PPARα activity to augment viral replication during CHC infection. Hence, reinstatement of PPARα activity may constitute an interesting treatment strategy to inhibit HCV replication. Several approved drugs for other clinical usages by targeting PPARα have displayed clinical promise as antiviral agents against HCV [85].

Resveratrol and Pterostilbene

Two natural compounds extracted from grapes and blueberries (resveratrol and its methylated form pterostilbene) as well as a derivative of the anti-cancer drug tamoxifen (*i.e.* toremifene) are good examples in this respect [87]. Bezafibrate, an antihyperlipidemic agent also expressed PPARα agonist activity in CHC-infected patients [88]. However, later on, it was noticed that bezafibrate antiviral potential was not related to a decrease in HCV viral load but rather to a significant decrease of hepatic enzymes and improved liver functions [89]. More recent studies indicate the efficacy of bezafibrate in the regulation of hepatic lipid metabolism and a decrease in HCV viral titers in cell culture [89].

Acyl-CoA: Cholesterol Acyltransferase (ACAT) Inhibitors

Mechanistic studies demonstrate that an inhibitor (avasimibe) of human acyl-CoA: cholesterol acyltransferase (ACAT; in nearly all mammalian cells, ACAT catalyzes the intracellular esterification of cholesterol and formation of cholesteryl esters) enzyme induces downregulation of microsomal triglyceride transfer protein expression and results in reduced Apo E and ApoB secretion [78]. Furthermore, a study demonstrates that avasimibe exhibits pan-genotypic antiviral activity by significantly impairing HCV LVPs assembly. Hence, it could be an effective antiviral treatment in combination with DAAs for HCV patients infected with hypercholesteremia as well [79].

A recent study notified HCV assembly and release downregulation capability of an MTP inhibitor amiodarone. However, prolonged amiodarone administration in combination with DAAs may elicit bradycardia in HCV-treated individuals [86, 90]. Different other VLDL pathway inhibitors are being evaluated in clinical trials for their potential use for dyslipidemia but their *in vitro* or *in vivo* efficacy against hepatitis C remains to be demonstrated. An antisense inhibitor of ApoB synthesis (*e.g.*, mipomersen) initially used for the treatment of hypercholesterolemia also exhibited potential blockade of HCV morphogenesis *in vitro* and required to be evaluated *in vivo* [91]. However, further clinical trials are eagerly awaited to determine the clinical antiviral efficacy of HCV assembly inhibitors [91].

Nanomedicine-Based Anti-HCV Agents

Nanomedicine has grabbed its attention very rapidly for the delivery of different therapeutic agents including anti-HCV immunization, and diagnostic and therapeutic agents in the last two decades [10]. The drugs, compounds, or agents are encapsulated or linked to nanoparticles (NPs) of different compositions including polymeric, lipid, or metallic NPs [10]. The current highly efficacious and pan-genotypic anti-HCV DAAs are still facing the barrier to safely reaching their target sites and consequently decreasing possible SAEs. Nanomedicines are also advantageous to reduce cytotoxicity as has been experienced with ribavirin (RBV) NPs associated reduced hemolytic anemia in treated individuals. The most important characteristic of NPs use is targeted liver drug delivery of anti-HCV drugs which was performed in the past through decoration of NPs surface with specific moieties like galactose (Gal), hyaluronic acid (HA), or vitamin E. These molecules either interact with receptors on hepatocytes (*e.g.*, HA and asialoglycoprotein receptors) or pass directly to the liver cells. Similarly, no vaccine is available to prevent HCV transmission risks, therefore nanotechnology also holds great potential for HCV vaccinology in the future by using conserved immune stimulant HCV parts to induce both humoral and cellular immune responses [10]. Herein, we will briefly overview to what extent the current advancement in nanotechnology could be helpful to develop safe, affordable, and effective anti-HCV drug delivery systems in near future.

Nanomedicine-Based anti-HCV Immunizing Nanoparticles

PEGylation of interferon (PEG-IFN) was the first application of nanotechnology to enhance the bioavailability, stability, safety, tissue or cell penetration, uptaking, and targeting of specific tissue and/or cells of any anti-HCV treatment [10]. It was also helpful to decrease the clearance rate of IFN and consequently resulted in a longer half-life. After that, extensive use of nanotechnology in the development and delivery of various anti-HCV agents including therapeutics, diagnostics, and immunizing products was carried out and continued with amazing forward steps in technology advancement both in extent and rate of anti-HCV nanomedicine which figure out the future of HCV therapeutics [10].

Nanovaccinology

Nanovaccinology (Also known as vaccine NPs) offers several benefits over traditional vaccine development strategies like rapid penetration of membrane barriers, protein antigen protection, and delivering them to target sites (*i.e.*, antigen-presenting cells; APCs) in a controlled environment which ultimately elicit prolonged immune responses [92]. Several vaccine NPs development approaches by using the carrier itself, homogenization of NPs with immunogens, encapsulating HCV antigen inside the NPs, or surface decoration of NPs with immunogen were adopted to deliver HCV NPs immunogens to induce an immune response or prevent virus spread [92].

Nanoparticles (NPs)

Polylactide-co-glycolide (PLGA), is an FDA-approved polymer, which can encapsulate different antigens and deliver them to APCs. HCV core and NS3 proteins are relatively conserved and play an important role in the induction of immune responses and clearance of HCV [92]. Recombinant core-NS3 (rC-N) fusion protein of HCV could induce T-cell mediated immune responses. rC-N/PLGA NPs were developed by linking the primary amine of rC-N and the carboxylic group of polymer NPs. These nano-vaccine particles were spherical with a particle size of 160 nm, had a polydispersity index (PDI) of 0.23, and exhibited higher penetration ability into the target cells [92].

NS2 gene of the HCV genome was physically conjugated to gelatin NPs, which had a particle size of 150 ± 2 nm and PDI of 0.09 [93]. NS2/gelatin NPs effectively enhanced the delivery of NS2 into *E. coli* bacteria to be amplified and expressed. This carrier could be used as a safe, non-viral vaccine against hepatitis C [93].

Triblock copolymers such as poly (d,l-lactic acid)-co-poly(ethylene glycol)-co-poly(d,l- lactic acid) (PLA–PEG–PLA) and poly(d,l-lactic-co-glycolic acid)-b-poly(ethylene glycol)-b poly(d,l-lactic-co-glycolic acid) (PLGA–PEG–PLGA) have been used as excellent carriers for genetic materials [94]. The presence of PEG improved copolymer hydrophilicity [95]. DNA encoding some regions of HCV GT-1b genes like NS2 (918–926 aa), NS4a (1694–1703 aa), C (30–43 aa), E2 (HVR390–401 aa), and E2 (408–414 aa) were incorporated into PLA–PEG–PLA, and PLGA–PEG–PLGA. These copolymers were able to deliver this multiple-epitope antigen gene to their target APCs and increased the humoral and cellular responses as compared with the naked gene. Similarly, the sustained release of multiple-epitope antigen genes from the micellar system enabled single-dose immunization with no side effects [94].

In one study, negatively charged plasmid DNA encoding HCV structural protein genes (*i.e.* core and E1/E2) was electrostatically complexed with cationic MPG cell-penetrating peptide [96]. MPG peptide was able to condensate DNA into small NPs at an N/P (nitrogen of peptide to the phosphate of DNA) ratio of 10:1. These NPs could protect the genes from degradation and at the same time facilitate their penetration into cells. Additionally, MPG/DNA could stimulate IgG1 and IgG2a levels higher than naked DNA [96].

Inorganic Nanoparticles (INPs)

Inorganic NPs were efficiently used to deliver immunogens of HCV such as gold NPs (AuNPs) and iron oxide (Fe_3O_4) NPs [97, 98]. AuNPs were mixed with pDNA encoding the HCV core gene and used as an approach for HCV nanovaccinology [98]. These NPs are highly conductive and can magnify the electric field. Upon electrical stimulation, NPs induce poration of the cell membrane to enable cellular uptake of the vaccine. Plasmonic AuNPs showed higher gene expression (100-fold than without NPs) and high levels of cellular and humoral immune responses against HCV [98].

Nano-system composed of dendrimers (hyper-branched polymers) can be used to deliver antiviral drugs [99, 100]. However, polyanionic dendrimers with a carbosilane structure can be used as prophylaxis against HCV spread by targeting the extracellular HCV and inhibiting its binding to target cells [101].

All the above-mentioned promising immunogen nanocarriers with a piece of evidence from literature about their ability to gradually release immunogen to elicit humoral immune responses in plasma and further cellular immunity after penetrating the cells suggest their further evaluation to clinical development against HCV. Furthermore, the gradual presentation of antigens to APCs enables single-dose immunization with no possible side effects and supports the body's immune system to grow immunological memory of the antigen. Similarly, antigen protection with these promising nanocarriers, and using multiple-epitope antigen genes in these NPs could be evaluated to strongly induce humoral and cellular immune responses against HCV in clinical trials.

Nanotechnology-based Anti-HCV Compounds

As the discovery and development of new anti-HCV drugs always remained a challenge for the investigators, a lot of efforts are being carried on to decrease the side effects of current regimens and most importantly to improve the drug delivery to target sites *via* new technologies like nanotechnology [102]. For this purpose, various types of polymeric, metallic, and lipid NPs were developed, utilized, and studied.

HA-decorated NPs

The first approach in this direction was the development of several hyaluronic acid (HA) and HA-decorated NPs to specifically target liver cells. HA is an abundant extracellular polysaccharide component in tissues that targets liver cells *via* binding with HA receptors (*i.e.* cluster determinant 44 'CD44' or hyaluronan receptor for endocytosis 'HARE') and then internalizes into the cells to deliver different drugs [102]. One of these HA-decorated AuNPs (52 nm, PDI = 0.09) was used to bind IFN-α *via* both hydrophobic and electrostatic forces and specifically delivered to hepatic cells [103]. Efficient binding between IFN and AuNPs resulted in sustained release of IFN-α for more than7 days. In addition to that, the polyanionic nature of HA prevents the adsorption of serum proteins, sterically inhibits the enzyme's negative effects on bound IFN, and imparts higher serum stability to the system. Adverse events associated with accompanied IFN, PEG-IFN, and even in combination with other anti-HCV agents were not observed following the use of these HA-decorated AuNPs [103].

Polymorphic Nanoparticles

RBV is still considered an integral part of some DAA combinations as an effective anti-HCV treatment strategy to cure HCV in some harder-to-treat HCV subpopulations. However, RBV cytotoxicity after extensive accumulation in red blood cells (RBCs) results in hemolytic anemia upon frequent use [104]. Modulation of RBV distribution by using various NPs resulted in decreased uptake by RBCs. RBV monophosphate (RMP, prodrug) stably loaded in a polymorphic nanocarrier composed of poly (D, L-lactic acid) (PLA) and arabinogalactan poly (L-lysine) (AG-PLL) was able to specifically deliver RBV to the hepatocytes without significant drug release in systemic circulation and subsequently no RBV accumulation in RBCs [104]. This RBV delivery to targeted liver cells was due to the polymer content of arabinogalactan (AG), which is a polysaccharide containing Gal side chains. Gal-decorated NPs specifically bind asialoglycoprotein receptors on hepatic cells, induce endocytosis, and release cargo inside the hepatic cells [104]. Another polymeric NPs based on polyglycerol adipate (PGA) has been reported as a liver-targeted RBV delivery system with reduced RBCs accumulation [105]. This approach exhibited that NPs uptake was significantly higher in HCV-infected cells than in non-viral-infected ones. Other NPs with different copolymer compositions (*e.g.*, Gal-decorated NPs and PHEAEDA- DPPE- GAL) have also been evaluated and resulted in improved entrapment efficiency of RBV prodrug due to its high hydrophobicity [105].

Despite DAA's development, other alternative drug moieties were also studied as an alternative therapeutic approach against HCV in the last decade. One such example was the development of peptide p41, which is a positively charged derivative of 18-mer C5A and was prepared by using arginine and lysine instead of the four moieties of C5A [106]. This modified peptide p41 was considered to have an equal ability to disrupt all HCV membrane lipids like 18-mer C5A. To protect this peptide from proteolysis and to reduce the positive charge-related cytotoxicity without affecting its antiviral efficacy, polymeric NPs (formed by electrostatic interaction between the cationic peptide p41 and anionic poly (amino acid)-based copolymer) were used. The same peptide electrostatically conjugated with other copolymers (PEG-b-PLD and PEG-b-PLE) was used as a trial to treat HCV and HIV coinfection in 2013 [107]. In 2015, another NPs composed of galactosylated PEG-b-PLE copolymers were used to specifically deliver p41 to HCV-infected hepatic cells *via* binding to asialoglycoprotein receptors present on hepatic cells [108]. These NPs significantly showed the inhibition of viral infection due to the virucidal activity of p41.

HCV Gene Therapy Based on Nanoviral Vectors

Anti-mRNA-based treatment strategies are extensively studied in the form of siRA and shRNA against HCV. Nanomedicine-based siRNAs and shRNAs were also designed and developed to evaluate their therapeutic potential by targeting certain enzymes and host factors, which regulate the HCV life cycle [108]. We have discussed in detail the host cellular factors which play an essential role in the regulation of the HCV life cycle in chapter 2. Herein we will highlight how the modulation of some of those by nano-based siRNA or shRNA may affect the HCV life cycle in host cells.

Protein kinase C-related kinase 2 (PRK2) is an enzyme responsible for the phosphorylation of HCV RdRp polymerase required for HCV replication [108]. Lipid-like material (Lipidoid), which results from the conjugation of amine to acrylamides, was used with cholesterol and PEG-ceramide to encapsulate PRK2-specific siRNA (*i.e.* siPRK2) and delivered to the hepatocytes. siPRK2 lipid NPs without any ligands were specifically uptaken by hepatocytes due to their lipid composition and effectively silenced PRK2 expression in hepatocytes [109]. Furthermore, these decorated NPs with PEG were multifunctional not only to prolong siRNA circulation time but also to reduce inflammatory responses accompanied by the use of lipid NPs. Another modulation of this siRNA *i.e.* (siPRK2/lipidoid) composed of epoxide-based lipidoids, diastearoyl phosphatidylcholine, cholesterol, and PEG-ceramide, was also assessed to interfere with HCV replication. Furthermore, galactosylation of siPRK2/lipidoid NPs improved PRK2 silencing in mouse liver up to 80% instead of 60% with nongalactosylated siPRK2/lipidoid NPs after systemic administration, and subsequently, rapid inhibition of HCV virus replication was noticed in HCV-xenograft mouse [108, 109].

Lipid Nanoparticles for siRNA Delivery

siRNA targeted against a conserved region of 5' UTR as well as core protein were encapsulated with unique NPs and evaluated to suppress HCV replication [110]. Liver-targeted cationic liposomes composed of 1,2-dioleoyl-3-trimethy lammonium propane (DOTAP) and cholesterol and further conjugated to VE (DC-VE) were used to deliver these siRNAs to their target sites. siRNA-5'UTR/DC-VE and siRNA-core 1/DC-VE NPs were efficiently delivered to hepatocytes and silenced liver-specific expression of 5' UTR luciferase and HCV core around 83% [110]. Other potential advantages of using this nanoviral vector include a decreased siRNA dose administration, and enhanced siRNA stability against serum nucleases with a broad safety spectrum on organ functions even in the blood system, making it a good tool for HCV siRNA delivery. Moreover, vitamin E (α-tocopherol) conjugated siRNAs can pass easily to hepatocytes [110].

Lipid Nanoparticles for shRNA Delivery

shRNAs represent an alternative to overcome chemically synthesized siRNA off-target effects, cytotoxicity, and limited delivery to their targeted sites [111]. shRNA encapsulated with lipid NPs composed of a mixture of various lipids (*e.g.*, PEG-lipid PEG-C-DMA, DLinDMA), cholesterol, and PEG was synthesized to target IRES domains of HCV and inhibit HCV replication. Single I.V administration of shRNAs/lipid NPs into HCV-infected mice exhibited efficient serum shRNA stability, enhanced uptake of NPs, and rapid inhibition of IRES-conjugated luciferase expression up to 90% in mouse hepatocytes. In addition to that, no significant changes in inflammatory responses were noticed because of lipid NPs induced modulation of shRNAs [111].

Nano-robots to Treat HCV

Nanozyme

Currently, the latest advancement in nanotechnology has transformed one step closer toward HCV therapy by designing a nano-robot that is programmed to specifically turn off the up-regulation of HCV genes and subsequently gene-encoding proteins [112]. This nano-robot which is also known as nanozyme is a colloidal NP and consists of an NPs core, the shell of DNA oligonucleotide, and a catalytically active enzyme in its composition. DNA oligonucleotide is complementary in this nanozyme to capture the target gene (*i.e.* HCV mRNA) and then send instructions to shell enzymes to cleave this target gene into two pieces and ultimately shut down HCV replication machinery. Other tailored nanozyme composed of AuNPs as a core and a shell consisting of DNA oligonucleotide complementary to target HCV RNA at 322-339 nucleotides and endoribonuclease (RNAase A) able to cleave HCV RNA were also evaluated for their anti-HCV therapeutic potential. This nanozyme conjugated with RNase activity showed that DNA complementary oligonucleotide target HCV mRNA gene and RNAse cleaved it into two pieces in a sequence- and site-specific manner resulting in a 99.9% decrease in HCV mRNA levels. Hence, this intracellular nanomachinery represents potential anti-HCV effects through substantial cooperative mechanisms along with good stability, safety, and target selectivity [112].

DNAzyme

A similar nano-robot was developed by using iron oxide NPs as a core and a shell composed of DNAzyme and myristoylated polyarginine peptide (MPAP) [113]. DNAzyme is an oligonucleotide sequence used in this nano-robot with the ability to target and cleave HCV mRNA from a specific region (*i.e.* NS3). NS3 gene of the HCV genome possesses both protease and helicase activities which are considered essential for HCV genome replication and translation. Subsequently, silencing or down-regulation of NS3 expression suppresses HCV replication. MPAP acts like a cell-penetrating peptide that enhances membrane penetration and cellular uptake [113]. Iron oxide NPs as a core facilitate tracking by using magnetic resonance imaging (MRI). DNAzyme/MPAP/iron oxide NPs efficiently delivered DNAzyme in haptic and kupffer cells and downregulated NS3 expression up to 91% with 1 mM NPs [114]. No cytotoxic effects or induction of immune responses were noticed with this DNAzyme. Hence both RNAzyme and DNAzyme could be considered potential antiviral tools against HCV as previous studies validate their potential to silence or down-regulate HCV genome replication [113].

Inorganic Nanoparticles: a Safe anti-HCV Drug Development Strategy

Inorganic nanotechnology based on trace elements found in the human body also showed promise to be a safe anti-HCV strategy [115]. For example, cuprous oxide (Cu_2O) NPs showed significant inhibition of HCV attachment and entry into HCVcc/Huh7.5.1 cells, while polyvalent binding to the virus surface, and shielding the virus binding sites to hepatic cell receptors and entry [116]. Hence, Cu_2O NPs were useful to reduce HCV infectivity having the least impact on its replication. Further evaluation of inorganic NPs is extensively needed as an anti-HCV approach to avoid many drug-related severe adverse events (SAEs) [116].

Nanomedicine-Based DAAs in Future

The extensive studies on nanomedicine technology while using all the above-mentioned systems insights into their bright future in novel HCV therapeutics development. Although no DAA- based nanomedicines have been reported and approved by the US FDA yet. DAAs are highly efficacious pan-genotypic regimens, are well tolerable, and produce fewer SAEs in treated individuals [117]. Although affordability and the emergence of RASs are still two big concerns with DAAs administration [117]. The benefits of nanomedicine research by adopting suitable drug delivery systems can be directed to develop certain nano-based DAAs in the future to improve their physicochemical properties, drug targeting, tissue distribution, as well as both pharmacokinetics and pharmacodynamics profile [118]. Furthermore, HCC occurrence or recurrence with DAAs usage in HCV-treated individuals have been reported in real-world clinical practice which mainly attributes to the time gaps between HCC treatment and DAAs administration [117]. It also represents an additional area to focus on where the development and evaluation of nano-based DAAs can contribute to reducing the risk of HCC recurrence and prevent the progression of CHC into other hepatic comorbidities [118].

HCV Vaccine Models-a Now or Never Situation in This Decade

The Global Health Sector Strategy on viral hepatitis (2016-2021) set an ambitious goal to eliminate HCV by 2030. To achieve this milestone, it is projected to reduce new HCV infections by 90% in 2030, which ultimately requires affordable access to effective prevention and treatment strategies all over the world [1]. Despite the highest clinical efficacy promise shown by the pan-genotypic DAAs to cure HCV-infected populations in real-life situations, to date, only 10% of HCV-infected individuals have received the treatment worldwide [1]. Hence, there is a huge demand to design and develop a protective or prophylactic HCV vaccine effective against all HCV GTs/subtypes worldwide to reduce the risk of infection transmission [1]. However, HCV vaccinology has always faced a lot of challenges to design and developing an effective vaccine due to the high genetic heterogeneity, genetic variability, and high mutation rate of HCV in infected individuals [2]. Furthermore, infection kinetics, variable immune responses against acute and chronic HCV infection, and immunological susceptibility to HCV reinfection also interrupt to design of a commercial preventive vaccine against HCV [2]. Efforts are underway in developing an effective HCV vaccine, although the progress is regrettably slow (Table **3**). However, there are potential lines of evidence that highlight its potential feasibility including; First, initial control of viremia during acute HCV infection coincides with the emergence of virus-specific B and T cell immune responses in blood, which persist for long-term (in particular $CD4^+$ T helper cells) and are strongly responsible for spontaneous clearance of acute infection. It is because of these immune responses that approximately 30% of acute HCV treatment-naive individuals clear the infection within 6 months of their first exposure. Second, the natural resolution of acute HCV infection may generate or memorize long-lasting immune responses that afford improved and durable virological control of HCV reinfection and significantly reduce the risk of CHC infection even occasionally against heterologous HCV strains. Prospective studies of HCV-infected individuals with potential injection drug use demonstrate that spontaneous clearance of prior infection reduces 60% of rates of HCV persistence following virus re-exposure. Hence, the availability and administration of a vaccine that may elicit immunity equivalent to that conferred by natural clearance of acute HCV infection would be reasonably efficacious in fractions of vulnerable HCV populations to prevent the transmission of HCV infection in the general population [2]. However, multiple studies reveal that naturally acquired HCV immunity is not always protective and reliable in preventing CHC reinfection in particular against heterologous virus strains, hence vaccine platforms effective against all HCV GTs/subtypes multiple epitopes should be pursued [119]. Third, the geographical distribution of HCV GTs/subtypes and quasispecies dynamics will also impact a proper HCV vaccine design [120]. Phylogenetic analysis of heterologous HCV strains from different regions indicates that HCV GTs-1 and 3 are highly prevalent worldwide with inter-genotypic or intra-genotypic host diversity while the remaining are primarily restricted to Africa and Asia [120]. It points out that an effective vaccine against HCV GT-1 and 3 infections would be of great value at least to prevent the transmission of new HCV infections of these GTs each year and will pave the ways to reduce the global healthcare burden while task-shifting the resources to treat other HCV GTs/subtypes with DAAs [2]. Furthermore, the vaccines for less prevented and regionally distributed HCV GTs/subtypes can be designed for their target deployment in at-risk populations. One rational approach that can be followed in this aspect was the successful eradication of poliovirus serotype 2 and 3 infections worldwide [2].

Potential Candidates for HCV Prophylactic Vaccines

Traditional Immunization Approaches

Multiple pieces of evidence for a large variety of candidate HCV vaccines inducing humoral and/or cellular immune responses have been evaluated in preclinical animal models [2]. Both prophylactic and/or protective/therapeutic (as an adjunct to HCV antiviral therapy) approaches were considered to design and develop an effective vaccine with the ability to induce vigorous and prolonged humoral and cellular immune responses against different HCV GTs to reduce virus spread between cells [2]. The journey started with traditional immunization approaches like whole proteins and virus-like particles, to newer DNA and recombinant viral vector-based strategies. However, the whole HCV virus (either attenuated or inactivated) was not recommended for vaccine design due to biohazard concerns [121]. Moreover, other vaccine strategies including recombinant proteins, synthetic peptides, dendritic cells, and virosome-based vaccines also grabbed the attention to design safe vaccines [2]. However, most of these approaches were focused on either targeting the envelope glycoproteins of HCV (E1 & E2) for the generation of neutralizing antibodies (nAbs) as well as induction of humoral immune responses or HCV nonstructural proteins (*e.g.*, NS3-NS5B) to vigorously induce the $CD4^+$ and $CD8^+$ T cell immune responses [122]. Several recombinant HCV protein vaccine models with dual approaches were also developed. An ample understanding of the HCV life cycle and valuable insights into some conserved immune system stimulant parts of the HCV genome (*i.e.* 5' and 3' UTRs) also sparked the investigators to engineer other possibilities for HCV vaccinations [2]. Interestingly very few of these vaccine models were evaluated for their protective efficacy in animal models (chimpanzees), with mixed findings (Table **3**). Only two of those vaccine models with some degree of effectivity while preventing CHC infection in chimpanzees were progressed to human clinical trials (Table **3**) [2].

Antibody-based Vaccine Model

The first Ab-based vaccine originally developed by Chiron Corporation (parent organization, Novartis®) consisted of recombinant E1 and E2 glycoproteins from HCV GT-1a virus adjuvanted with MF59 [123]. The elicited humoral responses by this vaccine significantly protected homologous challenge in chimpanzees;

however, the vaccine could not provide sufficient sterilizing immunity against heterologous infection except for delaying the onset of viremia and reducing the course of infection as compared to unvaccinated controls [124]. In healthy human volunteers, the vaccine regimens elicited both strong HCV-specific $CD4^+$ T-helper cell responses and in some recipients, cross-genotyping nAbs. Despite these encouraging findings, the follow-up trials of this vaccine model to further evaluate its efficacy are on hold and yet to proceed [125].

T-cell Based Vaccine Model

The second potential candidate vaccine is a T-cell-based vaccine model developed by Okairos Corporation (parent organization, Glaxo Smith Kline®) and consisting of a recombinant chimpanzee adenovirus (serotype 3) prime and modified vaccinia virus Ankara (MVA) boost encoding the NS3-5B proteins from HCV GT-1b virus [126]. The animal trial of this vaccine in chimpanzees immunized with an adenovirus prime followed by a plasmid DNA boost elicited long-lived $CD4^+$ and $CD8^+$ cell responses against virus nonstructural proteins. The heterologous infection resulted in a rapid recall of memory T cell responses in chimpanzees and a significant reduction of acute-phase viremia compared to historical controls [127]. Likewise, in healthy human volunteers, the vaccine broadly stimulated both multi-potent $CD4^+$ and $CD8^+$ cells' immune responses which resembled and were equivalent to those natural immune responses generated upon spontaneous clearance of primary infection. Based on these findings, the vaccine efficacy was tested in a group of HCV-infected high-risk IDUs in phase II clinical trials [128]. Some unique aspects of this clinical trial are remarkable. First, in the clinical trials, the vaccine efficacy was tested on the assumption that T cell-induced immunity alone could prevent or reduce persistent HCV infection in the absence of nAbs responses. Second, the feasibility to access HCV-infected IDUs to conduct rigorous vaccine research is not easy and demands substantial resources to maintain trial follow-up and engagement [129]. Although, the induction of T-cell immune responses was observed in the majority of volunteers; however, the vaccine could not succeed to reduce the incidences of chronic infection. The reasons for this failure are not yet understood.

New Hepacivirus Models for Vaccine Research

The major barrier to developing an effective HCV vaccine is the lack of an immunologically tractable animal model [2]. As mentioned earlier, HCV expresses a narrow and strict species tropism for humans, and the only permissive animal model after humans is the chimpanzee. However, that is not easily accessible and significant ethical concerns limit its use for vaccine research [2]. Several engineered mouse models which support the HCV life cycle were used to evaluate *in vivo* Abs activity. However, these models require the blockade of host immune responses to function, therefore, their use is not so fruitful for HCV vaccine research [2].

Based on a rational approach like an *in vivo* surrogate, a biologically similar and closely related infectious virus could be a plausible solution to overcome these challenges in HCV vaccine research.

Non-primate Hepacivirus (NPHV) Infection Model

The non-primate *Hepacivirus* (NPHV) naturally circulates in domestic horses and is the closest genetic relative of HCV and was first identified in 2011 [130]. Experimental NPHV infection of horses supports several features of HCV natural infection like the tendency to cause chronic disease, delayed seroconversion, and acute hepatic pathology [131]. One study demonstrates the spontaneous clearance of primary NPHV infection associated with immune protection against reinfection, similar to hepatitis C [132]. However, the difficulty in its frequent availability as an easily tractable animal, and some ethical concerns also limit its overall application [132]. From the experimental aspects, horse primary NPHV infection was noticed to be spontaneously cleared at high frequency, hence not favorable to study the vaccine assessment concepts related to the prevention of chronic infection as the primary endpoint [132].

Rodent Hepacivirus (RHV) Infection Model

A rodent *Hepacivirus* (RHV) with similar infection kinetics to HCV was discovered in the livers of feral Norway rats in New York City in 2014 [133]. The passage of an isolate of RHV into immune-competent laboratory mice and rats resulted in rapid hepatotropic viral infection [133]. Viremia was noticed to clear within several weeks in mice upon T cell-dependent immune responses; but, persisted at high levels in rats, the RHV's natural host [133]. Efforts were made to further adapt RHV to mice; however, the ability of chronic infection induction was only possible in those RHV strains lacking components of innate or adaptive immunity. Hence, limiting the use of RHV mice for vaccine concept testing [133].

In contrast, other infection characteristics like hepatic inflammation, innate immune sensing, spontaneous T cell dysfunction, and susceptibility to DAAs treatment in RHV rats revealed HCV-like patterns [133]. The use of a rat (-RHV) infection model for HCV vaccine research was recently demonstrated by two studies evaluating the effectiveness of T-cell immunization in preventing RHV persistence [134]. Administration of adenoviral vectors expressing the RHV NS3-5B proteins (similar to human HCV vaccine candidate) to rats generated $CD4^+$ and $CD8^+$ T cell responses and remarkably reduced the incidence of chronic infection after homologous challenge [134]. The protective immune response was T cell-dependent and was evident by the depletion of $CD4^+$ and $CD8^+$ T cells immediately before homologous infection that resulted in a substantially attenuated infection course [134]. Moreover, the inclusion of envelope glycoproteins (E1 and E2) as vaccine targets to elicit nAbs responses also enhanced protection from viral persistence; however, the mechanism of this effect is not yet known [134]. A recent follow-up study further demonstrates that infection with an RHV strain encoding mutations in dominant MHC class I epitopes that impair RHV-specific $CD8^+$ T cell function *in vitro* substantially reduce vaccine protection in naïve rats [135]. This finding highlights the importance of cross-reactivity between vaccine-induced T cell responses and infecting RHV strain. Surprisingly, vaccinated rats who had already cleared homologous infection were found to be protected against subsequent challenges with mutated RHV [135].

Table 3. Potential candidate prophylactic HCV vaccines tested in humans with their clinical phase development. GT; genotype. CD; cluster of differentiation.

Potential Candidate Vaccines Against HCV									
Vaccine Platform	**HCV Antigen**	**HCV Genotype**	**Tested Model**	**Immunogenicity**	**Clinical Trial Phase**	**Clinical Outcomes**	**Vaccine Protection**	**Challenges**	**References**
Recombinant protein	Core (C)	GT-1a	Humans	CD4 and CD8 T cells	Phase I	-	-	-	[136]
	E1	GT-1b	Humans	Anti-E1 antibodies, CD4 T cells	Phase I	-	-	-	[137]
	E1E2	GT-1a	Humans	Neutralizing antibodies, CD4 T cells	Phase I	-	-	-	[138, 139]

(Table 3) cont.....

Viral vector	NS3-NS5B	GT-1b	Humans	Heterotypic CD4 and CD8 T cells	Phase I	-	-	-	[140]
	NS3-NS5B	GT-1b	Humans	Heterotypic CD4 and CD8 T cells	Phase I	-	-	-	[128]
	NS3-NS5B fused to MHC class II-associated invariant chain	GT-1b	Humans	Heterotypic CD4 and CD8 T cells	Phase I	-	-	-	[141]
	NS3-NS5B	GT-1b	Humans	T cells	Phase I/II	-	Reduced peak viremia but did not protect against chronic infection upon natural exposure	-	[129]

This finding proposes that vaccine-elicited immunity can be enhanced or prolonged to prevent infection caused by genetically diverse *Hepacivirus* strains. However, the mechanism for this improvement is not yet clear along the contributory role of humoral immunity is also not well defined [134, 2].

The results of these two studies decipher the potential use of the rat RHV infection model to elucidate HCV vaccine concept testing related to protective immunity as well as evaluating mechanisms of HCV-like immunity [135]. However, *in vitro* models for measuring anti-RHV nAbs responses are not yet available and efforts are currently underway to design such a model that could be instrumental and helpful to figure out the obscure role of B cell or humoral immunity in protection against CHC infection [135]. One possible way out could be the administration of a vaccine against the RHV E1 and E2 envelope glycoproteins with a subsequent viral infection to raise nAb responses followed by to assess for protection [2]. The approaches like sera transfer and depletion studies can be used to swiftly determine vaccine efficacy. Since the RHV infection model was found susceptible to DAAs treatment, the efficacy of vaccine after therapeutic cure with DAAs can also be addressed with broad implications for CHC infection in general as well as in harder-to-cure HCV infected populations [2].

Limitations of the RHV Model

Some limitations of the RHV model are also noteworthy. First, there is currently only one available RHV strain for experimental study, precluding the evaluation of true and diverse heterologous immunity kinetics following vaccination [142]. However, it can be manageable by further isolation of multiple and genetically diverse RHV strains from wild rats or by choosing the strains that naturally acquired vaccine resistance. Furthermore, quasispecies dynamics of RHV during chronic infection like HCV is largely unknown so extra approaches to emulate the circulation of RHV as quasispecies need to be elucidated. Second, the limited access and affordability of immunological reagents for rats may hinder more detailed studies to understand immune mechanism dysfunction and vaccine failure in rats. Last but not least and most importantly, the difficulty in the translation of the findings in the rat RHV model to humans is also a major concern. The failure of recent T cell HCV vaccine trials in humans may augment this concern [142].

Controlled Human Infection Model (CHIM)

The limitations of a controlled animal infection model as described above with the specific scientific and practical challenges of conducting large-scale trials within at-risk populations urged the investigators to design a controlled human infection model (CHIM) to accelerate vaccine development [2]. The curative treatment of HCV infection with current DAAs further fueled this ongoing approach to be reasonably plausible. By adopting this approach, healthy human volunteers would be immunized first with a promising vaccine candidate or placebo and then exposed to a well-characterized and controlled strain of HCV to assess vaccine efficacy. The volunteers suffering from acute HCV infection will be typically benign and most probably will spontaneously clear the infection; however, the study volunteers developing clinically considerable findings of chronic infection would be rapidly treated with pan-genotypic DAAs to prevent long-term morbidity [2].

Advantages of CHIM

Indeed, the CHIM approach for future vaccine models has certain potential advantages [2]. The development of promising HCV vaccine candidates would be in a highly controlled scientific setting by identifying their efficacy very carefully and expeditiously in healthy individuals exposed to controlled HCV infection and then rapidly modulated with advanced settings for further testing in high-risk HCV infected populations (*e.g.*, IDUs, MSM, sex workers, HCV/HIV or HCV/HBV, HCV/CKD co-infected populations) if deems necessary. It would minimize the healthcare burden both in terms of tremendous costs and healthcare services and overcome crosscutting barriers associated with conducting HCV immunological studies in high-risk populations, who require extensive risk-reducing strategies (both in terms of cost and services) and often to mitigate significant social vulnerabilities that complicate linkage to HCV care and post-treatment monitoring and long-term follow-ups. Subsequently, a rich pool of potential candidates for HCV vaccines with scientific support data would be at the bottlenecks of HCV vaccine development by effectively sidestepping the limitations of the lack of large-patient groups [2].

Disadvantages of CHIM

However, multiple scientific and safety concerns will always be there with CHIM for HCV vaccine development. First, from the infection kinetics perspective, it is still not obvious that either a CHIM would adequately simulate natural HCV exposure events [2]. Inoculation of healthy study volunteers with a culture-derived HCV strain seems an unviable approach because these strains may possess multiple adaptive mutations that augment *in vitro* replication and upon study participants, the infection may induce unintended effects. Second, for the study of quasispecies dynamics of CHIM, the use of plasma-derived HCV from infected individuals would be required; however, the transfusion of plasma-derived HCV with the impurity of additional infectious pathogens may also misperceive study outcomes. Third, routes and dosage algorithms may impact the infectious course of CHIM in study participants in a controlled setting compared to a natural HCV course. Last, how the study outcomes derived from healthy volunteers would be reliably considered for high-risk HCV-infected populations, those that have intrinsically altered and complicated immune responses to HCV vaccination [2].

Limitations of CHIM Considering Vaccine Safety and Efficacy

In terms of vaccine safety and efficacy studies for a long duration, CHIM may have some major limitations [2]. As mentioned earlier the severity and chronicity of all HCV-associated comorbidities (*e.g.*, fibrosis, cirrhosis, and HCC) occur during or after chronic infection, the primary endpoint measures of vaccine effectiveness whether it prevents the development of persistent viremia, cannot be established until 3-6 months after virus exposure or during the acute infection period. It indicates that vaccine efficacy studies require a long follow-up period during which study participants may inadvertently transmit the virus to other individuals (*e.g.*, sexual partners). During the extensive and long follow-up period, study volunteers may be lost and it represents one of the major concerns that must be properly safeguarded to ensure a swift treatment in case chronic infection was to occur. Although the overall risk for the potential emergence of resistance is minimal with CHIM and can be effectively avoided by infecting study participants with a strain that is known to be sensitive, cross-resistance between DAAs treatment and CHIM exists and must be acknowledged during the study period [2].

Distinct Conceptualization and Translational Phases of HCV Vaccine Development

The current landscape of widescale availability of therapeutic cures for HCV in the form of pan-genotypic DAAs may mitigate ongoing HCV transmission and virus prevalence worldwide [1]. However, the lessons leveraged from the current ongoing COVID-19 pandemic management by promising vaccines signify the importance of the development of an effective vaccine to achieve the global HCV elimination goal by 2030 and, therefore must be pursued [143]. Despite many challenges to encounter, an exact and goal-centered strategy adopted for the development of anti-Covid-19 vaccines should be undertaken to widen the pool of potential HCV vaccine candidates and to swiftly evaluate their safety and efficacy in clinical studies [144]. The compensation for the lack of a true HCV animal model with the two most promising options (*i.e.*, RHV and CHIM) for testing new HCV vaccine concepts, as described above, could be influential to develop and trial an effective vaccine [2]. Both models seem self-sufficient while providing a mechanistic dissection for developing novel delivery vectors and vaccine targets as well as an avenue for evaluating vaccine safety and efficacy before engaging more complicated routes of high-risk population testing, respectively. The advantages of both models can be amalgamated by envisioning a rational approach to HCV vaccine design composed of distinct conceptualization and translational phases of development [2].

During the conceptualization phase, various vaccine strategies could be designed, engineered, and potentially evaluated for their capability to encounter diverse *Hepacivirus* infection challenges (either homologous or heterologous) in RHV [2]. After that, successful vaccine candidates can be modulated by the latest vaccinology tools for translational testing in a relatively small number of healthy volunteers in a CHIM. Although the adaptation of this 'conceptualization and translational phase' channel will narrow the spectrum for moving HCV vaccine development forward, its remarkable potential to generate the quality and quantity of candidates for HCV vaccines will open new horizons for meaningful progress in this arena and should be pragmatically pursued [2].

CONCLUSIONS

The 2020 Noble Prize in Physiology or Medicine was awarded to three extraordinary scientists, who paved the way for hepatitis C research and drug discovery, saving millions of lives worldwide. However, the design and development of effective, safe, and targeted drugs for HCV always remained an uphill task in front of researchers and investigators worldwide. This journey started from the evaluation of interferon-based regimens against HCV since the early nineties and is continued as we have a dense manual of IFN-free pan-genotypic DAAs to treat this silent epidemic. Anti-hepatitis C protein-specific oligonucleotides, RNA interference (RNAi), micro RNA (miRNA), phytochemicals, and some potential anti-hepatitis C vaccine models have been widely and extensively studied as an alternative or adjuvant therapeutic regimens for hepatitis C cure besides the advent and approval of once 'gold standard of hepatitis C care' (*i.e.* pegylated interferon (PEG-IFN) plus a nucleoside analog ribavirin (RBV)), and recently approved IFN-free DAA regimens. Some of these treatment strategies are still in the pipeline. Where the approval of the first small interference RNA (siRNA) therapy for a certain genetic disorder has urged the investigators to refocus this approach against hepatitis C because it represents the most thoroughly studied treatment approach against hepatitis C in the last two decades. Furthermore, some emerging approaches like host-targeting antivirals, nanoparticle-containing immunogens, and nanomedicine-based therapeutic agents are also in their full investigative form. There would always be a desperate demand for a prophylactic, protective, or minimum effective vaccine model to prevent and protect against the emergence and transmission of HCV from vulnerable and hidden retreatment failure of HCV populations. The development of controlled or HCV alike human infection models will open the ways to develop a minimum effective vaccine model against the most prevalent HCV GTs/subtypes worldwide to reduce infection transmission in healthy individuals. The transformational impact of the latest innovations in drug designing and development technologies, as seen during the Covid-19 pandemic, will also help to rationalize these approaches against HCV in the future.

REFERENCES

[1] Shahid I, Alzahrani AR, Al-Ghamdi SS, Alanazi IM, Rehman S, Hassan S. Hepatitis C Diagnosis: Simplified Solutions, Predictive Barriers, and Future Promises. Diagnostics 2021; 11: 7.

[2] Hartlage AS, Kapoor A, Hepatitis C. Hepatitis C Virus Vaccine Research: Time to Put Up or Shut Up. Viruses 2021; 13(8): 1596.
[PMID: 34452460]

[3] Shahid I, Ibrahim MM. All Oral Interferon-free Direct-acting Antivirals as Combination Therapies to Cure Hepatitis C. Curr Mol Med 2018; 18(7): 409-35.
[PMID: 30608042]

[4] AlMalki WH, Shahid I, Abdalla AN, Johargy AK, Ahmed M, Hassan S. Consensus small interfering RNA targeted to stem-loops II and III of IRES structure of 5′ UTR effectively inhibits virus replication and translation of HCV sub-genotype 4a isolates from Saudi Arabia. Saudi J Biol Sci 2021; 28(1): 1109-22.
[PMID: 33424405]

[5] Shahid I, Almalki WH, Ibrahim MM, *et al.* Characterization of *In vitro* inhibitory effects of consensus short interference RNAs against non-structural 5B gene of hepatitis C virus 1a genotype. Indian J Med Microbiol 2018; 36(4): 494-503.
[PMID: 30880695]

[6] Soobramoney C, Parboosing R. siRNAs and Viruses: The good, the Bad and the Way Forward. Curr

Mol Pharmacol 2022; 15(1): 143-58.
[PMID: 33881977]

[7] Lee EB, Sung PS, Kim JH, Park DJ, Hur W, Yoon SK. microRNA-99a Restricts Replication of Hepatitis C Virus by Targeting mTOR and de novo Lipogenesis. Viruses 2020; 12(7): E696.
[PMID: 32605105]

[8] Chang J, Nicolas E, Marks D, *et al.* miR-122, a mammalian liver-specific microRNA, is processed from hcr mRNA and may downregulate the high affinity cationic amino acid transporter CAT-1. RNA Biol 2004; 1(2): 106-13.
[PMID: 17179747]

[9] Crouchet E, Wrensch F, Schuster C, Zeisel MB, Baumert TF. Host-targeting therapies for hepatitis C virus infection: current developments and future applications. Therap Adv Gastroenterol 2018; 11: 1756284818759483.
[PMID: 29619090]

[10] Abd Ellah NH, Tawfeek HM, John J, Hetta HF. Nanomedicine as a future therapeutic approach for Hepatitis C virus. Nanomedicine (Lond) 2019; 14(11): 1471-91.
[PMID: 31166139]

[11] Aljowaie RM, Almajhdi FN, Ali HH, El-Wetidy MS, Shier MK. Inhibition of hepatitis C virus genotype 4 replication using siRNA targeted to the viral core region and the CD81 cellular receptor. Cell Stress Chaperones 2020; 25(2): 345-55.
[PMID: 32060691]

[12] Ansar M, Ashfaq UA, Shahid I, *et al.* Inhibition of full length hepatitis C virus particles of 1a genotype through small interference RNA. Virol J 2011; 8: 203.
[PMID: 21535893]

[13] Shahid I, AlMalki WH, AlRabia MW, *et al.* In vitro inhibitory analysis of consensus siRNAs against NS3 gene of hepatitis C virus 1a genotype. Asian Pac J Trop Med 2017; 10(7): 701-9.
[PMID: 28870347]

[14] Asad S, Ijaz B, Ahmad W, *et al.* Development of persistent HCV genotype 3a infection cell culture model in huh-7 cell. Virol J 2012; 9: 11.
[PMID: 22234052]

[15] Shahid I, Gull S, Ijaz B, *et al.* Stable Huh-7 cell lines expressing non-structural proteins of genotype 1a of hepatitis C virus. J Virol Methods 2013; 189(1): 65-9.
[PMID: 23352716]

[16] Prabhu R, Vittal P, Yin Q, *et al.* Small interfering RNA effectively inhibits protein expression and negative strand RNA synthesis from a full-length hepatitis C virus clone. J Med Virol 2005; 76(4): 511-9.
[PMID: 15977238]

[17] Yokota T, Sakamoto N, Enomoto N, *et al.* Inhibition of intracellular hepatitis C virus replication by synthetic and vector-derived small interfering RNAs. EMBO Rep 2003; 4(6): 602-8.
[PMID: 12740604]

[18] Kapadia SB, Brideau-Andersen A, Chisari FV. Interference of hepatitis C virus RNA replication by short interfering RNAs. Proc Natl Acad Sci USA 2003; 100(4): 2014-8.
[PMID: 12566571]

[19] Khaliq S, Jahan S, Ijaz B, *et al.* Inhibition of core gene of HCV 3a genotype using synthetic and vector derived siRNAs. Virol J 2010; 7: 318.
[PMID: 21073745]

[20] Zekri AR, Bahnassy AA, El-Din HM, Salama HM. Consensus siRNA for inhibition of HCV genotype-4 replication. Virol J 2009; 6: 13.
[PMID: 19173711]

[21] Krönke J, Kittler R, Buchholz F, *et al.* Alternative approaches for efficient inhibition of hepatitis C virus RNA replication by small interfering RNAs. J Virol 2004; 78(7): 3436-46.
[PMID: 15016866]

[22] Prabhu R, Garry RF, Dash S. Retraction Note: Small interfering RNA targeted to stem-loop II of the 5′ untranslated region effectively inhibits expression of six HCV genotypes. Virol J 2021; 18(1): 155.
[PMID: 34311743]

[23] Pan Q, Henry SD, Metselaar HJ, *et al.* Combined antiviral activity of interferon-alpha and RNA interference directed against hepatitis C without affecting vector delivery and gene silencing. J Mol Med (Berl) 2009; 87(7): 713-22.
[PMID: 19404587]

[24] Boyd SD. Everything you wanted to know about small RNA but were afraid to ask. Lab Invest 2008; 88(6): 569-78.
[PMID: 18427554]

[25] Fukuhara T, Matsuura Y. Role of miR-122 and lipid metabolism in HCV infection. J Gastroenterol 2013; 48(2): 169-76.
[PMID: 22965312]

[26] Chang J, Guo JT, Jiang D, Guo H, Taylor JM, Block TM. Liver-specific microRNA miR-122 enhances the replication of hepatitis C virus in nonhepatic cells. J Virol 2008; 82(16): 8215-23.
[PMID: 18550664]

[27] Thakral S, Ghoshal K. miR-122 is a unique molecule with great potential in diagnosis, prognosis of liver disease, and therapy both as miRNA mimic and antimir. Curr Gene Ther 2015; 15(2): 142-50.
[PMID: 25537773]

[28] Ono C, Fukuhara T, Li S, *et al.* Various miRNAs compensate the role of miR-122 on HCV replication. PLoS Pathog 2020; 16(6): e1008308.
[PMID: 32574204]

[29] Song K, Han C, Dash S, Balart LA, Wu T. MiR-122 in hepatitis B virus and hepatitis C virus dual infection. World J Hepatol 2015; 7(3): 498-506.
[PMID: 25848473]

[30] Chahal J, Gebert LFR, Gan HH, *et al.* miR-122 and Ago interactions with the HCV genome alter the structure of the viral 5′ terminus. Nucleic Acids Res 2019; 47(10): 5307-24.
[PMID: 30941417]

[31] Trebicka J, Anadol E, Elfimova N, *et al.* Hepatic and serum levels of miR-122 after chronic HCV-induced fibrosis. J Hepatol 2013; 58(2): 234-9.
[PMID: 23085648]

[32] Choi Y, Dienes HP, Krawczynski K. Kinetics of miR-122 expression in the liver during acute HCV infection. PLoS One 2013; 8(10): e76501.
[PMID: 24124569]

[33] Hou W, Tian Q, Zheng J, Bonkovsky HL. MicroRNA-196 represses Bach1 protein and hepatitis C virus gene expression in human hepatoma cells expressing hepatitis C viral proteins. Hepatology 2010; 51(5): 1494-504.
[PMID: 20127796]

[34] Zhou Y, Zhang P, Zheng X, *et al.* miR-155 regulates pro- and anti-inflammatory cytokine expression in human monocytes during chronic hepatitis C virus infection. Ann Transl Med 2021; 9(21): 1618.
[PMID: 34926662]

[35] Clément S, Sobolewski C, Gomes D, Rojas A, Goossens N, Conzelmann S. Activation of the oncogenic miR-21-5p promotes HCV replication and steatosis induced by the viral core 3a protein. Liver international : official journal of the International Association for the Study of the Liver 2019; 39(7): 1226-36.

[36] Calin GA, Sevignani C, Dumitru CD, *et al.* Human microRNA genes are frequently located at fragile sites and genomic regions involved in cancers. Proc Natl Acad Sci USA 2004; 101(9): 2999-3004. [PMID: 14973191]

[37] Kutay H, Bai S, Datta J, *et al.* Downregulation of miR-122 in the rodent and human hepatocellular carcinomas. J Cell Biochem 2006; 99(3): 671-8. [PMID: 16924677]

[38] Ninomiya M, Kondo Y, Kimura O, *et al.* The expression of miR-125b-5p is increased in the serum of patients with chronic hepatitis B infection and inhibits the detection of hepatitis B virus surface antigen. J Viral Hepat 2016; 23(5): 330-9. [PMID: 26924666]

[39] Thibault PA, Wilson JA. Targeting miRNAs to treat Hepatitis C Virus infections and liver pathology: Inhibiting the virus and altering the host. Pharmacol Res 2013; 75: 48-59. [PMID: 23541631]

[40] Tian H, He Z. miR-215 Enhances HCV Replication by Targeting TRIM22 and Inactivating NF-κB Signaling. Yonsei Med J 2018; 59(4): 511-8. [PMID: 29749134]

[41] Hayes CN, Chayama K. Why highly effective drugs are not enough: the need for an affordable solution to eliminating HCV. Expert Rev Clin Pharmacol 2017; 10(6): 583-94. [PMID: 28374641]

[42] Neumann AU, Lam NP, Dahari H, *et al.* Hepatitis C viral dynamics in vivo and the antiviral efficacy of interferon-alpha therapy. Science 1998; 282(5386): 103-7. [PMID: 9756471]

[43] Blanchard E, Belouzard S, Goueslain L, *et al.* Hepatitis C virus entry depends on clathrin-mediated endocytosis. J Virol 2006; 80(14): 6964-72. [PMID: 16809302]

[44] Burlone ME, Budkowska A. Hepatitis C virus cell entry: role of lipoproteins and cellular receptors. J Gen Virol 2009; 90(Pt 5): 1055-70. [PMID: 19264629]

[45] Shahid I, AlMalki WH, Hassan S, Hafeez MH. Real-world challenges for hepatitis C virus medications: a critical overview. Crit Rev Microbiol 2018; 44(2): 143-60. [PMID: 28539069]

[46] Pawlotsky JM. What are the pros and cons of the use of host-targeted agents against hepatitis C? Antiviral Res 2014; 105: 22-5. [PMID: 24583032]

[47] Xiao F, Fofana I, Heydmann L, *et al.* Hepatitis C virus cell-cell transmission and resistance to direct-acting antiviral agents. PLoS Pathog 2014; 10(5): e1004128. [PMID: 24830295]

[48] Zhu H, Wong-Staal F, Lee H, *et al.* Evaluation of ITX 5061, a scavenger receptor B1 antagonist: resistance selection and activity in combination with other hepatitis C virus antivirals. J Infect Dis 2012; 205(4): 656-62. [PMID: 22279172]

[49] Sulkowski MS, Kang M, Matining R, *et al.* Safety and antiviral activity of the HCV entry inhibitor ITX5061 in treatment-naive HCV-infected adults: a randomized, double-blind, phase 1b study. J Infect Dis 2014; 209(5): 658-67. [PMID: 24041792]

[50] Ji C, Liu Y, Pamulapati C, *et al.* Prevention of hepatitis C virus infection and spread in human liver chimeric mice by an anti-CD81 monoclonal antibody. Hepatology 2015; 61(4): 1136-44. [PMID: 25417967]

[51] Fofana I, Krieger SE, Grunert F, Glauben S, Xiao F, Fafi-Kremer S. Monoclonal anti-claudin 1 antibodies prevent hepatitis C virus infection of primary human hepatocytes. Gastroenterology 2010; 139(3): 953-64.
[http://dx.doi.org/10.1053/j.gastro.2010.05.073]

[52] Mailly L, Xiao F, Lupberger J, *et al.* Clearance of persistent hepatitis C virus infection in humanized mice using a claudin-1-targeting monoclonal antibody. Nat Biotechnol 2015; 33(5): 549-54.
[PMID: 25798937]

[53] Colpitts CC, Tawar RG, Mailly L, *et al.* Humanisation of a claudin-1-specific monoclonal antibody for clinical prevention and cure of HCV infection without escape. Gut 2018; 67(4): 736-45.
[PMID: 28360099]

[54] Mailly L, Wrensch F, Heydmann L, *et al. In vivo* combination of human anti-envelope glycoprotein E2 and -Claudin-1 monoclonal antibodies for prevention of hepatitis C virus infection. Antiviral Res 2019; 162: 136-41.
[PMID: 30599173]

[55] Shimizu Y, Yoneda K, Shirasago Y, *et al.* Human-rat chimeric anti-occludin monoclonal antibodies inhibit hepatitis C virus infection. Biochem Biophys Res Commun 2019; 514(3): 785-90.
[PMID: 31079928]

[56] Lupberger J, Zeisel MB, Xiao F, *et al.* EGFR and EphA2 are host factors for hepatitis C virus entry and possible targets for antiviral therapy. Nat Med 2011; 17(5): 589-95.
[PMID: 21516087]

[57] Sainz B Jr, Barretto N, Martin DN, *et al.* Identification of the Niemann-Pick C1-like 1 cholesterol absorption receptor as a new hepatitis C virus entry factor. Nat Med 2012; 18(2): 281-5.
[PMID: 22231557]

[58] Monrroy-Bravo H, Angulo J, Pino K, Labbé P, López-Lastra M, Soza A. Effect of ezetimibe in HCV viral load after liver transplantation. Ann Hepatol 2016; 15(5): 803-5.
[PMID: 27493122]

[59] Inoue K, Umehara T, Ruegg UT, *et al.* Evaluation of a cyclophilin inhibitor in hepatitis C virus-infected chimeric mice in vivo. Hepatology 2007; 45(4): 921-8.
[PMID: 17393519]

[60] Arai M, Tsukiyama-Kohara K, Takagi A, Tobita Y, Inoue K, Kohara M. Resistance to cyclosporin A derives from mutations in hepatitis C virus nonstructural proteins. Biochem Biophys Res Commun 2014; 448(1): 56-62.
[PMID: 24751518]

[61] Flisiak R, Pawlotsky JM, Crabbe R, Callistru PI, Kryczka W, Häussinger D. Once daily alisporivir (Debio025) plus pegIFNalfa2a/ribavirin results in superior sustained virologic response (SVR) in chronic hepatitis C genotype 1 treatment naive patients. J Hepatol 2011; 54.

[62] Pawlotsky JM, Flisiak R, Sarin SK, *et al.* Alisporivir plus ribavirin, interferon free or in combination with pegylated interferon, for hepatitis C virus genotype 2 or 3 infection. Hepatology 2015; 62(4): 1013-23.
[http://dx.doi.org/10.1002/hep.27960] [PMID: 26118427]

[63] Zeuzem S, Flisiak R, Vierling JM, *et al.* Randomised clinical trial: alisporivir combined with peginterferon and ribavirin in treatment-naïve patients with chronic HCV genotype 1 infection (ESSENTIAL II). Aliment Pharmacol Ther 2015; 42(7): 829-44.
[http://dx.doi.org/10.1111/apt.13342] [PMID: 26238707]

[64] Lawitz E, Godofsky E, Rouzier R, *et al.* Safety, pharmacokinetics, and antiviral activity of the cyclophilin inhibitor NIM811 alone or in combination with pegylated interferon in HCV-infected patients receiving 14 days of therapy. Antiviral Res 2011; 89(3): 238-45.
[http://dx.doi.org/10.1016/j.antiviral.2011.01.003] [PMID: 21255610]

[65] Hopkins S, Scorneaux B, Huang Z, *et al.* SCY-635, a novel nonimmunosuppressive analog of cyclosporine that exhibits potent inhibition of hepatitis C virus RNA replication in vitro. Antimicrob Agents Chemother 2010; 54(2): 660-72.
[http://dx.doi.org/10.1128/AAC.00660-09] [PMID: 19933795]

[66] Hopkins S, DiMassimo B, Rusnak P, *et al.* The cyclophilin inhibitor SCY-635 suppresses viral replication and induces endogenous interferons in patients with chronic HCV genotype 1 infection. J Hepatol 2012; 57(1): 47-54.
[http://dx.doi.org/10.1016/j.jhep.2012.02.024] [PMID: 22425702]

[67] Li YP, Gottwein JM, Scheel TK, Jensen TB, Bukh J. MicroRNA-122 antagonism against hepatitis C virus genotypes 1 6 and reduced efficacy by host RNA insertion or mutations in the HCV 5′ UTR. Proc Natl Acad Sci USA 2011; 108(12): 4991-6.
[http://dx.doi.org/10.1073/pnas.1016606108] [PMID: 21383155]

[68] Janssen HLA, Reesink HW, Lawitz EJ, *et al.* Treatment of HCV infection by targeting microRNA. N Engl J Med 2013; 368(18): 1685-94.
[http://dx.doi.org/10.1056/NEJMoa1209026] [PMID: 23534542]

[69] Tsai WC, Hsu SD, Hsu CS, *et al.* MicroRNA-122 plays a critical role in liver homeostasis and hepatocarcinogenesis. J Clin Invest 2012; 122(8): 2884-97.
[http://dx.doi.org/10.1172/JCI63455] [PMID: 22820290]

[70] Liu F, Shimakami T, Murai K, *et al.* Efficient Suppression of Hepatitis C Virus Replication by Combination Treatment with miR-122 Antagonism and Direct-acting Antivirals in Cell Culture Systems. Sci Rep 2016; 6(1): 30939.
[http://dx.doi.org/10.1038/srep30939] [PMID: 27484655]

[71] van der Ree MH, de Vree JM, Stelma F, *et al.* Safety, tolerability, and antiviral effect of RG-101 in patients with chronic hepatitis C: a phase 1B, double-blind, randomised controlled trial. Lancet 2017; 389(10070): 709-17.
[http://dx.doi.org/10.1016/S0140-6736(16)31715-9] [PMID: 28087069]

[72] Stelma F, van der Ree MH, Sinnige MJ, *et al.* Immune phenotype and function of natural killer and T cells in chronic hepatitis C patients who received a single dose of anti-MicroRNA-122, RG-101. Hepatology 2017; 66(1): 57-68.
[http://dx.doi.org/10.1002/hep.29148] [PMID: 28295463]

[73] Deng Y, Campbell F, Han K, *et al.* Randomized clinical trials towards a single-visit cure for chronic hepatitis C: Oral GSK2878175 and injectable RG-101 in chronic hepatitis C patients and long-acting injectable GSK2878175 in healthy participants. J Viral Hepat 2020; 27(7): 699-708.
[http://dx.doi.org/10.1111/jvh.13282] [PMID: 32096313]

[74] Herker E, Harris C, Hernandez C, *et al.* Efficient hepatitis C virus particle formation requires diacylglycerol acyltransferase-1. Nat Med 2010; 16(11): 1295-8.
[http://dx.doi.org/10.1038/nm.2238] [PMID: 20935628]

[75] Rojas Á, Del Campo JA, Clement S, *et al.* Effect of Quercetin on Hepatitis C Virus Life Cycle: From Viral to Host Targets. Sci Rep 2016; 6(1): 31777.
[http://dx.doi.org/10.1038/srep31777] [PMID: 27546480]

[76] Lu NT, Crespi CM, Liu NM, *et al.* A Phase I Dose Escalation Study Demonstrates Quercetin Safety and Explores Potential for Bioflavonoid Antivirals in Patients with Chronic Hepatitis C. Phytother Res 2016; 30(1): 160-8.
[http://dx.doi.org/10.1002/ptr.5518] [PMID: 26621580]

[77] Gane E, Stedman C, Dole K, *et al.* A Diacylglycerol Transferase 1 Inhibitor Is a Potent Hepatitis C Antiviral in Vitro but Not in Patients in a Randomized Clinical Trial. ACS Infect Dis 2017; 3(2): 144-51.
[http://dx.doi.org/10.1021/acsinfecdis.6b00138] [PMID: 27788579]

[78] Insull W Jr, Koren M, Davignon J, *et al.* Efficacy and short-term safety of a new ACAT inhibitor, avasimibe, on lipids, lipoproteins, and apolipoproteins, in patients with combined hyperlipidemia. Atherosclerosis 2001; 157(1): 137-44.
[http://dx.doi.org/10.1016/S0021-9150(00)00615-8] [PMID: 11427213]

[79] Hu L, Li J, Cai H, *et al.* Avasimibe: A novel hepatitis C virus inhibitor that targets the assembly of infectious viral particles. Antiviral Res 2017; 148: 5-14.
[http://dx.doi.org/10.1016/j.antiviral.2017.10.016] [PMID: 29074218]

[80] Neveu G, Barouch-Bentov R, Ziv-Av A, Gerber D, Jacob Y, Einav S. Identification and targeting of an interaction between a tyrosine motif within hepatitis C virus core protein and AP2M1 essential for viral assembly. PLoS Pathog 2012; 8(8): e1002845.
[http://dx.doi.org/10.1371/journal.ppat.1002845] [PMID: 22916011]

[81] Neveu G, Ziv-Av A, Barouch-Bentov R, Berkerman E, Mulholland J, Einav S. AP-2-associated protein kinase 1 and cyclin G-associated kinase regulate hepatitis C virus entry and are potential drug targets. J Virol 2015; 89(8): 4387-404.
[http://dx.doi.org/10.1128/JVI.02705-14] [PMID: 25653444]

[82] Kovackova S, Chang L, Bekerman E, *et al.* Selective Inhibitors of Cyclin G Associated Kinase (GAK) as Anti-Hepatitis C Agents. J Med Chem 2015; 58(8): 3393-410.
[http://dx.doi.org/10.1021/jm501759m] [PMID: 25822739]

[83] Gastaminza P, Cheng G, Wieland S, Zhong J, Liao W, Chisari FV. Cellular determinants of hepatitis C virus assembly, maturation, degradation, and secretion. J Virol 2008; 82(5): 2120-9.
[http://dx.doi.org/10.1128/JVI.02053-07] [PMID: 18077707]

[84] Huang H, Sun F, Owen DM, *et al.* Hepatitis C virus production by human hepatocytes dependent on assembly and secretion of very low-density lipoproteins. Proc Natl Acad Sci USA 2007; 104(14): 5848-53.
[http://dx.doi.org/10.1073/pnas.0700760104] [PMID: 17376867]

[85] Nahmias Y, Goldwasser J, Casali M, *et al.* Apolipoprotein B-dependent hepatitis C virus secretion is inhibited by the grapefruit flavonoid naringenin. Hepatology 2008; 47(5): 1437-45.
[http://dx.doi.org/10.1002/hep.22197] [PMID: 18393287]

[86] Cheng YL, Lan KH, Lee WP, Tseng SH, Hung LR, Lin HC. Amiodarone inhibits the entry and assembly steps of hepatitis C virus life cycle. Clinical science 2013; 125(9): 439-8.
[http://dx.doi.org/10.1042/CS20120594]

[87] Jiang L, Gu Y, Ye J, *et al.* Resveratrol prevents hepatic steatosis induced by hepatitis C virus core protein. Biotechnol Lett 2012; 34(12): 2205-12.
[http://dx.doi.org/10.1007/s10529-012-1034-0] [PMID: 22941371]

[88] Fujita N, Kaito M, Kai M, *et al.* Effects of bezafibrate in patients with chronic hepatitis C virus infection: combination with interferon and ribavirin. J Viral Hepat 2006; 13(7): 441-8.
[http://dx.doi.org/10.1111/j.1365-2893.2005.00718.x] [PMID: 16792537]

[89] Knop V, Bergk A, Schlosser B, *et al.* Bezafibrate maintenance therapy in patients with advanced chronic hepatitis C. Eur J Gastroenterol Hepatol 2013; 25(5): 594-600.
[http://dx.doi.org/10.1097/MEG.0b013e32835cc878] [PMID: 23325275]

[90] Renet S, Chaumais MC, Antonini T, *et al.* Extreme bradycardia after first doses of sofosbuvir and daclatasvir in patients receiving amiodarone: 2 cases including a rechallenge. Gastroenterology 2015; 149(6): 1378-1380.e1.
[http://dx.doi.org/10.1053/j.gastro.2015.07.051] [PMID: 26253303]

[91] Schaefer EAK, Meixiong J, Mark C, *et al.* Apolipoprotein B100 is required for hepatitis C infectivity and Mipomersen inhibits hepatitis C. World J Gastroenterol 2016; 22(45): 9954-65.
[http://dx.doi.org/10.3748/wjg.v22.i45.9954] [PMID: 28018102]

[92] Hekmat S, Aslani MM, Shafiee Ardestani M, *et al.* Preparation and characterization of PLGA

Nanoparticles containing recombinant core-NS3 Fusion protein of hepatitis C virus as a nano-vaccine candidate. Vaccine Rep 2016; 3(8): 48-53.
[http://dx.doi.org/10.29252/vacres.3.8.9.48]

[93] Sabet S, George MA, El-Shorbagy HM, *et al.* Gelatin nanoparticles enhance delivery of hepatitis C virus recombinant NS2 gene. PLoS One 2017; 12(7): e0181723.
[http://dx.doi.org/10.1371/journal.pone.0181723] [PMID: 28746382]

[94] Lee H, Jeong JH, Park TG. PEG grafted polylysine with fusogenic peptide for gene delivery: high transfection efficiency with low cytotoxicity. Journal of controlled release : official journal of the Controlled Release Society 2002; 79(1-3): 283-91.
[http://dx.doi.org/10.1016/S0168-3659(02)00002-0]

[95] Yang Y, Kuang Y, Liu Y, *et al.* Immunogenicity of multiple-epitope antigen gene of HCV carried by novel biodegradable polymers. Comp Immunol Microbiol Infect Dis 2011; 34(1): 65-72.
[http://dx.doi.org/10.1016/j.cimid.2010.02.003] [PMID: 20542567]

[96] Mehrlatifan S, Mirnurollahi SM, Motevalli F, Rahimi P, Soleymani S, Bolhassani A. The structural HCV genes delivered by MPG cell penetrating peptide are directed to enhance immune responses in mice model. Drug Deliv 2016; 23(8): 2852-9.
[http://dx.doi.org/10.3109/10717544.2015.1108375] [PMID: 26559939]

[97] Yang Y, Kuang Y, Yuan D, Cao LL, Wang BN, Li MY. Investigation of HCV multi-epitope gene vaccine loaded by CTS-Fe3O4. Sichuan da xue xue bao Yi xue ban = Journal of Sichuan University Medical science edition 2011; 42(6): 757-88.

[98] Draz MS, Wang YJ, Chen FF, Xu Y, Shafiee H. Electrically Oscillating Plasmonic Nanoparticles for Enhanced DNA Vaccination against Hepatitis C Virus. Adv Funct Mater 2017; 27(5): 1604139.
[http://dx.doi.org/10.1002/adfm.201604139] [PMID: 29180949]

[99] Thomas T, Foster G. Nanomedicines in the treatment of chronic hepatitis C? focus on pegylated interferon alpha-2a. Int J Nanomedicine 2007; 2(1): 19-24.
[http://dx.doi.org/10.2147/nano.2007.2.1.19] [PMID: 17722508]

[100] Giannitrapani L, Soresi M, Bondì ML, Montalto G, Cervello M. Nanotechnology applications for the therapy of liver fibrosis. World J Gastroenterol 2014; 20(23): 7242-51.
[http://dx.doi.org/10.3748/wjg.v20.i23.7242] [PMID: 24966595]

[101] Sepúlveda-Crespo D, Jiménez JL, Gómez R, *et al.* Polyanionic carbosilane dendrimers prevent hepatitis C virus infection in cell culture. Nanomedicine 2017; 13(1): 49-58.
[http://dx.doi.org/10.1016/j.nano.2016.08.018] [PMID: 27562210]

[102] Assmann V, Fieber C, Herrlich P, *et al.* CD44 is the principal mediator of hyaluronic-acid-induced melanoma cell proliferation. J Invest Dermatol 2001; 116(1): 93-101.
[http://dx.doi.org/10.1046/j.1523-1747.2001.00236.x] [PMID: 11168803]

[103] Lee MY, Yang JA, Jung HS, *et al.* Hyaluronic acid-gold nanoparticle/interferon α complex for targeted treatment of hepatitis C virus infection. ACS Nano 2012; 6(11): 9522-31.
[http://dx.doi.org/10.1021/nn302538y] [PMID: 23092111]

[104] Pathak A, Vyas SP, Gupta KC. Nano-vectors for efficient liver specific gene transfer. Int J Nanomedicine 2008; 3(1): 31-49.
[PMID: 18488414]

[105] Sharma D, Parihar S, Chaudhary K. A Critical Review on Nanoscience Advancement: In Treatment of Viral Infection. Journal of Drug Delivery and Therapeutics 2021.

[106] Cheng G, Montero A, Gastaminza P, *et al.* A virocidal amphipathic α-helical peptide that inhibits hepatitis C virus infection *in vitro*. Proc Natl Acad Sci USA 2008; 105(8): 3088-93.
[http://dx.doi.org/10.1073/pnas.0712380105] [PMID: 18287023]

[107] Cho NJ, Dvory-Sobol H, Xiong A, Cho SJ, Frank CW, Glenn JS. Mechanism of an amphipathic alpha-helical peptide's antiviral activity involves size-dependent virus particle lysis. ACS Chem Biol

2009; 4(12): 1061-7.
[http://dx.doi.org/10.1021/cb900149b] [PMID: 19928982]

[108] Zhang J, Garrison JC, Poluektova LY, Bronich TK, Osna NA. Liver-targeted antiviral peptide nanocomplexes as potential anti-HCV therapeutics. Biomaterials 2015; 70: 37-47.
[http://dx.doi.org/10.1016/j.biomaterials.2015.08.014] [PMID: 26298393]

[109] Moon JS, Lee SH, Han SH, *et al.* Inhibition of hepatitis C virus in mouse models by lipidoid nanoparticle-mediated systemic delivery of siRNA against PRK2. Nanomedicine 2016; 12(6): 1489-98.
[http://dx.doi.org/10.1016/j.nano.2016.02.015] [PMID: 27013134]

[110] Duan L, Yan Y, Liu J, *et al.* Target delivery of small interfering RNAs with vitamin E-coupled nanoparticles for treating hepatitis C. Sci Rep 2016; 6(1): 24867.
[http://dx.doi.org/10.1038/srep24867] [PMID: 27113197]

[111] Dallas A, Ilves H, Shorenstein J, *et al.* Minimal-length Synthetic shRNAs Formulated with Lipid Nanoparticles are Potent Inhibitors of Hepatitis C Virus IRES-linked Gene Expression in Mice. Mol Ther Nucleic Acids 2013; 2(9): e123.
[http://dx.doi.org/10.1038/mtna.2013.50] [PMID: 24045712]

[112] Moazed D. Small RNAs in transcriptional gene silencing and genome defence. Nature 2009; 457(7228): 413-20.
[http://dx.doi.org/10.1038/nature07756] [PMID: 19158787]

[113] Ryoo SR, Jang H, Kim KS, *et al.* Functional delivery of DNAzyme with iron oxide nanoparticles for hepatitis C virus gene knockdown. Biomaterials 2012; 33(9): 2754-61.
[http://dx.doi.org/10.1016/j.biomaterials.2011.12.015] [PMID: 22206595]

[114] Saito G, Swanson JA, Lee KD. Drug delivery strategy utilizing conjugation via reversible disulfide linkages: role and site of cellular reducing activities. Adv Drug Deliv Rev 2003; 55(2): 199-215.
[http://dx.doi.org/10.1016/S0169-409X(02)00179-5] [PMID: 12564977]

[115] Hang X, Peng H, Song H, Qi Z, Miao X, Xu W. Antiviral activity of cuprous oxide nanoparticles against Hepatitis C Virus in vitro. J Virol Methods 2015; 222: 150-7.
[http://dx.doi.org/10.1016/j.jviromet.2015.06.010] [PMID: 26116793]

[116] Turnlund JR. Human whole-body copper metabolism. Am J Clin Nutr 1998; 67(5) (Suppl.): 960S-4S.
[http://dx.doi.org/10.1093/ajcn/67.5.960S] [PMID: 9587136]

[117] Khaliq S, Raza S. Current Status of Direct Acting Antiviral Agents against Hepatitis C Virus Infection in Pakistan. Medicina (Kaunas) 2018; 54(5): 80.
[http://dx.doi.org/10.3390/medicina54050080] [PMID: 30400604]

[118] Ventola CL. Progress in Nanomedicine: Approved and Investigational Nanodrugs. P & T : a peer-reviewed journal for formulary management 2017; 42(12): 742-55.

[119] Prince AM, Brotman B, Lee DH, *et al.* Protection against chronic hepatitis C virus infection after rechallenge with homologous, but not heterologous, genotypes in a chimpanzee model. J Infect Dis 2005; 192(10): 1701-9.
[http://dx.doi.org/10.1086/496889] [PMID: 16235167]

[120] AlMalki WH, Shahid I, Abdalla AN, Johargy AK, Ahmed M, Hassan S. Virological surveillance, molecular phylogeny, and evolutionary dynamics of hepatitis C virus subtypes 1a and 4a isolates in patients from Saudi Arabia. Saudi J Biol Sci 2021; 28(3): 1664-77.
[http://dx.doi.org/10.1016/j.sjbs.2020.11.089] [PMID: 33732052]

[121] Semmo N, Lucas M, Krashias G, Lauer G, Chapel H, Klenerman P. Maintenance of HCV-specific T-cell responses in antibody-deficient patients a decade after early therapy. Blood 2006; 107(11): 4570-1.
[http://dx.doi.org/10.1182/blood-2005-11-4522] [PMID: 16717132]

[122] Bassett SE, Thomas DL, Brasky KM, Lanford RE. Viral persistence, antibody to E1 and E2, and

hypervariable region 1 sequence stability in hepatitis C virus-inoculated chimpanzees. J Virol 1999; 73(2): 1118-26.
[http://dx.doi.org/10.1128/JVI.73.2.1118-1126.1999] [PMID: 9882313]

[123] Houghton M. Prospects for prophylactic and therapeutic vaccines against the hepatitis C viruses. Immunol Rev 2011; 239(1): 99-108.
[http://dx.doi.org/10.1111/j.1600-065X.2010.00977.x] [PMID: 21198667]

[124] Meunier JC, Gottwein JM, Houghton M, *et al.* Vaccine-induced cross-genotype reactive neutralizing antibodies against hepatitis C virus. J Infect Dis 2011; 204(8): 1186-90.
[http://dx.doi.org/10.1093/infdis/jir511] [PMID: 21917891]

[125] Logan M, Law J, Wong JAJX, *et al.* Native Folding of a Recombinant gpE1/gpE2 Heterodimer Vaccine Antigen from a Precursor Protein Fused with Fc IgG. J Virol 2017; 91(1): e01552-16.
[http://dx.doi.org/10.1128/JVI.01552-16] [PMID: 27795422]

[126] Park SH, Shin EC, Capone S, *et al.* Successful vaccination induces multifunctional memory T-cell precursors associated with early control of hepatitis C virus. Gastroenterology 2012; 143(4): 1048-1060.e4.
[http://dx.doi.org/10.1053/j.gastro.2012.06.005] [PMID: 22705008]

[127] Folgori A, Capone S, Ruggeri L, *et al.* A T-cell HCV vaccine eliciting effective immunity against heterologous virus challenge in chimpanzees. Nat Med 2006; 12(2): 190-7.
[http://dx.doi.org/10.1038/nm1353] [PMID: 16462801]

[128] Swadling L, Capone S, Antrobus RD, *et al.* A human vaccine strategy based on chimpanzee adenoviral and MVA vectors that primes, boosts, and sustains functional HCV-specific T cell memory. Sci Transl Med 2014; 6(261): 261ra153.
[http://dx.doi.org/10.1126/scitranslmed.3009185] [PMID: 25378645]

[129] Page K, Melia MT, Veenhuis RT, *et al.* Randomized Trial of a Vaccine Regimen to Prevent Chronic HCV Infection. N Engl J Med 2021; 384(6): 541-9.
[http://dx.doi.org/10.1056/NEJMoa2023345] [PMID: 33567193]

[130] Scheel TKH, Kapoor A, Nishiuchi E, *et al.* Characterization of nonprimate hepacivirus and construction of a functional molecular clone. Proc Natl Acad Sci USA 2015; 112(7): 2192-7.
[http://dx.doi.org/10.1073/pnas.1500265112] [PMID: 25646476]

[131] Pfaender S, Cavalleri JMV, Walter S, *et al.* Clinical course of infection and viral tissue tropism of hepatitis C virus-like nonprimate hepaciviruses in horses. Hepatology 2015; 61(2): 447-59.
[http://dx.doi.org/10.1002/hep.27440] [PMID: 25212983]

[132] Pfaender S, Walter S, Grabski E, *et al.* Immune protection against reinfection with nonprimate hepacivirus. Proc Natl Acad Sci USA 2017; 114(12): E2430-9.
[http://dx.doi.org/10.1073/pnas.1619380114] [PMID: 28275093]

[133] Billerbeck E, Wolfisberg R, Fahnøe U, *et al.* Mouse models of acute and chronic hepacivirus infection. Science 2017; 357(6347): 204-8.
[http://dx.doi.org/10.1126/science.aal1962] [PMID: 28706073]

[134] Hartlage AS, Murthy S, Kumar A, *et al.* Vaccination to prevent T cell subversion can protect against persistent hepacivirus infection. Nat Commun 2019; 10(1): 1113.
[http://dx.doi.org/10.1038/s41467-019-09105-0] [PMID: 30846697]

[135] Atcheson E, Li W, Bliss CM, *et al.* Use of an Outbred Rat Hepacivirus Challenge Model for Design and Evaluation of Efficacy of Different Immunization Strategies for Hepatitis C Virus. Hepatology 2020; 71(3): 794-807.
[http://dx.doi.org/10.1002/hep.30894] [PMID: 31400152]

[136] Drane D, Maraskovsky E, Gibson R, *et al.* Priming of CD4+ and CD8+ T cell responses using a HCV core ISCOMATRIX™ vaccine: A phase I study in healthy volunteers. Hum Vaccin 2009; 5(3): 151-7.
[http://dx.doi.org/10.4161/hv.5.3.6614] [PMID: 19246990]

[137] Leroux-Roels G, Depla E, Hulstaert F, *et al.* A candidate vaccine based on the hepatitis C E1 protein: tolerability and immunogenicity in healthy volunteers. Vaccine 2004; 22(23-24): 3080-6. [http://dx.doi.org/10.1016/j.vaccine.2004.02.002] [PMID: 15297058]

[138] Frey SE, Houghton M, Coates S, *et al.* Safety and immunogenicity of HCV E1E2 vaccine adjuvanted with MF59 administered to healthy adults. Vaccine 2010; 28(38): 6367-73. [http://dx.doi.org/10.1016/j.vaccine.2010.06.084] [PMID: 20619382]

[139] Law JLM, Chen C, Wong J, *et al.* A hepatitis C virus (HCV) vaccine comprising envelope glycoproteins gpE1/gpE2 derived from a single isolate elicits broad cross-genotype neutralizing antibodies in humans. PLoS One 2013; 8(3): e59776. [http://dx.doi.org/10.1371/journal.pone.0059776] [PMID: 23527266]

[140] Barnes E, Folgori A, Capone S, *et al.* Novel adenovirus-based vaccines induce broad and sustained T cell responses to HCV in man. Sci Transl Med 2012; 4(115): 115ra1. [http://dx.doi.org/10.1126/scitranslmed.3003155] [PMID: 22218690]

[141] Esposito I, Cicconi P, D'Alise AM, *et al.* MHC class II invariant chain adjuvanted viral vectored vaccines enhances T cell responses in humans. Sci Transl Med 2020; 12(548): eaaz7715. [http://dx.doi.org/10.1126/scitranslmed.aaz7715] [PMID: 32554708]

[142] Hartlage AS, Walker CM, Kapoor A. Priming of Antiviral CD8 T Cells without Effector Function by a Persistently Replicating Hepatitis C-Like Virus. J Virol 2020; 94(10): e00035-20. [http://dx.doi.org/10.1128/JVI.00035-20] [PMID: 32102885]

[143] Martinez MA, Franco S. Impact of COVID-19 in Liver Disease Progression. Hepatol Commun 2021; 5(7): 1138-50. [http://dx.doi.org/10.1002/hep4.1745] [PMID: 34533001]

[144] Boettler T, Newsome PN, Mondelli MU, *et al.* Care of patients with liver disease during the COVID-19 pandemic: EASL-ESCMID position paper. JHEP Reports 2020; 2(3): 100113. [http://dx.doi.org/10.1016/j.jhepr.2020.100113] [PMID: 32289115]

CHAPTER 11

Global Health Sector Strategy (2016-2021) Toward Ending Hepatitis-C: Promises, Policies, and Progress

Abstract: The worldwide prevalence of the hepatitis C virus takes a heavy toll on lives, communities, and health systems. Every year more than 4 million peoples die from hepatitis C-related liver cancers and cirrhosis- a mortality tool comparable to that of HIV and tuberculosis. It needs for a global health sector strategy stems from the scale and complexity of the hepatitis C epidemic, along with growing recognition of its massive public health burden, and the huge opportunities for action. It is a golden time now to establish a coherent public health hepatitis C response that prioritizes effective interventions, promotes service delivery approaches that ensure quality and equity to test and treat every hepatitis C infected individual, takes programs to achieve the sustained impact of hepatitis C diagnostics and therapeutics at the population level, and establishes clear stakeholder responsibility and accountability. There are unprecedented opportunities to act while ending the hepatitis C epidemic and are feasible with the tools and approaches currently available and in the pipeline. For the greatest impact, these opportunities should be combined and tailored for specific populations, locations, and settings. New opportunities and health sector policies provide a ray of hope for the elimination of hepatitis C as a public health threat. In this book chapter, we will highlight the goals, aims, opportunities, and barriers to a coherent public health policy for hepatitis C effective interventions at screening, diagnostic, and therapeutic scale in general and vulnerable hepatitis C infected populations and their consensus implementations to healthcare systems.

Keywords: Cost-effective analysis, Cohesive health policies, Delivery approaches, Delivering for equity, Focused action, Financing for sustainability, GHSS 2016-2021, Healthcare systems, HCV elimination goal, HCV research development, Innovation for acceleration, Priority actions, Progress status, Policy impact, Progress toward impact, Primary care program, Service coverage targets, Strategy implementation, Strategic directions, WHO progress.

Imran Shahid and Qaiser Jabeen

INTRODUCTION

"Human immunodeficiency virus (HIV), viral hepatitis B and C, and sexually transmitted infections (STIs) are major public health threats worldwide [1]".All these infections account for more than 2.3 million mortalities per year, which represents 14% of all deaths from infectious and parasitic infections, digestive diseases, and cancer [2]. An estimated 1 million new individuals are being reported per day infected with these infections and 1.2 million among those are developing cancer each year. New data estimates that 9.4 million people are receiving DAAs treatment to cure CHC infection, an almost 10-fold increase from the baseline of 1 million at the end of 2015 and before the establishment of the global health sector strategy GHSS; 2016-2021) that defines the goals, objectives, strategies, and their implementation to achieve HCV elimination by 2030 [3]. This scale-up of HCV treatment has been proven sufficient to reverse the trend of increasing mortality from HCV infection from the first time. For example, Egypt and Georgia, the two bright examples to follow and implement universal HCV diagnosis and access to treatment strategies defined by GHSS have resulted in declining mortality rates and new infection incidences [3]. However, improved data both in terms of viral screening and treatment access, indicate that the number of people dying from hepatitis B and C worldwide remains daunting at 1.1 million per year [4]. Interestingly, these communicable infections share common modes of transmission and determinants and call for a common public health approach along the continuum of prevention, diagnosis, treatment, and care. However, key differences exist in their status in 2021, with important lessons learned to design policies and strategies and to find opportunities for their implementation to achieve universal health coverage [2, 5].

In 2016, WHO member states established three aligned global health sector strategies on HIV, viral hepatitis, and STIs, respectively, to guide actions over the period 2016-2021 (*i.e.* GHSS 2016-2021) towards eliminating them as public health threats by 2030 [6 - 8]. The strategies share a common goal to progress towards universal health coverage and the 2030 agendas for sustainable development. Furthermore, the strategies were organized around a common framework that promoted synergy across the diseases and with other programmatic health priorities. At that time, the pace of progress was uneven and insufficient to meet global targets by 2030. The global response to hepatitis C was gaining momentum, but access to testing and treatment remained far below needs, and mortality was increasing. "Key and vulnerable populations were not adequately reached with essential interventions, and many opportunities for joint action were being missed. The report called for accelerating progress with integrated and people-centered approaches to end epidemics as public health threats by 2030 [8]".

THE MAIN GOALS OF GHSS (2016-2021) AND MAJOR GAPS

"The GHSS (2016-2021) covered the first six years of the post-2015 health agenda, building on the prevention and control of viral hepatitis infection along with the framework for global action on two resolutions of viral hepatitis adopted by the world health Assembly in 2010 and 2014 respectively [8]". The strategy addressed all five hepatitis viruses (hepatitis A, B, C, D, and E), with a particular focus on hepatitis B and C, owing to the relative public health burden they represent. One of the main goals of this strategy describes the elimination of viral hepatitis C as a major public health threat by 2030. For this purpose, short and long terms targets were set for 2020 and 2030 along with potential pragmatic strategies to achieve these targets [8]. As the implementation period for the GHSS for HIV, viral hepatitis, and STIs ended in 2021, it is the time of accountability for the main achievements and gaps to date and to highlight actions to take forward toward eliminating these diseases as public health threats by 2030 [8].

The estimates of a recent progress report published by WHO indicate that if we lose focus now, the progress achieved so far will plateau with the risk of resurgence [8]. According to the report, many gaps need to fill, most global 2020 targets have been missed, and accelerated actions are needed to reach the sustainable development goals in the next decade. For example, since the adaptation and implementation of GHSS 2016-2021, 21% more people infected with HCV infection have been diagnosed and 62% of those diagnosed receive treatment [5]. The price reduction has made HCV treatment an affordable high-impact intervention, but coverage needs to increase nearly sixfold in the next decade to reach the 2030 targets for elimination [9, 10]. Furthermore, Key and vulnerable populations were not adequately reached with essential interventions (*e.g.*, HCV screening and diagnosis), and many opportunities for joint action (POC HCV testing and treatment) were missed. Many countries are organizing strategies and planning frameworks to eradicate HCV; however, most are missing important opportunities to integrate and link services and responses to provide people-centered services that also leverage efficiency at the primary healthcare and health system levels [8, 9].

This book chapter overviews the main achievements since the establishment of GHSS 2016-2021toward ending viral hepatitis (in particular HCV) by 2030, addressing specific gaps in implementation, and bringing innovation to scale up HCV diagnosis, linkage to care, and the cascade of care to get the ambitious goal of HCV elimination worldwide. Furthermore, it provides new estimates on the disease burden of hepatitis C, which will enable a more informed global response as part of the next phase of strategies for the period 2022-2030 [10].

GHSS (2016-2021) VISION, GOAL, TARGETS, STRATEGIC DIRECTIONS, AND PRIORITY ACTIONS FOR HCV ELIMINATION BY 2030

The global vision of GHSS 2016-2021 deciphers a world where HCV transmission is negligible and everyone having hepatitis C has affordable access to simplified diagnostic solutions and approach safe, effective prevention, care, and treatment services [8, 10]. Keeping this in mind, GHSS set some short-term targets for 2020 and long-term targets for 2030 while decreasing new incidences of HCV infection, increasing diagnosis and treatment, decreasing mortality rates, and accessing service coverage to eliminate HCV worldwide (Fig. **1**) [8, 11]. The strategy included both impact (*i.e.* incidence and mortality) and service coverage targets. It was emphasized that countries can potentially contribute to eliminating hepatitis C as a major public health threat if they act with enough resolve to achieve a set of ambitious targets for 2020 and 2030. To achieve the 2030 agenda for Sustainable Development, action is required in five areas, referred to as "strategic directions". "Under each of the strategic directions, specific actions should be taken by countries, WHO, and partners". This strategy outlines those priority actions to be taken by countries and by WHO. The proposed actions are intended to guide country efforts, with countries selecting and implementing those actions that are most appropriate to their respective hepatitis epidemics, national priorities, and country contexts, taking into consideration national policies, jurisdiction, and legislation [8, 11]. Fig. (**1**) outlines the five strategic directions of the GHSS on HCV, 2016-2021.

"Each of the strategic directions addresses a specific set of questions as; strategic direction 1 deals with that what is the situation?" It focuses on the need to understand the HCV epidemic and response as a basis for advocacy, political commitment, national planning, resource mobilization, allocation, implementation, and program improvement [8, 11]. Strategic direction 2 informs about what services should be delivered. It addresses the first dimension of universal health coverage by describing the essential package of high-impact interventions that need to be delivered along the continuum of hepatitis C services to reach the country and global targets, and which should be considered for inclusion in national health benefit packages. Strategic direction 3 focuses on how can these services be delivered. It addresses the second dimension of universal health coverage by identifying the best methods and approaches for delivering the continuum of hepatitis C services to different populations and in different locations to achieve equity, maximize impact and ensure quality. Strategic direction 4 informs how can the costs of delivering the package of services be met. It addresses the third dimension of universal health coverage by identifying sustainable and innovative models for financing hepatitis C responses and approaches for reducing costs so that people can access the necessary services without incurring financial hardship (Fig. **1**) [8, 11].

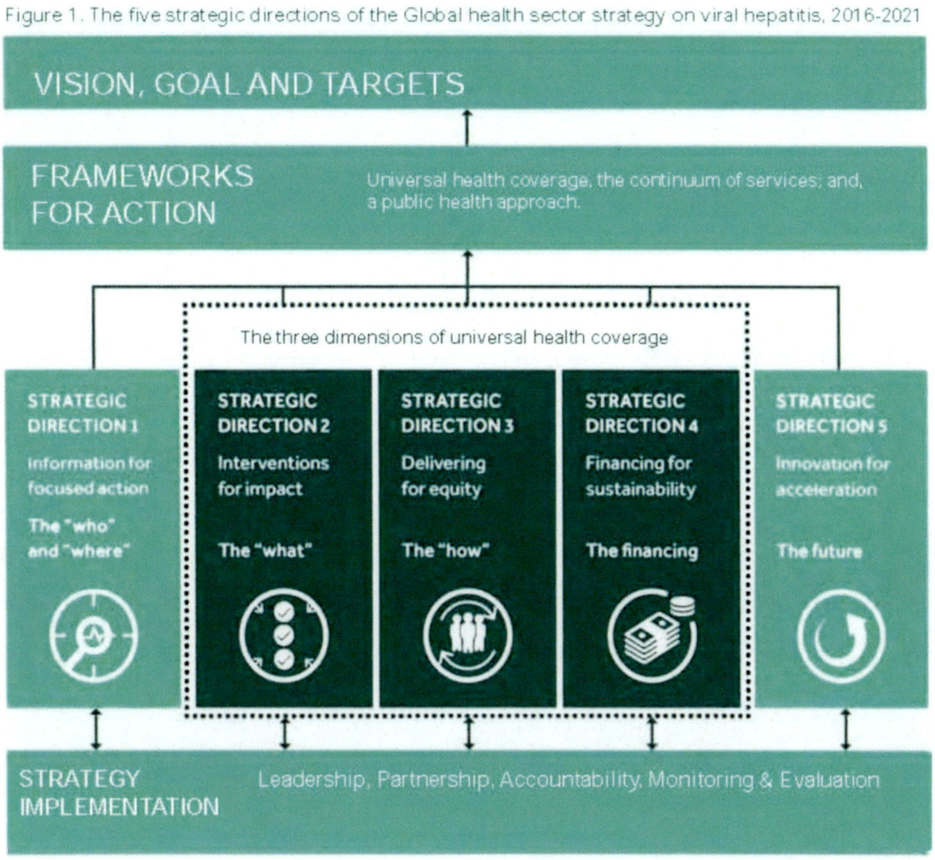

Fig. (1). The five strategic directions of GHSS (2016-2021) on viral hepatitis to implement while achieving the HCV elimination goal by 2030 [11].

Strategic direction 5 explicit how can the trajectory of the response be changed. It identifies where there are major gaps in knowledge and technologies, and where innovation is required to shift the trajectory of the hepatitis C response in order for those responses to be accelerated and in order for the 2020 and 2030 targets to be achieved. Each strategic direction then further defines, suggests, or recommends priority actions for countries and WHO to achieve GHSS 2020 and 2030 targets respectively.

Strategic Direction 1 Priority Actions

1. Know your hepatitis C epidemic and response in order to implement tailored investments.
2. Implement evidence-based national hepatitis C plans [11].

Strategic Direction 2 Priority Actions

1. Individuals diagnosed with HCV infection should receive the full range of hepatitis C services they need [11].
2. Define an essential benefit package for HCV-infected individuals.
3. Essential interventions for preventing hepatitis C transmission by treating with DAAs.
4. Improving blood safety.
5. Enhancing infection prevention and control in health care settings.
6. Preventing mother-to-child transmission of hepatitis C.
7. Providing harm-reduction services.
8. Promoting Safer Sex.
9. Ensuring access to safe food and water.
10. Diagnosing hepatitis C infection.
11. Enhancing hepatitis C treatment and chronic care.

Strategic Direction 3 Priority Actions

1. All people should receive the HCV diagnostics and care services they need, and such services should be of adequate quality and delivery for equity [11].
2. Tailor services for different populations and locations.
3. Link and integrate HCV services with other health services.
4. Strengthen of community-based services.
5. Involve people living with HCV.
6. Ensure the quality of interventions and services.
7. Strengthen human resources for HCV.
8. Ensure access to good quality and affordable HCV medicines, diagnostics, and other commodities.
9. Promote an enabling environment.

Strategic Direction 4 Priority Actions

1. HCV-infected individuals should receive the HCV services they need without experiencing financial hardship [11].
2. Increase investments through innovative financing and new funding approaches.
3. Address financial and other barriers to access and provide financial risk protection.

4. Reduce prices and costs, and remove inefficiencies.

Strategic Direction 5 Priority Actions

1. Elimination of HCV epidemics will require new technologies and approaches [11].
2. Optimize HCV Prevention.
3. Optimize testing and diagnostics.
4. Optimize medicines and treatment regimens.
5. Optimize service delivery.

KEY COMPONENTS OF GHSS (2016-2021) STRATEGY IMPLEMENTATION

Effective implementation of the GHSS (2016-2021) depends on concerted actions from all stakeholders in the health sector response to HCV [11]. "Success requires strong leadership and partnerships to ensure policy and program coherence". Within the health sector, linkages across different disease-specific and cross-cutting programs need to be established and strengthened [11]. The following priority actions were suggested to perform for the successful implementation of the GHSS strategy for HCV.

1. Collaboration with partners and stakeholders.
   1.1 Multilateral and bilateral donor and development agencies, funds, and foundations.
   1.2 Civil society engagement.
   1.3 Technical partners' involvement and integration.
2. Monitoring, evaluating, and reporting.
   2.2 Monitoring and reporting progress toward global goals and targets.
   2.3 Monitoring and evaluating the response at the country level.
   2.4 WHO's framework for results-based management.
3. Implementing the strategy at the national level.
4. Accountability.
5. Costing estimates for implementing the strategy.

COUNTRY TARGETS OF GHSS (2016-2021) FOR HCV ELIMINATION BY 2020 AND 2030 AND THEIR PROGRESS STATUS:

Informed by global goals and targets, GHSS stressed that countries should be developed as soon as practicable ambitious national goals and targets for 2020 and beyond, taking into consideration the country context, including the nature and dynamics of country hepatitis C epidemics, populations affected, structure and capacity of the health care and community systems, and resources that could be mobilized (Table **1**) [10, 11]. Targets should be feasible and developed based on country realities, the best possible data available on hepatitis C situations, trends, and responses, and monitored through a set of standard and measurable indicators. The targets should apply to everyone. These targets were set to choose as a universal healthcare plan against hepatitis C either in resource-replete nations or in resource-poor countries and apply to everyone at risk of hepatitis C infection including; children, adolescents, and adults; rich and poor; women and men; and all populations affected and at-risk. According to GHSS, by 2020, three million people would have been treated for CHC infection and the number of new cases of chronic hepatitis infection would have been reduced by 30% compared with the number of new cases in 2015 [10]. By 2030, the incidence of chronic hepatitis infection will have been reduced by 90% and there will be universal access to key prevention and treatment services [10, 11]. Table **1** presents the impact and service coverage targets of the GHSS (2016-2021) for HCV elimination by 2020 and 2030 [11].

Table 1. The impact and service coverage targets of the GHSS (2016-2021) for HCV elimination by 2020 and 2030 [10].

Target Area	Baseline 2015	2020 Targets	2030 Targets
Impact targets			
Incidence: New cases of chronic viral hepatitis C infections	Between 6 and 10 million infections are reduced to 0.9 million infections by 2030 (80% decline in hepatitis C virus infections)	30% reduction	90% reduction
Mortality: Viral hepatitis B and C deaths	1.4 million deaths reduced to less than 500 000 by 2030 (65% for both viral hepatitis B and C)	10% reduction	65% reduction
Service coverage targets			
Blood safety	39 countries do not routinely test all blood donations for transfusion-transmissible infections 89% of donations screened in a quality-assured manner	95% of donations screened in a quality-assured manner	100% of donations are screened in a quality-assured manner
Safe injections: percentage of injections administered with safety-engineered devices in and out of health facilities	5%	50%	90%

(Table 1) cont.....

Harm reduction: number of sterile needles and syringes provided per person who injects drugs per year	20	200	300
Viral hepatitis C diagnosis	<5% of chronic hepatitis infections diagnosed	30%	90%
Viral hepatitis C treatment	<1% receiving treatment	3 million people have received hepatitis C virus treatment	80% of eligible persons with chronic hepatitis C virus infection treated

GLOBAL PROGRESS REPORT 2021 FOR ACCOUNTABILITY OF GHSS (2016-2021) FOR HCV ELIMINATION

This report publishes new estimates for HCV by providing a more accurate baseline for the forthcoming decades of progress towards eliminating hepatitis C by 2030 [8, 10]. The report also measures the progress of the six-year achievements of GHSS (2016-2021) regarding the implementation of its vision, goal, strategic directions, and priority actions adopted by the member states as well as suggests actions to bridge the remaining gaps and actions for impact to achieve Sustainable development by 2030 [8, 10]. Table **2** presents the impact and service coverage targets (2016-2021) of GHSS for hepatitis C and provides an update on the achievement of these targets by the end of 2020.

Table 2. The impact and service coverage targets of the GHSS (2016-2021) for HCV elimination by 2020 and the current status of achievement by the end of 2020 [10].

Impact	
Targets (by 2020 and 2030)	**Status**
• 30% reduction in new cases of chronic viral hepatitis B and C infections by 2020, 90% reduction by 2030 • 10% reduction in viral hepatitis B and C deaths by 2020, 65% reduction by 2030	• 1.5 million [1.3 million 1.8 million] people were newly infected with chronic hepatitis C infection in 2019 • 290 000 [230 000 580 000] people died from hepatitis C infection-related causes in 2019
Service coverage	

(Table 2) cont.....

• 95% of blood donations screened in a quality-assured manner by 2020, 100% screened by 2030 • 50% of injections administered with safety-engineered devices in and out of health facilities by 2020, 90% by 2030 • 200 sterile needles and syringes provided per person who injects drugs per year by 2020, 300 by 2030 • 30% of chronic viral hepatitis B and C infections diagnosed by 2020, 90% by 2030 • 80% of eligible people with chronic hepatitis B and C virus infection treated by 2030, respectively	• Only baseline data available: 97% of donations screened with quality assurance in 2015 • 3.9% reuse of injection equipment in 2017 • 33 syringes or needle sets per person who injects drugs per year in 2017 • 15.2 million [11.2 million 19.0 million] people living with hepatitis C knew their hepatitis C status in 2019 • 9.4 million [7.5 million 11.7 million] people diagnosed with hepatitis C infection had been treated using direct-acting antiviral drugs between 2015 and 2019

HCV accounts for a significant global disease burden and high mortality from cirrhosis and HCC. According to this report, 58 million people were living with CHC virus infection worldwide in 2019 [11]. New estimates show that about 1.5 million people newly acquire HCV infection each year (Figs. **3** and **4**) [4]. Viral hepatitis caused 1.1 million deaths in 2019, 96% of which were caused by HBV and C virus. Most of these deaths result from chronic hepatic diseases and hepatic cancers (Fig. **3**). The greatest burden of hepatitis C infection is concentrated by geography and population, with 80% of the global burden of hepatitis C infection in the 10 most severely affected countries [4, 10]. In 2018, 500,000 new cases of HCC were caused by hepatitis B and C viruses. People from economically disadvantaged regions, displaced people and migrants, and rural populations are more severely affected (Table **3**). Further, IDUs are a major contributor to the hepatitis C epidemic globally. Other affected population groups include HCPs exposed through needle-stick injuries, people in prisons and closed settings, and gay men and other men who have sex with men [4, 11].

Table 3. The coinfections and comorbidities risks related to hepatitis C and other major infectious diseases [10].

Disease Summary of evidence	
HIV and viral hepatitis	2.3 million people are coinfected with HIV and hepatitis C virus
HIV and viral hepatitis	1. Among people living with HIV, untreated hepatitis coinfection promotes more rapid progression of hepatitis B and/or C related liver disease, hepatocellular cancer, and untimely death, undermining the gains of effective HIV treatment. 2. HIV coinfection doubles the risk of mother-to-child transmission of viral hepatitis. 3. More than half of all people coinfected with HIV and hepatitis C are people who inject drugs. 4. Men living with HIV who have sex with men are at substantially higher risk of hepatitis C infection.

Fig. (**2**) illustrates the deaths related to HIV, viral hepatitis (B and C), and STIs among all deaths related to infectious and parasitic diseases, digestive diseases, and cancer, 2019.

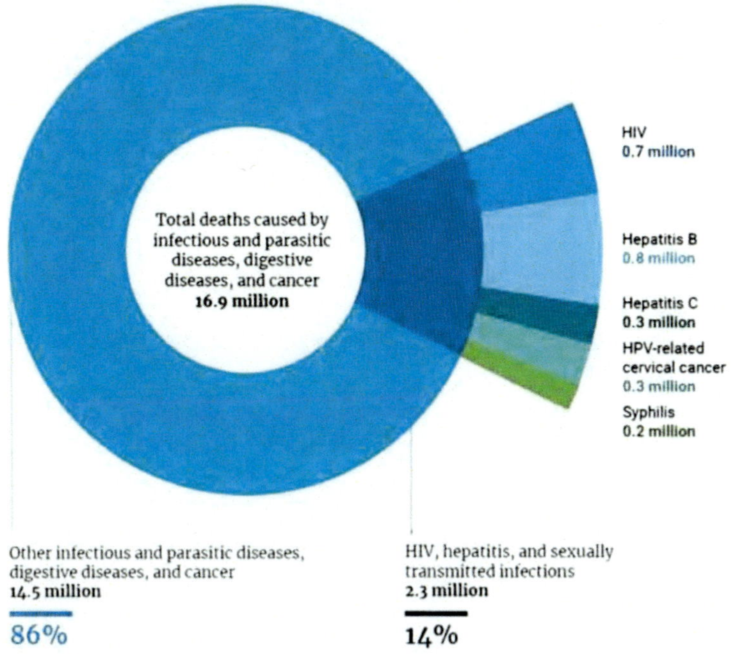

Fig. (2). Total deaths caused by four worldwide prevalent infections (HCV, HBV, HIV, and STIs) and associated comorbidities-related mortalities by 2019 [10].

PROGRESS TOWARD IMPACT

The Progress View of the WHO Strategic and Technical Committee on HIV and Viral Hepatitis (STAC-HIVHEP)

The WHO strategic and technical committee on HIV and viral hepatitis (STAC-HIVHEP) meets biennially to provide the WHO director-general with independent strategic and technical advice on WHO's program of work on the two epidemics (*i.e.* HIV and viral hepatitis). In October 2021, the STAC-HIVHEP reviewed the GHSS on HIV, viral hepatitis, and STIs 2016-2021, focusing on elements to be highlighted in the forthcoming 2022-2030 strategies [5, 10]. The STAC-HIVHEP strongly supported WHO's commitment to pursue elimination targets for all three health strategies. Success, it said, requires stronger political will, adequate financing, and ensuring that programs reach populations at higher risk, including through stronger community engagement and by upholding people's right to health. Greater health equity is a priority, and integration can be used to greater effect. The STAC- HIVHEP also called on WHO to support countries to use all options to reduce prices for vaccines, diagnostics, and drugs for preventing and treating HIV, viral hepatitis, and other STIs. The committee reports the global responses to the HIV, viral hepatitis, and STI epidemics at different junctures [5, 10, 12].

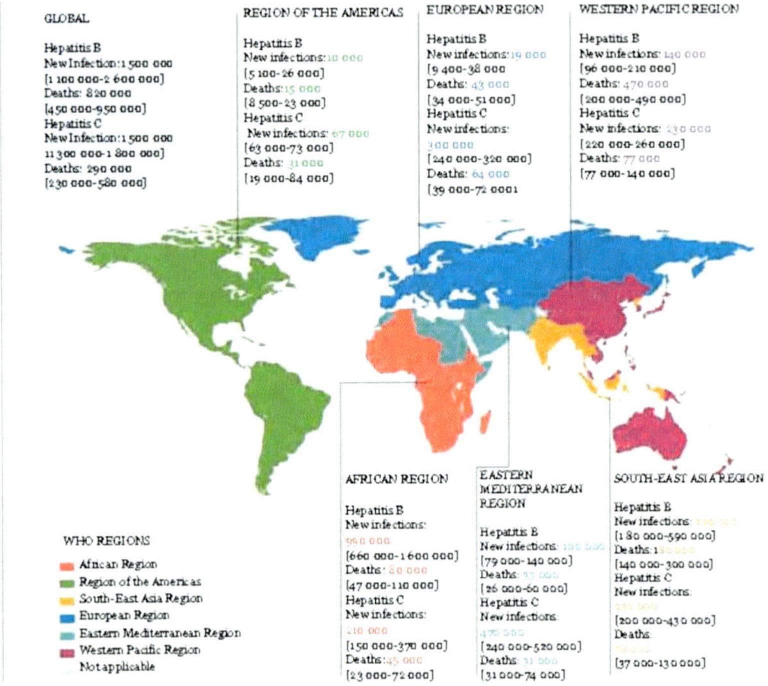

Fig. (3). New infections of hepatitis B and C and deaths in WHO member states by 2019 [10].

External Review of Progress by STAC-HIVHEP in Implementing the GHSS (2016-2021) for Viral Hepatitis

The committee reports that the incidence of viral hepatitis B and C infection appears to be declining with 3 million people newly infected, especially for HBV, with the 2020 targets of the Sustainable Development Goals being reached, but massive testing and treatment scale-up is needed to reduce the unacceptably high mortality of 1.1 million and reach the 2030 targets [5, 10]. There are major opportunities to prevent both HBV and C infections and to treat and cure HCV infections. The committee further reported proven prevention, diagnostic and treatment tools, and methods exist for all three epidemics, and a growing number of countries are using them effectively. Strategic information systems are improving, and differentiated services are more common. Scaled-up vaccination has steeply reduced the prevalence of HBV infection among children younger than five years (to 0.9% in 2019), although birth dose coverage has not increased sufficiently. Treatment cures exist for HCV and are being used successfully (notably in Egypt, Georgia, Mongolia, and Pakistan), and the prices of treatments for HBV and HCV (including generic DAAs) have fallen steeply in many countries [5, 13].

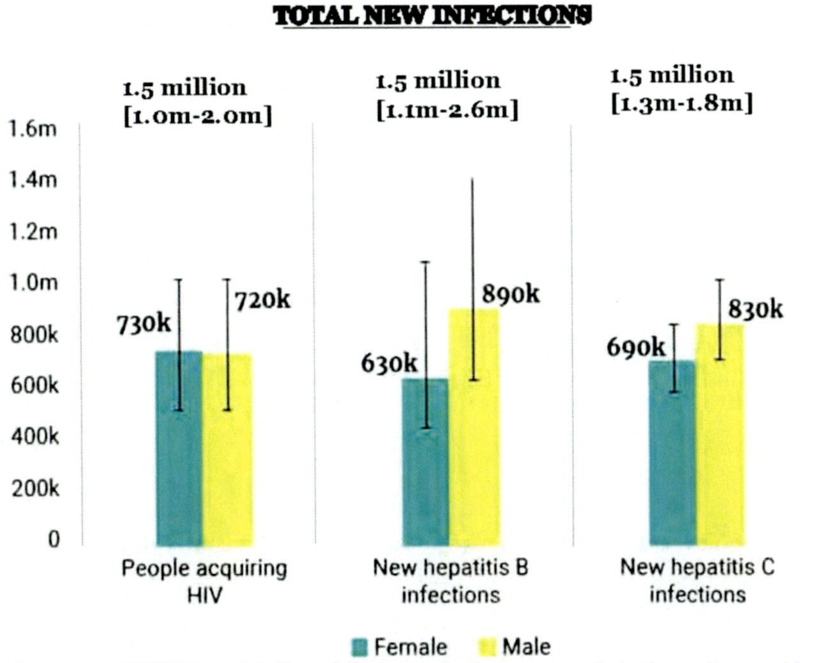

Fig. (4). New cases of HIV, hepatitis B, and C virus infection per year in both genders worldwide by 2019-2020 [10].

Weaknesses in the GHSS Strategic Plan and Its Implementation

In contrast, the committee noticed certain weaknesses in the strategic plan and its implementation strategies that may create big hurdles to achieving HCV elimination goals by 2030 [5, 10, 13]. For example, only a fraction of people living with HCV infection are being diagnosed and treated. Globally, only about 5 million people received hepatitis C treatment in 2017. The new estimates bring us to 9.4 million people receiving hepatitis C treatment achieving the 2020 targets, but this is still far from our goal of 40 million to reach 2030 targets. Although a global reporting system was set up in 2018, country reporting is still limited and up-to-date data are lacking. Improved strategic information is vital to mobilize funding, set priorities, and monitor and evaluate programs. One plausible justification for this interruption and delay might be the ongoing Covid-19 pandemic that caused widespread service disruption and highlighted ongoing inequalities and inequities in who can access, afford and use life-saving services and medicines [5, 10]. "Diagnostic and treatment gaps persist, especially for key populations, and legal and policy barriers still pose hindrances, and funding shortfalls are a common problem [5, 11]".

PROGRESS ACHIEVED UNDER EACH GHSS TOWARD IMPACT, SERVICE COVERAGE TARGETS, AND STRATEGIC DIRECTIONS

WHO global progress report on HIV, viral hepatitis, and STIs 2021

The WHO global progress report on HIV, viral hepatitis, and sexually transmitted infections, 2021 accounts for the accountability of GHSS 2016-2021 actions for impact (Fig. **5**) [5]. According to the report, there has been significant progress in many areas during this strategy (*i.e.* GHSS 2016-2021) implementation period. For example, in respect of worldwide viral hepatitis elimination, solid progress has been demonstrated against HBV based on prevention and increasing immunization rates. The 2020 targets for viral hepatitis B prevention are on track, and the global target of HBsAg prevalence of below 1% for 2020 among children younger than five years is one of the first 2020 targets of the health-related sustainable development goals to be met [11, 14]. However, most global impact targets for 2020 have been missed because of several reasons. Like, progress in reducing the prevalence of hepatitis B infection among children younger than five years is not matched with equal progress in addressing hepatitis B and C infection among adults. Further, although mortality from hepatitis C is declining for the first time, supported by a 10-fold increase in treatment for HCV compared with the strategy baseline, treatment coverage remains 13% (21% diagnosed and 62% treated) in relation to need [8, 14]. Treatment for hepatitis B is progressing much too slowly despite affordable treatments, as is hepatitis C prevention and harm reduction among PWIDs [14]. Fig. (**5**) presents progress and the accountability ratings for progress achieved under each of the GHSS toward impact and service coverage targets and towards implementing the priority actions under each of the five strategic directions of the strategies along with the areas of improvement in missing global impact targets.

The report also demonstrates that progress was already insufficient before the emergence of the Covid-19 pandemic, which further deterred progress in many countries [6, 15]. Ultimately, a doubling of progress would be needed to achieve the sustainable development goal trajectory. It means that to get back on track to GHSS 2016-2021, we will have to prevent 2 million people from dying each year and prevent 1 million people from becoming newly infected with HIV, viral hepatitis (both B and C types), and STIs each day [15]. However, the unprecedented global health crisis due to the Covid-19 pandemic has been a stark reminder that disease-specific action and universal health coverage goals are mutually reinforcing and must be advanced together through a people-centered public health approach [6, 15].

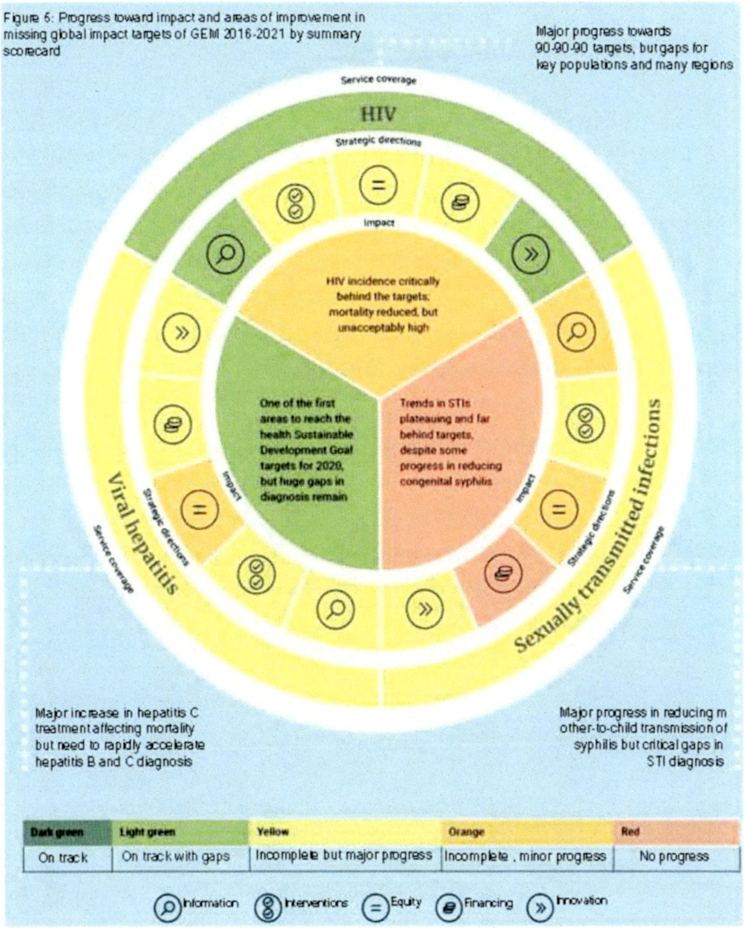

Fig. (5). A schematic illustration deciphering the summary scorecard of accountability for the GHSS 2016-2021 progress [10].

At the end of 2020, the responses to HCV in the perspective of increased diagnosis and treatment, linkage to care, accessible care cascade models, and post-treatment monitoring were at very different stages of progress, and much can be learned across the implementation of the strategies to optimize opportunities through primary health care as the critical platform to ensure universal access to prevention, testing, treatment, and care of HCV over the next decade [15]. Urgent and decisive action is necessary now and over the next decade to sustain progress, prevent a resurgence, and accelerate action to eliminate HCV by 2030 as part of broader global health goals [10, 15].

GHSS (2016-2021) Progress on Viral Hepatitis in 2020

Global targets aim to reduce the number of people newly infected with HBV and C virus by 30% by 2020 and 90% by 2030 respectively [5]. New estimates for 2019 show that 1.5 million people were newly infected with chronic hepatitis B infection and 1.5 million with CHC infection (Fig. **6A**). The 10-fold scale-up of hepatitis C treatment during the strategy implementation period has led to a stabilization of mortality for the first time, although the annual number of people acquiring hepatitis C infection at 1.5 million and dying from this at 290 000 remains unacceptably high [11, 16]. Global targets call for a 10% reduction in the number of people dying from HBV and C by 2020 and a 65% reduction by 2030. New estimates show that 1.1 million people died from viral hepatitis in 2019. A huge scale-up and simplification of hepatitis diagnosis and treatment are required to achieve the targets for reduced mortality by 2030 [11, 16].

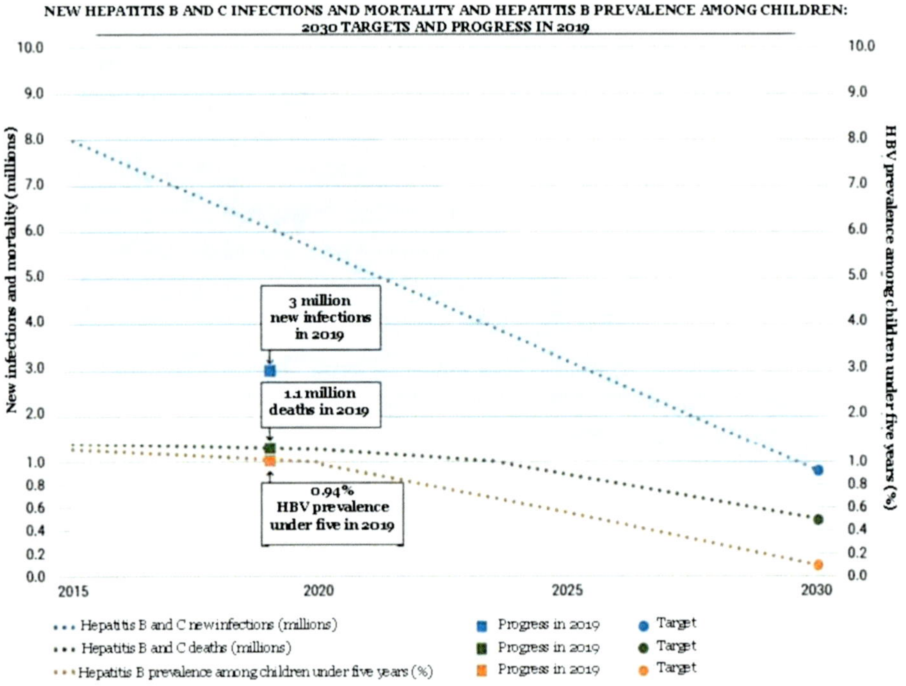

Fig. (6A). Global estimates of new HBV and HCV incidences and mortalities and prevalence of HBV among children by 2030 and current progress in 2019 [10].

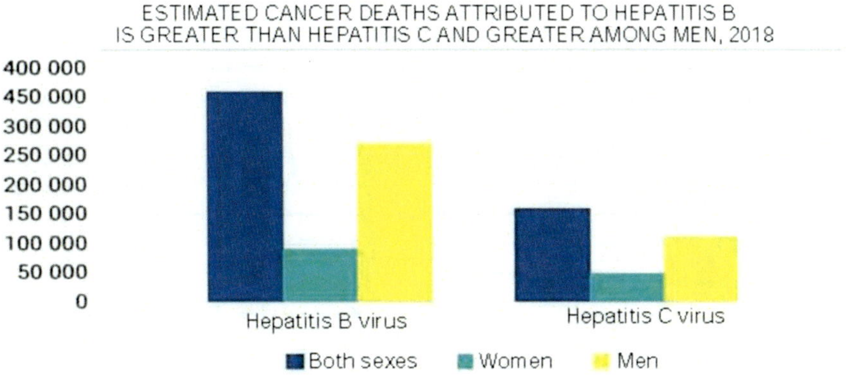

Fig. (6B). A comparison of estimated mortalities due to HBV-associated cancers to HCV-induced HCC in both sexes [10].

Increasing WHO Member States Having National Hepatitis Strategic Plan

The momentum to address viral hepatitis is growing. Only 17 countries had national hepatitis strategic plans in 2012, but this had increased to 124 by 2019 [10, 16]. However, progress in service delivery has been insufficient. Only 21% of people living with CHC infection know their status. 9.4 million people chronically infected with HCV were cumulatively receiving treatment at the end of 2019, a 10-fold increase from 1 million people receiving treatment at the end of 2015, yet treatment coverage is only 13% of the people in need. DAA treatment cure for CHC infection offers great potential for eliminating hepatitis C and associated diseases as public health threats by 2030 [10]. A collective effort is needed to address gaps in the coverage of testing and treatment of hepatitis C and in harm-reduction services for PWIDs to achieve global goals. Fig. (**6A** and **B**) illustrates new hepatitis B and C infections and mortality, hepatitis B prevalence among children, and estimated cancer deaths attributable to hepatitis B and C. While Fig. (**7**) depicts the hepatitis C service cascade (both in terms of HCV diagnosis and treatment by WHO region, 2019 [10, 11, 16].

PROGRESS BY STRATEGIC DIRECTION

As mentioned earlier the three GHSS for HIV, viral hepatitis, and STIs are organized around a common synergetic framework of five strategic directions to advance progress towards universal access (as deciphered in figure 11.1), the WHO progress report, 2021 enumerates progress achieved in delivering the priority interventions and policies of GHSS for HIV, viral hepatitis and STIs [10, 16]. It also highlights key achievements and gaps and recommends priority actions to advance progress toward global goals. The analysis is based and mainly focused on disease-specific actions as well as cross-cutting priorities that can be addressed through integrated efforts [10].

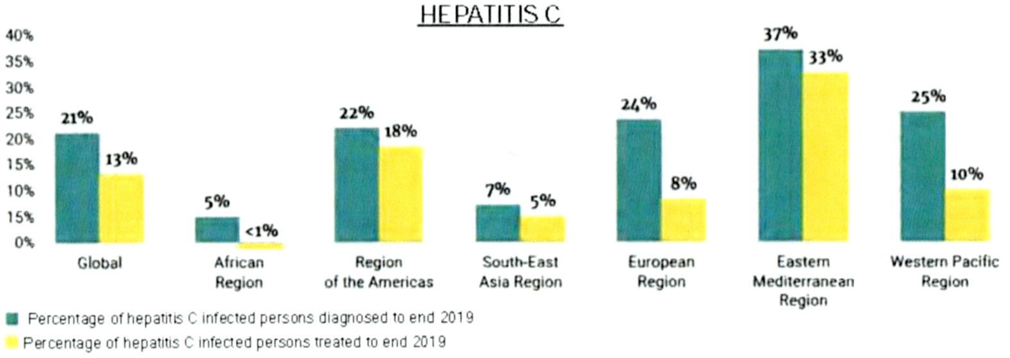

Fig. (7). A comparative analysis of the HCV cascade of care both in terms of HCV diagnosis and treatment by WHO region to the end of 2019 [10].

Progress Toward Information for Focused Actions

Data availability and use are improving. New global and regional disease burden estimates are now available for hepatitis C, which will inform future investments. Nevertheless, substantial gaps remain in the quality and scope of country-level surveillance systems for HCV infections [10]. WHO has also supported countries in implementing guidelines for person-centered data and electronic district-level health information systems for HIV and worked closely with the Global Fund to fight AIDS, Tuberculosis, and Malaria to promote district-level data use. The data summary work is now being extended from the aggregate to the individual level and will include data modules for hepatitis C [10, 17, 18]. Table **4** shows the progress toward information for focused action and priority actions to fill gaps that remain in surveillance systems and facility-level reporting for viral hepatitis [10].

Table 4. Information for focused action - global accountability 2020.

Viral Hepatitis
1- Global reporting for viral hepatitis has been established, and the number of reporting countries has increased from 42 in 2018 to 130 countries in 2019. Updated global and regional estimates have been developed in collaboration with partners, including the CDA Foundation, Imperial College, the Institute for Health Metrics and Evaluation, and the University of Bristol. 2- The first global costing of the viral hepatitis response has been developed showing a need of US$ 6 billion per year and included in the costing for universal health coverage.
Key considerations • Improved granular generation, review, and use of data are improving services using common health information platforms. • Gaps remain in surveillance systems and facility-level reporting for viral hepatitis and STIs.

(Table 4) cont.....

Priority actions
• Strengthen country-level surveillance capacity for viral hepatitis and STIs, with concerted investment in line with the recommended 5 10% of program funds invested in strategic information for action. • Invest in person-centered data and monitoring, especially for prevention, to link people at risk to services, retain them in services and support them to remain negative. • Strengthen digital health data capacity, including guidance on data interoperability and security. • Standardize analytical data reviews and build data analysis capacity, especially at decentralized levels for improving programs. • Take an integrated approach to strengthen data availability and quality on the populations most severely affected and at risk of infection, including population size estimates and integrated biobehavioural surveys. • Joint efforts to strengthen routine data systems and use data to improve health services and inform program priorities and design. • Use data to drive decision-making and ensure that no one is left behind, including by strengthening community-led monitoring that is owned and used by programs working closely with the people who are most marginalized and in need to improve access and quality and holding service providers and decision-makers accountable.

Progress Toward Interventions for Impact

Recent evolutions in decentralized, simplified, and integrated service delivery models, further catalyzed by the Covid-19 pandemic, are showing how existing health system resources can be used more effectively to respond to people's needs and preferences [10, 17]. Such people-centered approaches need to be used fully to accelerate progress over the next decade. However, many gaps remain like primary prevention is lagging behind as available diagnostics and treatment for viral hepatitis (in particular HCV) are not accessible to many people and investment and political support for harm-reduction services are critically lacking in many regions [18, 19]. Table **5** shows the progress toward interventions for impact and priority actions to fill gaps to expand, decentralize, integrate, and simplify access to diagnostics and treatment so that the services can be delivered at the same site [10].

Table 5. Interventions for impact - global accountability 2020.

Viral Hepatitis
1- Pangenotypic direct-acting antiviral drugs, effective against all six genotypes of the hepatitis C virus, are available, providing an effective cure. Coverage of hepatitis C treatment has increased 10-fold since 2015 to 9.4 million people receiving treatment; yet overall, only 10% of people globally know their hepatitis B status, and 21% for hepatitis C and even fewer are receiving treatment. 2- Some champion countries are expanding access to hepatitis C diagnosis and treatment through public health approaches or targeting micro-elimination in the most affected subpopulations or locations.

(Table 5) *cont.....*

Priority actions
• Reinvigorate primary prevention, including condom use, to prevent the sexual transmission of HIV and STIs, with a focus on the populations most severely affected and at higher risk of infection, and integration with sexual and reproductive health services. • Continue to differentiate and adapt service delivery by making it more people-centered to meet the needs of different population groups, bringing prevention, testing and treatment closer to home and including leveraging adaptations from the COVID-19 response. • Expand, decentralize, integrate and simplify access to diagnostics, so that services can be delivered at the same site, with the use of affordable and quality rapid diagnostic tests, including self-tests, serological and molecular point-of-care, and near-point-of-care tests, and promote greater task sharing. • Expand the provision of harm reduction in an integrated and comprehensive manner. • Make use of existing opportunities to accelerate the triple elimination of mother-to-child transmission of HIV, syphilis, and hepatitis B virus through an integrated approach that builds on a comprehensive antenatal care platform that also incorporates eliminating cervical cancer. • Strengthen the response to antimicrobial drug resistance, including through improved use of data to reduce loss to follow-up. • Integrate HIV, viral hepatitis, and STI services within a broader health systems approach, including with noncommunicable diseases and cancer prevention and care and primary health care initiatives.

Progress Toward Delivering Equity

The most marginalized, vulnerable, and underserved populations, who face the highest rates of infection, often have the poorest access to services. Persistent stigma, inequalities, criminalization, violence, and other sociostructural barriers are preventing response efforts from reaching the people and communities who need them most [17, 19]. To achieve impact, the most vulnerable and marginalized people must be guaranteed their right to health. The gaps are most acute for key populations, such as MSM, PWIDs, sex workers, transgender people, and people in prisons [20 - 22]. Some of these populations are also disproportionately affected by hepatitis C. More than half the people who inject drugs have had HCV infection at some point in their lifetime [19]. Modeled projections suggest that eliminating the increased risk of hepatitis C transmission among PWIDs would prevent about 40% of new hepatitis C infections from 2018 to 2030 [21, 22]. Key populations often have coinfections with STIs and viral hepatitis. A rights-based and people-centered response, planned and delivered with leading participation by affected populations, will be essential to achieve true universal health coverage [16, 23]. Table **6** figures out the possible ways to deliver equity both in diagnosis and cure of HCV to achieve global elimination goals. Many of the fragments of the populations who are most severely affected by HCV are also those that face the greatest challenges in accessing necessary services [16]. Gay men and other MSM, people in prisons and other closed settings, PWIDs, sex workers, and transgender people are confronted with social and structural barriers that affect their health, safety, and access to services. Their marginalization, in turn, influences epidemic dynamics and diminishes the effectiveness of the response [16, 22]. Conservative cultural and gender norms, pervasive stigma and discrimination, and legal barriers also continue to hinder access to health services. Several countries have taken recent steps to review and reform punitive laws and practices, supported by advocacy and engagement by communities [16]. These efforts must be sustained, and all countries should work towards decriminalizing behavior such as drug use and possession for personal use, sex work, same-sex sexual relationships and sexual orientation, and non-conforming gender identities. They must strive to eliminate the unjust application of civil law and regulations against people who practice these types of behavior to create equitable and enabling environments for an effective public health response. The key and vulnerable populations may vary but the interventions are synergistic [16, 23].

Table 6. Delivering for equity - global accountability 2020.

Viral Hepatitis
1- There are major gaps in hepatitis B and C testing and treatment in all populations, specifically among economically disadvantaged regions, rural and displaced populations, and key populations. 2- Community awareness and advocacy related to viral hepatitis, including eliminating the hepatitis C virus among people who inject drugs, is increasing; however, access to services remains low. 3- There have been major price reductions in hepatitis diagnostics and treatment and yet many middle-income countries are unable to benefit from these prices as a result of patent-related barriers.
Key considerations • Harm reduction coverage for people who inject drugs remains low 40% of countries report having operational needle and syringe programs, and 64% of countries reported having operational opioid substitution therapy programs as of mid-2020. • There has been progressing in decriminalizing behavior such as drug use, sex work, and same-sex relations in some countries, but several countries continue to have laws, regulations, or policies that are barriers to effective service.
Priority actions
• Design and deliver services that are people-centered and decentralized in accordance with WHO's the operational framework for primary health care, leveraging the experience of HIV programs and extending them to a wider group of economically disadvantaged and vulnerable populations; and engaging communities. • Strengthen the focus on young people, including young people from key populations. • Expand the provision of prevention, harm reduction, testing, and treatment of HIV, viral hepatitis, and STIs in an integrated and comprehensive manner. • Address stigma and discrimination, including within healthcare settings and by focusing on the healthcare workforce. • Decriminalize behavior such as drug use, sex work, same-sex sexual relationships, sexual orientation, and nonconforming gender identities.

Progress Toward Financing for Sustainability

In 2019, WHO and partners developed the first comprehensive global resource needs estimates for the hepatitis response in the context of universal health coverage. The study found that investing an additional US$ 58.7 billion from 2016 to 2030, would avert 4.5 million premature deaths by 2030 and eliminate viral hepatitis as a public health threat in 67 LMICs that account for the majority of HBV and C infections [10, 16, 19]. The rapid declines in the prices of commodities, supported by increased competition from generic products, are making this investment feasible for more countries. LMICs can now aim to achieve a price as low as US$ 60 per person for a 12-week course of hepatitis C treatment with WHO-prequalified generic sofosbuvir and daclatasvir (Fig. **8**) [16, 19]. An increasing number of champion countries are giving priority to financing and delivering viral hepatitis interventions as part of national universal health coverage frameworks [21]. Supported by government commitment, updated national strategic plans, and simplified guidelines, countries are making hepatitis treatment more widely available by implementing a wide range of access strategies. Approaches include expanding generic competition, addressing patent-related barriers, conducting central price negotiations and pooled procurement, and ensuring timely product registration and quality assurance processes [16, 21]. However, many countries are not benefitting from these prices, and great variations in prices and patent barriers continue to persist among countries. In particular, high prices in upper-middle-income countries because of patents remain a major barrier to scale-up. For example, in 2019, the lowest generic price for sofosbuvir was US$ 15 per 28-day supply in India for a WHO-prequalified product [16, 21]. In the Russian Federation, which is not included in the voluntary licensing agreement with the originator company, the price of sofosbuvir was US$ 1099 per 28-day supply [9, 16]. Expanding access to simple, affordable, and quality-assured hepatitis C diagnostics is also urgently needed so that countries can screen large numbers of people, identify people who need treatment, and provide appropriate care [9, 16]. Continuing to pursue various strategies to reduce prices will be essential to make hepatitis services more widely available to everyone in need [9]. Further, investing in scaling up hepatitis diagnostics and treatment will also bring longer-term returns and remove an avoidable strain on the health system. A hepatitis C virus transmission modeling exercise in Pakistan projected that the health system would recover the investment in elimination through savings in healthcare costs from prevented cases of cirrhosis and liver cancer in less than three years [12].

Fig 8. Trends in drug prices for a) Lowest prices of direct-acting antiviral drugs per 28-day supply

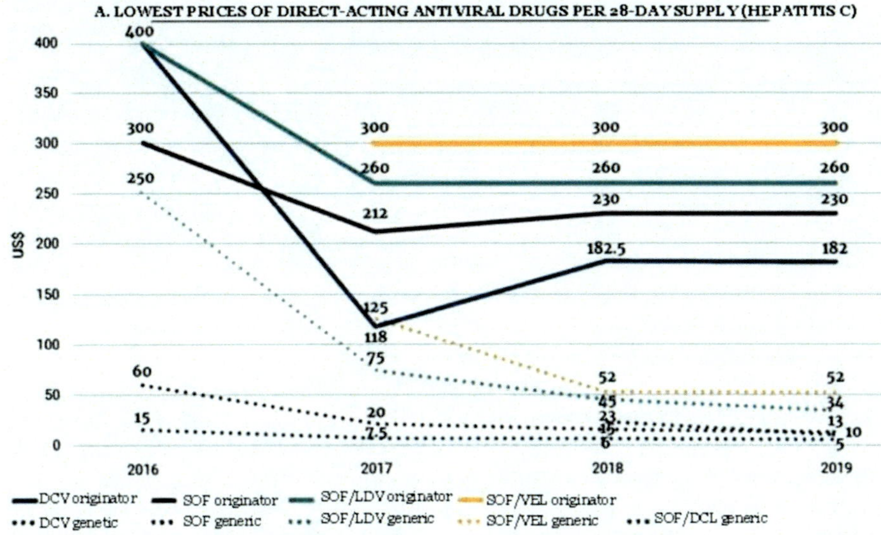

Fig. (8). The trends in decreasing the prices of brand DAAs per 28-day supply from 2016 to 2019 [10].

Integrated resource planning and removing price and regulatory barriers will improve access and efficiency. More countries are demonstrating domestic commitments to finance hepatitis C as part of their efforts to progress toward universal health coverage [10, 16, 24]. Further, major declines in the prices of medicines and other health commodities, specifically for HCV are making a public health scale-up of diagnostics and treatment more affordable. For a sustainable response, global efforts at disease-specific resource mobilization must continue to be complemented by more integrated approaches at the country level to mobilize and allocate resources efficiently through the health system; and ensure that everyone can receive services without incurring financial hardship - thus attaining universal health coverage as delivered through a primary care framework [24]. However, the macroeconomic and fiscal implications of Covid-19 and the response to it will affect domestic as well as donor resources in the coming years, increasing the challenge everywhere but especially in LMICs [6]. Table **7** enlists the major achievements in financing sustainability to achieve the global goal of HCV elimination by 2030 [10].

Progress Toward Innovation for Acceleration

Innovations with cross-cutting relevance can catalyze the overcoming of barriers and move the response to viral hepatitis (*e.g.*, in particular, HCV) closer to the strategy targets [10, 16, 25]. Ongoing research in basic science, new tools and technologies (*e.g.*, HCV-self testing and digital diagnostics), and service delivery approaches (*e.g.*, mobile molecular labs to diagnose hepatitis C) are critical to enhancing the efficiency, quality, and impact of the response [25]. In addition, innovative methods are needed to tackle social and structural determinants related to hepatitis C-associated disease areas to ensure that prevention efforts do not stall. Wider diffusion of innovation is necessary to bring successful approaches to scale to achieve public health impact. Furthermore, the potential of innovative approaches must be fully leveraged and brought to scale to achieve wider public health impact [10, 16, 25].

Table 7. Financing for sustainability - global accountability 2020.

Viral Hepatitis
1- Resource needs and cost effectiveness data are available. The first global costing of the viral hepatitis response has been developed, showing a need of US$ 6 billion per year and included in costing for universal health coverage; however domestic and international investments are lagging behind. 2- In the absence of a donor fund for viral hepatitis, many countries that have established a national viral hepatitis program have leveraged domestic resources in the form of either direct government budgetary allocations to national programs or via reimbursement through national health insurance schemes. 3- There have been major declines in drug prices for hepatitis C, expanding access significantly. 4- Reductions in the prices of diagnostics and simplification of approaches provide major opportunities for increased efficiency in expanding testing.
Priority actions
• Maximize the use of available resources by using data to focus resources on the populations and geographies with the greatest burden and lowest coverage. • Continue to advocate for including medicines and diagnostics for HIV, viral hepatitis, and STIs within the scope of publicly funded and guaranteed services as part of the government's commitment to making progress toward universal health coverage. • Leverage task sharing as a pragmatic response to address health worker shortages and expand the decentralized provision of testing, care, and treatment, especially for the hepatitis B and C response, to lower-level health facilities and using existing non-specialist and primary health care workforce. • Leverage efficiency in procurement and supply chain mechanisms, including through improved joint analytics and data sharing between patient and logistics data systems. • Leverage existing international financing opportunities through partners such as the Global Fund and continue to strengthen investment cases.

Table **8** enlists the strategies for the strong focus on cross-cutting innovations in the next decade of HCV diagnosis and treatment to achieve the global goal of HCV elimination by 2030 [10].

Table 8. Innovation for acceleration - global accountability 2020.

Viral Hepatitis
1- Progressive simplification in diagnostics and treatment algorithms and service delivery models for hepatitis C virus. 2- Implementation innovations to simplify diagnostics and their delivery and access are needed as part of primary health care approaches. Innovation needs further development and quality products including core antigen for hepatitis C virus as a rapid diagnostic test but even simply having high-quality hepatitis B surface antigen tests.
Key considerations • Strong focus on cross-cutting innovations, such as differentiated and community-led models accelerated during COVID-19. • Availability of new technologies to scale up diagnostics, such as triple HIV, syphilis, and hepatitis B tests; point-of-care nucleic acid tests for hepatitis B and C virus; and self-testing for hepatitis B, hepatitis C, and STIs. • Greater use of virtual platforms and digital tools, especially to reach young people.
Priority actions
• Leverage the potential of innovative service delivery approaches, including through self-management and care approaches and community-led delivery, building on lessons learned from the COVID-19 response. • Leverage the potential of digital tools, including for demand creation, service delivery, and monitoring and evaluation. • Ensure continued investment in research in priority areas such as vaccines for HIV, hepatitis C virus, gonorrhea, and HSV and a functional cure for hepatitis B. • Seek opportunities for innovative approaches to address the social determinants of health.

CONCLUSIONS

Despite major progress over the past decade, the 2020 targets for HCV prevention, diagnosis, and treatment were off-track in major areas even in many countries before the Covid-19 pandemic. The ambition of the next decade to eliminate viral hepatitis C as a public health threat by 2030 is enormous yet feasible. It will require collective efforts toward universal health coverage and global health security, leveraging resilience and innovation in the global response to Covid-19. The public health response to viral hepatitis C offers many opportunities to join forces to accelerate towards achieving the 2030 elimination targets. "Joint action can create synergy across health and community systems to ensure the widest possible access to high-quality services for all populations in need and advance the goals of universal health coverage by identifying additional to prevent and eliminate silent epidemics in the future like hepatitis C".

REFERENCES

[1] Gower E, Estes C, Blach S, Razavi-Shearer K, Razavi H. Global epidemiology and genotype distribution of the hepatitis C virus infection. J Hepatol 2014; 61(1) (Suppl.): S45-57. [http://dx.doi.org/10.1016/j.jhep.2014.07.027] [PMID: 25086286]

[2] Schinazi R, Halfon P, Marcellin P, Asselah T. HCV direct-acting antiviral agents: the best interferon-free combinations. Liver international : official journal of the International Association for the Study of the Liver 2014; 34(Suppl 1): 69-78.
[http://dx.doi.org/10.1111/liv.12423]

[3] Shahid I, Alzahrani AR, Al-Ghamdi SS, Alanazi IM, Rehman S, Hassan S. Hepatitis C Diagnosis: Simplified Solutions, Predictive Barriers, and Future Promises. Diagnostics 2021; 11: 7.

[4] Jin F, Dore GJ, Matthews G, *et al.* Prevalence and incidence of hepatitis C virus infection in men who have sex with men: a systematic review and meta-analysis. Lancet Gastroenterol Hepatol 2021; 6(1): 39-56.
[http://dx.doi.org/10.1016/S2468-1253(20)30303-4] [PMID: 33217341]

[5] Boettler T, Newsome PN, Mondelli MU, *et al.* Care of patients with liver disease during the COVID-19 pandemic: EASL-ESCMID position paper. JHEP Reports 2020; 2(3): 100113.
[http://dx.doi.org/10.1016/j.jhepr.2020.100113] [PMID: 32289115]

[6] Martinez MA, Franco S. Impact of COVID□19 in Liver Disease Progression. Hepatol Commun 2021; 5(7): 1138-50.
[http://dx.doi.org/10.1002/hep4.1745] [PMID: 34533001]

[7] Global Health Estimates 2019: deaths by cause, age, sex, by country and by region, 2000 2019. Geneva, World Health Organization. 2020. Available from: https://www.who.int/data/gho/data/themes/mortality-and-global-health-estimates

[8] Thirteenth General Programme of Work 2019 2023. Geneva: World Health Organization. 2019. Available from: https://apps.who.int/iris/ bitstream/handle/10665/324775/WHO-PRP-18.1-eng.pdf

[9] Transforming our world: the 2030 Agenda for Sustainable Development, 2015. United Nations General Assembly, Seventieth Session (document A/RES/70/1). 2015. Available from: https://www.un.org/ga/search/view_doc.asp?symbol=A/ RES/70/1&Lang=E

[10] Global progress report on HIV, viral hepatitis and sexually transmitted infections, 2021. Accountability for the global health sector strategies 2016 2021: actions for impact. Geneva: World Health Organization. 2021. Available from: https://www.who.int

[11] Accelerating access to hepatitis C diagnostics and treatment: overcoming barriers in low- and middle-income countries. Geneva: World Health Organization. 2021. Available from: https://www.who.int/publications/i/item/9789240019003

[12] Pakistan's investment in hepatitis may see return within years. Geneva: World Health Organization. 2018. Available from: https://www.who.int/ hepatitis/news-events/towards-hepatitis-eliminat-on-pakistan/

[13] Tordrup D, Hutin Y, Stenberg K, *et al.* Additional resource needs for viral hepatitis elimination through universal health coverage: projections in 67 low-income and middle-income countries, 2016 30. Lancet Glob Health 2019; 7(9): e1180-8.
[http://dx.doi.org/10.1016/S2214-109X(19)30272-4] [PMID: 31353061]

[14] European Centre for Disease Prevention and Control. Public health guidance on HIV, hepatitis B and C testing in the EU/EEA An integrated approach. Stockholm: ECDC. 2018. Available from: https://www.ecdc.europa.eu

[15] Progress report on access to hepatitis C treatment: focus on overcoming barriers in low- and middle-income countries, March 2018. Geneva, Switzerland: World Health Organization. 2018. Available from: https://www.who.int

[16] Activist Guide to Hepatitis C Virus Diagnostics. Available from: https://www.hepcoalition.org/advocate/advocacy-tools/article/activist-guide-to-hepatitis-c-virus-diagnostics

[17] U.S. Department of Health and Human Services. 2020. Viral Hepatitis National Strategic Plan for the United States: A Roadmap to Elimination (2021 2025). Washington, DC. 2020. Available from:

https://www.hhs.gov

[18] WHO guidelines on hepatitis B and C testing. Geneva: World Health Organization. 2017. Available from: https://www.who.int

[19] World Health Organization. (2016). Global health sector strategy on viral hepatitis 2016-2021. Towards ending viral hepatitis. World Health Organization. 2016. Available from: https://apps.who.int/iris/handle/10665/246177

[20] HCV Guideline Committee of the New York State Department of Health AIDS Institute (NYSDOH AI). Treatment of Chronic HCV with Direct-Acting Antivirals. Baltimore (MD): Johns Hopkins University. 2020. Available from: https://www.ncbi.nlm.nih.gov/books/NBK559965/

[21] Monitoring and evaluation for viral hepatitis B and C: recommended indicators and framework: technical report. Geneva: World Health Organization. 2016. Available from: http://apps.who.int/iris/bitstream/10665/204790/1/9789241510288_eng.pdf

[22] Guidance on prevention of viral hepatitis B and C among people who inject drugs. Geneva: World Health Organization. 2012. Available from: http://apps.who.int/iris/bitstream/10665/75357/1/9789241504041_eng. pdf?ua=1

[23] WHO guideline on the use of safety-engineered syringes for intramuscular, intradermal and subcutaneous injections in health care settings. Geneva: World Health Organization. 2016. Available from: http://apps.who.int/iris/ bitstream/10665/204790/1/9789241510288_eng.pdf

[24] Evon DM, Simpson K, Kixmiller S, *et al.* A randomized controlled trial of an integrated care intervention to increase eligibility for chronic hepatitis C treatment. Am J Gastroenterol 2011; 106(10): 1777-86.
[http://dx.doi.org/10.1038/ajg.2011.219] [PMID: 21769136]

[25] Ho SB, Bräu N, Cheung R, *et al.* Integrated care increases treatment and improves outcomes of patients with chronic hepatitis C virus infection and psychiatric illness or substance abuse. Clin Gastroenterol Hepatol 2015; 13(11): 2005-14.
[http://dx.doi.org/10.1016/j.cgh.2015.02.022] [PMID: 25724704]

CHAPTER 12

WHO Hepatitis C Elimination Goal by 2030: Feasible or not?

Abstract: To put an end to hepatitis C from the world, the quality and equity of hepatitis C screening, diagnosis, and treatment must be accessible to everyone infected with the virus, regardless of age, sex, racism, nationalism, and religious differences. If several key strategies are successfully implemented, countries could collectively meet the WHO target of reducing new HCV infections by around 80% by 2030, compared with 2015. But even with successful implementation, the target of reducing HCV mortality by 65% would take until 2032, according to recent data. To evaluate the power of several interventions those help to reach these goals, several transmission models with data from affected countries that comprise hepatitis C patients demographics, virus prevalence in vulnerable populations, current dynamics of prevention programs, the natural history of hepatitis C and its prevalence, and percentages of deaths caused by hepatitis C must be considered. In addition to that, the models to project what it would take to reach the targets would need to change and improve blood safety and infection control, vertical transmission of hepatitis C infection, extending harm reduction services for PWIDs, expanded testing, and increased treatment with DAAs, with intensive improvements in public health care sectors and strong political will in third-world countries where hepatitis C is almost endemic would be required. In this book chapter, we are focusing on the achievements of the GHSS 2016-2021 plan for hepatitis C with their probable implementations in WHO member states as well as cross-cutting priority actions for the next decade.

Keywords: Community engagement, Diagnostic burnout, Digital health, HCV self-testing, HCV micro-elimination model, HCV macro-elimination model, Hepatitis C elimination, Linkage to care, Monitor outcome, Mobile diagnostic units, National framework, Potential program integration, Reflex HCV testing, Scale-up HCV testing, Task-shifting, Universal DAAs coverage, Virus surveillance.

INTRODUCTION

Hepatitis C remains a deadly viral infection since its discovery in 1989 to yet, although the DAAs breakthrough and plausible achievements of WHO viral hepatitis elimination targets by implementing the recommendations of GHSS 2016-2021 on viral hepatitis in member states have raised the hopes to eliminate

Imran Shahid and Qaiser Jabeen

this silent epidemic by 2030 or beyond [1]. As described earlier in chapter 11, although much progress has been made in distinctive areas of HCV screening, diagnosis, treatment, and monitoring in the last decade, many countries are still off-track to implement these tools, strategies, and policies in their national healthcare plan to curb HCV in the next decade. Consequently, an estimated 58 million people are still living with CHC and only 9.8 million get treatment since the approval of breakthrough all-oral IFN-free DAAs to treat all HCV GTs/subtypes infected patients. Furthermore, the distant obstructions while considering in the context of the ongoing Covid-19 pandemic also outpaced HCV diagnosis to find missing million from vulnerable HCV populations as well as to provide treatment who is in need [1]. The pandemic has also interrupted screening campaigns and routine health visits that confirm HCV diagnoses and identify new cases, as part of efforts to reduce people's risk of exposure to the SARS-CoV-2 virus. Indeed, the global viral hepatitis C response has been profoundly impacted by the Covid-19 pandemic [2]. The pandemic has not only paused HCV community outreach, education, screening, and linkage to care programs, but the lack of personal protective equipment (PPE), overwhelmed health systems, and looming austerity budgets threaten to roll back even the limited progress achieved since the debut of the HCV cure. The syndemic of blood-borne infectious disease, substance misuse, and overdose continues to take lives and shows signs of worsening as a result of the Covid-19 crisis [1]. Even before the pandemic shuttered economies across the globe, the HCV response had been woefully underfunded, with less than 10 percent of needs met. Political apathy, the challenges of mobilizing highly marginalized and criminalized communities for advocacy, limited licenses for affordable generics that exclude LMICs, and slow registration for generic production by both originator companies and national governments continue to be barriers to expanded access and scale-up. While our understanding of Covid-19 continues to evolve, as of press time, elevated liver enzymes have been observed among people who have recovered from Covid-19 infection [1]. This highlights the ongoing, and often unmet, need for life-long liver health and function monitoring for all those with current or past viral hepatitis C, cirrhosis, or other hepatic conditions [1].

Despite the expanded rollout of generic, curative treatments with pangenotypic DAAs, political apathy, less than 10% of the necessary funding, and diagnostics barriers have been sabotaging efforts to meet global HCV elimination targets [2, 3]. Enormous amounts of public funding and health resources have been reallocated to respond to Covid-19 around the world, compounding the complications of providing essential services, let alone scaling up the hepatitis C response [1 - 4]. Subsequently, staggering rates of new infections continue to outpace annual cures, and low treatment uptake and high mortality derail efforts to meet WHO 2030 targets [1, 4]. Of course, to achieve WHO set global targets to eliminate HCV, diagnosis of new HCV infections is crucial for early detection and treatment and to prevent onward transmission of the virus. Chapter 11 of the book comprehensively discusses the framework of GHSS 2016-2021 on HCV and its achievements with cross-cutting barriers to overcome in this decade to smoothly achieve HCV elimination targets by 2030. Fig. (**1**) illustrates the continuum of viral hepatitis services and the retention cascade in an ideal healthcare system. Modeled studies predict that we need to treat 5 million people every year, worldwide, to achieve HCV elimination by 2030. However, different disease modeling suggests that only 11 countries are on track to achieving elimination by 2030 which are treating more than five patients for every new infection, and countries with higher cure rates for new infections (5:1 or more) are projected to achieve elimination by 2030 or sooner [1 - 4].

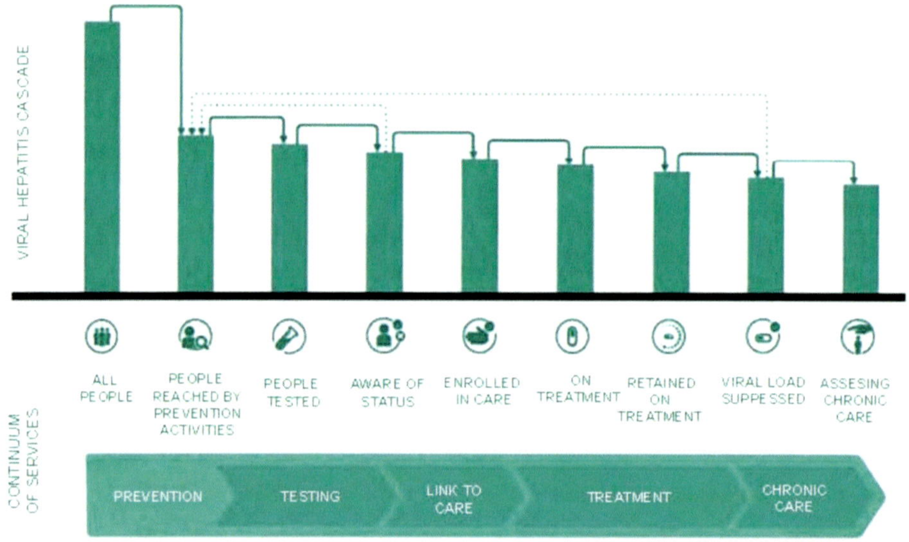

Fig. (1). The continuum of viral hepatitis services and the retention cascade [5].

To reach the 2030 targets, we need to accelerate progress, address specific gaps in implementation, and bring innovation in strategies to scale-up HCV diagnosis and treatment in this decade [1, 2]. Fig. (**2**) depicts the key measures to adopt while achieving both macro and micro-elimination of hepatitis C worldwide. Furthermore, barriers to diagnostics and treatment are also needed to overcome while identifying those and discussing strategies according to the available resources and considering their local and international contexts as they differ in each country. Social determinants of health (*e.g.*, stigma, racial disparity, marginalization, and criminalization) are also needed to end which prevents newly diagnosed populations from linkage to care, treatment adherence, and post-treatment follow-ups (Fig. **3**) [1, 2].

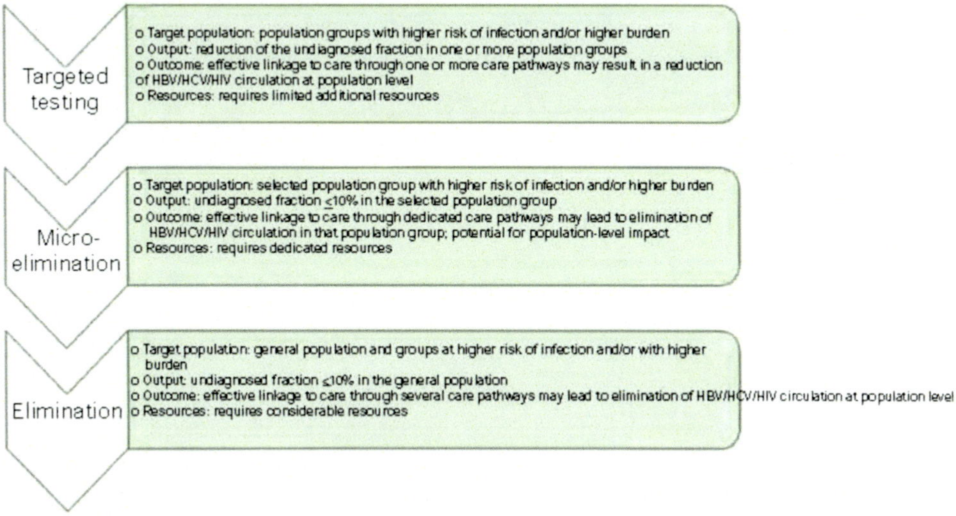

Fig. (2). Prioritizing population groups to achieve HCV elimination targets [6].

This book chapter overviews to what extent the GHSS strategies would be proven helpful to eliminate viral hepatitis C by 2030, what type of strategies and improvements we require to integrate specialized hepatic care with primary care to escalate HCV diagnosis and treatment in remote areas, and harder-to-reach HCV risk populations. Finally, how the lessons learned from rapid management responses to the Covid-19 pandemic and resource distribution, utilization, health system integration, and task-shifting to rationalize for hepatitis C pandemic [1, 3].

IS HCV ELIMINATION POSSIBLE BY 2030?------PLAUSIBLE QUALMS AND JUSTIFICATIONS

To put an end to hepatitis C worldwide, needle exchange programs (NSPs) in vulnerable HCV populations should be expanded to prevent new HCV incidences, and licensing and pricing barriers to manufacture generics of one of the existing brands of HCV DAAs should be overcome so that the expensive treatment can be given to everyone who needs regardless of the prioritize of the treatment (*e.g.*, HCV disease stage (cirrhosis, fibrosis scaling, *etc.*)). In addition, primary care physicians need to take a greater role in treating patients with HCV [3 - 6].

Disease	High-risk groups and potential programme integration
Hepatitis B	o Infants of infected mothers (delivery units, maternal and child health [under-5 and immunization] clinics) o Children in endemic regions (maternal and child health [under-5 and immunization] clinics) o Sexual transmission in adults (STI and HIV clinics) o People who inject drugs (harm reduction and drug treatment services) o Health-care workers (occupational health)
Hepatitis C	o People who have received unsafe therapeutic injections/blood products (health promotion) o People who inject drugs (harm reduction and drug treatment services) o Men who have sex with men (STI and HIV clinics) o Health-care workers (occupational health)

Source: Adapted from: Mihigo R, Nshimirimana D, Hall A, Kew M, Wiersma S, Clements CJ. Control of viral hepatitis infection in Africa: are we dreaming? Vaccine. 2013;31 (2):341-6.

Fig. (3). High-risk populations and programs for integration to promote hepatitis B and C testing [6].

HCV Must be a Sufficient Priority for Healthcare Management Worldwide

On the flip side of the coin, unfortunately, HCV is simply not a sufficient priority for healthcare management and research funding for international healthcare stakeholders and policymakers [3 - 6]. Despite being the seventh leading cause of death in the world and killing more people every year than HIV, road traffic accidents, or diabetes viral hepatitis (all five types of viral hepatitis) accounts for less than 1% of the National Institutes of Health research budget in the USA. Both two viruses (hepatitis B and C) cause 80% of liver cancers globally and were the primary cause of an almost 40% increase in liver cancer in the United States from 2003 to 2012 [4 - 6]. HBV can be prevented with vaccination. Some 60,000 deaths from HBV-related disease can be eliminated if 90% of the patients with chronic infection will be diagnosed and brought to care and if 80% are treated optimistically [5]. Interestingly, the United States has done a decent job by vaccinating children with 90% coverage; however, only about 25% of adults older than 19 years have been vaccinated. This can be overcome by offering hepatitis B vaccines in pharmacies, which could help reach a wider swath of the US population [6].

HCV can be Cured with Pan-genotypic DAAs

HCV can be cured with pan-genotypic DAAs, although treatment is underutilized because of its expense — (still, the prices are in thousand of US$ dollars despite the manufacturing and dispensing of the generic version of DAAs in many countries) per course of therapy [4]. However, these regimens are so efficacious that when we see their benefits compared to their costs, it seems quite plausible compared to the rest of what we do in HCV medicine. A novel solution to ensuring that more people are treated with HCV DAAs, the manufacturers can be convinced to bid on giving a limited license to sell one or more of their brand products as cheap generic versions (already successfully implemented in India, Pakistan, and Egypt that corresponds to three hot spot nations in HCV prevalence worldwide) [7]. No DAAs come off patent until 2029, which means the cost of those products will continue to delay treatment for many individuals who need to be targeted to stop the spread of hepatitis C. The delay will lead to billions of dollars in medical costs and lost lives. If nothing changes, and to achieve a goal of a 90% reduction in HCV incidence by 2030, we will have to work out the ways to NSPs and access to opioid agonist therapy, because worldwide injection IDUs account for 23% of new HCV infections from an estimated 1.7 million new infections in 2015 [8].

Top-level Coordination is Required to Escalate HCV Screening and Treatment

Top-level coordination is required to eliminate HCV worldwide among health policymakers, procurement agencies for HCV diagnostics and medicine procurement, and healthcare providers to identify and implement settings for greater screening for HCV and manage treatment for infected ones [9 - 11]. It will also involve screening out harder-to-reach illegal immigrants and homeless IDUs in remote areas as well as incarcerated individuals and offering treatment to those who test HCV positive [9, 10]. To get more services to patients — especially the more vulnerable HCV populations (PWIDs, MSM, and sex workers) — the country's government should find a way to build a comprehensive program to offer insured or reimbursed HCV care and support services, such as case management and transportation. Similarly, a system of the same flexibility and breadth would be needed to reach the marginalized populations suffering from hepatitis C [10 - 12].

Expanding HCV Diagnosis and Cascade of Care are Must

Expanding diagnosis and treatment of hepatitis C will mean bringing more physicians into the mix both in specialty hospitals, clinics, primary healthcare services, and in community health care (Fig. **4**). In this scenario, both infectious disease specialists and expert clinicians must partner with primary care providers (PCPs) and their professional organizations to increase the capacity to treat hepatitis C in primary care [11, 12]. Acute hepatitis C does not necessarily mean complications if managed timely. Only 20% to 25% of patients with CHC infection may develop cirrhosis after 2 or 3 decades [3]. But for patients who do develop those complications, management can be more difficult which is why many physicians, especially those in small and rural practices, do not have the inclination or resources to care for those patients. Some worldwide highly recognized and well-efficient models such as the University of New Mexico's ECHO program could help primary care practices to manage HCV patients [10 - 12]. It is also recommended that any program for viral hepatitis C management should establish referral systems for medically complex patients (Fig. **4**) [13].

INTERVENTIONS TO PROMOTE UPTAKE OF HEPATITIS TESTING AND LINKAGE TO CARE

USE OF DRIED BLOOD SPOT (DBS) SPECIMENS FOR SEROLOGY AND NUCLEIC ACID TESTING

Topic	Recommendations*
Serological testing	• The use of DBS specimens for HBsAg and HCV antibody serology testing[1] may be considered in settings where: - there are no facilities or expertise to take venous whole blood specimens; **or** - RDTs are not available or their use is not feasible; **or** - there are persons with poor venous access (e.g. in drug treatment programmes, prisons). *Conditional recommendation, moderate (HBV)/low (HCV) quality of evidence*
Detection of viraemia (nucleic acid testing)	• The use of DBS specimens to test for HBV DNA and HCV RNA for diagnosis of HBV and HCV viraemia[1], respectively, may be considered in settings where: - there is a lack of access to sites or nearby laboratory facilities for NAT, or provision for timely delivery of specimens to a laboratory, or - there are persons with poor venous access (e.g. in drug treatment programmes, prisons). *Conditional recommendation, low (HBV)/moderate (HCV) quality of evidence*

Topic	Recommendations*
Uptake of testing and linkage to care	• All facility- and community-based hepatitis testing services should adopt and implement strategies to enhance uptake of testing and linkage to care. ***Strong recommendation, moderate quality of evidence*** • The following evidence-based interventions should be considered to promote uptake of hepatitis testing and linkage to care and treatment initiation. *(Conditional recommendations)* - **Peer and lay health worker support in community-based settings** *(moderate quality of evidence)*. - **Clinician reminders** to prompt provider-initiated, facility-based HBV and HCV testing in settings that have electronic records or analogous reminder systems *(very low quality of evidence)*. - **Provision of hepatitis testing as part of integrated services** within mental health/substance use services *(very low quality of evidence)*.

*The GRADE system (Grading of Recommendations, Assessment, Development and Evaluation) was used to categorize the strength of recommendations as strong or conditional (based on consideration of the quality of evidence, balance of benefits and harms, acceptability, resource use and programmatic feasibility) and the quality of evidence as high, moderate, low or very low.

1 well-functioning laboratory specimens referral network and system for return of results should be in place to maximize the impact of DBS specimens. There are currently few assays where the manufacturer's instructions state that DBS specimens are validated for use. Therefore, currently use of DBS specimens would be considered 'off-label'.

Fig. (4). Interventions to promote uptake of HCV testing and linkage to care in highly endemic areas and many LMICs having poor health infrastructure and lack of confirmatory HCV diagnostic platforms [6].

HCV Surveillance Data are Essentially Required But Lacking in the WHO Member States

Another obstacle to eliminating hepatitis C as a public health problem is virus surveillance, as HCV infections are largely asymptomatic until the individuals progress toward chronic stages of the infection [15, 16]. We need to have a surveillance system in place to detect the cases, and then, once they are detected, we need a system in place to treat them (Fig. **5**) [15 - 17]. There are very few places in the world that have funded such a system, and unfortunately, many WHO member states lack a good hepatitis C surveillance system in place [16, 17]. Virological surveillance is crucial for immigrants, particularly those from Asia and Africa, where most people are infected with hepatitis B and C [16 - 19]. When these individuals move to European and American countries, they are only tested for HCV but then they are not eligible for medical care, so cannot get treatment [19]. There is so much transmission of hepatitis C in Asian and African countries [19]. If we really want to prevent new HCV incidences, we need to consider things like funding for HCV diagnosis and treatment in countries with large numbers of illegal migrants and homeless shelter seekers [18 - 20].

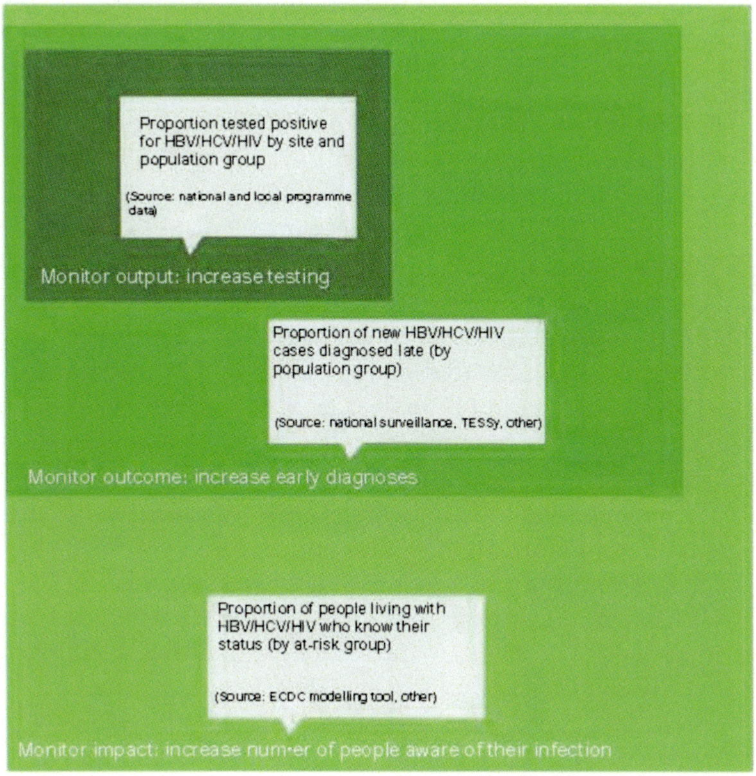

Fig. (5). Key steps to monitor and evaluation of HCV testing programs and virus surveillance [14]. HBV; Hepatitis B virus, HCV; Hepatitis C virus, HIV; Human immunodeficiency virus, ECDC; European Center for Disease and Control.

Social Determinants of Health must be Addressed to Enhance HCV Diagnosis and Care

Stigma regarding HCV infection is another barrier to the management of the disease [21]. New incidences of HCV infections are primarily and continuously reported in IDUs, but IDUs are suffering from discrimination regarding HCV treatment in many parts of the world, and people don't want to invest a lot of money in them [21]. To alleviate this discrimination and to surmount the healthcare burden both in terms of treatment facilities and cost while treating HCV-infected IDUs, much better comprehensive drug and alcohol addiction programs are of prime importance nowadays [14, 21]. Furthermore, diagnostic algorithms and treatment programs for incarcerated people are also needed to approve and updated because a lot of IDUs with suspected HCV infection are in prison [13]. It is one of the sole platforms where we can do HCV diagnosis and treatment for all of them, but it costs money, and many LMICs and even resource-replete nations don't spend money on inmates to do that [14, 21].

Diagnostic Burnout: A Potential Threat to Off-Track HCV Elimination

Diagnostic burnout would also be a problem for resource-rich countries with high treatment uptake among people known to have HCV while failing to diagnose new infections and running out of diagnosed patients to treat [15, 21, 22]. Modeling studies forecast that Brazil, Spain, and Portugal could soon reach the stage where there are no more diagnosed patients available to treat. It means that annual HCV cures in those nations will exceed annual new infections in order to achieve hepatitis C elimination soon or by 2030 [21, 23]. However, this category of nations will reach 'diagnostic burnout' before 2030, which may ultimately derail national HCV elimination efforts. It may evolve into another barrier for the nations that are on track to achieving elimination by 2030 and must become more familiar with the issue and think through the diagnostic burnout problem [21]. It may happen because the individuals who have been treated are mainly diagnosed at the hospitals or polyclinics when they are very sick with CHC infection or advanced hepatic comorbidities [24 - 27]. Furthermore, countries, that are off-track to HCV elimination targets and where new HCV infection incidences are more than treatment will need to adopt decentralized testing and treatment services to identify missing millions of hepatitis C individuals with no symptoms and who live in rural, semi-urban, or remote areas. If this approach is not shifted, the harder-to-reach vulnerable populations will be hidden reservoirs of HCV transmission in this decade and new infections will continue to proliferate [24 - 27]. Subsequently, we will not be able to treat new infections and prevent the progression of advanced hepatic diseases and ultimately HCV-associated hepatic mortalities [21]. Fig. (**6**) explains the importance of knowing your infection status or virus surveillance and tailoring HCV diagnostics to integrate the allocation of resources.

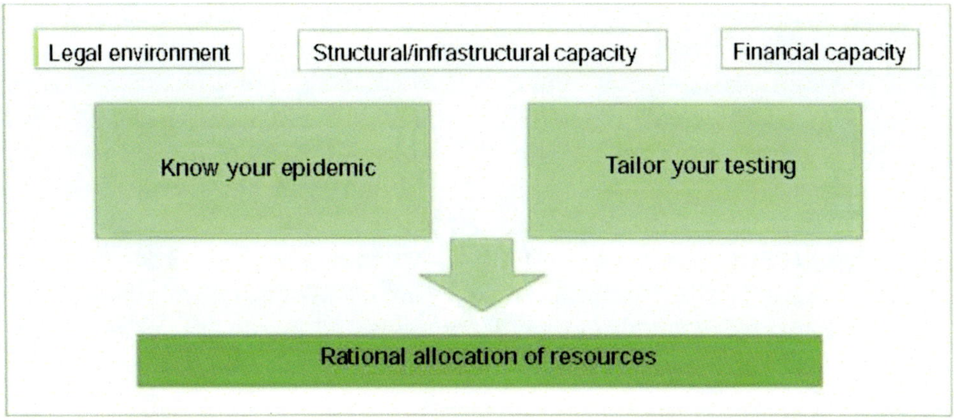

Fig. (6). A key strategy to expand HCV testing in LMICs and harder-to-reach HCV communities [14].

CURRENT PROGRESS OF HCV ELIMINATION BY THE WHO MEMBER STATES

Progress in the African Region

Despite the challenges, WHO efforts while implementing GHSS 2016-2021 in member states have paved the way to prevent new HCV incidences, as well as significant progress, has been made both in HCV diagnosis and treatment [20]. Herein, we will take a glance at WHO's achievements against HCV elimination in various regions of the world with priority actions. Table **1** enlists the data at a glance, 2019-2020 with progress highlights and priority actions for the African region.

Egyptian HCV Elimination Model

Egypt, which has the highest prevalence rate of hepatitis C in the world in 2015, is carrying out an unprecedented campaign to detect and treat the HCV disease in a bid to eliminate it by 2022 [20]. It aims to test the entire adult population of about 50 million people. Nearly 4.4 percent of adult Egyptians are infected and about 40,000 die of the disease every year, making it the country's third leading cause of death, according to the World Bank [20, 28]. In Egypt, many individuals were infected decades ago when poorly sterilized needles were used as part of a national treatment campaign against schistosomiasis, a disease caused by parasitic worms. Most donated blood is still not effectively screened, according to a recent World Bank report [20]. At least 11.5 million people have been screened in the new campaign, with 5 percent testing positive. Due to a lack of health clinics, some churches, mosques, and youth centers also offer blood tests [20]. Unless the population is tested and treated in a single campaign, the disease won't be eliminated, if the campaign only tests and treat parts of the population... then those who weren't treated might infect others [4]. According to this 100 Million Healthy Lives program, 50 million individuals (*i.e.*, 80% of the targeted 62.5 million population) were screened for HCV during the 7 months of the initiation of the campaign [4, 20]. Of those, 4.6% tested anti-HCV Abs positive, of whom 76.5% had an active infection. All confirmed HCV-infected patients were administered SOF plus DCV (400/60 mg daily) with or without RBV for 12 or 24 weeks duration based on the patient's cirrhosis status (present or absent) and disease staging (*i.e.*, compensated or decompensated cirrhosis). SVR rates were achieved at 98.8% in treated individuals [20, 28].

Table 1. HCV elimination progress in the African region in accordance with GHSS (2016-2021) for viral hepatitis [6].

Viral hepatitis **(prevalence)**	Incident cases of hepatitis B infection 990 000 [660 000 1 600 000] Incident cases of hepatitis C infection 210 000 [150 000 370 000] People dying from hepatitis B infection 80 000 [47 000 110 000] People dying from hepatitis C infection 45 000 [23 000 72 000]
Viral hepatitis **(progress toward elimination)**	1- Twenty-eight countries had national hepatitis strategic plans in 2018. 2- Access to diagnosis and treatment is still limited. 3- Hepatitis reporting has improved significantly in the Region since the mid-term report but major gaps remain. 4- Egypt has initiated support for planning toward eliminating viral hepatitis in sub-Saharan African countries, a leading example of South-to-South support. 5- Joint approaches to viral hepatitis and HIV coinfection provide opportunities, given the reductions in prices for hepatitis B and C treatment.
Viral hepatitis **(priority actions)**	• Invest in integrated data systems and streamline the governance of data reviews and use. • Continue to scale up differentiated service delivery, leveraging the innovations from the COVID-19 response. • Intensify efforts to reach men at higher risk of HIV infection. • Advance integrated people-centered health services across diseases, with greater decentralization, task sharing, and community engagement as part of universal health coverage. • Continue to advocate for domestic investment and innovative financing mechanisms; especially to address the chronic funding gaps for viral hepatitis and STIs.

WHO Progress Toward Eliminating HCV in the Region of America

The countries in the American region have led the approaches to eliminate vertical transmission of HIV and deliver the service cascade for key populations in the last decade [20]. In this decade, the region in the Americas will intend to fill the gaps in the service cascade for three infectious diseases (HIV, viral hepatitis, and STIs) and task-shifting of the services to be utilized for HCV diagnosis and treatment [20]. Table **2** enlists the progress data at a glance, 2019-2020, and priority actions for the region of America.

Table 2. HCV elimination progress in the region of America [6].

Viral hepatitis **(prevalence)**	Incident cases of hepatitis B infection 10 000 [5 100 26 000] Incident cases of hepatitis C infection 67 000 [63 000 73 000] People dying from hepatitis B infection 15 000 [8 500 23 000] People dying from hepatitis C infection 31 000 [19 000 84 000]
Viral hepatitis **(progress toward elimination)**	1- Previously adopted preventive interventions, including vaccination and blood safety, have enabled the regional elimination of early childhood transmission of hepatitis B (hepatitis B surface antigen) 2- A total of 23 countries had national hepatitis strategic plans in 2020 versus 10 in 2015. 3- However, access to diagnosis and treatment is still limited, and few people living with hepatitis B and hepatitis C virus have been diagnosed. 4- High prices of commodities and complex patent protection schemes that limit access to generics continue to pose barriers.
Viral hepatitis **(priority actions)**	• Expand integrated testing and treatment services, such as the joint elimination of mother-to-child transmission of HIV and syphilis as part of maternal and child health, common platforms for HIV and STI testing, and mental health. • Facilitate access to commodities by taking a joint approach to addressing market and patent barriers. • Expand the roll-out of differentiated approaches for HIV, including multi-month dispensing of medicines, the expanded role of lay providers, and the use of telemedicine. • Improve surveillance and information systems, especially on viral hepatitis and STIs. • Strengthen surveillance of antimicrobial resistance for N. gonorrhoeae and align treatment guidelines with local susceptibility patterns.

Progress in the South-East Asian Region

The South-East Asia Region has some of the world's leading programs for key populations and community-based responses for hepatitis C.However, financing for viral hepatitis C needs to be sustained and expanded toward universal health coverage [20]. Furthermore, community-led interventions for improving health outcomes across the region have been improved. For example, in Nepal, a community-based intervention leveraged existing sites providing opioid substitution therapy for PWIDs and provided HCV screening and linkage to treatment. The role of communities has also been well recognized in other areas such as in advocacy for access to medicines for hepatitis C [25 - 27]. During the Covid-19 pandemic, community-based organizations played critical roles in providing immediate, short-term mitigation efforts [28]. Nevertheless, these experiences also underscore the need for reconsidering social protection arrangements, addressing structural barriers, and providing support to communities to ensure sustained ownership and involvement [29]. Table **3** shows HCV elimination progress in this region with priority actions for this decade.

Table 3. Progress of HCV elimination program in the South-East Asia Region [6].

Viral hepatitis **(prevalence)**	Incident cases of hepatitis B infection 260 000 [180 000 590 000] Incident cases of hepatitis C infection 230 000 [200 000 430 000] People dying from hepatitis B infection 180 000 [140 000 300 000] People dying from hepatitis C infection 38 000 [37 000 130 000]
Viral hepatitis **(progress toward elimination)**	1- Eight countries in the Region have national hepatitis strategic plans. 2- There have been strong gains in coverage of hepatitis B vaccination, and four countries in the Region have achieved 2020 control targets through immunization. 3- The prevalence of hepatitis B infection has declined significantly. There has been slow progress in scaling up access to hepatitis diagnosis and treatment, and mortality has not yet declined. 4- Funding for viral hepatitis remains inadequate, and the prices of commodities vary across countries.
Key considerations: Three countries Maldives, Sri Lanka, and Thailand have been validated as achieving the elimination of mother-to-child transmission of HIV and syphilis. Access to harm reduction in the Region is low.	
Viral hepatitis **(priority actions)**	• Enhance the coverage of prevention and testing services with linkage to treatment. • Reinvigorate programs with increased focus on key populations and people at higher risk. • Address barriers to accessing services, including stigma and discrimination. • Give priority to hepatitis, HIV, and STI within universal health coverage and with improved financing and investment cases. • Advance a triple elimination framework to end mother-to-child transmission of HIV, hepatitis B, and syphilis. • Utilize price advantages fully, since the costs of health commodities vary greatly in the Region. • Strengthen surveillance and disease burden estimates with better collection and utilization of data. • Maximize the potential of decentralized approaches, including the private sector, to achieve universal health coverage.

Progress in European Region

The major advances in hepatitis C program planning have been noticed in many European countries, but the estimated number of people acquiring HIV has been increasing. Gaps in testing and treatment for HCV need to be filled rapidly in the European Region (Table 4) [20]. Expanding access to hepatitis C treatment through country funding and local production of the generic DAAs has significantly reduced the healthcare burden in Belarus [20]. An estimated 100, 000 people live with CHC infection in Belarus. Most new cases occur among the working-age population, and hepatic cirrhosis caused by CHC is the most common indication for liver transplantation in Belarus. Since 2018, the government of Belarus has funded DAAs for people with CHC infection across the country [20].

Table 4. Highlights and priority actions to eliminate HCV in the Europen region [6].

Viral hepatitis **(prevalence)**	Incident cases of hepatitis B infection 19 000 [9 400 38 000] Incident cases of hepatitis C infection 300 000 [240 000 320 000] People dying from hepatitis B infection 43 000 [34 000 51 000] People dying from hepatitis C infection 64 000 [39 000 72 000]
Viral hepatitis **(progress toward elimination)**	1- A total of 33 countries in the Region have national hepatitis strategic plans. 2- The scale-up of diagnostics and treatment has been slow. 3- There are major gaps in hepatitis data.
Key considerations: • Harm reduction continues to be a low priority in some countries. • The costs of medicines and diagnostics remain high in middle-income countries that face patent-related barriers.	
Viral hepatitis **(priority actions)**	• Catch-up plan for COVID-19-related slowdown in progress on key interventions. • Tailor prevention to key populations, with an integrated people-centered approach across disease areas. • Take an integrated approach to address harm reduction and mental health for key populations. • Use PrEP as an opportunity for better STI screening and treatment in key populations. • Strengthen civil society involvement in the regional response. • Decentralize and simplify HIV testing. • Scale up early antiretroviral therapy provision with optimized regimens and improved quality of care. • Strengthen hepatitis surveillance and monitoring and evaluation to better understand the situation and progress. • Increase the number of countries with funded national plans for hepatitis. • Simplify hepatitis testing strategies and treatment and improve access to treatment. • Strengthen STI surveillance.

The country also updated its national protocol for diagnosis, treatment, and care for people with CHC and developed a 10-year plan for expanding access to hepatitis C treatment from 2019 to 2028 [20]. In 2019, 6000 courses of the pangenotypic DAA regimens of SOF and DCV were procured through the state budget and distributed to health facilities. Among 6074 people treated in 2018–2019 with known treatment outcomes, 6062 (99.8%) had successful treatment outcomes. With a strong commitment to ensuring the sustainability of state-funded hepatitis-related activities, the government of Belarus also established local production of generic DAAs.As of 1 September 2018, the cost of a 12-week treatment regimen was about US$ 706, lower than some other countries in the region. The Ministry of Health continues to work to further reduce costs in cooperation with the pharmaceutical industry, representatives of patient organizations, infectious diseases specialists, and international partners [20].

Progress Toward HCV Elimination in Eastern Mediterranean Region

The countries in the Eastern Mediterranean region are finding ways to scale-up HCV screening and diagnosis in harm reduction centers and harder-to-reach populations in remote areas [20]. Some countries have adopted GHSS 2016-2021 on viral hepatitis in their national action plan and strictly implemented those recommendations in their healthcare services to have an opportunity to move toward HCV elimination by 2030. However, efforts are needed to expand and transfer the impact of these population-based approaches to correctional populations and vulnerable HCV populations in rural areas. Table **5** enlists the WHO's progress toward HCV elimination in the Eastern Mediterranean region with priority actions [20].

Egyptian Model of Scaling-up HCV Diagnosis and Treatment

Egypt is one of the countries with the largest burden of HCV infection in the world [4, 20]. It has made significant advances since 2018 toward eliminating hepatitis C, supported by strong government commitment, local generic manufacturing, and price reductions obtained through negotiations with manufacturers [30]. During 2017–2018, Egypt conducted a massive countrywide effort to screen the entire population aged 18 years and older and provide treatment free of charge to everyone with an infection [4, 20]. Nearly 60 million people had been tested by late 2019, and 4 million had started treatment [4, 20]. This constitutes one of the largest public health efforts to date towards eliminating hepatitis C in LMICs countries worldwide. Egypt now plans to support countries in the African Region in their scale-up efforts [30, 31].

Pakistan Following Micro-elimination Approaches to Eliminate Hepatitis C

In Pakistan, the Hepatitis Control Program has initiated micro elimination projects in the highly prevalent HCV areas of the country [32]. Such a demonstration was initiated in one district of the country's largest province, Punjab [20, 32]. Within this district, a total population of 29,500 people, concentrated in five villages, was selected with the aim of testing 95% of the population 12–80 years old [20, 32]. During a three-week pretest phase in 2019, health education sessions were conducted at the community level, 96% of the target population was screened for HBV and C virus, and people diagnosed were linked to treatment [20, 32]. The efforts were backed by strong political commitment and local ownership. The experience provides lessons for pursuing hepatitis micro elimination efforts in other geographical areas of Pakistan and other countries [20, 32].

Table 5. WHO efforts and priority actions to eliminate HCV in the Eastern Mediterranean Region including highly endemic HCV areas (*e.g.* Egypt, Pakistan) [6].

Viral hepatitis **(prevalence)**	Incident cases of hepatitis B infection 100 000 [79 000 140 000] Incident cases of hepatitis C infection 470 000 [240 000 520 000] People dying from hepatitis B infection 33 000 [26 000 60 000] People dying from hepatitis C infection 31 000 [31 000 74 000]
Viral hepatitis **(progress toward elimination)**	1- Strategic information systems for hepatitis data are slowly improving, and two countries have conducted serological surveys. 2- There has been strong momentum and progress with major initiatives in champion countries such as Egypt and Pakistan; however, programs in most countries remain weak with limited funding. 3- Coverage of the hepatitis B virus vaccine has increased to exceed 80% for the third dose, but birth dose coverage is low. 4- Diagnosis and treatment of hepatitis B and C infection are low. 5- Many countries have achieved reductions in the price of direct-acting antiviral drugs for hepatitis C infection through price negotiations and local manufacturing.
Key considerations: There has been progress in harm reduction, with favorable policies adopted in Egypt and Pakistan, but overall coverage of harm reduction among people who inject drugs in the Region remains very low.	

(Table 5) cont.....

Viral hepatitis **(priority actions)**	• Expand the use of people-centered and differentiated service delivery models and targeted interventions for prevention, diagnosis, and treatment for key populations. • Expand access to hepatitis diagnosis and treatment, including with a focus on micro elimination in high-burden populations, and continue to pursue price reduction strategies and public health approaches for scale-up. • Renew the focus on STIs through greater integration with HIV and other health program areas and efforts to mobilize resources. • Promote domestic funding and mobilize catalytic cross-cutting funding. • Make joint efforts to strengthen strategic information for HIV, viral hepatitis, and STIs as part of broader health management information system strengthening, including with support for electronic data collection and promoting data use through improved analytics and visualization dashboards.

Progress Toward HCV Elimination in the Western Pacific Region

The Western Pacific Region has made major progress in expanding access to services for people with HBV and C infection, largely from domestic funding and substantial reductions of DAAs prices [20]. Such responses to HCV, in particular, have opportunities in national financing for universal health coverage. Table **6** enlists the current scenario of HCV infection in Western Pacific Region along with WHO progress and future priority actions [20].

Table 6. WHO progress and future priority actions to eliminate HCV from Western Pacific Region [6].

Viral hepatitis **(prevalence)**	Incident cases of hepatitis B infection 140 000 [96 000 210 000] Incident cases of hepatitis C infection 230 000 [220 000 260 000] People dying from hepatitis B infection 470 000 [200 000 490 000] People dying from hepatitis C infection 77 000 [77 000 140 000]
Viral hepatitis **(progress toward elimination)**	1- National action plans are in place in 20 countries, strategic information action plans in seven countries, and investment cases, including disease burden and economic analysis, have been developed in 13 countries. 2- The coverage of hepatitis services is expanding through domestic funding in 19 countries. 3- Drug prices have been reduced substantially, and hepatitis medicines have been included in national health insurance in China and Mongolia. Malaysia applied TRIPS flexibilities to expand access to hepatitis C medicines. 4- Hepatitis services are being scaled up at the primary healthcare level in 10 countries. 5- Public private partnership service delivery models are being rolled out in Papua New Guinea.
Key considerations: One country has achieved elimination of mother-to-child transmission of HIV and syphilis.	

(Table 6) cont.....

Viral hepatitis **(priority actions)**	• Maximize opportunities for integrating services based on local epidemiology and context, including across reproductive health services, HIV, viral hepatitis and TB services, and non-communicable diseases, and decentralize integrated services to the primary health care level. • Pursue high-level advocacy for domestic financing and multisectoral collaboration, including the private sector, and promote an integrated health financing approach. • Promote the active involvement of communities for advocacy, stigma and discrimination reduction, and service delivery. • Integrate strategic information into existing systems and simplify data collection to improve quality and increase use.

China ---- Unblocking the Barriers of High DAA Prices to Achieve Universal Coverage for HCV Medicines

In 2015, access to treatment was limited for China's estimated 96 million people living with hepatitis B and C virus [10, 20]. The price of hepatitis C medicines was US$ 10 000 for a cure [20]. DAAs are not universally and equitably reimbursed through health insurance throughout the world, so most people are paying out of pocket [33]. To address this major barrier in China, WHO supported the government and stakeholders in performing economic analysis and health technology assessment of new medicines and facilitated round-table discussions on intellectual property rights and sharing of DAA price information from other countries [33]. The government continued its pursuit of universal coverage in successive years by including hepatitis B and C medicines in the national reimbursement drug list and centrally pooled procurement [33]. In early 2021, hepatitis C treatment cost is US$ 1500–2000 for a cure in China with a reduction of 20% [20]. The reduction in prices enables these medicines to be covered by national health insurance, providing affordable care to many more people living with CHC [33].

LOOKING AHEAD IN THIS DECADE TO ACHIEVE HCV ELIMINATION BY 2030

Despite major progress over the past decade both in HCV diagnostic solutions, the development and approvals of the pan-genotypic DAAs to cure hepatitis C, and the establishment of GHSS 2016-2021 to eliminate hepatitis C by 2030, the 2020 targets were off-track in major areas even before the Covid-19 pandemic in many countries [20]. The ambition of this decade to eliminate hepatitis C as a public health threat by 2030 is enormous yet feasible [20, 21]. However, collective efforts towards universal health coverage and global health security, leveraging the resilience and innovation seen in the global response to Covid-19 as well as the integration and task-shifting of the services to achieve this ambitious goal are of utmost importance [22 - 24].

The Covid-19 pandemic has exposed the deep social, economic, and gender inequalities that make some people more vulnerable to disease and determine their health outcomes [20, 21]. The population groups most severely affected by hepatitis C also encounter the greatest stigma, discrimination, and marginalization, and face difficulty in accessing the services they need. In some ways, they are tracer populations for the progress of inclusive and innovative universal health coverage that reaches beyond health facilities into communities [20 - 22].

Expansion of HCV Service Delivery

The massive expansion in service delivery that will be required in this decade must be matched by efforts to tackle the structural barriers that undermine the response to hepatitis C outcomes (Fig. 7) [16, 34]. To get close to elimination, all countries must continue to go beyond health service delivery to address the social and structural determinants of health and equitably serve the populations most severely affected and at higher risk of HCV infection [52]. Communities must be fully resourced to play their role in reaching those who are hard to reach, delivering services, advocating for change, and holding decision-makers accountable [20, 35]. People-centered health services mean tailoring services to people but also involving them in a new partnership in their delivery [16, 34, 35].

Task-Shifting to Utilize Existing Resources for HCV Elimination

Shifting towards elimination is always going to require a leap forward in our approaches [16, 17]. The lessons from the Covid-19 response provide a historical opportunity to foster greater solidarity and innovation in the response to the hepatitis C epidemic in this decade [1, 19]. Disease-specific responses and the goals of primary health care, universal health coverage, and health security are mutually reinforcing and need to be advanced through integrated health systems approach (Fig. **8**) [36]. Closer links between hepatitis C services with related communicable and non-communicable disease services can make the intervention more efficient and improve their coverage and quality [36]. Joint efforts to strengthen clinical and laboratory platforms, logistics management, information systems, and human resource planning offer many opportunities to jointly strengthen health systems that will be resilient, adaptable, and equitable, including addressing future hepatitis C break-outs (Fig. **8**) [36].

	National framework for viral hepatitis testing	National testing policy
		National hepatitis strategic plan (including testing)
		National regulatory mechanisms (for diagnostic products, staff and services)
		National reference laboratory
	Building capacity for testing services	Human resource management
		Inventory management (procurement and supply chain)
		Storage and transportation
		Equipment management
		Laboratory information management systems
	Product selection	Monitoring testing algorithms
		Post-marketing surveillance of diagnostics
	Assuring the quality of testing services	Quality management system
		Quality control
		Personnel and training
	Assuring the safety of testing services	Facilities and safety

Adapted from Asia Pacific strategy for strengthening health laboratory services (2010-2015). Manila/Delhi: WHO; 2010 (http://www.searo.who.int/about/administration_structure/cds/BCT_Asia_Pacific_Strategy10-15.pdf, accessed 06 February 2017). Development of national health laboratory policy and plan. Manila/Delhi: WHO; 2011 (http://www.wpro.who.int/health_technology/documents/docs/Nationalhealthlab2_0F38.pdf?ua=1, accessed 06 February 2017)

Fig. (7). Key elements for consideration of a national hepatitis plan to expand and implement hepatitis C testing services [6].

Achieving this requires learning from the fragility and solidarity of global health experience with the Covid-19 pandemic and ensuring renewed political commitment and sustainable financing to take the response to hepatitis C to the next level [36]. Such a response must be anchored in the principles of human rights and social justice. By acting decisively now, we can emerge stronger from the challenge of this silent epidemic of hepatitis C and use this momentum to reach the goals of the 2030 agenda for sustainable development [36].

WHO GLOBAL HEALTH SECTOR STRATEGY 2022-2030 FOR HEPATITIS C ELIMINATION

As the GHSS 2016 2021 for viral hepatitis C reaches the end of its implementation period in 2021, WHO will lead a consultative process to develop the next phase of the strategies to guide action towards eliminating these HCV infections as a public health threat by 2030 [20]. Taking into account the progress achieved in the last decade and the remaining gaps in achieving 2030 goals, the process will define the way forward for countries and WHO actions in this decade. Although many of the core public health interventions and target populations of the strategies remain relevant, there have been contextual shifts that must be considered in the next phase [20]. The Covid-19 pandemic has strongly affected public health worldwide, drawing attention to the risks of unprepared health systems, exposing the social determinants of health, and spurring innovations [20]. The new strategies will ensure that the global response to hepatitis C responds to these shifts to deliver health for all [20].

Key Features of GHSS 2022-2030 for Viral Hepatitis Elimination by 2030

The new strategies will also take into account epidemiological and technological developments since 2016, such as updated estimates of the burden of disease, the availability of new diagnostics and medicines, and advances in service delivery approaches [20]. They will also consider the evolving global landscape of shifts in domestic and donor funding and align with political commitments. WHO 2022-2030 strategies will promote synergy with other global hepatic strategy processes (*e.g.*, UNAIDS post-2021 global AIDS strategy) and the new strategy under development for the Global Fund. To strengthen accountability, the strategies will include interim targets for 2025 as milestones toward 2030 goals [20]. WHO's technical leadership, normative guidance and country support remain critical for member states and partners to implement the next phase. The new strategies will ensure that WHO remains well-positioned to provide leadership on achieving the 2030 targets for hepatitis C as part of the broader goals of primary health care and universal health coverage [20].

The strategy development process will include consultations with member states, partners, civil society, communities, and other stakeholders and public online consultations in the official WHO languages [20]. These consultations will be held during 2021, with a view to presenting the final strategies for consideration by the World Health Assembly in May 2022. The current strategies will remain active until that time [20].

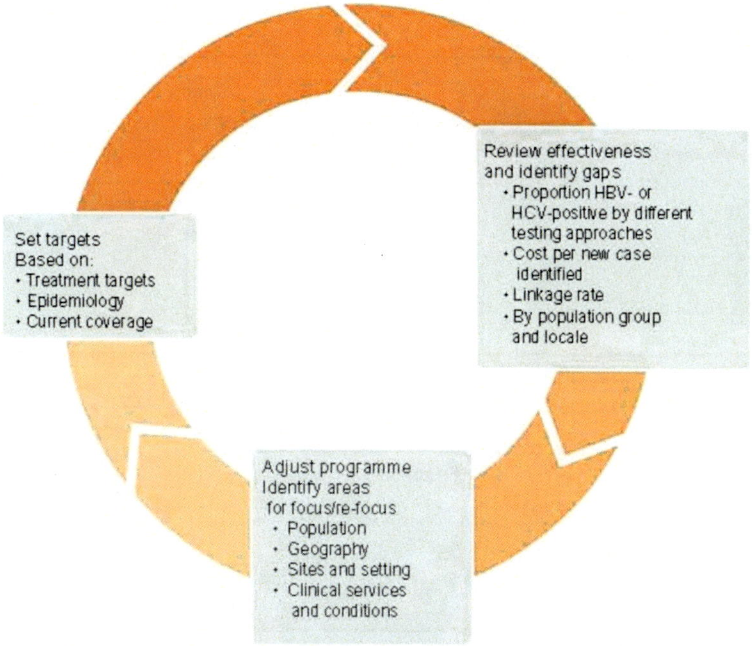

Fig. (8). Key approaches to assess, select, and evaluate hepatitis C testing algorithms [6].

Gaps to Need Fill and Steps to Address These Gaps in WHO Strategies by 2030

GHSS 2016-2021 targets for hepatitis C elimination and relevant strategies defined fast track actions that WHO must be undertaken to support countries to accelerate progress in the fight against hepatitis C since its implementation period [20]. Much has been done during that time; however, due to the unprecedented and devastating impact of the Covid-19 pandemic on halting healthcare services, disrupting HCV diagnosis, and impeding deliveries of treatment, many targets of GHSS could either be partially implemented or not put forward in WHO member states from 2016 to 2021 [5, 36]. Those must be considered for the establishment and implementation of WHO's final strategies to achieve the global goal of HCV elimination by 2030. Table **7** highlights the major gaps that remain in 2020 and identifies suggested steps to address these gaps for WHO global health sector strategies 2022-2030. Ultimately, the rationale of these priorities could be used in this decade for fast-track HCV diagnosis and treatment worldwide or in LMICs where healthcare infrastructure and facilities are scarce to respond to every HCV-positive patient [5, 36].

Table 7. The gaps left in GHSS 2016-2021 for viral hepatitis and key measures to address those gaps by 2030 in WHO member states [6].

Global health sector strategy	WHO action with significant gaps in 2020	Suggested steps to address the gap by 2030
Viral hepatitis	Support countries with tools and technical assistance.	Strengthen partner technical support and support from WHO regional offices.
	Support countries in fully implementing WHO's injection safety policy and global campaign.	Highlight injection safety in the next phase of the global health sector strategies.
	Provide advocacy and technical support to countries to mobilize commitment to harm reduction.	Address barriers to harm reduction as a cross-cutting priority in the next phase of the global health sector strategies.
	Provide guidance on quality assurance and quality improvement systems.	Assess approaches to improve quality assurance and improvement in countries.
	Provide policy and technical guidance aimed at building a competent workforce.	Develop guidance on differentiated human resources support for hepatitis services.
	Provide technical support to countries to forecast the need for essential hepatitis commodities.	Initiate forecasting for hepatitis C commodities in the 2021 forecasting meeting for drug and diagnostics stakeholders and partners.
	Support regulatory authorities in pre-market assessment and registration of new hepatitis medicines and diagnostics, with post-market surveillance.	Strengthen post-market surveillance to support regulatory authorities.
	Consider in the next phase of the global health sector strategies.	Assess the quality and performance of commercially available hepatitis diagnostics.

GLOBAL MESSAGES AND ACTIVIST LESSONS

Key priorities in WHO cross-cutting actions for this decade mainly include; advancing community engagement and community-led services, exploring the potential of digital health to reach young people, and self-testing for infectious diseases to maintain services for key populations [20]. Table **8** enlists some cross-cutting actions with their implementation status in 2020 as well as recommendations for catch-up actions to 2030.

Community Engagement and Community-led Service Delivery to Vulnerable and Harder-to-Reach HCV Populations

HCV diagnostics and treatment algorithms are transforming rapidly with an increasing number of new diagnostics, devices, medicines, and other technologies that can be self-administered and self-managed, often supported by digital innovations [4]. Community-based and peer-led approaches bring services closer to people in need and deliver them in an environment of trust (Table **8**). They empower individuals with a wider choice of interventions, including greater possibilities for self-care and autonomy [37 - 39]. They also empower communities to play a lead role in advocacy, priority-setting, and designing services to meet their needs and promote accountability (Fig. **9**) [20].

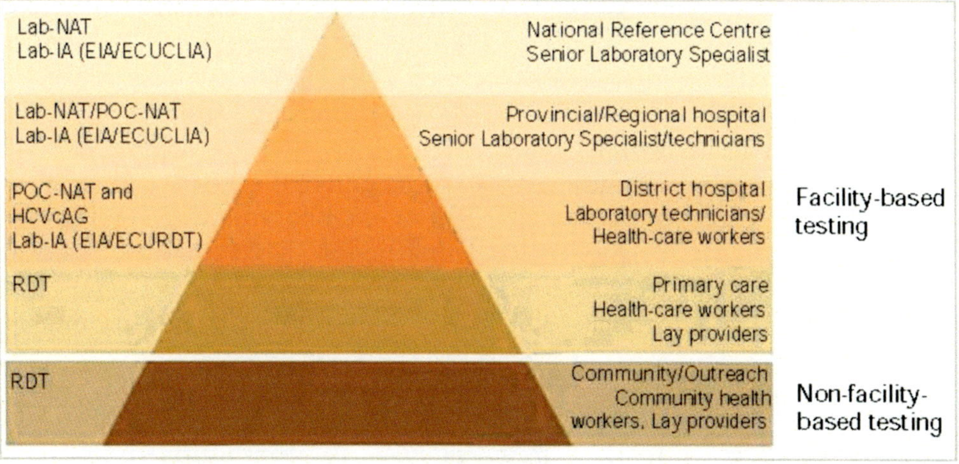

Fig. (9). A tiered testing service, with a test format menu and staff qualifications [6]. CLIA: chemiluminescence immunoassay, ECL; electrochemiluminescence, EIA; enzyme immunoassay, RDT; rapid diagnostic test, Lab-NAT; laboratory-based nucleic acid testing, POC-NAT; nucleic acid at point of care, HCVcAG; Hepatitis C Core antigen.

In response to the Covid-19 pandemic, community-based organizations worldwide stepped up efforts to identify and expand innovative ways to continue to reach people with essential services in contexts of lockdowns and stay-home measures, physical distancing requirements, difficulties in accessing health-care services, and supply disruptions [37, 38]. Community-based organizations delivered essential supplies such as ART therapy and harm-reduction services directly within communities and to people's homes, expanded the use of self-testing for hepatitis C and self-management approaches, and used telehealth and social media to provide information and support, often integrating Covid-19 messaging in their work [38].

Several of these approaches were already being successfully used before the Covid-19 pandemic for hepatitis C infection diagnosis and management [1, 52, 53]. Their expanded use in the context of a public health crisis (*e.g.*, the Covid-19 pandemic) has clearly demonstrated how community engagement plays a major role in delivering people-centered services to populations that are hard to reach [2, 39]. Community-led service delivery is integral to effective primary health care and an essential complement to facility-based services. The innovations introduced in Community engagement and community-led service delivery during the Covid-19 pandemic must be sustained and leveraged to reach larger numbers of the people most severely affected and at higher risk – to achieve the goals of eliminating hepatitis C as a public health threat by 2030 [40, 41]. Community-led and community-based responses require greater investment with stronger links to primary health care and its focus on building people-centered, resilient and sustainable health systems that uphold the right to health, promote social justice, empower individuals and communities and address the determinants of health (Table **8**) [42]. Countries are encouraged to further scale up innovative community-led approaches as they strive towards elimination, in accordance with the pathways described in the WHO/UNICEF operational framework for primary health care (Fig. **9**) [30]. Young people, in particular, have emerged as critical gatekeepers in pioneering and sustaining community-led innovations and should be further supported in consolidating their leadership into the next phase of WHO targets to reset the responses to hepatitis C back on track [37, 39].

Exploring the Potential of Digital Health to Maintain Hepatitis C Surveillance Data and to Reach Young HCV-Infected Populations

Young IDUs are a potential source of new HCV incidences worldwide and in particular in the European nations. Furthermore, this fraction of HCV affected population has poor knowledge of available prevention measures and healthcare services [43].Young people also report concerns around confidentiality, provider attitudes, and feelings of stigma and shame as barriers to accessing services (Table **8**) [44].

In South Africa, faced with the Covid-19 pandemic, a project providing sexual and reproductive health services to adolescent girls and young women 15–24 years old rapidly adapted its service delivery to the Covid-19 context [45]. STIs infections have been reported most in young people in South Africa. By using social media, chatbots, and messaging apps, the project ensured that young people continued to have access to information and educational materials in times of lockdown [46]. The project decentralized service delivery to mobile clinics and community delivery points and expanded the use of telehealth for screening, consultations, and psychosocial support [20]. They also sent electronic prescriptions and postal self-testing or self-sampling kits for HIV, chlamydia, syphilis, and gonorrhea, with follow-up through telemedicine [47].The project found that young clients responded positively to having a wider choice of service delivery options for sample collection, diagnosis, receiving results, initiating treatment, and notifying partners. It also found high utilization of social media for information, screening, and follow-up, demonstrating the potential to extend these adaptations in the future [48].

Table 8. Recommended priority actions for this decade by WHO for Viral Hepatitis Elimination by 2030 and their current progress in 2020 [6].

Priorities	Status in 2020	Catch-up actions to 2030
Actions identified in the mid-term review (2019)		
1. Leverage common disaggregated data platforms	Electronic district-level data systems have been implemented in most countries, with regular data reviews to improve programs. However, gaps remain in facility-level reporting for viral hepatitis and STIs and in the security and interoperability of data systems.	• Strengthen digital health data, including guidance on data interoperability, security, and unique identifiers. • Conduct standardized analytical reviews and build capacity to use data at decentralized levels to improve programs. • Consider agile, small-scale surveys across the three disease areas that can assess trends and progress in specific populations.
2. Scale up point-o--care diagnostics and self-testing	The availability of diagnostics for HIV, viral hepatitis, and STIs is improving, supported by recent innovations. However, there are many missed opportunities to leverage common platforms for service delivery and common learnings, such as in the case of self-testing across all three disease areas.	• Make self-testing available for all three disease areas, especially to reach the key and vulnerable populations and men. • Strengthen joint diagnostic platforms that can be leveraged across all three disease areas and more widely across the health.
3. Achieve triple elimination of mother-to-child transmission of HIV, hepatitis B virus, and syphilis and explore extending the elimination focus to children	There has been major progress in aligning guidelines and processes and validating the first set of countries for dual and triple elimination. Fifteen countries have already been validated as having eliminated the mother-to-child transmission of HIV and/or syphilis as public health threats, and two additional countries are preparing to submit country data to join the path toward elimination. Stronger incentives to align countries in the full path towards elimination would strengthen the approach, together with further inclusion of hepatitis B.	• Strengthen approaches and incentives to involve countries in the full path towards elimination, including in larger countries with a higher burden of disease. • Scale up the triple elimination of mother-to-child transmission and, where feasible, expand approaches to validate adult elimination, such as for hepatitis C virus infection. • Develop strategies to expand the focus on eliminating vertical transmission to eliminating infections among children across the diseases.

(*Table 8*) *cont.....*

4. Improve access to drugs and diagnostics	The price reductions have been remarkable for hepatitis C medicines in the past three years and HIV over the last two decades. These need to be extended and efforts made to include the costs of expanding coverage of these within national health plans, including any health insurance entities, and to provide the needed financing across all three disease areas as part of universal health coverage. In addition, developing an end-t--end process for antiretroviral medicines for children, early infant diagnosis, and using multi-disease platforms can improve the effectiveness of interventions.	• Include drug and diagnostics cost increasingly in-country health financing, for example for HIV and viral hepatitis in Rwanda's health insurance program and hepatitis B in China's insurance programs. This also enables further reductions as prices are aligned, for example between hepatitis B virus and HIV. • Promote South-to-South support, for example, Egypt's support for eliminating hepatitis C more widely in Africa. • Strengthen subnational use of unique identifiers to better match patient numbers with drug and diagnostic stocks. • Facilitate drug development for new gonorrhea treatment and options for syphilis treatment and availability of STI drugs and diagnostics at the primary health care level.
5. Protect against the threat of antimicrobial resistance	There have been strong improvements in HIV medicines with regard to antimicrobial resistance supported by a global action plan. Cross-cutting antimicrobial resistance actions across HIV, STIs, and TB could be strengthened.	• Improve surveillance and monitoring of antimicrobial resistance for HIV and STIs. • Improve data used to reduce loss to follow-up on life-long HIV treatment. • Align actions to address antimicrobial resistance for HIV and STIs and coordinate with cross-cutting management of antimicrobial resistance.
6. Strengthen joint responses to HIV, viral hepatitis, and STIs with TB and other key comorbidities	There has been major progress in the provision of testing and treatment, but TB remains the major cause of death among people living with HIV. Programs in many countries in sub-Saharan Africa remain separate in terms of management, supply chains, and monitoring.	• Review integration of HIV and TB programs, especially in sub-Saharan Africa, while continuing strong progress in aligning testing and treatment. • Align joint monitoring approaches in terms of the use of health information system platforms such as DHIS-2, program reviews, and ongoing data use to improve services.

(Table 8) cont.....

7. Integrate sexual and reproductive health and rights	Many countries have pioneered important approaches in relation to key and vulnerable populations, but progress has met significant barriers. Renewed efforts are required to secure sexual and reproductive rights for all.	• Extend activities across all three disease areas and mainstream key components in universal health care approaches, where the tracer is often progressed in key and vulnerable populations. • Integrate STI prevention and care services into HIV, adolescent health, antenatal care, sexual and reproductive health services, and primary health care. • Further integrate sexual and reproductive health rights including STIs into existing programs, including those supported by the Global Fund and the United States President's Emergency Plan for AIDS Relief (PEPFAR).
8. Address social and structural determinants	The failure to achieve HIV incidence reduction targets and STI targets highlights the need to address social, behavioral, and structural determinants more directly in the next decade to progress toward elimination.	• Support national prevention programs with strong leadership to tackle social and structural determinants, since many countries suggest these have not been adequately supported at the highest level • Develop activities across the Triple Billion targets, leveraging the increasing WHO emphasis on social and structural determinants.
Actions identified to leverage innovations and lessons from the COVID-19 response		
9. Maximize the use of differentiated and people-centered service delivery options	Many of the policies have been developed, but they gained additional impetus in implementation in response to the COVID-19 pandemic. This momentum needs to be further leveraged to build back a stronger response to HIV, viral hepatitis, and STIs.	• Extend flexibility in policies, such as multi-month dispensing of antiretroviral medicines to six months, and require differentiated care policies to be in place. • Strengthen the use of person-centered data and digital health to further implement people-centered service delivery.
10. Strengthen community, engagement, community-based service delivery, and community-led monitoring	Community engagement has been a critical part of the response, but communities have increasingly taken on additional responsibilities to integrate prevention, testing, and treatment with innovative approaches in response to the COVID-19 pandemic.	• Integrate community-level services to bring together prevention, testing, and treatment. • Develop direct, simplified service delivery that goes beyond health facilities, using community networks and workplaces to reach the most vulnerable populations, adolescent girls and young women and men.

The task-shifting and rationalization of these approaches could also be possible for hepatitis C in this decade while involving minor training and capacity building of a wide range of healthcare workers as well as by recruiting volunteers from the colleges and universities by providing continued medical and community health education (Table **8**) [49, 50]. Furthermore, people with ongoing HCV infection or most affected by these diseases should also be consulted and included in the design, leadership, and decision-making in the HCV response. In addition to that, people with lived experience, such as peer educators, may play a critical role in screening and increasing the number of patients cured [49, 50].

Expansion of Self-Testing for Key HCV-Infected Populations

A key lesson learned from Thailand during the Covid-19 pandemic resulted in a decline of 50–75% in clients testing for HIV and STIs in major HIV and STI service delivery centers [4, 20]. To maintain access to sexual health services while respecting physical distancing and occupational safety regulations during the pandemic, Thailand's key population–led health services program introduced self-sampling for STIs at major key population-led health clinics for the first time. The uptake of self-sampling was high, and the rate of acceptance of STI self-sampling increased from 48% in May 2020 to 78% by July 2020. Thailand also adopted other services to the Covid-19 context, such as extending PrEP prescriptions from three to six months for continuing clients, delivering medication and supplies discretely, and using telehealth consultations [20, 21].

Such adaptations provide greater accessibility and acceptability of services for populations in need and can be sustainable over the long term for other infectious diseases like hepatitis C (Table **8**) [4, 19].A meta-analysis of data from 11 studies from different countries found that self-collection of samples nearly tripled the overall uptake of STI testing services compared with the clinician-based collection, offering an important additional strategy to increase service uptake for hepatitis C in the future [33].

Acceleration of Progress Within Primary Healthcare and Frameworks of Universal Health Coverage for Hepatitis C

The responses to HIV, viral hepatitis, and STIs play an important role in advancing the global goals of universal health coverage and primary health care [34, 35]. Similarly, increased investment in the key components of primary health care drives progress towards disease-specific goals and people-centered care as critically important elements of the push for universal health coverage [20, 36]. With universal health coverage as the goal, strengthening primary health care while continuing with disease-specific approaches can ensure optimal opportunities for people-centered services and greater efficiency through strengthened integration (Table **8**) [20, 37, 39]. Primary health care covers the range of disease prevention, health promotion, treatment, rehabilitation, and palliation care that are needed throughout a person's lifespan, delivered as close as feasible to people's everyday environment [51 - 53]. WHO's vision for primary health care seeks to achieve healthy lives and well-being for all by building people-centered, resilient, and sustainable primary health care–based health systems that uphold the right to health, empower individuals and communities, and address the determinants of health through multisectoral policy and action [54 - 56].

Propagation of Universal Health Coverage Framework for HCV

Universal health coverage means that all people have access to the health services they need, when and where they need them, without financial hardship. Effective control of disease is therefore integral to progress towards universal health coverage [57]. The GHSS 2016-2021 for viral hepatitis (in particular for HCV) recognize universal health coverage as an overarching guiding framework and contributes towards its progressive realization; in turn, progress towards universal health coverage enables a comprehensive response to hepatitis C [58]. People-centered and resilient health systems that deliver primary health care are essential to achieve universal health coverage. Countries and international partners must commit themselves to orient health systems towards primary health care for accelerated progress on universal health coverage and the health-related sustainable development goals to eliminate hepatitis C [59].

The global response to hepatitis C is anchored by accelerating progress within the frameworks of universal health coverage and primary health care (Table **8**) [60]. Joint efforts to eliminate hepatitis C are important steps toward advancing universal health coverage and primary health care through disease-specific action [61]. These include strengthening cross-cutting surveillance and information systems, deploying multi-disease diagnostic technologies, strengthening self-care and self-management approaches, addressing common price and patent-related barriers, integrating disease-specific financing into universal health coverage packages, empowering communities, and addressing common social determinants of health [62]. For many countries, integrating primary health care for hepatitis C across a wide range of policies, strategies, activities, and services is lacking and requires a substantial transformation of how health-related policies and actions across disease areas are given priority, funded, and implemented [34 - 36]. Each country must progress towards universal health coverage and primary health care in accordance with local contexts and priorities [57]. Countries must assess, set priorities for, optimize, and sequence their actions as part of national health sector planning for hepatitis C (Fig. **10**) [62].

These processes should occur in the context of an inclusive planning process with community participation that includes the most vulnerable, disadvantaged, and marginalized people, and care must be taken to ensure that greater integration does not compromise the focus on hepatitis C-specific responses that serve these populations [62].

	Considerations	Strategic information	Monitoring and evaluation
Who?	Which populations should be targeted for testing? Are there any particular groups who are disproportionately affected by the infection? Are there legal barriers to targeting these groups (e.g. criminalisation of transmission or risk behaviours)? Are there any barriers for these groups to access care and treatment after testing positive?	National surveillance/ prevalence studies: undiagnosed fraction rate of late diagnosis infection prevalence/ incidence number of recently acquired/acute infections number newly diagnosed	Overall and for each target group: people living with HBV, HCV or HIV who know their status testing coverage rate positivity rate number/proportion of first -time testers number/proportion diagnosed late
What?	Which infections will be covered by the testing programme? Does the testing programme offer opportunities for other public health interventions or case-finding/ contact tracing?	National surveillance/ prevalence studies: prevalence of co-infections overlapping risks	Number/proportion of new diagnoses and rates of co-infection detected
Where?	In which setting(s) will the testing take place? Is there evidence of the acceptability and feasibility of testing in this setting for the target population? Are there any restrictions on who can carry out testing in this setting (e.g. legal or regulatory)? What will the geographical coverage of the testing programme be (e.g. local, regional or national)? Is there an established clinical pathway for those testing positive in this setting?	Acceptability and feasibility of testing in this setting (for staff and clients) Legal environment Structural/organisational barriors to testing in this setting Accessibility of setting for the target population	Number of individuals tested by setting and risk group Positivity rate by setting Return rates of testing kits (self-sampling) Rate of linkage to care
When	What is the timescale for implementing the programme? How long will the testing programme last? Are there any barriers that may delay implementation (e.g. changes to testing guidelines)?	Review of relevant case studies Possibility of a pilot to inform cost, resource and positivity rate projections	Programme sustainability, as measured by specific success indicators over time Spread of programme Integration of testing implementation into guidelines
How	How will the testing programme be implemented? What funding is available to implement the testing programme, and is the funding sustainable? Which stakeholders need to be involved to ensure the testing programme is successful (clinicians, nurses, community organisations)? Who will carry out the testing (e.g. clinicians, nurses, lay providers)? Are there any legal or regulatory barriers as to who can carry out testing tasks (e.g. offering tests, obtaining samples, carrying out point-of-care tests)? Is education or training required for the people How? who will perform the test or be tested? Which diagnostic technologies will be used? How will the target population be recruited to the testing programme? How frequently should the target population be tested? Will the testing be integrated into existing services, or will additional infrastructure be required? How will the testing programme be promoted? How will timely linkage to care be ensured if an individual tests positive? How and where will reactive results be confirmed? How will programme results be disseminated (local/national engagement)?	Review of relevant case studies and evidence of successful implementation of similar programmes OptTEST tools for implementing indicator condition-guided testing (HIV), addressing legal and regulatory barriers to testing, addressing stigma and assessing cost—effectiveness Financial assessment Possibility of a pilot to inform cost, resource and positivity rate projections	Cost per new diagnosis Cost per positive test Overall cost of programme Coverage of the programme Acceptability of the testing programme Testing uptake and offer rate, overall and by risk group Testing positivity rate Scope of HIV testing programme interventions (includes community-based testing, self-testing, lay provider testing)

Fig. (10). Key considerations in developing a national HCV testing program [14].

CONCLUSIONS

Eliminating hepatitis C as a public health problem by 2030 is feasible, but it will take substantial efforts, hard work, resources, and policy changes. We now have innovative diagnostic tools to prevent and treat hepatitis C, as new DAAs for CHC can cure the infection in more than 95% of patients. The treatment for hepatitis C is remarkably effective, but it's also extremely expensive. Even though the DAAs are still expensive in many parts of the world, they are so effective that they save an enormous amount of money compared to most healthcare interventions. Right now, steep progress has been seen in the administration of DAAs to treat HCV since their first-time approval as 10% of HCV patients will get treatment worldwide by 2020. Although, this pace of HCV treatment by DAAs is still slow, nevertheless, now we have the opportunity to cure HCV. This would be valuable to reduce the plausible causes of HCC because something like 80% of liver cancer comes from hepatitis B and C. By curing HCV, we now have the opportunities to prevent an enormous amount of liver cancers to save healthcare intervention resources and treatment costs. Eradicating hepatitis C completely does not seem feasible in this decade or by 2030 but, rather, making its status as a public health problem may disappear. Because there will always be the hidden and missing HCV-undiagnosed people bringing it back. Surprisingly, even the availability of an effective prophylactic or protective HCV vaccine would still take two generations to disappear it. We should be very conscious of the fact that eliminating hepatitis C as a public health problem is not going to be easy, and be fair to what is feasible and highly feasible in a clear table format based upon real-world calculations, statistics, and data.

REFERENCES

[1] Martinez MA, Franco S. Impact of COVID-19 in Liver Disease Progression. Hepatol Commun 2021; 5(7): 1138-50.
[http://dx.doi.org/10.1002/hep4.1745] [PMID: 34533001]

[2] Boettler T, Newsome PN, Mondelli MU, *et al.* Care of patients with liver disease during the COVID-19 pandemic: EASL-ESCMID position paper. JHEP Reports 2020; 2(3): 100113.
[http://dx.doi.org/10.1016/j.jhepr.2020.100113] [PMID: 32289115]

[3] Heffernan A, Cooke GS, Nayagam S, Thursz M, Hallett TB. Scaling up prevention and treatment towards the elimination of hepatitis C: a global mathematical model. Lancet 2019; 393(10178): 1319-29.
[http://dx.doi.org/10.1016/S0140-6736(18)32277-3] [PMID: 30704789]

[4] Shahid I, Alzahrani AR, Al-Ghamdi SS, Alanazi IM, Rehman S, Hassan S. Hepatitis C Diagnosis: Simplified Solutions, Predictive Barriers, and Future Promises. Diagnostics (Basel, Switzerland). 2021; 11: 7.

[5] World Health Organization. (2016). Global health sector strategy on viral hepatitis 2016-2021. Towards ending viral hepatitis. World Health Organization. Available from: https://apps.who.int/iris/handle/10665/246177.

[6] WHO guidelines on hepatitis B and C testing. Geneva: World Health Organization; 2017. Available

from: https://www.who.int.

[7] Qu LX, Shi Y, Chen KY, Wang W, Ren H. Analysis of integrated HCV surveillance in Shanghai, 2014-2019. Zhonghua liu xing bing xue za zhi = Zhonghua liuxingbingxue zazhi. 2021; 42(4): 626-31.

[8] Wilder J, Saraswathula A, Hasselblad V, Muir A. A Systematic Review of Race and Ethnicity in Hepatitis C Clinical Trial Enrollment. J Natl Med Assoc 2016; 108(1): 24-9. [http://dx.doi.org/10.1016/j.jnma.2015.12.004] [PMID: 26928485]

[9] Grubyte S, Urboniene J, Nedzinskiene L, Jancoriene L. The Epidemiological Patterns of Hepatitis C in Lithuania: Changes in Surveillance from 2005 to 2018. Medicina (Kaunas) 2021; 57(10): 1120. [http://dx.doi.org/10.3390/medicina57101120] [PMID: 34684157]

[10] Chen Y, Shen Z, Morano JP, *et al.* Bridging the epidemic: a comprehensive analysis of prevalence and correlates of HIV, hepatitis C, and syphilis, and infection among female sex workers in Guangxi Province, China. PLoS One 2015; 10(2): e0115311. [http://dx.doi.org/10.1371/journal.pone.0115311] [PMID: 25723548]

[11] Rio C, Springer SA. Hepatitis C in the United States: One Step Forward, Two Steps Back. Am J Public Health 2021; 111(5): 768-9. [http://dx.doi.org/10.2105/AJPH.2021.306251] [PMID: 33826392]

[12] Sarin SK, Kumar M, Eslam M, *et al.* Liver diseases in the Asia-Pacific region: a Lancet Gastroenterology & Hepatology Commission. Lancet Gastroenterol Hepatol 2020; 5(2): 167-228. [http://dx.doi.org/10.1016/S2468-1253(19)30342-5] [PMID: 31852635]

[13] Saine ME, Szymczak JE, Moore TM, *et al.* Determinants of stigma among patients with hepatitis C virus infection. J Viral Hepat 2020; 27(11): 1179-89. [http://dx.doi.org/10.1111/jvh.13343] [PMID: 32500618]

[14] European Centre for Disease Prevention and Control. 2018. https://www.ecdc.europa.eu

[15] Pol S, Lair-Mehiri L, Vallet-Pichard A. Is elimination of HCV realistic by 2030: France. Liver international : official journal of the International Association for the Study of the Liver. 2021; 41 Suppl 1: 45-9.

[16] Kattakuzhy S, Gross C, Emmanuel B, *et al.* Expansion of Treatment for Hepatitis C Virus Infection by Task Shifting to Community-Based Nonspecialist Providers. Ann Intern Med 2017; 167(5): 311-8. [http://dx.doi.org/10.7326/M17-0118] [PMID: 28785771]

[17] Draper BL, Htay H, Pedrana A, Yee WL, Howell J, Pyone Kyi K, *et al.* Outcomes of the CT2 study: A 'one-stop-shop' for community-based hepatitis C testing and treatment in Yangon, Myanmar. Liver international : official journal of the International Association for the Study of the Liver. 2021; 41(11): 2578-89.

[18] Martinello M, Hajarizadeh B, Grebely J, Dore GJ, Matthews GV. Management of acute HCV infection in the era of direct-acting antiviral therapy. Nat Rev Gastroenterol Hepatol 2018; 15(7): 412-24. [http://dx.doi.org/10.1038/s41575-018-0026-5] [PMID: 29773899]

[19] Oru E, Trickey A, Shirali R, Kanters S, Easterbrook P. Decentralisation, integration, and task-shifting in hepatitis C virus infection testing and treatment: a global systematic review and meta-analysis. Lancet Glob Health 2021; 9(4): e431-45. [http://dx.doi.org/10.1016/S2214-109X(20)30505-2] [PMID: 33639097]

[20] Global progress report on HIV, viral hepatitis and sexually transmitted infections, 2021. Accountability for the global health sector strategies 2016 2021: actions for impact. Geneva: World Health Organization; 2021. Available from: https://www.who.int

[21] Activist Guide to Hepatitis C Virus Diagnostics. https://www.hepcoalition.org/advocate/advocacy-tools/article/activist-guide-to-hepatitis-c-virus-diagnostics

[22] Komaromy M, Duhigg D, Metcalf A, *et al.* Project ECHO (Extension for Community Healthcare

Outcomes): A new model for educating primary care providers about treatment of substance use disorders. Subst Abus 2016; 37(1): 20-4.
[http://dx.doi.org/10.1080/08897077.2015.1129388] [PMID: 26848803]

[23] Wiktor S. How feasible is the global elimination of HCV infection? Lancet 2019; 393(10178): 1265-7. [http://dx.doi.org/10.1016/S0140-6736(18)32750-8] [PMID: 30704788]

[24] Johnston L, Ahmad F, Stephens B, Dillon JF. The eradicate-C study-curing people who are actively injecting drugs of hepatitis C: the first step to elimination. J Hepatol 2017; 66(1): S312. [http://dx.doi.org/10.1016/S0168-8278(17)30945-5]

[25] Rajkumar N. Raising awareness and advocacy to improve access to HCV screening, diagnosis and treatment in Manipur. London: World Hepatitis Alliance 2020. https://www.worldhepatitis alliance.org/missing-millions/casestudy/raising-awareness-and-advocacy-to-improve-access-to-hcv-screening-diagnosis-and-treatment-in-manipur

[26] Cambridge Economic Policy Associates Ltd. 2018.https://unitaid.org/assets/Update-of-the-mid- term-evaluation-of-the-hiv-hcv-drug-affordability-project.pdf

[27] Community advocacy and policy. New York: amfAR; 2021. https://www.amfar.org/treat-asia-community-advocacy-policy

[28] Reza-Paul S, Lazarus L, Haldar P, *et al.* Community action for people with HIV and sex workers during the COVID-19 pandemic in India. WHO South-East Asia J Public Health 2020; 9(2): 104-6. [http://dx.doi.org/10.4103/2224-3151.294302] [PMID: 32978341]

[29] Benjarattanaporn P, Janyam S, Phuengsamran D, *et al.* Protecting sex workers in Thailand during the COVID-19 pandemic: opportunities to build back better. WHO South-East Asia J Public Health 2020; 9(2): 100-3.
[http://dx.doi.org/10.4103/2224-3151.294301] [PMID: 32978340]

[30] WHO, UNICEF. Operational framework for primary health care: transforming vision into action. Geneva: World Health Organization; 2020 (https://www.who.int/publications/i/ item/9789240017832).

[31] Newton-Levinson A, Leichliter JS, Chandra-Mouli V. Sexually transmitted infection services for adolescents and youth in low- and middle-income countries: perceived and experienced barriers to accessing care. J Adolesc Health 2016; 59(1): 7-16.
[http://dx.doi.org/10.1016/j.jadohealth.2016.03.014] [PMID: 27338664]

[32] Unitaid SA. Department of Health, University of Witwatersrand. Engaging young Africans in STI and HIV care: what is the reality, what are the opportunities? 23rd International AIDS Conference, Virtual.

[33] Ogale Y, Yeh PT, Kennedy CE, Toskin I, Narasimhan M. Self-collection of samples as an additional approach to deliver testing services for sexually transmitted infections: a systematic review and meta-analysis. BMJ Glob Health 2019; 4(2): e001349.
[http://dx.doi.org/10.1136/bmjgh-2018-001349] [PMID: 31139454]

[34] From Alma-Ata towards universal health coverage and the Sustainable Development Goals. Global Conference on Primary Health Care. Astana, Kazakhstan, 25 26 October 2018. Geneva: World Health Organization; 2018 (https://www. who.int/teams/primary-health-care/conference/declaration)

[35] Political declaration of the high-level meeting on universal health coverage. United Nations General Assembly, Seventy-fourth session. (document A/RES/74/2), 18 October 2019. New York: United Nations; 2019 (https://documents-dds-ny. un.org/doc/UNDOC/GEN/N19/311/84/PDF/N1931184. pdf?OpenElement)

[36] Tordrup D, Hutin Y, Stenberg K, *et al.* Additional resource needs for viral hepatitis elimination through universal health coverage: projections in 67 low-income and middle-income countries, 2016 30. Lancet Glob Health 2019; 7(9): e1180-8.
[http://dx.doi.org/10.1016/S2214-109X(19)30272-4] [PMID: 31353061]

[37] Accelerating access to hepatitis C diagnostics and treatment: overcoming barriers in low- and middle-income countries. Geneva: World Health Organization; 2021 (https://www.who.int/

publications/i/item/9789240019003).

[38] Pakistan's investment in hepatitis may see return within years. Geneva: World Health Organization; 2018 (https://www.who.int/ hepatitis/news-events/towards-hepatitis-elimination-pakistan/ en).

[39] Grebely J, Bruggmann P, Treloar C, Byrne J, Rhodes T, Dore GJ. Expanding access to prevention, care and treatment for hepatitis C virus infection among people who inject drugs. Int J Drug Policy 2015; 26(10): 893-8.
[http://dx.doi.org/10.1016/j.drugpo.2015.07.007] [PMID: 26254497]

[40] Bloodborne viral and sexually transmissible infections in Aboriginal and Torres Strait Islander people: annual surveillance report 2015. https://kirby.unsw.edu.au/sites/default/files/hiv/resources/atsip2015_v3.pdf

[41] Guidance for post-market surveillance of in vitro diagnostics. Geneva: World Health Organization; 2015 (http://www.who.int/diagnostics_laboratory/postmarket/150210_pms_ivds_guidance.pdf?ua=1).

[42] Kondili LA, Aghemo A, Andreoni M. Challenges on the achievement of World Health Organization goals for HCV elimination in Italy: need for a Regional programmatic approach on screening and linkage to care. Commentary. Ann Ist Super Sanita 2021; 57(3): 201-4.
[PMID: 34554113]

[43] Li J, Shang X, Liang Y, Yang W, Wang Z, Ji H. Assessment of the Hepatitis C Surveillance System in Henan, China: 2014~2016. BioMed Res Int 2018; 2018: 1-8.
[http://dx.doi.org/10.1155/2018/8942152] [PMID: 30356439]

[44] Schackman BR, Leff JA, Barter DM, *et al.* Cost-effectiveness of rapid hepatitis C virus (HCV) testing and simultaneous rapid HCV and HIV testing in substance abuse treatment programs. Addiction 2015; 110(1): 129-43.
[http://dx.doi.org/10.1111/add.12754] [PMID: 25291977]

[45] Cipriano LE, Zaric GS, Holodniy M, Bendavid E, Owens DK, Brandeau ML. Cost effectiveness of screening strategies for early identification of HIV and HCV infection in injection drug users. PLoS One 2012; 7(9): e45176.
[http://dx.doi.org/10.1371/journal.pone.0045176] [PMID: 23028828]

[46] Urbanus AT, van Keep M, Matser AA, *et al.* Is adding HCV screening to the antenatal national screening program in Amsterdam, the Netherlands, cost-effective? PLoS One 2013; 8(8): e70319.
[http://dx.doi.org/10.1371/journal.pone.0070319] [PMID: 23950920]

[47] Miners AH, Martin NK, Ghosh A, Hickman M, Vickerman P. Assessing the cost-effectiveness of finding cases of hepatitis C infection in UK migrant populations and the value of further research. J Viral Hepat 2014; 21(9): 616-23.
[http://dx.doi.org/10.1111/jvh.12190] [PMID: 24215210]

[48] Martin NK, Hickman M, Miners A, Hutchinson SJ, Taylor A, Vickerman P. Cost-effectiveness of HCV case-finding for people who inject drugs *via* dried blood spot testing in specialist addiction services and prisons. BMJ Open 2013; 3(8): e003153.
[http://dx.doi.org/10.1136/bmjopen-2013-003153] [PMID: 23943776]

[49] Brogueira P, Costa A, Miranda A, *et al.* Improve screening of HCV infection by targeting high prevalence aged groups: analysis of a cohort of HCV and HIV co-infected patients. J Int AIDS Soc 2014; 17(4) (Suppl. 3): 19601.
[http://dx.doi.org/10.7448/IAS.17.4.19601] [PMID: 25394105]

[50] Kim DD, Hutton DW, Raouf AA, *et al.* Cost-effectiveness model for hepatitis C screening and treatment: Implications for Egypt and other countries with high prevalence. Glob Public Health 2015; 10(3): 296-317.
[http://dx.doi.org/10.1080/17441692.2014.984742] [PMID: 25469976]

[51] Ministry of Health and Population [Egypt], El-Zanaty and Associates [Egypt], ICF International. Egypt Demographic and Health Survey 2014. Cairo, Egypt and Rockville, Maryland, USA: Ministry

of Health and Population and ICF International; 2015.

[52] Ho SB, Bräu N, Cheung R, *et al.* Integrated care increases treatment and improves outcomes of patients with chronic hepatitis C virus infection and psychiatric illness or substance abuse. Clin Gastroenterol Hepatol 2015; 13(11): 2005-2014.e3, 3.
[http://dx.doi.org/10.1016/j.cgh.2015.02.022] [PMID: 25724704]

[53] Evon DM, Simpson K, Kixmiller S, *et al.* A randomized controlled trial of an integrated care intervention to increase eligibility for chronic hepatitis C treatment. Am J Gastroenterol 2011; 106(10): 1777-86.
[http://dx.doi.org/10.1038/ajg.2011.219] [PMID: 21769136]

[54] Norman J, Walsh NM, Mugavin J, *et al.* The acceptability and feasibility of peer worker support role in community based HCV treatment for injecting drug users. Harm Reduct J 2008; 5(1): 8.
[http://dx.doi.org/10.1186/1477-7517-5-8] [PMID: 18298862]

[55] Jones L, Bates G, McCoy E, Beynon C, McVeigh J, Bellis M. A systematic review of the effectiveness and cost-effectiveness of interventions aimed at raising awareness and engaging with groups who are at an increased risk of hepatitis B and C infection final report. Liverpool: Centre for Public Health, Faculty of Health and Applied Social Sciences, Liverpool John Moores University 2012.

[56] Sahajian F, Excler G, Bailly F, *et al.* Hepatitis C screening practices among private practitioners: impact of an information campaign. Gastroenterol Clin Biol 2004; 28(8-9): 714-9.
[http://dx.doi.org/10.1016/S0399-8320(04)95061-0] [PMID: 15646538]

[57] Impact of Physician Directed Education on Patient Compliance With Hepatitis C Therapy (OPTIMAL). Chronic Liver Disease Foundation; 2014. (https://clinicaltrials.gov/ct2/show/NCT01405027).

[58] Zhou K, Fitzpatrick T, Walsh N, *et al.* Interventions to optimise the care continuum for chronic viral hepatitis: a systematic review and meta-analyses. Lancet Infect Dis 2016; 16(12): 1409-22.
[http://dx.doi.org/10.1016/S1473-3099(16)30208-0] [PMID: 27615026]

[59] Bruggmann P, Litwin AH. Models of care for the management of hepatitis C virus among people who inject drugs: one size does not fit all. Clin Infect Dis 2013; 57(Suppl 2) (Suppl. 2): S56-61.
[http://dx.doi.org/10.1093/cid/cit271] [PMID: 23884067]

[60] Islam MM, Topp L, Conigrave KM, *et al.* Linkage into specialist hepatitis C treatment services of injecting drug users attending a needle syringe program-based primary healthcare centre. J Subst Abuse Treat 2012; 43(4): 440-5.
[http://dx.doi.org/10.1016/j.jsat.2012.07.007] [PMID: 22938915]

[61] Lloyd AR, Clegg J, Lange J, *et al.* Safety and effectiveness of a nurse-led outreach program for assessment and treatment of chronic hepatitis C in the custodial setting. Clin Infect Dis 2013; 56(8): 1078-84.
[http://dx.doi.org/10.1093/cid/cis1202] [PMID: 23362288]

[62] WHO, UNODC, UNAIDS technical guide for countries to set targets for universal access to HIV prevention, treatment and care for injecting drug users. Geneva: World Health Organization; 2012 revision (http://apps.who.int/iris/bitstream/10665/77969/1/9789241504379_eng.pdf?ua=1).

APPENDICES

APPENDIX A

ALP	alkaline phosphatase
ALT	alanine aminotransferase
ANC	antenatal clinic
APRI	aminotransferase/platelet ratio index
ART	antiretroviral therapy
ARV	antiretroviral (drug)
AST	aspartate aminotransferase
CDC	U.S. Centers for Disease Control and Prevention
CHB	chronic hepatitis B
CI	confidence interval
CLIA	chemiluminescence immunoassay
CrCl	creatinine clearance
DAA	direct-acting antiviral (drug)
DALY	disability-adjusted life year
DBS	dried blood spot (specimen)
ECL	electrochemiluminescence immunoassay
eGFR	estimated glomerular filtration rate
EIA	enzyme immunoassay
ELISA	enzyme-linked immunosorbent assay
FBC	full blood count
FDA	U.S. Food and Drug Administration
FIB-4	fibrosis-4 score
GDP	gross domestic product
gGT	gamma glutamyl transpeptidase
GHTF	Global Harmonization Task Force
GHSS	Global Health Sector Strategy
GRADE	Grading of Recommendations Assessment,
HBcAg	hepatitis B core antigen
HBeAg	hepatitis B e antigen
HBIG	hepatitis B immunoglobulin
HBsAg	hepatitis B surface antigen

Imran Shahid and Qaiser Jabeen

HBV hepatitis B virus
HCC hepatocellular carcinoma
HCV hepatitis C virus
HCVcAg hepatitis C virus core antigen
HDV hepatitis D virus
HIC high-income country
HIV human immunodeficiency virus
ICER incremental cost-effectiveness ratio
IFN interferon
IQR interquartile range
IVD in vitro diagnostic (medical device)
LMICs low- and middle-income countries
LoD limit of detection
LY life year
M&E monitoring and evaluation
MSM men who have sex with men
MTCT mother-to-child transmission
NAT nucleic acid testing
NGO nongovernmental organization
NIT non-invasive test
NPV negative predictive value
NRTI nucleos(t)ide reverse transcriptase inhibitor
OR odds ratio
OST opioid substitution therapy
PCR polymerase chain reaction
PEG-IFN pegylated interferon
PICO population, intervention, comparison, outcomes
PITC provider-initiated testing and counseling
AIDS acquired immunodeficiency syndrome
CDC Centers for Disease Control and Prevention
COVID-19 coronavirus disease 2019
FDA U.S. Food and Drug Administration
IDU injection drug use
PMTCT prevention of mother-to-child transmission
PPV positive predictive value

PQ (WHO) prequalification
PWID people who inject drugs
QA quality assurance
QALY quality-adjusted life year
QC quality control
QI quality improvement
RBV ribavirin
RCT randomized controlled trial
RDT rapid diagnostic test
RNA ribonucleic acid
RR relative risk
SOP standard operating procedure
SSA sub-Saharan Africa
STI sexually transmitted infection
SVR sustained virological response
TDF tenofovir
ULN upper limit of normal
D+o/p/r dasabuvir + ombitasvir/paritaprevir/ritonavir
UNAIDS Joint United Nations Programme on HIV/AIDS
UNICEF United Nations Children's Fund
WHO GHP WHO Global Hepatitis Programme
NIH National Institutes of Health
OR odds ratio
OUD opioid use disorder
POC point-of-care
RFI Request for Information
RNA ribonucleic acid
SARS-CoV-2 severe acute respiratory syndrome coronavirus 2
SSP syringe services program
STD sexually transmitted disease
STI sexually transmitted infection
SUD substance use disorder
VA Veterans Affairs
WHO World Health Organization
UMIC upper-middle-income country

Ab Antibody

Ag Antigen

fmol/L femtomole(s) per liter

FS Fingerstick

IU/mL International unit per milliliter

LLoD Lower limit of detection

MSM Men who have sex with men

ND No data

OST Opioid substitution therapy

PCR Polymerase chain reaction

POC Point-of-care

PQ Prequalification (For HCV, PQ is approved for diagnosis only, not SVR as LLoD has not yet been determined).

R&D Research and development

SVR Sustained virological response

TK To come

uL unit of liquid volume equal to one millionth of a liter, or 1 mm3

VL Viral load

BBV Blood-borne virus

GP General practitioner

NSP Needle and syringe program

PEP Post-exposure prophylaxis

PHC Primary healthcare

PrEP Pre-exposure prophylaxis

TasP Treatment as prevention

APPENDIX B

Acceptability. The degree to which given intervention is acceptable to the target population in relation to the effect of an intervention.

Accessibility. The degree to which given intervention is accessible to the target population (availability of good health services within reasonable reach and when needed).

Audit: Quality improvement process that aims to improve the care of patients by reviewing practices against criteria such as existing policy or guidelines and modifying practices where necessary.

Campaign: Series of activities and efforts to increase awareness and/or to promote initiatives. Campaigns can be conducted nationally or locally. For HIV testing national campaigns generally focus on increasing awareness, while local campaigns generally advertise local testing activities.

Checkpoint: Community-based center for detection of HIV and other sexually transmitted infections targeted at gay men other men who have sex with men, and transgender women.

Clinical decision-making tool: Clinical decision-making uses a combination of experience knowledge, and assessment tools to make effective clinical decisions. Clinical decision-making tool for HBV, HCV, or HIV testing is any strategy that aids staff in deciding who should get tested, *e.g.* patient-completed risk-assessment questionnaire or reminding staff to offer to test.

Community-based testing services: Programmes and services that offer voluntary free, and anonymous HBV, HCV, and/or HIV testing outside formal health facilities designed to target specific communities. For this guidance, such services include the following:

Community-based drug and harm-reduction service facilities: Provide community-based testing in a fixed location and specifically target people who use drugs. Typically though not universally, they maintain a low threshold for attendance and adopt a client perspective on service provision to make user access as simple as possible. Services at these facilities may include needle and syringe exchange programs, opioid substitution therapy, and other forms of drug treatment, as well as additional services such as HBV, HCV, and HIV testing, health-promotion activities, and social services.

Community-based outreach activities: Generic term covering several types of service delivery in the community that does not occur at a fixed site. They include services provided by mobile units and vans street outreach by community health workers, and regular satellite services sited in community-based facilities. Outreach services are often able to reach people who are not in contact with other health services by targeting them where they live or places they access. Such services play important role in identifying their needs and referring them to community-based facilities or public healthcare services.

Community-based testing facilities: Provide client-initiated (voluntary) testing services at a fixed location outside formal health facilities. These sites may also provide additional services such as counseling and health promotion activities. Community-based testing sites in EU/EEA are mainly focused on MSM and typified by peer-driven services (*e.g.* checkpoints).

Comparative study: Study designed to compare two or more groups or interventions (*e.g.* types of testing offered or test timings); statistical measure often provided for comparison.

Cost-effectiveness: Cost-effectiveness analysis is an aide to decision making that measures the ratio of costs of a program or intervention to effects it has on a defined outcome. For HIV testing this is defined as the threshold for HIV screening associated with favorable cost-effectiveness ratios when undiagnosed HIV prevalence rates are ≥0.1%.

Emergency department: Treatment facility specializing in providing medical and/or surgical care to patients who present to hospital often in need of immediate/urgent care. Most are open access with no requirement for the referral.

Feasibility: The degree to which it is possible to implement an intervention in terms of time money, or other circumstances.

Homelessness: A homeless person is an individual without permanent housing who may live on the streets stay in a shelter, mission, single-room occupancy facility, abandoned building or vehicle or live in any other unstable or non-permanent situation.

Incremental cost-effectiveness ratio (ICER): Measure used in cost-effectiveness studies to represent the value of intervention compared against an alternative (comparator). ICER is calculated by dividing the difference in total costs of two interventions by the measure of health outcome *e.g.* quality-adjusted life-year (QALY, see below). ICER determines whether a new intervention is an efficient use of resources.

Indicator condition guided-testing: For HIV the testing approach where HIV tests are routinely offered to all patients presenting with AIDS-defining illness or HIV indicator condition including STI, malignant lymphoma, cervical/anal dysplasia or cancer, herpes zoster infection, hepatitis B or hepatitis C infection, ongoing mononucleosis-like illness, unexplained leukocytopenia or thrombocytopenia, and dermatitis/exanthema.

Inpatient department: Hospital department where patients stay while they receive treatment.

Integrated testing: Provision of testing for more than one infection at the same time. For example HIV testing may be provided alongside testing for infections such as hepatitis B, hepatitis C, STIs, or TB.

Key populations: Include both most at-risk and vulnerable groups of people in a given population.

Late presentation: Occurs when the person is tested and diagnosed too late to either prevent avoidable harm or for treatment to be fully effective. For hepatitis late presentation is defined as persons presenting for care with chronic hepatitis B and C and significant fibrosis (≥ F3 assessed by either APRI score > 1.5, FIB-4 > 3.25, Fibrotest > 0.59 or alternatively transient elastography (FibroScan) > 9.5 kPa or liver biopsy ≥ METAVIR stage F3) with no previous antiviral treatment [4]. For HIV, late presentation is defined as persons presenting for care with a CD4 count below 350 cells/mL or presenting with an AIDS-defining event regardless of CD4 cell count.

Lay provider: Person providing healthcare in a community setting trained to deliver specific services such as blood-borne testing services, but has not completed formal professional healthcare training.

Low-threshold service: Service that places few restrictions on access and adopts client perspective on service provision to make utilization as accessible as possible for users.

Migrants: Individuals who change their country of usual residence irrespective of the reason for migration or legal status. Generally a distinction is made between short-term or temporary migration, covering movements between three and 12 months, and long-term or permanent migration, referring to change of country of residence for one year or more. For this guidance, migrants are individuals who originate from a country of intermediate or high endemicity for HBV/HCV/HIV or belong to local migrant communities known to have a high prevalence or incidence of HBV/HCV/HIV.

Opt-out testing: Testing modality where patients are informed they will be tested as part of routine care but may decline testing by objecting to the test.

Outpatient department: Hospital department that diagnoses and treats patients without requiring an overnight stay.

Outreach: Type of health service that mobilizes health workers to provide services to a population away from the location where providers usually work.

Partner notification/contact tracing: Process where individuals potentially exposed to infection are informed of exposure and offered testing and other interventions dependent upon specific infection. When contact is of a sexual or injecting nature this process is also referred to as partner notification. Partner notification is a voluntary process in which a trained provider asks a person diagnosed with HBV, HCV, or HIV about their sexual partners, at-risk drug-injecting partners, and household contacts as appropriate for diagnosis. With the individual's consent, the provider then offers, facilitates, or provides advice on testing for relevant infections to these partners and contacts, as well as linking them to preventive interventions such as vaccination (HBV) or post-exposure prophylaxis (PEP) for HIV. The identity of a diagnosed person is not revealed to contact by the provider unless consent has been given to do so. Web-based partner notification is an approach delivered via websites that allow users to send emails, e-cards, or text messages to inform partners anonymously.

Post-exposure prophylaxis (PEP): Use of antiretroviral therapy following exposure to HIV infection to try to prevent the establishment of infection.

Prevalence: Prevalence measures the proportion of individuals in the defined population with a specific disease (or specific characteristic) at a certain point in time. High intermediate, and low prevalence rates may be defined for HCV, HBV, and HIV to guide testing strategies after taking local epidemiology and other circumstances into account. Present guidance applies the following definitions of prevalence rates based on several published thresholds:

- **Intermediate HBV and HCV prevalence:** When HBsAg seroprevalence or HCV antibody seroprevalence in the general population is between 2% and 5%. For both HBV and HCV the high prevalence is ≥5%.
- **High HIV prevalence:** When HIV prevalence consistently exceeds 1% in the general population.

Pre-exposure prophylaxis (PrEP): Antiretroviral therapy-based HIV prevention strategy to prevent or at least reduce risk of HIV infection in adults who have not been infected with a virus but are at high risk of infection.

Primary care: Healthcare provided by general practitioners (GPs) nurses, and ancillary healthcare workers and first point of contact for healthcare for the majority of the population.

Provider-initiated testing: Voluntary testing offered to eligible individuals by healthcare providers.

People who inject drugs (PWID): People who inject non-medically sanctioned psychotropic (or psychoactive) substances. These drugs include but are not limited to opioids amphetamine-type stimulants, cocaine, hypnosedatives, and hallucinogens. The injection may be through intravenous, intramuscular, subcutaneous, or other injectable routes.

Quality-adjusted life year (QALY): Composite measure of health adjusted to reflect length and quality of life. One QALY equates to one year of life in perfect health. For an individual requiring an intervention QALY would be the weighted value of each year remaining to the patient with a quality of life score (on a 0 to 1 scale). In cost-effectiveness studies, QALYs are used to assess the effectiveness of a new intervention against the baseline intervention.

Rapid diagnostic test (RDT): Test that provides the result with a short turnaround time typically with oral fluid or finger-prick blood sample. RDTs are employed for point-of-care rapid tests and self-testing.

Reflex testing: Occurs when a positive test automatically initiates performance of another test typically to improve diagnostic sensitivity or presence of active infection. For this document, reflex testing refers to performing HCV nucleic acid test (NAT) on the same sample as a positive antibody screening test to detect active HCV infection.

Retesting: People who should be retested after a defined period. This includes HIV HBV, and HCV-negative people with recent (to cover the window period) or ongoing risk of exposure and people with inconclusive HBV/HCV/HIV status.

Risk group testing: Testing strategy targeted at groups identified as being at higher risk of infection. Identification of these groups depends on local epidemiology and typically includes men who have sex with men (MSM) prisoners, sex workers, people who inject drugs (PWID), and migrants.

Self-sampling: When individual collects a blood or saliva sample from themselves typically outside a healthcare setting, using a suitable kit. The sample is then delivered to a designated laboratory for processing. Results are usually delivered by phone, text message, or online, with referral mechanisms in place to ensure linkage to treatment and care as appropriate.

Self-testing: When an individual collects a blood or saliva sample then uses a rapid diagnostic kit to process the sample, obtain results and interpret them according to instructions provided with the kit. The kit typically includes linkage information to care as appropriate.

Sex workers: Individuals who receive money or goods in exchange for sexual services and consciously define those activities as income generating even if they do not consider sex work to be their occupation.

Task sharing: Rational redistribution of tasks and increased scope of work among different cadres of healthcare providers including trained lay providers.

Testing coverage: Extent to which testing program covers potential need usually measured as the proportion of persons tested in a given population.

Testing uptake: Rate of acceptance of testing by individuals offered a test in a given population.

Testing strategy: Describes testing approach to attain a specific objective that takes into consideration prevalence in the population tested.

Traditional and non-traditional settings: For HIV testing traditional settings are specialist healthcare settings where HIV testing is provided, including dedicated STI and sexual health clinics, antenatal services, and infectious disease units. Non-traditional settings are non-specialist for HIV testing such as general practice, community settings, and hospital outpatient departments.

Trans* people: Trans is an overarching term referring to those people whose internal perception of their own gender (gender identity) and/or a gender expression differs from the sex they were assigned at birth. The term trans includes but is not limited to men and women with transsexual pasts and people who identify as transsexual transgender, transvestite/cross-dressing, androgyne, polygender, genderqueer, agender, gender variant, or with any other gender identity and/or expression that is not standard male or female and express their gender through their choice of clothes, presentation or body modifications, including undergoing multiple surgical procedures.

Treatment as prevention (TasP): The impact of antiretroviral therapy to reduce the HIV viral load to undetectable levels effectively preventing onward transmission.

Universal testing: Strategy of offering HIV tests to everyone regardless of individual risk. Settings where this strategy may be particularly relevant, include hospital departments and general practice. In certain settings, such as antenatal services, universal testing may be opt-out (see above).

Window period: For tests designed to detect a specific disease the window period is the between first exposure to infection and the point in time after when the test can give the definitive (accurate and reliable) result.

AASLD/IDSA: American Association for the Study of Liver Diseases/Infectious Diseases Society of America.

ActiTest: A noninvasive test to determine the extent of liver inflammation damage, and scarring; however, it is not widely available outside high-income countries. This test is assessed on FibroTest and must be analyzed using BioPredictive diagnostics services. The test was developed using French public funding, then granted exclusive licensing to FibroTest.

Acute Infection: A recently acquired infection which may have mild or no symptoms; acute HCV infection may result in some inflammation to the liver.

ALP: Alkaline phosphatase an important liver enzyme used in determining your liver health.

ALT; SGPT: Alanine aminotransferase or serum glutamic pyruvic transaminase liver enzymes used in determining your liver health.

Antibody: Part of a person's immune system that responds to viruses bacteria, and other harmful substances.

APRI: Aspartate aminotransferase (AST) to platelet ratio index a formula used to determine the level of liver disease.

ART: Antiretroviral therapy a combination of antiretroviral drugs to suppress HIV and to stop HIV from progressing.

ARV: Antiretroviral drugs in the context of HIV, these medications suppress viral activity by preventing the virus from reproducing.

Assay: A diagnostic test performed to determine the presence of an infectious disease (qualitative assay) and if present the amount (quantitative assay).

AST; SGOT: Aspartate aminotransferase or serum glutamic oxaloacetic transaminase a liver enzyme made in the heart, intestines, and muscle used in determining your liver health.

cAG: HCV core antigen the viral protein of HCV, which can be found in the bloodstream within two weeks of infection. This type of confirmation test detects whether a person is currently infected with the virus.

CD4: Cluster of differentiation 4 a type of protein found in immune cells such as T cells, a type of white blood cells that lead the fight against infections. HIV infects the CD4 cells and then uses them to make copies of the virus. The CD4 count test calculates the total white blood cells and the proportion of cells that are CD4 positive. CD4+ cell count is used to monitoring the health of the immune system and antiretroviral treatment success. If the count drops lower than 200 cells per millionth of a liter, the person is at higher risk of opportunistic infections. Current WHO treatment guidelines indicate a person should start treatment at the time of diagnosis, regardless of CD4+ cell count. This improves the health of the person living with HIV and helps reduce the amount of the virus in the blood (viral load) and other bodily fluids to undetectable levels, which prevents transmission.

CDC: Centers for Disease Control and Prevention the U.S. agency that develops and applies disease prevention and control programs, as well as environmental health, health promotion, and health education activities.

CE-marked: Conformité Européenne a certification mark that shows the compliance to safety, health, and environmental protections for products within the European Economic Area.

Chronic Infection: An infection that can last for weeks months, or a lifetime, causing more damage to the affected tissue or organs.

Cirrhosis: Serious liver scarring or damage that can lead to liver failure.

CKD: Chronic kidney disease a condition where the kidneys' ability to filter harmful waste and excess fluid from the blood deteriorates over time.

CL: Compulsory license a license granted by a governmental administrative or judicial body to a third party to manufacture or use a patented product, such as medication, without the consent of the patent holder. A CL is an effective strategy to enable generic competition and reduce the price of patented medicines. The the patent holder is remunerated such as through royalty payments.

Community: A form of self-organization of a group of people with one or several characteristics that unite people living in nearby locations, foster relations between them, and share culture and values within the scope of these relations. A community can be defined by the following people, location, and relationship.

DAA: Direct-acting antivirals all-oral, highly effective medications for treating hepatitis C in usually 8 or 12 weeks. People with cirrhosis or other conditions may need to be treated longer to achieve sustained virological response, or when the virus is undetectable. DAAs can achieve sustained virological response in over 95% of patients, and the latest regimens treat all genotypes of the virus with similar results.

DBS: Dried blood spot blood sample obtained by pricking the finger or heel that is preserved and dried on filter paper. DBS can be easily shipped from a remote testing site to a lab for analysis.

DCV: Daclatasvir (also abbreviated as DAC); a direct-acting antiviral that is taken with sofosbuvir once daily with or without food for 12 or 24 weeks.

Diagnostic Burnout: The phenomenon in which countries are treating mainly patients known to have HCV and are failing to diagnose new infections. In this case countries will run out of diagnosed patients to treat, HCV transmission will continue to proliferate, and new infections will go undiagnosed, leading to advanced liver disease and liver-related deaths.

EASL: European Association for the Study of the Liver.

EDL: Essential Diagnostics List WHO guidance and reference on the tests and medical devices needed to diagnose the most common conditions as well as a number of global priority diseases. The EDL helps countries decide on the type and categories of diagnostics depending on their epidemiology, testing strategies, human resources, and healthcare and laboratory infrastructure.

EIA: Enzyme immunoassay antibody tests used in labs that detect antibodies in blood samples.

ESLD: End-Stage Liver Disease chronic liver failure, often as a result of cirrhosis.

FDC: Fixed-dose combination two or more drugs contained in a single dosage form, such as a capsule or tablet.

FibroScan: An ultrasound machine for your liver that measures liver stiffness scarring, and damage as well as the accumulation of fat in the liver.

FibroTest: A noninvasive blood test that can measure the degree of liver damage in a person; it requires results to be analyzed by BioPredictive software.

FIB-4: An inexpensive noninvasive calculation to determine the amount of liver scarring by using patient's age, platelet count, AST, and ALT.

Fingerstick: Also known as fingerprick a method of collecting a small amount of blood by pricking a finger with a lancet, or a sharp needle-like instrument.

Genedrive: A portable point-of-care confirmatory test, using plasma, for the detection of HCV RNA. It is designed for use in low-resource settings and delivers results in 90 minutes.

Genotype: Abbreviated as GT different subtypes of HCV, or a way to put HCV into categories based on similar genes. HCV has six genotypes, labeled 1 through 6. There are also subtypes labeled with letters, for example, genotypes 1a and 1b. Genotypes respond differently to medicines that treat and cure HCV, but pangenotypic (all genotypes) DAAs have similar SVR rates for all genotypes.

GGT: Gamma-glutamyl transferase an important liver enzyme used in determining your liver health.

G/P: Glecaprevir and pibrentasvir DAA taken once daily, as three pills, with food, that treats all genotypes of HCV in 8 weeks for people with no cirrhosis, or 12 or 16 weeks for people with compensated cirrhosis or other complications. It has been approved by the FDA for children and adolescents aged 12 and older who weigh at least 99 pounds (44 kilograms).

HBIG: Hepatitis B immune globulin an injection used to protect against hepatitis B within 24 hours of exposure.

HBV: Hepatitis B virus a highly contagious virus that infects the liver transmitted through blood, semen, and vaginal fluid. You can protect yourself against hepatitis B by getting vaccinated or having an injection of HBIg within 24 hours of exposure.

HCC: Hepatocellular carcinoma liver cancer, occurring most often in people with chronic liver diseases.

HCV: Hepatitis C virus a virus transmitted through blood, although small amounts have been found in semen and vaginal fluid, that causes hepatitis C, a liver infection that causes inflammation and tissue damage. There is no preventative vaccine, but all-oral DAAs can now effectively cure HCV. Untreated HCV can lead to severe liver damage and liver cancer.

HIV Self Test A simple blood test that a person can use on themselves to test for HCV; expected to become available in 2020.

HICs: High-income countries.

HIV: Human immunodeficiency virus a virus that weakens the immune system, ultimately leading to acquired immunodeficiency syndrome (AIDS).

IL28B CC genotype: The IL28B gene is involved in the immune response to certain viruses, including HCV. There are three IL28B subtypes (genotypes) CC, CT, and TT. People with the CC genotype have a stronger immune response to HCV infection than people with the CT or TT genotypes. In the pegylated interferon treatment era, IL28B genotype determined the type and possibly length of HCV treatment.

INHSU: International Symposium on Hepatitis Care in Substance Users.

Invasive Test: Any type of medical test that requires the use of instrumentation to physically enter the body such as a liver biopsy.

IP: Intellectual property refers to the concept of ownership over an idea or design, in which the person or entity that developed that idea or design is given exclusive right over it for a period of time, usually 20 years under international agreements. No one can copy or reuse the idea or design without the owner's permission. Common forms of intellectual property include patents copyrights, trademarks, industrial design rights, geographical indications, and trade secrets. In international law, legal mechanisms, such as compulsory licenses and patent oppositions, exist to gain access and manufacturer technological advancements, such as medicines, in order to create less expensive, generic versions.

LGBTQ+: Lesbian, gay, bisexual, transgender, queer/ questioning, and others an umbrella acronym that encompasses a spectrum of gender and sexual identities but is not comprehensive as the terminology is evolving and changing.

LED: Ledipasvir a direct-acting antiviral that is taken with sofosbuvir as two drugs in one pill, taken daily, with or without food, for 8 to 24 weeks. It is used for people with genotypes 1, 4, 5, and 6 who are over 12 years old.

LFT: Liver function test a group of blood tests used to detect, evaluate, and monitor liver disease or damage.

LMIC: Low-and middle-income countries.

LoD: Limit of detection in chemistry, the smallest amount of a microorganism or genetic material from a virus in a sample that can be reliably detected in optimal conditions. LoD is a step in determining the sensitivity of a test.

MAT: Medication-assisted treatment which uses medications such as buprenorphine, methadone, and naltrexone, often combined with counseling and behavioral therapy to treat opioid use disorders also referred to as OST.

MIC: Middle-income country.

Mixed Infection: People who are infected with more than one HCV genotype. This is most likely to happen to people who received blood products or blood transfusions many years ago or in a place where the blood supply was not checked for HCV people on kidney dialysis, or people who inject drugs with shared unsterilized equipment.

MSM: Gay bisexual, and other men who have sex with men.

Multiplexing: Testing for more than one infection at the same time on one device such as HIV, HBV, and HCV.

NAT: Nucleic acid amplification test a highly sensitive laboratory process used to detect genetic material, such as RNA of HCV. The NAT uses repeated chemical reactions (polymerase chain reaction) to make multiple copies of the HCV RNA that is trying to be detected. In this way, it is easier to detect tens of thousands of copies of a gene than only a few copies.

ND: No data.

NHANES: National Health and Nutrition Examination Survey a survey conducted by the CDC assessing the health and nutritional status, including the hepatitis epidemiology of adults and children in the United States. There are limitations because it did not include homeless people, incarcerated people, nursing home residents, people living on Native American reservations, or active military personnel, and it did not show wide geographic representation. Information on members of additional racial and ethnic groups was classified as "other".

Noninvasive Test: Medical test that does not require a medical instrument to physically enter in the body such as using ultrasound.

NSEP: Needle syringe exchange programs.

OST: Opioid substitution therapy which uses medications such as buprenorphine, methadone, and naltrexone, is often combined with counseling and behavioral therapy to treat opioid use disorders also referred to as MAT.

Pangenotypic: DAA treatments that can effectively cure all HCV genotypes at nearly the same rates.

PCR: Polymerase chain reaction the process during a nucleic acid amplification test to detect genetic material, such as HCV RNA, by making multiple copies of the HCV RNA that is trying to be detected. The PCR HCV RNA test determines how much of the virus (or viral load) is in the bloodstream.

PEG-IFN: Pegylated interferon an older treatment regimen requiring regular injections, combined with oral doses of ribavirin, between 12 to 48 weeks; no longer recommended by WHO, AASLD/IDSA, or EASL. Countries without access to direct-acting antivirals or prisons may still be using pegylated interferon.

PLHIV: People living with HIV preferred to use the people-centered term instead of the abbreviation.

PoC: Point-of-care test diagnostic testing conducted at the time and place of patient care, such as community clinics, harm reduction sites, and prisons.

Polyvalency: One machine can do different tests but uses a different sample and not always at the same time.

PT: Prothrombin time measurement for how long it takes for blood to clot.

PWID: People who inject drugs preferred to use the people-centered term instead of the abbreviation.

Qualitative RNA: Viral load test that checks whether there is RNA genetic material such as from HCV, in the bloodstream. The test result is either positive (the virus is detectable) or negative (no virus can be detected).

Quantitative RNA: Viral load test that measures the amount of RNA genetic material such as from HCV, in the bloodstream. These tests, while not available in every country, are also used to monitor HCV treatment to see if it is working.

R&D: Research and development.

RBV: Ribavirin oral treatment for hepatitis C, given as pills or capsules, twice a day. The dose depends on a person's weight. Ribavirin can increase cure rates in people with cirrhosis and is sometimes added to DAAs, although it causes side effects, such as anemia, insomnia, fatigue, irritability, and depression. Ribavirin is not recommended for men and women who are planning a pregnancy because it causes birth defects. Male partners of women who become pregnant or are nursing should use condoms for six months after completing HCV treatment.

RDT: Rapid diagnostic test antibody tests designed for use at the point of care.

Reagent: Chemical ingredients that are added to test a patient's sample to see if a reaction occurs. A change in color intensity in light, or other differences may occur. The change is measured against a known change or control and then calculated for a test result.

Reagent cartridge: A container with prefilled reagents to be loaded inside a diagnostics device.

Reflex testing: When additional tests are automatically ordered after a specific test result. For HCV if a patient has a positive antibody test, confirmatory tests (HCV RNA or core antigen) would be automatically ordered.

Reinfection: When a person who has been successfully treated such as for HCV, becomes infected again. HCV RNA testing is recommended for people with ongoing behaviors that may put them at risk of HCV infection. Access to sterile injection equipment, OST, and comprehensive prevention and harm reduction services is necessary to prevent reinfection.

RVD: Ravidasvir (also abbreviated as RAV) taken with sofosbuvir as a generic regimen that is under study in clinical trials, which may be used to treat all genotypes. It is taken once daily for 12 weeks or 24 weeks for people with compensated cirrhosis.

Sensitivity: True positive rate a test's ability to correctly identify people with an infection, such as HCV. High sensitivity closer to 100% helps avoid missing an HCV infection and determines the quality of a test.

Serological tests: Also known as screening or antibody tests generally used as the first step in a testing strategy due to the relatively lower cost. These tests detect antibodies or a viral antigen, and which people may have an active infection. They can be conducted with rapid diagnostic tests or laboratory-based enzyme immunoassays.

Serum: Clear and watery part of the blood that separates when the blood clots or is centrifuged (spun at high speeds).

SOF: Sofosbuvir an HCV-fighting DAA that must be used with other drugs. In combination with other DAAs, it can treat all genotypes in patients 18 years old and older; sofosbuvir with or without ribavirin can be used to treat genotypes 2 and 3 in patients 12 17 years old (2018 WHO Guidelines). Sofosbuvir is taken once daily, with or without food, for 12 to 24 weeks, depending on a person's liver damage, other health conditions, and treatment experience.

Specificity: True negative rate the test's ability to correctly identify people without HCV. High specificity closer to 100% helps avoid misinforming a person about being infected when they are not and determines the quality of a test.

SRA: Stringent Regulatory Authority a quality assurance policy to ensure certain requirements are met at a manufacturing facility for medicines or medical devices. This includes a list of countries with a national drug regulatory authority that are members observers, or associates of the International Conference on Harmonization of Technical Requirements for Registration of Pharmaceuticals for Human Use (ICH). The SRA aligns with the Global Fund Quality Assurance Policy for Pharmaceutical Products which took effect on July 1, 2009.

Steatosis: Accumulation of fat in the liver; sometimes referred to as fatty liver.

STI: Sexually transmitted infection.

SVR: Sustained virological response a person has no detectable HCV after treatment has been completed.

Throughput: Rate of production or amount, of tests that can be run through a diagnostics system at a time.

VEL: Velpatasvir combined with sofosbuvir as the fixed-dose combination that treats all HCV genotypes, taken once daily, with or without food, for 12 weeks. People who have advanced (or decompensated) cirrhosis will need to add ribavirin twice daily.

Virological testing: Also known as confirmatory testing uses NAT. Laboratory processes to detect genetic material (DNA or RNA) of a virus and determine if the infection is active and to decide whether to start a patient on treatment. It is also used to confirm sustained virological response (for HCV) or effective suppression of the virus (for HBV).

VL: Voluntary license a patent holder allows another pharmaceutical company to manufacture a generic version of their medication. The patent holder sets conditions and may receive a fee or royalty. In effect, voluntary licenses permit patent holders/originator companies to control the market by limiting the countries that are licensed to produce and sell generics. Countries that are not included in licensing agreements must buy more expensive drugs from the originator companies. Voluntary licenses can also include other restrictions, such as the number of people who can be treated, whether drugs can be coformulated, and which suppliers must be used for the active pharmaceutical ingredients needed to make the medication.

WHO PQ: World Health Organization Prequalification a process conducted by the WHO using unified standards to assess the quality, safety, and efficacy of medicines, active pharmaceutical ingredients, medical products, and quality control laboratories. It is not a prescriptive list; rather, this standard can help countries consider medicines and medical devices that meet high-quality standards to procure for their national programs.

HB surface antigen (HBsAg): HBV envelope protein often produced in excess and detectable in the blood in acute and chronic HBV infection.

HB core antigen (HBcAg): HBV core protein. The core protein is coated with HBsAg and therefore not found free in serum.

HB e antigen (HBeAg): Viral protein found in the high replicative phase of HBV. HBeAg is usually a marker of high levels of replication with wild-type viruses but is not essential for viral replication.

HB surface antibody (anti-HBs): Antibody to HBsAg. Develops in response to hepatitis B vaccination and during recovery from hepatitis B denoting past infection and immunity.

HB core antibody (anti-HBc): Antibody to HBV core (capsid) protein. Anti-HBc antibodies are non-neutralizing antibodies and are detected in both acute and chronic infections.

anti-HBc IgM: Subclass of anti-HBc. Detected in recent HBV infection but can be detected by sensitive assays in chronic HBV infection.

HBVe antibody (anti-HBe): Antibody to HBeAg. Detected in persons with lower levels of HBV replication but also in HBeAg-negative disease (i.e. HBV that does not express HBeAg).

HBV DNA: HBV viral genomes that can be detected and quantified in serum by nucleic acid testing (NAT).

Anti-HCV antibody: Antibody to HCV which can be detected in the blood usually within two or three months of HCV infection or exposure. The terms HCV antibody and anti-HCV antibody are equivalent, but in the guidelines of this book, both are used throughout.

HCV RNA: HCV viral genomes that can be detected and quantified in serum by nucleic acid testing (NAT).

HCV core antigen (HCVcAg): Nucleocapsid peptide 22 [p22] of HCV which is released into plasma during viral assembly and can be detected from early on and throughout the course of infection.

Chronic HBV infection: Persistence of HBsAg for at least six months. The persistence of HBsAg in two specimens six months apart is frequently used in clinical practice to confirm chronic hepatitis B infection.

Chronic HCV infection: The presence of viraemic HCV RNA or HCVcAg in association with positive serology for HCV antibody.

Viraemic infection: Hepatitis B or C infection associated with the presence of virus in the blood (as measured by HBV DNA or HCV RNA) and often referred to as active, ongoing, or current infection.

Occult HBV infection: HBsAg negative but HBV DNA positive although at very low levels (invariably <200 IU/mL). Most are also anti-HBc positive.

Cirrhosis: An advanced stage of liver disease characterized by extensive hepatic fibrosis nodularity of the liver, alteration of liver architecture, and disrupted hepatic circulation.

Decompensated cirrhosis: Clinical features are portal hypertension (ascites, variceal hemorrhage, and hepatic encephalopathy) coagulopathy, or liver insufficiency (jaundice). Other clinical features of advanced liver disease/cirrhosis may include hepatomegaly, splenomegaly, pruritus, fatigue, arthralgia, palmar erythema, and edema.

Hepatocellular carcinoma (HCC): Primary cancer of the liver arising from the hepatocytes and may be a complication of chronic hepatitis B or C infection.

HCV sustained virological response (SVR): Undetectable HCV RNA in the blood at a defined time point after the end of treatment usually at 12 or 24 weeks (SVR12 or 24)

HCV non-response: Detectable HCV RNA in the blood throughout treatment.

HCV relapse: Undetectable HCV RNA during treatment and/or at end of treatment but subsequent detectable HCV RNA following treatment cessation.

HCV viral breakthrough: Undetectable HCV RNA during treatment followed by detectable HCV RNA despite continued treatment.

HBV treatment failure: May be primary or secondary. Primary antiviral treatment failure may be defined as failure of an antiviral drug to reduce HBV DNA levels by ≥1x log10 IU/mL within 3 months of initiating therapy. Secondary antiviral treatment failure may be defined as a rebound of HBV DNA levels of ≥1 x log10 IU/mL from the nadir in persons with an initial antiviral treatment effect (≥1 x log10 IU/mL decrease in serum HBV DNA).

Serological assays: Assays that detect the presence of either antigens or antibodies typically in serum or plasma but also in capillary/venous whole blood and oral fluid. These include rapid diagnostic tests (RDTs), and laboratory-based immunoassays, *e.g.* enzyme immunoassays (EIAs), chemiluminescence immunoassays (CLIAs), and electrochemiluminescence immunoassays (ECLs).

Rapid diagnostic test (RDT): Immunoassays that detect antibodies or antigens and can give a result in less than 30 minutes. Most RDTs can be performed with capillary whole blood collected by finger-stick sampling.

Enzyme immunoassay (EIA): Laboratory-based serological immunoassays that detect antibodies antigens, or a combination of both.

Nucleic acid testing (NAT): A molecular technology for example, polymerase chain reaction (PCR) or nucleic acid sequence-based amplification (NASBA) that can detect very small quantities of viral nucleic acid (RNA or DNA), either qualitatively or quantitatively.

Multiplex or multi-disease testing: Refers to testing using one specimen in the same test device (or reagent cartridge) that can detect other infections (*e.g.* HIV, syphilis, hepatitis C, hepatitis B).

Clinical/diagnostic sensitivity of a test: The ability of a test to correctly identify those with the infection or disease (i.e. true positives/true positives + false negatives).

Clinical/diagnostic specificity of a test: The ability of a test to correctly identify those without the infection or disease (i.e. true negatives/true negatives + false positives). Sensitivity and specificity are usually expressed as point estimates accompanied by confidence intervals.

Positive predictive value (PPV): The probability that when a person's test result is positive they truly have the infection/disease.

Negative predictive value (NPV): The probability that when a person's test result is negative they truly do not have the infection/disease. Predictive values are influenced by the prevalence of the disease in the population.

Analytical sensitivity/Limit of detection (LoD): The lowest concentration of measurement that can be consistently detected in 95% of specimens tested under routine laboratory conditions. It defines the analytical sensitivity in contrast to the clinical or diagnostic sensitivity.

Testing algorithm: The combination and sequence of specific assays used within hepatitis B and C testing strategies.

Testing approach: In the context of the guidelines mentioned in this book the testing approach describes both "who to test" i.e. different populations, and "where to test" i.e. different settings. Testing approaches include general population testing, focused testing of high-risk groups, "birth-cohort" testing, or of antenatal clinics. These can be delivered through either health-facility or community-based testing.

Testing strategy: A general sequence of assays for a specific testing objective or approach taking into consideration the presumed disease prevalence in the population being tested. A one-assay serological testing strategy involves a single serological assay. A two-assay serological testing strategy involves two different serological assays used sequentially.

Key populations: Groups of people who due to specific high-risk behaviors, are at increased risk for HIV infection irrespective of the epidemic type or local context. This may also apply to HBV and/or HCV infection. Key populations often have legal and social issues related to their behaviors that increase their vulnerability to HIV, HBV, and HCV infection. These guidelines refer to the following groups as key populations men who have sex with men (MSM); people who inject drugs (PWID); people in prisons and other closed settings; sex workers; and transgender people.

Vulnerable populations: Groups of people who are particularly vulnerable to HBV/HCV infection in certain situations or contexts. These guidelines refer to the following groups as vulnerable populations migrant and mobile workers, and indigenous populations.

General population testing: This approach refers to routine testing throughout the entire population without attempting to identify high-risk behaviors or characteristics. It means that all members of the population should have potential access to the testing program.

"Birth cohort" testing: This approach means routine testing among easily identified age or demographic groups (i.e. specific "birth cohorts") known to have a high HCV prevalence due to past generalized exposures that have since been identified and removed.

Antenatal clinic testing: This approach means routine testing of pregnant women especially in settings where there is an intermediate or high seroprevalence to identify women in need of antiviral treatment for their own health and additional interventions to reduce mother-to-child transmission (MTCT).

Community-based testing: Includes using outreach (mobile) approaches in general and key populations; home-based testing (or door-to-door outreach); testing in workplaces places of worship, parks, bars, and other venues; in schools and other educational establishments; as well as through campaigns.

Facility-based testing: Includes testing in primary care clinics inpatient wards, and outpatient clinics, including specialist dedicated clinics such as HIV, STI, and TB clinics, in the district, provincial or regional hospitals and their laboratories, and in private clinical services.

Integration The co-location and sharing of services and resources across different disease areas. In the context of hepatitis B or C infection, this may include the provision of testing, prevention, care, and treatment services alongside other health services, such as HIV, tuberculosis (TB), sexually transmitted infections (STI), antenatal clinic (ANC), contraceptive and other family planning services.

Decentralization: The process of delegating significant authority and resources to lower levels of the health system (provincial regional, district, sub-district, primary health care, and community.

Task-shifting/sharing: The rational redistribution of tasks from "higher-level" cadres of healthcare providers to other cadres such as trained lay providers.

Lay provider: Any person who performs functions related to healthcare delivery and has been trained to deliver services but has received no formal professional or paraprofessional certificate or tertiary education degree.

Linkage to care: A process of actions and activities that support people testing for HBV/HCV to engage with the prevention treatment, and care services as appropriate for their hepatitis B and C status.

SUBJECT INDEX

Imran Shahid and Qaiser Jabeen

E

F

G

H

I

J

K

L

Made in the USA
Las Vegas, NV
15 November 2026

b8166ec4-26b0-455d-adaa-0dd37fc4a438R01